KU-821-455

Books are to be returned on or before

Pharmaceutical Inhalation Aerosol Technology

DRUGS AND THE PHARMACEUTICAL SCIENCES

Executive Editor

James Swarbrick

PharmaceuTech, Inc.
Pinehurst, North Carolina

Advisory Board

DRUGS AND THE PHARMACEUTICAL SCIENCES

A Series of Textbooks and Monographs

1. Pharmacokinetics, *Milo Gibaldi and Donald Perrier*
2. Good Manufacturing Practices for Pharmaceuticals: A Plan for Total Quality Control, *Sidney H. Willig, Murray M. Tuckerman, and William S. Hitchings IV*
3. Microencapsulation, *edited by J. R. Nixon*
4. Drug Metabolism: Chemical and Biochemical Aspects, *Bernard Testa and Peter Jenner*
5. New Drugs: Discovery and Development, *edited by Alan A. Rubin*
6. Sustained and Controlled Release Drug Delivery Systems, *edited by Joseph R. Robinson*
7. Modern Pharmaceutics, *edited by Gilbert S. Banker and Christopher T. Rhodes*
8. Prescription Drugs in Short Supply: Case Histories, *Michael A. Schwartz*
9. Activated Charcoal: Antidotal and Other Medical Uses, *David O. Cooney*
10. Concepts in Drug Metabolism (in two parts), *edited by Peter Jenner and Bernard Testa*
11. Pharmaceutical Analysis: Modern Methods (in two parts), *edited by James W. Munson*
12. Techniques of Solubilization of Drugs, *edited by Samuel H. Yalkowsky*
13. Orphan Drugs, *edited by Fred E. Karch*
14. Novel Drug Delivery Systems: Fundamentals, Developmental Concepts, Biomedical Assessments, *Yie W. Chien*
15. Pharmacokinetics: Second Edition, Revised and Expanded, *Milo Gibaldi and Donald Perrier*
16. Good Manufacturing Practices for Pharmaceuticals: A Plan for Total Quality Control, Second Edition, Revised and Expanded, *Sidney H. Willig, Murray M. Tuckerman, and William S. Hitchings IV*
17. Formulation of Veterinary Dosage Forms, *edited by Jack Blodinger*
18. Dermatological Formulations: Percutaneous Absorption, *Brian W. Barry*
19. The Clinical Research Process in the Pharmaceutical Industry, *edited by Gary M. Matoren*
20. Microencapsulation and Related Drug Processes, *Patrick B. Deasy*
21. Drugs and Nutrients: The Interactive Effects, *edited by Daphne A. Roe and T. Colin Campbell*
22. Biotechnology of Industrial Antibiotics, *Erick J. Vandamme*
23. Pharmaceutical Process Validation, *edited by Bernard T. Loftus and Robert A. Nash*

ADDITIONAL VOLUMES IN PREPARATION

Pharmaceutical Inhalation Aerosol Technology

Second Edition, Revised and Expanded

edited by
Anthony J. Hickey
University of North Carolina
Chapel Hill, North Carolina, U.S.A.

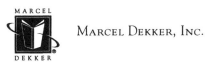

MARCEL DEKKER, INC.   NEW YORK · BASEL

Library of Congress Cataloging-in-Publication Data
A catalog record for this book is available from the Library of Congress.

ISBN: 0-8247-4253-2

This book is printed on acid-free paper.

Headquarters
Marcel Dekker, Inc., 270 Madison Avenue, New York, NY 10016, U.S.A.
tel: 212-696-9000; fax: 212-685-4540

Distribution and Customer Service
Marcel Dekker, Inc., Cimarron Road, Monticello, New York 12701, U.S.A.
tel: 800-228-1160; fax: 845-796-1772

Eastern Hemisphere Distribution
Marcel Dekker AG, Hutgasse 4, Postfach 812, CH-4001 Basel, Switzerland
tel: 41-61-260-6300; fax: 41-61-260-6333

World Wide Web
http://www.dekker.com

The publisher offers discounts on this book when ordered in bulk quantities. For more information, write to Special Sales/Professional Marketing at the headquarters address above.

Foreword

It is hard to believe that in ten short years since the publication of *Pharmaceutical Inhalation Aerosol Technology* the number of chapters would be increased two-thirds in order to bring the second edition up to date. But it is true! For one who had the privilege of experiencing the heady days, nearly a half century ago, during the development of early metered-dose inhalers (MDIs), the accelerated pace of development in inhalation technology during the past decade has been truly astonishing.

In the early days, we didn't have the foggiest idea of how much of the drug discharged from our MDIs actually deposited in the lung: we only knew that those patients were getting relief for their asthma. Today, using recently developed mathematical models that are based on lung morphology and aerosol physics, we can estimate with reasonable certainty the amount of drug delivered from an inhaler that is expected to be deposited in the lung. New methods of imaging appropriately labeled drug discharged from inhalers provide exquisite pictures of the distribution and accurate estimate of the quantity of drug deposited in the lung. Greater understanding of the cell biology of the lung and of the pharmacodynamics and pharmacokinetics of drug in the lung helps us understand what happens, and the rate at which it happens, to drug deposited there.

Methods of aerosol generation—ultrasound, electrohydrodynamics, hydrostatic pressure extrusion of liquid through small orifices—that, just ten years ago, might have been considered laboratory curiosities or perhaps only implemented as laboratory prototype generators, are now in late-stage development as handheld inhalers. In addition, precision dry-powder inhalers are in late-stage development. Chlorofluorocarbon (CFC)-free MDIs, often more efficient than their CFC counterparts, are on the market. The dream of delivering insulin by inhalation to eliminate injection in the treatment of diabetes is coming to fruition. Inhaled insulin, delivered by precision dry-powder inhalers and from metered aqueous–aerosol inhalers, is in late-stage clinical trials with very encouraging results. Ten years ago, gene implantation from inhaled aerosol was only beginning to be talked about. Today it is being explored in clinical trials as treatment for cystic fibrosis. Proteins and peptides comprise a growing number of drugs coming from the biotech industry that are now being developed as aerosol dosage forms.

Keeping pace with this technological development, the science and understanding of formulation factors that govern aerosol generation, of factors governing pulmonary deposition, and of the chemical and biological fate of drug deposited in the respiratory tract are burgeoning. For one experienced in the development of pharmaceutical aerosols, this second addition of *Pharmaceutical Inhalation Aerosol Technology* provides, in a compact way, a useful overview of new developments in the technology. This volume will be particularly useful for the many people entering this increasingly exciting field—pharmaceutical scientists, engineers, and clinicians. It will provide them with a jump start to bring them up to speed in this rapidly expanding field.

Charles G. Thiel
3M Drug Delivery Systems Division, Retired
Maplewood, Minnesota, U.S.A.

Foreword to the First Edition

The metered-dose aerosol inhaler is not only a most convenient system for the delivery of therapeutically active drugs but it has proven to be a life-saving device for many asthmatics. This system has made it possible for millions of asthma sufferers to lead normal lives. The convenience of self-administering a dose of drug accurately and quickly has made the metered-dose aerosol the dosage form of choice for the delivery of drugs to the respiratory system. From epinephrine to albuterol, from triamcinolone to flunisolide, from proteins and peptides to hormones, this dosage form has proven its value.

This volume covers the subject of inhalation technology from start to finish and is a welcome addition to the literature in this area. The reader can quickly become aware of the many ramifications of aerosol inhalation therapy along with the underlying principles for the deposition of particles in the lungs.

Ever since the introduction of the first metered-dose inhaler in the early 1950s, this dosage form has been readily prescribed by the physician and readily accepted by the patient. This text extends our knowledge in this rapidly growing field and will enable the pharmaceutical scientist to develop existing and new drugs in a suitable aerosol system.

John J. Sciarra
Arnold and Marie Schwartz College of Pharmacy
Long Island University
Brooklyn, New York, U.S.A.

Preface

When the first edition of *Pharmaceutical Inhalation Aerosol Technology* was published there was a clear need for a concise review of the state-of-the-art technology for those entering the field. During the previous 25 years this had been a relatively dormant field for innovation outside of large corporations, which clearly dominated the market for these products. As the 1990s began, it was clear that interest in the potential of aerosols for the treatment of both local and systemic diseases was increasing. This seemed an ideal time to produce a specialized book in this field. By the end of the 1990s it would not be an overstatement to say that a revolution had occurred. Many new and some existing companies began to focus on aerosols. Hundreds of new openings for personnel were created, and the literature flourished with new and ever more interesting discoveries regarding the administration of drugs as aerosols to the lungs.

In this current climate of discovery and increased commercial activity the time is right for this second edition. In this volume I have tried to incorporate all of the old, yet still relevant topics, and I have included new sections that cover material that was either in the early days of evaluation or unheard of in 1992.

In Part One, chapters have been included covering cell biology and pharmacokinetics. Historically, the pharmacokinetics of locally acting drugs administered in low doses was thought to be an irrelevancy. With the burgeoning interest in the systemic action of drugs intended either for local activity, such as corticosteriods, or for remote activity, such as insulin–the pharmacokinetics of disposition is now key in the development of aerosol products. Needless to say, with this interest in the disposition of drugs from the lungs, the mechanisms of transport must be elucidated and the tools of cell biology will be necessary to achieve this goal.

Part Two remains largely the same as in the first edition. The fundamentals of aerosol science have changed little in the last decade. However, the original focus was on the pressure-packaged metered-dose inhaler. Environmental concerns over ozone depletion and global warming and the need for alternative formulation strategies for biological molecules have driven the development of new dry-powder inhalers and handheld aqueous aerosol inhalers. These were discussed briefly in the first edition and are now given separate sections.

Part Three is the most extensively modified in the second edition. In the early 1990s asthma was the only disease that was being treated systematically with aerosols. Throughout the decade the concept of treating diabetes with insulin aerosols, cystic fibrosis by gene transfection, and infectious diseases with antimicrobials gained ground. Many of these approaches have yet to be commercial or therapeutic success stories, but by the time this book is in print they may be available to the clinician. Consequently, sections on these topics have been added.

It is worth reiterating a sentiment from the first edition. The literature is replete with publications advancing the frontiers of knowledge. This text is intended to be an overview of the state of the art of the technology. I leave it to others to edit prospective, scientifically detailed books. To remind the readers how far we have come, and how quickly, a concluding chapter is included that reviews the past decade and speculates on the future.

On a personal note, it was most gratifying to see how well the original volume was received. To those of you who read the book, some of whom have thanked me for collating the materials, I owe you a debt of gratitude for applying this knowledge and making it worthwhile. I hope you find this new edition as useful and informative.

Anthony J. Hickey

Contents

Contents

Contributors

Abeer M. Al-Ghananeem, Ph.D. College of Pharmacy, University of Kentucky, Lexington, Kentucky, U.S.A.

Paul J. Atkins, Ph.D. Oriel Therapeutics, Inc., Research Triangle Park, North Carolina, U.S.A.

Andrew R. Clark, Ph.D. Nektar Therapeutics, Inc., San Carlos, California, U.S.A.

Peter A. Crooks, Ph.D. College of Pharmacy, University of Kentucky, Lexington, Kentucky, U.S.A.

Timothy M. Crowder, Ph.D. Oriel Therapeutics, Inc., Research Triangle Park, North Carolina, U.S.A.

Michelle Dawson Department of Chemical Engineering, Johns Hopkins University, Baltimore, Maryland, U.S.A.

Myrna B. Dolovich, P.Eng. Departments of Medicine and Radiology, McMaster University, Hamilton, Ontario, Canada

David A. Edwards, Ph.D. Department of Engineering and Applied Science, Harvard University, Cambridge, Massachusetts, U.S.A.

Jennifer Fiegel Department of Chemical Engineering, Johns Hopkins University, Baltimore, Maryland, U.S.A.

W. H. Finlay, Ph.D. Department of Mechanical Engineering, University of Alberta, Edmonton, Alberta, Canada

Igor Gonda, Ph.D. Acrux Limited, West Melbourne, Victoria, Australia

Justin Hanes, Ph.D. Department of Chemical Engineering, Johns Hopkins University, Baltimore, Maryland, U.S.A.

Yah-el Har-el Department of Chemical Engineering, Johns Hopkins University, Baltimore, Maryland, U.S.A.

Anthony J. Hickey, Ph.D., D.Sc. School of Pharmacy, University of North Carolina, Chapel Hill, North Carolina, U.S.A.

F. Charles Hiller, M.D. University of Arkansas for Medical Sciences, Little Rock, Arkansas, U.S.A.

Günther Hochhaus, Ph.D. Department of Pharmaceutics, University of Florida, Gainesville, Florida, U.S.A.

Manish Issar Department of Pharmaceutics, University of Florida, Gainesville, Florida, U.S.A.

Patricia Khan Department of Pharmaceutics, University of Florida, Gainesville, Florida, U.S.A.

Keng H. Leong, Ph.D. Diodetec, Allison Park, Pennsylvania, U.S.A.

Jonathan Man Department of Engineering and Applied Science, Harvard University, Cambridge, Massachusetts, U.S.A.

Cary Mobley Department of Pharmaceutics, University of Florida, Gainesville, Florida, U.S.A.

A. Bruce Montgomery Corus Pharma Inc., Seattle, Washington, U.S.A.

Ralph Niven, Ph.D. Discovery Laboratories, Inc., Redwood City, California, U.S.A.

Christophe Sirand BLM Associates, Inc., Greenwich, Connecticut, U.S.A.

Junghae Suh Department of Chemical Engineering, Johns Hopkins University, Baltimore, Maryland, U.S.A.

David C. Thompson, Ph.D.   School of Pharmacy, University of Colorado Health Sciences Center, Denver, Colorado, U.S.A.

Nicolas Tsapis   Department of Engineering and Applied Science, Harvard University, Cambridge, Massachusetts, U.S.A.

André X. Valente   Department of Engineering and Applied Science, Harvard University, Cambridge, Massachusetts, U.S.A.

Jean-Pierre Varlet   Valois S.A., Le Neubourg, France

Dennis M. Williams, Pharm.D.   School of Pharmacy, University of North Carolina, Chapel Hill, North Carolina, U.S.A.

Pharmaceutical Inhalation Aerosol Technology

1

Physiology of the Airways

Anthony J. Hickey

University of North Carolina, Chapel Hill, North Carolina, U.S.A.

David C. Thompson

University of Colorado Health Sciences Center, Denver, Colorado, U.S.A.

INTRODUCTION

The airways represent a unique organ system in the body. Their structure allowing air to come into close contact with blood is one of the principal adaptations permitting the existence of terrestrial life. This adaptation also makes the airways useful as a route of administration of drugs in the inhaled, or aerosol, form. This chapter provides an overview of the physiology of the airways, excluding the nasopharyngeal regions of the airways. Aspects considered relevant to the practical and theoretical application of inhaled substances are emphasized.

ANATOMY OF THE AIRWAYS

The airways (constituting the lungs) may be viewed as a series of dividing passageways originating at the trachea and terminating at the alveolar sacs.

In the context of aerosol design and delivery, such a "static" overview represents a satisfactorily simple model. However, many factors beyond the anatomy of the airways are relevant to the therapeutic use of aerosols.

Structure

The airways are often described as the *pulmonary tree*, in that their overall form resembles a tree. The tree trunk is analogous to the trachea of the airways that bifurcates to form main bronchi. These divide to form smaller bronchi that lead to individual lung lobes, three lobes on the right side and two on the left side. Inside each lobe, the bronchi undergo further divisions to form new generations of smaller caliber airways, the bronchioles. This process continues through the terminal bronchioles (the smallest airway not involved with an alveolus), the respiratory bronchioles (which exhibit alveoli protruding from their walls), and alveolar ducts and terminates in the alveolar sacs. In the classic model of the airways (as described by Weibel [1]), each airway divides to form two smaller "daughter" airways (Fig. 1); as a result, the number of airways at each generation is double that of the previous generation. The model proposes the existence of 24 airway generations in total, with the trachea being generation 0 and the alveolar sacs being generation 23.

In passing from the trachea to the alveolar sacs, two physical changes occur in the airways that are important in influencing airway function. Firstly, the airway caliber decreases with increasing generations, for example, tracheal diameter 1.8 cm versus alveolar diameter 0.04 cm (Fig. 2). This permits adequate penetration of air to the lower airways for a given expansion of the lungs. Secondly, the surface area of the airways increases with each generation, to the extent that the total area at the level of the human alveolus is on the order of 140 m^2 [2]. The alveolus is the principal site of gas exchange in the airways, a function compatible with the increased surface area that promotes extensive and efficient diffusional gas exchange between the alveolar space and the blood in alveolar capillaries (vide infra). The relatively small change in cross-sectional area that occurs over the 19 generations of airways between the trachea and the terminal bronchiole (from 2.5 to 180 cm^2) [3] fosters the rapid, bulk flow of inspired air down to the terminal bronchiole. By contrast, the cross-sectional area increases greatly in the four generations between the terminal bronchiole and the alveolar sac (from 180 to 10,000 cm^2) [3], which results in a significant decrease in the velocity of airflow to the extent that the flow velocity fails to exceed that of diffusing oxygen molecules [4]. Accordingly, diffusion assumes a greater role in determining the movement of gases in these peripheral airways.

The various levels of the airways may be categorized functionally as being either conducting or respiratory airways. Those airways not participating in gas

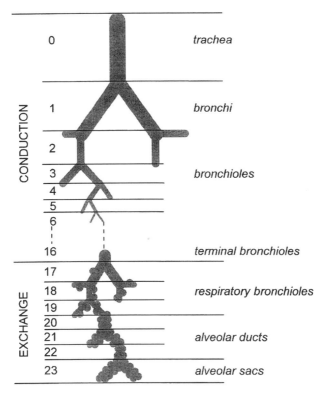

FIGURE 1   Model of airway according to Weibel. (Modified from Ref. 1.)

exchange constitute the conducting zone of the airways and extend from the trachea to the terminal bronchioles. This region is the principal site of airway obstruction in obstructive lung diseases, such as asthma. The respiratory zone includes airways involved with gas exchange and comprises respiratory bronchioles, alveolar ducts, and alveolar sacs. As such, conducting and respiratory zones of the airways may be distinguished simply by the absence or presence of alveolar pockets (which confer the gas exchange function). Regions within each zone may be classified further on a histological basis. For example, the contribution of cartilage to the airway wall is one means of differentiating the trachea from bronchi and bronchioles because cartilage exists as incomplete rings in the trachea, regresses to irregularly shaped plates in bronchi, and is absent from bronchioles. Also, respiratory bronchioles may be discriminated from terminal bronchioles by the presence of associated alveoli.

Other histological changes are evident downward throughout the pulmonary tree, and the cellular profile of each region has distinctive effect on

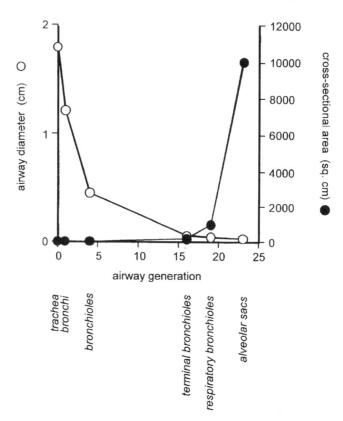

FIGURE 2 Graph of airway diameter and cross-sectional area as a function of airway generation.

functional aspects of the airways under physiological and pathophysiological conditions.

Epithelium

The epithelium of the airways is a continuous sheet of cells lining the lumenal surface of the airways. It separates the internal environment of the body (i.e., subepithelial structures) from the external environment (i.e., airway lumen). The lumenal surface of the epithelium is, therefore, exposed to inhaled substances, such as gases, particulates, or aerosols. Connecting adjacent epithelial cells are specialized tight junctional processes [5,6] that limit the penetration of inhaled substances by the intercellular route of administration. Under normal or physiological conditions, larger molecules must past through the epithelial cell. Therefore, the epithelium serves the important function of limiting access of inhaled substances to the internal environment of the body. Under pathophysiological conditions, the epithelium may be damaged, leading to enhanced penetration of substances present in the airway lumen [7].

The airway epithelium comprises a variety of cell types (Table 1), the distribution of which confers different functions on the airway region. Extending from the trachea to the terminal bronchus, the lumenal surface of the airways are lined by ciliated cells. Mucus, a viscous fluid containing mucin glycoproteins and proteoglycans, floats on a watery layer of periciliary fluid (or sol) and covers the lumenal surface of the epithelium. The secretions fulfill four important functions. Firstly, they protect the epithelium from becoming dehydrated. Secondly, the water in the mucus promotes saturation of inhaled air. Thirdly, the mucus contains antibacterial proteins and peptides, such as defensins and lysozyme, that serve to repress microbial colonization of the airways [8,9]. Fourthly, the mucus is involved in airway protection from inhaled xenobiotics or chemicals. Coordinated beating of the epithelial cilia propels the blanket of mucus toward the upper airways and pharynx, where the mucus may be either swallowed or ejected. The rate of mucus propulsion varies according to the airway region such that movement in the smaller airways is slower than in the larger airways, a situation that arises from the proportionately larger number of ciliated cells in the larger airways and the higher ciliary beat frequency in the larger airways [10]. Syllogistically, this process is advantageous, given that many small airways

TABLE 1   Cells of the Airway Epithelium

Cell	Putative function
Ciliated columnar	Mucus movement
Mucous (goblet)	Mucus secretion
Serous	Periciliary fluid; mucus secretion
Clara (nonciliated epithelial)	Xenobiotic metabolism; surfactant production
Brush	Transitional form of ciliated epithelial cell
Basal	Progenitor for ciliated epithelial and goblet cells
Dendritic	Immunity
Intermediate	Transitional cell in differentiation of basal cell
Neuroendocrine (Kultschitsky or APUD)	Chemoreceptor; paracrine function
Alveolar type I	Alveolar gas exchange
Alveolar type II	Surfactant secretion; differentiation into type I cell
Alveolar macrophage	Pulmonary defense
Mast	Immunoregulation

Source: Refs. 100–102.

converge on the larger, more central airways, whose mucus clearance rate would have to be greater to accommodate the large volumes of mucus being delivered by the smaller distal airways. This process of the movement of mucus up the pulmonary tree, known as the mucociliary escalator, serves the defensive function of clearing from the lung inhaled particles that become trapped in the mucus.

The significance of mucous trapping of aerosolized particles is emphasized by the fact that radiolabeled aerosols have been used in the measurement of mucociliary transport [11]. Mucus clearance from the airways is also enhanced by coughing, which rapidly propels the mucus toward the pharynx. Failure to clear mucus from the airways as a result of ciliary dysfunction or mucus hypersecretion (as may occur in cystic fibrosis or chronic bronchitis) can result in airway obstruction and infection. Such a situation may adversely affect the therapeutic activity of an inhaled drug by increasing the thickness of the mucus layer through which the drug must diffuse to reach its site of action and retard penetration of the aerosolized particles throughout the airways as a result of mucus plugging of the airway lumen. Goblet cells (and mucous glands) are not present in airways distal to the bronchi [12], and therefore a mucus layer does not line the peripheral airways.

Alveolar type I cells represent the principal cell type lining the lumenal surface of the alveoli [10,13], and it is through these cells that gases must diffuse for oxygen and carbon dioxide exchange to occur with blood in the pulmonary capillaries. Alveolar type II cells are also present in the alveoli. Cuboidal in nature, these cells possess microvilli and serve the important function of secreting surfactant [10], a mixture of carbohydrates, proteins, and lipids essential in reducing alveolar surface tension, which diminishes the work of alveolar expansion during inspiration. In addition, type II cells serve as progenitor cells in the regeneration of the alveolar epithelium. For example, type II cells differentiate into type I cells after type I cell damage [10,14].

Epithelium of the central and peripheral airways have the capacity to produce and release proinflammatory mediators, such as arachidonic acid metabolites, nitric oxide, cytokines, and growth factors, and thereby modulate the progression of airway diseases [15]. In addition, substances released from central airway epithelium can influence the ability of adjacent smooth muscle to contract [16].

Smooth Muscle Cells

Smooth muscle is separated from the epithelium by the lamina propria, a region of connective tissue containing nerves and blood vessels. In the trachea, the smooth muscle connects the open ends of the incomplete cartilage rings and therefore constitutes only a fraction of the circumference of this component of the airways. Further down the pulmonary tree, through the bronchi and bronchioles, the contribution of the smooth muscle to the airway wall increases to the point of completely encircling the airway. Contraction or relaxation of the smooth muscle has a direct influence on airway caliber and thereby affects airflow in the airways. Bronchoconstriction is the result of smooth muscle contraction and is the principal cause of airway obstruction in reversible obstructive airway diseases, such as asthma. The tone or state of contraction of airway smooth muscle is subject to control by neurotransmitters released from innervating nerves, hormones, or mediators released from activated inflammatory cells.

Gland Cells

Located in the submucosa of cartilage-containing airways and in the lamina propria of the trachea are glands that secrete mucus into the airway lumen [17]. Each mucous gland consists of four regions: the ciliated duct, collecting duct, mucous tubules, and secretory tubules [18]. The ciliated duct opens to the lumen of the airways and is lined by ciliated epithelial cells. It merges with the collecting duct, the walls of which comprise columnar cells. Mucous cells line the mucous tubules that lead from the collecting duct. Serous cells (which contribute to the more liquid component of mucus) line the blind-ended serous tubules that are located at the distal ends of the mucous tubules. Several secretory tubules feed into the collecting duct. Mucus is secreted via the collecting and ciliated ducts into the lumen of the airways. Goblet cells, located in the epithelium of the larger central airways, secrete mucus directly into the airway lumen [19]. The number and/or size of mucous glands and goblet cells increases in disease states, such as chronic bronchitis [8,19], leading to conditions of mucus hypersecretion.

Nerves

The airways are innervated by afferent and efferent nerves that respectively serve sensory and effector functions in the central nervous system regulation of airway function (Table 2, Fig. 3) [20]. Slowly adapting receptors (or pulmonary stretch receptors) are located in the smooth muscle of the central airways (trachea to larger bronchi), respond to airway stretch, and are thought to be involved in the reflex control of ventilatory drive. Rapidly adapting receptors (or irritant receptors) ramify within the epithelium of the central airways and are sensitive to chemical or irritant stimuli (e.g., inflammatory mediators), mechanical stimuli, and interstitial edema. Activation of these receptors results in an increase in the rate or depth of breathing and in bronchoconstriction mediated through a central nervous system reflex in efferent cholinergic nerve activity. Inhalation of foreign substances, such as particulates, can activate these receptors to elicit reflex bronchoconstriction. Afferent C-fibers are tachykinin-containing nerves that ramify within the epithelium and between smooth muscle cells [21]. Chemical (e.g., inflammatory mediators), particulate, and mechanical stimuli activate

TABLE 2 Innervation of the Airways

Nerve type	Putative function
Afferent	
Slowly adapting receptor (pulmonary stretch receptor)	Breuer-Hering reflex (inhibition of inspiration; prolongation of expiration)
Rapidly adapting receptor	Responds to airway irritants, mechanical stimuli, interstitial edema
C-fiber	Responds to airway irritants, mechanical stimuli
Neuroepithelial body	Responds to hypoxia
Efferent	
Adrenergic	Vasoconstriction
Cholinergic	Bronchoconstriction, mucus secretion
Nonadrenergic noncholinergic inhibitory	Bronchodilation, mucus secretion

afferent C-fibers to cause rapid, shallow breathing or apnea and to evoke central reflex bronchoconstriction through increased efferent cholinergic nerve activity [20,22]. Under conditions of cholinoceptor blockade, central reflex bronchodilation through activation of efferent nonadrenergic noncholinergic nerves may be observed [23]. Stimulation of afferent C-fibers can result in the release of tachykinins at the site of stimulation and alter airway function independent of the central nervous system, e.g., by inducing mucosal edema [24]. These nerves are thought to be important sensory modalities for conveying retrosternal discomfort induced by inhaled irritants. Neuroepithelial bodies are located in the epithelium of the central airways and are intimately associated with the endings of nerves, which are primarily afferent in nature [20,24]. Each neuroepithelial body comprises groups of neuroendocrine cells that contain biogenic amines, such as serotonin, and peptides, such as calcitonin gene-related peptide (cGRP) [25]. Hypoxia induces the release of these biologically active substances, which can then activate the sensory nerve endings to elicit a central reflex or act locally on adjacent tissues, such as blood vessels or airway smooth muscle [20,25]. Cholinergic nerves are carried to the airways in the vagus nerve and innervate airway smooth muscle and submucosal glands. The neurotransmitter acetylcholine, released from cholinergic nerves, promotes bronchoconstriction [26] and mucus secretion [27,28]. Nonadrenergic noncholinergic inhibitory nerves, also carried in the vagus nerve, are the sole bronchodilator innervation of airway smooth muscle [29]. These nerves may also inhibit airway mucus

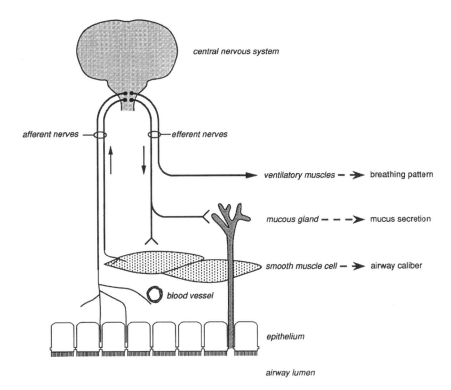

FIGURE 3 Role of afferent and efferent nerves in altering airway function. Stimulation of afferent (or sensory) nerves, such as afferent C-fibers, rapidly adapting receptors or slowly adapting receptors, results in an increase in electrical impulse traffic to the central nervous system. Depending on the afferent nerve activated, processing and integration in the central nervous system may result in an increase in the activity of (a) efferent motor nerves governing muscles that regulate breathing (i.e., affect rate and depth of ventilation) or (b) efferent autonomic nerves, such as cholinergic and nonadrenergic noncholinergic inhibitory nerves, that modify mucus secretion or airway caliber through changes in smooth muscle tone. Afferent C-fibers may also serve an efferent function insofar as impulses can spread throughout the C-fiber network from the site of C-fiber stimulation to result in the release of tachykinins (such as substance P and neutokinin A). These released substances may then act on blood vessels to increase permeability or on smooth muscle to increase vascular permeability and elicit bronchoconstriction, respectively.

secretion [30]. Adrenergic nerves do not innervate human airway smooth muscle [31] and have little effect on mucus secretion in human airways [28,31].

Defensive Cells

Alveolar macrophages are migrating mononuclear cells present in the interstitium and lumenal surface of the alveoli [32]. These cells phagocytize (envelop and, when possible, enzymatically degrade) foreign substances, particles, or microorganisms in the alveoli, after which they remain in the alveolus or migrate to the mucociliary escalator or into lymph tissue. Upon activation, macrophages release a variety of enzymes and biologically active mediators [33,34] that may influence airway function. The synthesis and release of matrix metalloproteinases (MMPs) by activated alveolar macrophages can contribute to lung tissue remodeling [35,36].

Mast cells are located in the walls of the central and peripheral airways and may be found free the lumen of the airways [37]. Activation by antigen cross-bridging of surface antibodies elicits cellular degranulation of the mast cell and the release of biologically active preformed and newly generated mediators. Also released are proteases, including chymase and tryptase, which can modify airway function by degrading biologically active proteins and peptides [38]. In addition, tryptase activates protease-activated receptors (PARs), leading a variety of unanticipated biological actions, such as induction of airway smooth muscle proliferation [39,40]. Mast cells serve an important role in the response of the airways to challenge by antigens (or allergens).

Blood Supply

The cardiovascular system can be divided into two components (as shown in Fig. 4): the pulmonary circulation and the systemic circulation. The pulmonary circulation carries deoxygenated blood from the right ventricle to the lungs and returns oxygenated blood from the lungs to the left atrium. Emerging from the right ventricle is the main pulmonary artery, which branches to form smaller pulmonary and intrapulmonary arteries. This pulmonary arterial tree undergoes further rapid subdivision in parallel with the pulmonary tree to form pulmonary capillaries, a fine network of blood vessels present in intimate contact with the alveolus. The capillaries drain into postcapillary venules that unite to form small veins and, distally, larger veins. These drain into the pulmonary vein, which returns blood from the lungs to the left atrium. The systemic circulation carries oxygenated blood from the left ventricle to the tissues of the body and returns deoxygenated blood from the body to the right atrium. Arteries and arterioles carry blood to capillary networks within tissues, and venules and veins return blood from tissues to the heart. There are several important differences between the systemic and pulmonary circulations.

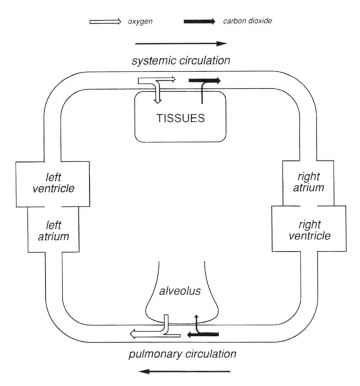

FIGURE 4 Cardiovascular system in the body. Oxygen diffuses from the oxygen-rich environment of the alveolus into the deoxygenated blood of the pulmonary circulation. The newly oxygenated blood returns by the pulmonary vein to the left atrium and ventricle; contraction of the latter provides the driving force for circulation of oxygen-rich blood to the organs and tissues of the body. Cells of the body use oxygen for energy-producing processes that result in the formation of carbon dioxide. Depleted of oxygen and richer in carbon dioxide, blood leaving the tissues returns by the venous circulation to the right atrium. The right ventricle pumps the carbon dioxide-rich blood into the pulmonary circulation from whence the carbon dioxide may diffuse into the alveolus. Arrows indicate the direction of blood flow.

First, blood pressure is lower in the pulmonary circulation than in the systemic circulation; for example, mean pressures in the pulmonary artery (emerging from the right ventricle) and aorta (artery emerging from the left ventricle) are 15 and 100 mmHg, respectively. As a result, the walls of the various pulmonary arterial vessels are thinner and are invested with less smooth muscle than their systemic counterparts, presumably as a consequence of the differences in stress borne by the vessel walls. Secondly, the pulmonary vessels are subject to different transmural pressures than are systemic vessels, such as those caused by changes in pressure in the alveolus and thoracic cavity, together with the stresses applied to the vessel wall through movement of adherent lung tissue. For example, during inspiration, alveoli expand and tend to compress the pulmonary capillaries, which are located in the walls of the alveoli. At the same time, large vessels are subject to distention caused by the negative intrapleural pressure during inspiration.

Blood vessels supplying the conducting or central airways (i.e., the bronchial circulation) are part of the systemic circulation. By contrast, the blood supply to airways of the respiratory zone involve the pulmonary circulation. The separation of these vascular networks can be almost complete. For example,

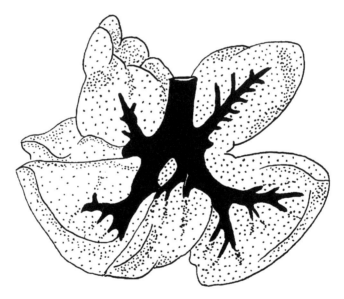

FIGURE 5 Diagram of staining of the bronchial circulation in the cat. The bronchial and pulmonary circulations of the cat were perfused separately with aerated physiological salt solution containing bovine serum albumin (4% wt/vol) maintained at 37°C. Perfusates from the bronchial and pulmonary circulations were collected from cannulae positioned in the right and left ventricles, respectively. Infusion of Evans blue dye (30 mg/Kg) into the systemic circulation resulted in deep blue staining of the central airways (black) with no staining of the parenchymal tissues (dotted). Further, 75–80% of the dye was collected from the cannula from the right heart.

in the cat, with separately perfused systemic (bronchial) and pulmonary circulations, infusion of Evans blue dye into the systemic circulation results in staining of the central airways (distal trachea to fourth-generation intralobar bronchus) and no staining of parenchymal tissue (Fig. 5). From 75% to 80% of the dye returns to the right ventricle, a result consistent with this circulations being part of the systemic circulation. The remainder of the dye returns to the left ventricle. This result, taken together with the absence of staining of parenchymal tissue, suggests that part of the bronchial circulation drains into the venous return of the pulmonary circulation. Recent studies demonstrate the ability to independently perfuse these two circulations in larger animals [41]. In studying the absorption of an aerosol from the central versus the peripheral airways, it is therefore prudent to be cognizant of the nature of the circulation serving the site of expected deposition and sample from the appropriate sites, namely, right ventricle or left ventricle.

ZONES OF THE AIRWAYS

The different zones of the airways, conducting and respiratory zones, possess different physiological functions and are distinguished by their roles in the exchange of gases.

Conducting Zone

Conducting airways do not contribute to the gas exchange and can be considered to be merely a conduit between the external environment and the respiratory zone (vide infra). The volume of air accommodated by the conducting airways represents the anatomic dead space and is air not directly available for gas exchange. Aside from serving as a conduit to the respiratory zone, the conducting airways perform two other functions: gas buffering and humidification.

The dead space (the volume of airway not involved indirectly in gas exchange) confers a buffering capacity on the airways, in that, for each breath, air taken in from the external environment or alveolar air must mix with dead-space air. This process, although decreasing the efficiency with which oxygen is delivered to and carbon dioxide is removed from the alveolar space (e.g., dead-space oxygen concentration will be determined by the oxygen concentration of air inhaled from the external environment and of that in the alveolar space that was shunted into the dead space in the previous breath), serves to even out the alveolar gas concentrations by preventing dramatic swings in alveolar gas concentrations that would occur if the alveolar air were exchanged completely during each breath. It should be recognized that the volume of the dead space is not insignificant. For example, in a normal tidal breath of 500–600 mL, 150 mL represents dead-space volume.

Inhaled air is humidified in the conducting airways through exposure to fluids lining these airways, a process that results in the delivery to the alveoli of air that is in isotonic equilibrium of 99.5% or greater relative humidity at body temperature.

Respiratory Zone

The relationship between the respiratory system and the cardiovascular system is ideally suited for the process of gas exchange between the alveolus and the blood. Pulmonary capillaries (diameter = 6–15 μm) are located in the walls of each alveolus (diameter = 250 μm) [42]. Many capillaries are in close association with each alveolus, leading to a large "common" area for gas or solute exchange estimated to be 50–120 m^2 in an adult human. In traversing the air–blood barrier, gases in the alveolus must cross the alveolar epithelium, the capillary endothelium, and their basement membranes before reaching the blood, a distance in all of approximately 500 nm [42]. In some regions of the alveolus, an interstitial space (containing connective tissue elements) separates the basement membranes of the alveolar epithelium and the capillary endothelium, and it is in these loci that solutes and liquid exchange have been hypothesized to occur [43]. The large area for absorption, together with the short transit distances, optimizes the process of diffusion of gases between the alveolar space and blood. Adjacent epithelial cells lining the alveolus are connected by a tight junction that limits the intercellular passage of solutes [7,44]. Pulmonary endothelial cells are also joined by tight junctions, although the nature of these junctional processes differs from that in the epithelium, insofar as interruption of the junctions in the endothelium may occur and permit the intercellular passage of large solutes to and from the interstitium [44]. Lipophilic solutes readily diffuse across epithelial and endothelial cells. Other solutes pass through the alveolar epithelium and capillary by transcellular paths (e.g., pores, transcytosis) in a manner related inversely to their size and lipophobicity [44].

FUNCTION OF THE AIRWAYS
Gas Exchange

The principal function of the airways is to permit exchange of gases between blood and the atmosphere that surrounds us, specifically the supply of oxygen to the blood and the removal of carbon dioxide from the blood. This is accomplished by: (1) exchanging gases between the external environment and the alveolar space through breathing or ventilation, and (2) exchanging gases between the alveolar space and the blood by diffusional processes. These two processes are optimized by the structural features of the pulmonary tree. Firstly, the caliber of the airways decreases from the trachea to the alveolus, thereby reducing the dead-space volume. For a given tidal volume (volume of air inspired), decreasing the dead-space volume enhances exchange of atmospheric gases with alveolar gases and results in higher levels of oxygen in the alveolar space and enhanced removal of carbon dioxide from the alveolar space. Secondly, the large surface area shared by the alveoli and the pulmonary capillaries and the short transit distance required for the passage of gases between the alveolar space and the blood enhance gas diffusion.

The direction and extent of passage of gases between the blood in the pulmonary capillary and the alveolar space is determined principally by the gas concentration or partial pressure gradient between these two sites. For example, the partial pressure of oxygen in the alveolus (104 mmHg) normally exceeds that in the deoxygenated blood of the pulmonary capillaries (40 mmHg), and therefore oxygen tends to diffuse from the alveolus to the blood (Fig. 2). The opposite is true for carbon dioxide, which has a higher partial pressure in the blood of pulmonary capillaries (45 mmHg) than in the alveolus (40 mmHg), resulting in the diffusion of this gas from the blood into the alveolus. Under optimal conditions for gas exchange, all alveoli would be well ventilated and all pulmonary capillaries would be well perfused. However, not all alveoli are ventilated equally; similarly, not all pulmonary capillaries are perfused to the same degree. An alveolus may be well ventilated, but the associated capillaries may be poorly perfused or not perfused, a situation that may occur as a result of thrombosis, embolization, or compression of pulmonary vessels by high alveolar pressures. The volume of air ventilating unperfused alveolar units during each breath is the alveolar dead space. This volume, together with the anatomic dead space, is known as the physiological dead space. An alveolus may be poorly ventilated (as a result of bronchoconstriction, mucus obstruction, or atelectasis [peripheral airway closure]), and the associated capillaries may be well perfused. In this situation, deoxygenated blood coursing through the pulmonary capillaries is not subject to oxygenation and forms part of a physiological shunt that delivers inadequately oxygenated (or deoxygenated) blood to the left heart. Low alveolar or pulmonary arterial oxygen concentrations induce vasoconstriction [45], which diverts blood away from underventilated alveoli. This process could be viewed as an intrinsic one serving to optimize ventilation–perfusion relationships. Mismatching of ventilation and perfusion can result in less efficient gas exchange between the alveolus and blood. Under normal conditions, ventilation–perfusion of the airways is adequate to maintain the important function of gas exchange and is a composite of the previously mentioned situations.

Acid–Base Balance

Carbon dioxide is continually produced by cellular aerobic metabolism of glucose and fatty acids. Carbon dioxide diffuses down its concentration gradient from the cell to the blood, which carries it to the lungs. It can interact with water to form carbonic acid (H_2CO_3), a process catalyzed by carbonic anhydrase, an enzyme present in erythrocytes. Carbonic acid can then dissociate to liberate bicarbonate ion (HCO_3^-) and hydrogen ion (H^+) as follows:

$$CO_2 + H_2O \rightarrow H_2CO_3 \rightarrow HCO_3^- + H^+$$

This process reverses in the lung, where hydrogen ion and bicarbonate ion combine to form carbonic acid, which then breaks down to form water and carbon dioxide, the latter diffusing into the alveolar space down its concentration gradient for removal by ventilation.

A close relationship exists in the blood between carbon dioxide levels and hydrogen ion concentrations such that increases in carbon dioxide cause increases in blood hydrogen ion levels and, as a result, decreases in blood pH. Ventilation has a direct influence on blood carbon dioxide concentrations and thereby affects blood pH as shown:

$$\uparrow \text{ventilation} \rightarrow \downarrow [\text{blood } CO_2] \rightarrow \downarrow [\text{blood } H^+]$$
$$\rightarrow \uparrow \text{blood pH} \rightarrow \text{respiratory alkalosis}$$

$$\downarrow \text{ventilation} \rightarrow \uparrow [\text{blood } CO_2] \rightarrow \uparrow [\text{blood } H^+]$$
$$\rightarrow \downarrow \text{blood pH} \rightarrow \text{respiratory acidosis}$$

Alterations in ventilation, therefore, influence blood pH. Impaired ventilation, as may occur during central nervous system depression or airway obstruction, can result in respiratory acidosis. Conversely respiratory alkalosis can be caused by hyperventilation, as might occur during ascent to high altitude or by fever. In general, renal mechanisms function to compensate for inordinate respiratory alternations in blood pH. In addition, feedback control mechanisms exist in the body that alter respiration in the face of changes in blood pH. For example, changes in blood pH as a consequence of nonrespiratory mechanisms (such as may occur in severe diarrhea, altered renal function, and ingestion of acids or bases) or respiratory mechanisms may be returned toward normal (pH = 7.4) by altering the rate and depth of ventilation. Increases in blood hydrogen ion (and carbon dioxide) concentration stimulate carotid chemoreceptors (located in the bifurcation of the common carotid arteries) to elicit a central nervous system reflex in ventilation. A decrease in the blood concentration of hydrogen ions depresses ventilation through the same central nervous system reflex. In addition, ventilation is also regulated by chemoreceptors in the medulla of the brainstem sensitive to changes in hydrogen ion and carbon dioxide concentrations in the cerebrospinal fluid.

Endocrine

Cells of the lung produce and secrete substances that may exert a local action (i.e., autocrine or paracrine function) or, through passage into the pulmonary circulation, a systemic action (i.e., endocrine function). Prostacyclin, a potent vasodilator and inhibitor of platelet aggregation, is generated by pulmonary endothelium [46]. Antigenic challenge of sensitized airways induces the release of bronchoactive and vasoactive mediators from the airways, including histamine, prostaglandins, and leukotrienes [47], that, aside from exerting local bronchoconstrictor and vascular actions, can spill over into the pulmonary circulation to have actions in organs other than the lungs.

Metabolism

In passage through the pulmonary circulation, a variety of blood-borne substances are subject to metabolism by enzymes associated with the pulmonary endothelium (Table 3). The metabolic processes appear to be very selective, as exemplified by the ability of the lung to metabolize norepinephrine but not other catecholamines, such as epinephrine and dopamine. For many of the compounds, uptake into the endothelial cell is required before enzymatic degradation occurs, and it is the substrate selectivity of these processes that appear to govern metabolic selectivity. Substances that are taken up into the endothelial cells include 5-hydroxytryptamine, norepinephrine, and prostaglandins E_2 and $F_{2\alpha}$. The external surface of the endothelium bears several enzymes that serve to inactivate or biotransform blood-borne substances. These include phosphate esterases, which metabolize the adenosine phosphate compounds, and angiotensin-converting enzyme, which cleaves bradykinin to inactive fragments. The latter enzyme has been extensively studied, primarily because it is responsible for the bioactivation of angiotensin I to angiotensin II (a potent vasoconstrictor) and because the lungs represent the principal site of this conversion. Other peptidases have been identified on the pulmonary endothelium, but their physiological relevance remains to be established [48]. A fair amount is known about the metabolic properties of the pulmonary endothelium, in large part because of the relative ease of studying the pulmonary circulation, and the ability to study endothelium grown in cell culture. Considerably less is known about the metabolic properties of the airway epithelium, save that related to neutral endopeptidase or endothelin-converting enzyme activity [49–51]. In both areas, more research is needed to allow a more comprehensive understanding about how the lung metabolizes substances perfused through or depositing in it. In the context of aerosol administration to

TABLE 3 Fate of Substances Passing Through the
Pulmonary Circulation

Removal
  5-Hydroxytryptamine
  Norepinephrine
  Prostaglandins E_2, $F_{2\alpha}$
  Leukotrienes C_4, D_4
  Adenosine monophosphate, diphosphate, triphosphate
  Bradykinin
  Tachykinins
  Endothelin
Unaffected
  Epinephrine
  Dopamine
  Isoproterenol
  Histamine
  Prostaglandin A_2
  Prostacyclin
  Oxytocin
  Vasopressin
  Angiotensin II
Activation
  Angiotensin I

Source: Refs. 50, 51, 103–111.

the peripheral airways, it should be evident from the foregoing that compounds delivered to the alveoli and absorbed into the pulmonary circulation will be subject to endothelial metabolic processes.

EVALUATION OF AIRWAY PHYSIOLOGY AND FUNCTION

Previously, the anatomy and physiology of the airways were considered. In clinical practice, the assessment of pulmonary function is important in diagnosis of the airway disease, in determination of appropriate therapy, and in evaluation of the success of therapy.

Measures of Pulmonary Volumes

Spirometry is the measurement of the volume of air moving into or out of the airways. In this process, various ventilatory maneuvers are undertaken that

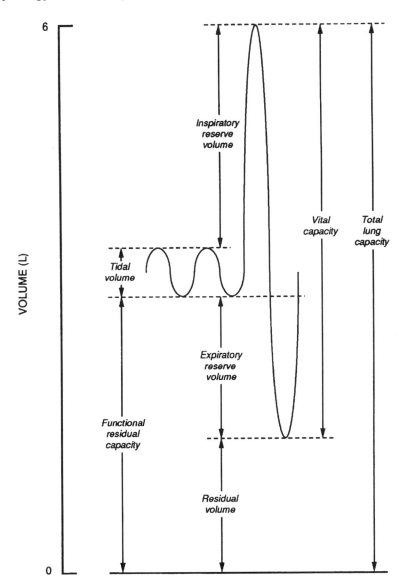

FIGURE 6   Spirometric representation of lung volumes.

permit an estimation of pulmonary volumes and capacities (Fig. 6). Such measurements are valuable for diagnosis of airway disease because pathological conditions can modify specific pulmonary volumes. Definitions of the specific lung volumes are provided in Table 4. Measurements of lung volumes are

TABLE 4   Definitions of Lung Volumes

Volume	Definition
Tidal volume (TV)	Air inspired or expired during a normal breath
Inspiratory reserve volume (IRV)	Volume maximally inspired after a normal tidal inspiration
Expiratory reserve volume (ERV)	Volume maximally expired after a normal tidal expiration
Residual volume (RV)	Volume remaining in the airways after completion of a maximal expiratory effort
Inspiratory capacity	Volume inspired maximally after a normal expiration; $= TV + IRV$
Functional residual capacity (FRC)	Volume remaining in the airways after a normal expiration; $= ERV + RV$
Vital capacity	Volume maximally expired from the lungs after a maximal inspiration; $= IRV + TV + ERV$
Total lung capacity	Volume in the airways after a maximal inspiration; $= IRV + TV + ERV + RV$

Lung volumes can be determined by spirometry and reflect the volume of air remaining in the airways after various inspiratory or expiratory maneuvers. Lung capacities encompass two or more lung volumes (as shown by the provided formulas).

generally normalized for a subject's body size (weight, height, or surface area), age, and gender. This process permits a comparison with standardized or predicted lung volumes, thereby allowing identification of lung pathophysiologies using a simple procedure. Some examples of the way in which airway disorders alter lung volumes are described in the following. During an episode of airway obstruction (as in asthmatic bronchospasm), expiration of air is difficult, and air becomes trapped in the lower airways. This results in an increase in the residual volume and functional residual capacity and a decrease in vital capacity. In conditions that adversely affect respiratory muscles, such as poliomyelitis and spinal cord injuries, voluntary control of inspiratory or expiratory movement is diminished (or absent) and vital capacity is reduced.

Measures of Airway Caliber

The diameter, or caliber, of the airways is of great value in the investigation or diagnosis of obstructive airways diseases. Techniques used to evaluate airway caliber generally center on analysis of the rate of expiratory airflow, because airway obstruction tends to diminish expiratory flow.

1. *Peak flow measurements.* Perhaps the simplest measurement of expiratory airflow involves the use of a peak flowmeter. Subjects inspire maximally (i.e., to total lung capacity) and expire rapidly and maximally to residual volume into the mouthpiece of the instrument that provides a measurement of the peak expiratory flow. These instruments are simple to operate and often are provided to asthmatic patients for self-measurement and documentation of their ventilatory function.

2. *Forced expiratory flow measurements.* Spirometric techniques are used to measure the time course of expired volumes. The same ventilatory

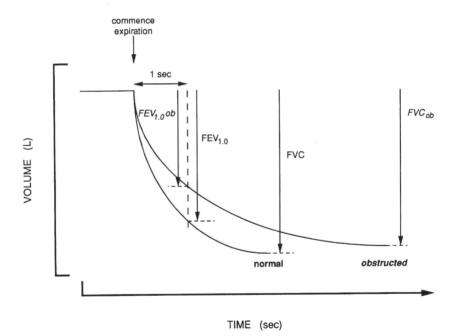

FIGURE 7 Forced expiratory flow maneuvers in normal and obstructed airways. A maximal expiratory effort from total lung capacity results in a rapid expiration of air from the lungs, the volume of which is equivalent to the forced vital capacity (FVC) and the rate of which is dependent on the caliber of the airways. The volume of air expired in the first second of a maximal expiratory effort is the $FEV_{1.0}$. In subjects with obstructed airways, air flow is retarded as reflected in a smaller $FEV_{1.0}$ ($FEV_{1.0}$ob) than in subjects with normal airways ($FEV_{1.0}$).

maneuvers are conducted as those described for peak flow measurements. The subject exhales rapidly and maximally into the mouthpiece of the spirometer. This results in a trace similar to that shown in Fig. 7. The volume expired in the first second is termed the forced expiratory volume ($FEV_{1.0}$), and the total volume expired is the forced vital capacity (FVC). $FEV_{1.0}$ may be normalized to account for the body size, sex, and age of the subject and thereby permit comparison with "normal" estimates. Alternatively, the ratio $FEV_{1.0}$: FVC can be calculated. In subjects with normal airways, this ratio is approximately 0.8; under conditions of airway obstruction, the ratio is less than 0.8.

3. *Airway resistance and dynamic lung compliance.* Measurement of expiratory flow represents a simple, noninvasive means of estimating airway caliber. However, these measurements are relatively insensitive to changes in peripheral airway caliber. More complicated measures of caliber include airway resistance (R_L) and dynamic lung compliance (C_{dyn}). Airway resistance is thought to measure the caliber of the larger airways, such as the bronchi and bronchioles. Dynamic lung compliance measures the elasticity of the peripheral airways and is given as the change in volume of the lungs for a given change in pressure distending the alveoli. Measurement of these parameters in subjects involves highly specialized equipment (e.g., whole-body plethysmograph and pneumotachygraph) and can be invasive, i.e., requiring the placement of an intraesophageal balloon for intrathoracic pressure measurements. A precise description of the means of estimating these parameters is beyond the scope of the present discussion, but interested readers are directed to Ref. 52.

AEROSOL DEPOSITION AND AIRWAY PHYSIOLOGY

In considering the mechanisms of aerosol deposition within the lung and the factors that may influence them, it is of some importance to consider first the anatomy and air velocities within the respiratory tract. The temporal aspects of the passage of air through the various anatomic regions and the point during the breathing cycle are also relevant factors.

The angles of branching, the diameter and lengths of different elements of the airways, and the pulmonary air spaces must be visualized in an arbitrary and oversimplified form to make practical use of anatomic data. Some of the details of the divisions of the respiratory system that have been assumed by Landahl [53] and the anatomic flow rate and transitional features in these areas are shown in Table 5.

TABLE 5 Schematic Representation of the Respiratory Tract

Region	Diameter (cm)	Length (cm)	Velocity (cm sec^{-1})	Passage time (sec)
Mouth	2	7	100	0.07
Pharynx	3	3	45	0.07
Trachea	1.4	11	150	0.07
Bronchi				
Primary	1.0	6.5	190	0.03
Secondary	0.4	3	200	0.015
Tertiary	0.2	1.5	100	0.015
Quaternary	0.15	0.5	22	0.02
Terminal bronchioles	0.06	0.3	2	0.15
Respiratory	0.05	0.15	1.4	0.1
Alveolar ducts	0.02	0.02	—	—
Alveolar sacs	0.03	0.03	—	—

Source: Refs. 53, 81.

For a particular minute volume, the actual rate of airflow throughout the ventilatory cycle varies from zero to a maximum and back to zero. Thus, because air velocity and time of air transit within the system determine the effectiveness of particle deposition, it is evident that this must vary over a considerable range within the cycle.

At least two regions of the respiratory tract are ventilated at different rates. Of the total inspired air, 40% ventilates 17% of the lung, and the remaining 60% ventilates the other 83% of the lung. As a consequence of such unequal distribution of ventilation, air velocity and times of air passage vary, producing different probabilities of deposition of the inhaled particles from one site to another at the same structural depth.

The volume of the nasopharyngeal chamber and airways is 150 mL, that is, dead-space volume. Thus, with a resting tidal volume of 600 mL, only 75% of the air reaches the pulmonary air spaces. There is evidence to suggest that sequential breathing patterns occur that result in poorly ventilated regions [54–56].

The complexity of the anatomic and dynamic factors involved in deposition can readily be appreciated from the brief outline of factors involved.

The physiological factors that influence aerosol deposition in the lung have been investigated experimentally [57–62] and theoretically [63–70]. Flow rates within the lung affect deposition. Airway obstruction [71], breathing rate [72,73], and breath holding [74–76] determine these rates. Because species variations

[77,78] and the state of the lung, whether healthy or diseased [77,79], influence the physiological factors, they are being investigated, with a view to establishing predictable patterns in deposition.

The nature of particle deposition forces and their relationship to aerodynamic particle size have been the subject of many studies and reports. A variety of models for aerosol deposition in the respiratory tract have been proposed. The most notable are those of Findeisen [80], Landahl [53,81], and Weibel [1].

Rohrer [82] measured the diameter and length of the elements of the bronchial tree and constructed a dimensional model on which he based his reasoning on flow resistance in the human airways.

Findeisen was the first to examine the problem of respiratory deposition of aerosols in physical–mathematical terms. After dividing the airways into nine successive sections, starting with the trachea, he assumed a constant rate of respiration (frequency = 15 breaths/min, tidal volume = 200 mL) from which the air velocities and times of air passage through successive zones were calculated. With these parameters, the average angles of branching from one order to the next could be postulated. Landahl modified the assumed anatomic arrangement in some respects. In this model, the airways were divided into 12 sections by including the mouth and pharnyx and two order of alveolar ducts. The parameters adopted in this model were a tidal volume of 450 mL, a breathing frequency of 15 breaths/min, pauses of half seconds at the beginning and middle of each cycle, and a constant respiration rate of 300 mL/sec. The local velocities and times of air passage through the successive sections were obtained using this flow rate and a variety of breathing frequencies and tidal volumes in Landahl's calculation of respiratory deposition. In all cases, the inspiratory and expiratory phases were assumed to consist of a constant airflow rate. Work based on this model has been performed by Beeckmans [83].

Weibel [1] criticized the Findeisen–Landahl model as being based on insufficient clinical data, and, thus, the dimensions of even the proximal airways were not correct. The zones consisting of different branching factors were also criticized as inadequately representing the pulmonary architecture. Weibel proposed two alternative models; the first emphasized the regular features of the airways, and the second accounted for some irregularities. The fundamental geometry of dichotomy was the basis for these models; this refers to the average adult lung and includes the airway of the conductive, transitory, and respiratory zones as well as the blood vessels (alveolar capillaries) of the respiratory zone.

Experimental data on the deposition of aerosols in vivo have been described by Lippman and colleagues [84–86]. Lippman noted that, among normal subjects and nonbronchitic smokers, each individual has a characteristic and reproducible deposition pattern with respect to particle size. This contrasts with the great variation from subject to subject among cigarette smokers and patients with lung disease. Other studies pertaining to alveolar penetration, deposition, and mixing have been performed [83,87]. Deposition studies directed at particles with minimal settling and diffusional deposition tendencies, that is, 0.1–1.0 μm, have been described by Davies and colleagues [88,89]. Particulate deposition by the nasal airways has been reported [90–92], as has deposition by mouth inhalation [93]. Other studies have emphasized deposition of highly diffusive aerosols [75].

In 1966, the Task Group on Lung Dynamics examined the models and experimental data in the literature and described the deposition of aerosols in three areas of the lung: the nasopharyngeal, tracheobronchial, and pulmonary regions [94]. The investigators' major concern was the deposition of hazardous aerosols. The Task Group's predictive model uses Findeisen's simplified anatomy and his impaction and sedimentation equations [80]. For diffusional deposition, the equations of Gormley and Kennedy [95] were adopted, and the nasal route of entry was assumed. For a tidal volume of 1,450 mL, there were relatively small differences in estimated deposition over a wide range of geometric standard deviations ($1.2 < g < 4.5$). The comparison of this model with earlier predictive models indicated that Landahl's model was the closest but overestimated alveolar deposition for particles with aerodynamic diameters larger than 3.5 μm. The major conclusion of the Task Group was that regional deposition within the respiratory tract may be estimated using a single aerosol measurement: the mass median diameter. Subsequently, investigators [96,97] have reaffirmed the importance of the geometric standard deviation, taken in conjunction with the mass median diameter, in-mouth breathing, for describing the character of the aerosol. This may be of particular relevance because of the heterodisperse nature of therapeutic aerosols [98]. The degree of polydispersity of an aerosol, which may be described by the geometric standard deviation, has been shown to influence significantly aerosol deposition in the respiratory tract. Models have been developed for mouth inhalation, where the complex nasal filtration and deposition does not occur [98,99].

From the Task Group model, it was suggested that particles must have a diameter less than 10 μm before deposition occurs in regions below the nasopharnyx. Aerosols with diameters between 1 and 5 μm are deposited primarily in the tracheobronchial and pulmonary regions, and aerosols with diameters less than 1 μm are deposited predominately in the pulmonary region. This guide to the deposition of aerosol particles may be explained in terms of physicochemical parameters governing aerosol particle behavior. Dr. Gonda discusses these issues in Chap. 3.

REFERENCES

1. Weibel ER. Morphometry of the Human Lung. Berlin: Springer Verlag, 1963.
2. Gehr P, Bachofen M, Weibel ER. Respir Physiol 1978; 32:121.
3. Bouhuys A. In: Bouhuys A, ed. Breathing: Physiology, Environment and Lung Disease. New York: Grune and Stratton, 1974:25.
4. Weibel ER. In: Weibel ER, ed. The Pathway for Oxygen. Cambridge, MA: Harvard University Press, 1984:272.
5. Inoue S, Hogg J. Lab Investig 1974; 31:68.
6. Williams MC. In: Schraufnagel DE, ed. Electron Microscopy of the Lung [Lung Biology in Health and Disease, Vol. 48]. New York: Marcel Dekker, 1990:121.
7. Godfrey RWA. Microsc Res Tech 1997; 38:488.
8. Finkbeiner WE. Respir Physiol 1999; 118:77.
9. Schutte BC, McCray PB, Jr. Annu Rev Physiol 2002; 64:709.
10. Gail DB, Lenfant CJM. Am Respir Dis 1983; 127:366.
11. Morrow PE. Arch Intern Med 1973; 131:101.
12. Tyler WS. Am Rev Respir Dis 1983; 128:S32.
13. Crapo JD, Young SL, Fram EK, Pinkerton KE, Barry BE, Crapo RO. Am Rev Respir Dis 1983; 128:S42.
14. Voekler DR, Mason RJ. In: Massaro D, ed. Lung Cell Biology [Lung Biology in Health and Disease, Vol. 41]. New York: Marcel Dekker, 1989:487.
15. Mills PR, Davies RJ, Devalia JL. Am Rev Respir Crit Care Med 1999; 160:S38.
16. Spina D. Am Rev Respir Crit Care Med 1998; 158:S141.
17. Reid L. Thorax 1960; 15:132.
18. Meyrick B, Sturgess JM, Reid L. Thorax 1969; 24:729.
19. Rogers DF. Eur J Respir J 1994; 7:1690.
20. Widdicombe JG. Resp Physiol 2001; 125:3.
21. Lundberg JM, Hökfelt T, Martling C-R, Saria A, Cuello C. Cell Tissue Res 1984; 235:251.
22. Coleridge JCG, Coleridge HM. Rev Physiol Biochem Pharmacol 1984; 99:1.
23. Michoud M-C, Jeanneret-Grosjean A, Cohen A, Amyot R. Am Rev Respir Dis 1988; 138:1548.
24. McDonald DM, Bowden JJ, Baluk P, Bunnett NW. Adv Exp Med Biol 1996; 410:453.
25. Cutz E, Jackson A. Respir Physiol 1999; 115:201.
26. Widdicombe JG. Physiol Rev 1963; 43:1.
27. Ueki I, German VF, Nadel JA. Am Rev Respir Dis 1980; 121:351.
28. Baker B, Peatfield AC, Richardson PS. J Physiol (Lond) 1985; 365:297.
29. Diamond L, Altiere RJ. In: Kaliner MA, Barnes PJ, eds. The Airways: Neural Control in Health and Disease. New York: Marcel Dekker, 1989:343.
30. Rogers DF. Respir Physiol 2000; 125:129.
31. Richardson JB. In: Lichenstein LM, Austen KF, eds. Asthma: Physiology, Immunopharmacology and Treatment. New York: Academic Press, 1977:237.
32. Crapo JD, Barry BE, Gehr P, Bachofen M, Weibel ER. Am Rev Respir Dis 1982; 125:332.
33. Sibile Y, Reynolds HY. Am Rev Respir Dis 1990; 141:471.

34. Laskin DL, Laskin JD. Toxicology 2001; 160:111.
35. Shapiro SD. Am J Respir Crit Care Med 1999; 160:S29.
36. Parks WC, Shapiro SD. Respir Res 2001; 2:10.
37. Cutz E, Orange RP. In: Lichenstein LM, Austen KF, eds. Asthma: Physiology, Immunopharmacology and Treatment. New York: Academic Press, 1977:51.
38. Caughey GH. Am J Respir Crit Care Med 1991; 4:387.
39. Abraham WM. Am J Lung Cell Mol Physiol 2002; 282:L193.
40. Cocks TM, Moffatt JD. Pulm Pharmacol Ther 2001; 14:183.
41. Serikov VB, Fleming NW. J Appl Physiol 2001; 91:1977.
42. Simionescu M. Metabolic Activities of the Lung. Ciba Foundation Symposium 78. New York: Excerpta Medica, 1980:11.
43. Murray JF. In: Murray JF, ed. The Normal Lung: The Basis for Diagnosis and Treatment of Disease. Philadelphia: W. B. Saunders, 1986:283.
44. Effros RM. In: Crystal RG, West JB, eds. The Lung: Scientific Foundations. Vol. I. New York: Raven Press, 1991:1163.
45. Marshall C, Marshall B. J Appl Physiol 1983; 55:711.
46. Gryglewski RJ. Metabolic Activities of the Lung. Ciba Foundation Symposium 78. New York: Excerpta Medica, 1980:147.
47. Wasserman SI. J Allergy Clin Immunol 1983; 72:101.
48. Ryan JW. Am J Physiol (Lung Cell Mol Physiol) 1989; 257:1.
49. Baraniuk JN, Ohbuko K, Kwon OK, Mak J, Ali M, Favies R, Twort C, Kaliner M, Barnes PJ. Eur Respir J 1995; 8:1458.
50. Martins MA, Shore SA, Drazen JM. Int Arch Allergy Appl Immunol 1991; 94:325.
51. Battistini B, Dussault P. Pulm Pharmacol Ther 1998; 11:79.
52. Miller WF, Scacci R, Gast LR. Laboratory Evaluation of Pulmonary Function. New York: J. B. Lippincott, 1987.
53. Landahl HD. Bull Math Biophys 1950; 12:43.
54. Bums CB, Taylor WR, Ingram RH. J Appl Physiol 1985; 59:1590.
55. Frazer DG, Weber KC, Franz GN. Respir Physiol 1985; 61:277.
56. Maxwell DL, Cover D, Hughes JMB. Respir Physiol 1985; 61:255.
57. Ferron GA. J Aerosol Sci 1977; 8:251.
58. Ferron GA. J Aerosol Sci 1977; 8:409.
59. Schlesinger RB, Bohning DE, Chan TL, Lippman M. J Aerosol Sci 1977; 8:429.
60. Chan TL, Lippman M. Am Ind Hyg Assoc J 1980; 41:399.
61. Chan TL, Schrenck RM, Lippman M. J Aerosol Sci 1980; 11:447.
62. Martonen TB. J Aerosol Sci 1983; 14:11.
63. Horsfield K. Bull Math Biol 1976; 38:305.
64. Lee W-C, Wang C-S. In: Walton WH, ed. Inhaled Particles. Vol. IV. Oxford, UK: Pergamon Press, 1976:49.
65. Gerrity TR, Lee PS, Hass FJ, Marinelli A, Werner P, Lourenco RV. J Appl Physiol 1979; 47:867.
66. Yeh HC, Schum GM. Bull Math Biol 1980; 42:461.
67. Yeh HC, Schurn GM, Duggan MT. Anat Rec 1979; 195:483.
68. Davies CN. J Aerosol Sci 1980; 11:213.
69. Yu CP, Diu CK. J Aerosol Sci 1983; 14(5):99.

70. Rudolph G. J Aerosol Sci 1984; 15:195.
71. Dubois AB, Botelho SY, Comroe JH. J Clin Investig 1956; 35:327.
72. Emmett PC, Aitken RJ, Muir DCF. J Aerosol Sci 1979; 10:123.
73. Williams TJ. Br J Dis Chest 1982; 76:223.
74. Palmes ED, Wang C-S, Goldring RM, Altschuler B. J Appl Physiol 1973; 34:356.
75. Yu C-P, Thiagarajen C. J Aerosol Sci 1979; 10:11.
76. Lawford P, McKenzie D. Br J Dis Chest 1982; 76:229.
77. Brain JD, Sweeney TD, Tryka AF, Skomik WA, Godleski JJ. J Aerosol Sci 1984; 15:217.
78. Taylor SM, Pare PD, Schellenberg RR. J Appl Physiol 1984; 56:958.
79. Stahlhofen W, Gebhart J, Heyder J, Scheuch G, Juraske P. J Aerosol Sci 1984; 15:215.
80. Findeisen W. Arch Ges Physiol 1935; 236:367.
81. Landahl HD. Bull Math Biophys 1950; 12:161.
82. Rohrer F. In: West JB, ed. Translations in Respiratory Physiology. Stroudsburg, PA: Dowden, Hutchinson and Ross, 1955:3.
83. Beeckmans JM. Can J Physiol Pharmacol 1965; 43:157.
84. Lippman M. In: Mercer TT, Morrow PE, Stober W, eds. Assessment of Airborne Particles. Rochester Third International Conference on Environmental Toxicity. Springfield, IL: Charles C. Thomas, 1970:449.
85. Lipman M, Albert RE. Am Ind Hyg Assoc J 1969; 30:257.
86. Lippman M, Albert RE, Petersen HT. In: Walton WH, ed. Inhaled Particles. Vol. III. Oxford, UK: Pergamon Press, 1971:105.
87. Altschuler B, Palmes ED, Yarmus L, Nelson N. J Appl Physiol 1959; 14:321.
88. Davies CN. In: Mercer TT, Morrow PE, Stober W, eds. Assessment of Airborne Particles. Rochester Third International Conference on Environmental Toxicity. Springfield, IL: Charles C. Thomas, 1970:371.
89. Davies CN, Heyder J, Subba-Ramu MC. J Appl Physiol 1972; 32:591.
90. George AC, Breslin AJ. Health Phys 1967; 13:375.
91. Hounam RF, Black A, Walsh M. In: Walton WH, ed. Inhaled Particles. Vol. 111. Oxford, UK: Pergamon Press, 1971:71.
92. Heyder J, Rudolph G. In: Walton WH, ed. Inhaled Particles. Vol. IV. Oxford, UK: Pergamon Press, 1977:107.
93. Gonda I, Byron PR. Drug Dev Ind Pharmacol 1978; 4:243.
94. Task Group on Lung Dynamics, Health Phys 1966; 12:173.
95. Gormley PG, Kennedy M. Proc R Ir Acad 1949; 52A:163.
96. Gonda I. The International Symposium on Deposition and Clearance of Aerosols in the Human Respiratory Tract, Bad Gleichenberg, Austria, GAF, IGAM, May 22–23.
97. Morrow PE. Chest 1981; 80:809.
98. Mercer TT, Goddard RF, Flores RL. Ann Allergy 1968; 26:18.
99. Gonda I. J Pharm Pharmacol 1981; 33:692.
100. Jeffery PK. Am Rev Respir Dis 1983; 128:S14.
101. Scheuermann DW. Microsc Res Tech 1997; 37:31.
102. Holt PG, Schon-Hegrad MA, Phillips MJ, McMenamin PG. Clin Exp Allergy 1989; 19:597.

103. Ferreira SH, Vane JR. Br J Pharmacol Chemother 1967; 30:417.
104. Schuster VL. Ann Rev Physiol 1998; 60:221.
105. Thomas DP, Vane JR. Nature 1967; 216:335.
106. Ryan JW, Ryan US. Fed Proc 1977; 36:2683.
107. Hyman AL, Spannhake EW, Kadowitz PJ. Am Rev Respir Dis 1978; 117:111.
108. Sole MJ, Dobrac M, Schwartz L, Hussain MN, Vaughn-Neil EF. Circulation 1979; 60:160.
109. Ferreira SH, Greene LJ, Salgado MCO, Krieger EM. Metabolic Activities of the Lung. Ciba Foundation Symposium 78. Amsterdam: Excerpta Medica, 1980:129.
110. Piper PJ, Tippins JR, Samhoun MN, Morris HR, Taylor GW, Jones CM. Bull Eur Physiopathol Respir 1981; 17:571.
111. de Nucci G, Thomas R, D'Oleans-Juste P, Antunes E, Walder C, Warner TD, Vane JR. Proc Natl Acad Sci (USA) 1988; 85:9797.

2

Pharmacology of Therapeutic Aerosols

David C. Thompson
University of Colorado Health Sciences Center, Denver, Colorado, U.S.A.

INTRODUCTION

In the treatment of disease, aerosol administration represents a valuable means by which a therapeutic agent may be delivered. This route possesses many advantages over other routes of administration for the treatment of specific disease states, particularly those associated with the lungs. However, aerosol administration also exhibits unique limitations. To appreciate fully the usefulness or potential of aerosols as a means of drug delivery, it is important that the advantages and disadvantages of aerosols for this task be considered. This chapter deals with the pharmacology (including pharmacokinetics and pharmacodynamics) of aerosolized drugs in the airways. The impact of airway histology and physiology as they pertain to the action of an aerosolized drug are also considered.

PHARMACODYNAMICS

A drug may be described simply as a chemical substance that affects the activity of living processes. As a therapeutic agent, the drug serves to prevent, treat, or reverse an undesirable physiological or pathophysiological process. In general, the action of a drug results from an interaction of the drug molecule with a macromolecular structure associated with a cell, the consequence of which is a change in cellular function and, relatedly, in physiological function. In such a process, a drug may act to inhibit or mimic the actions of an endogenously produced chemical or to modify the response of cellular components to the actions of endogenously produced chemicals. Specific sites at which drugs act to produce an observable response include receptors (macromolecular sites at which chemicals interact to influence cellular function) and enzymes. A chemical is considered to be an agonist when it interacts with a receptor to produce a response, be it an increase or a decrease in cellular activity, whereas a chemical is considered to be an antagonist when it interacts with a receptor to block the response induced by an agonist. Accordingly, the observed effect of an antagonist relies on its capacity to inhibit the actions of other substances on cellular function.

The physiological actions of a drug are determined by: (1) the receptors or enzymes on which the drug acts, (2) the cells on which the receptors are located, and (3) the access of drug to cells on which the appropriate receptors are located. A cell may possess more than one receptor sensitive to the actions of a drug, although, in general, a drug exhibits concentration dependence in its selectivity for receptors, and, therefore, selection of appropriate doses of a drug is important in obtaining the desired therapeutic and physiological action. Nevertheless, the selectivity or specificity of many drugs and chemicals is sufficient to provide a basis upon which receptors may be described. However, it is important to recognize that receptors are not unique to specific cells. Consequently, an agonist or antagonist can influence the biological activity of all tissues comprising cells that express the appropriate receptor, provided it has equivalent and free access to the receptors.

PHARMACOKINETICS

The passage of a drug from the outlet of a nebulizer or metered-dose inhaler to its therapeutic or biological site of action is governed by many factors, which may be grouped empirically into two categories: (1) physical factors, which determine the deposition of drug from the mouth and onto the surface of the airway lumen, and (2) pharmacokinetic factors, which influence the amount of drug passing from the airway lumen to the target cell or tissue, i.e., the site at which the drug acts in producing a therapeutic action.

Physical Factors

In general, the impaction of all inhaled aerosol particles on the lumenal surface of the airways is governed by physical forces, such as gravity, inertia, and diffusion [1] (see Chap. 3 for details). Other factors that may be modified to influence aerosol deposition include the following.

Aerosol Particle Size

The influence of particle size on the deposition pattern of a drug in the lung is summarized as follows [2]:

Selection of an appropriate monodisperse (i.e., uniform particle size) aerosol may permit the administration of a drug to the central or peripheral airways, a process that may be of benefit in targeting drugs for local or systemic actions. In general, however, aerosols used in therapy are polydisperse (i.e., consist of a range of particle sizes) and, therefore, distribute throughout the airways. Nevertheless, it should be recognized that 10% or less of an administered aerosol dose will attain the airways, with the remainder depositing on the mouth or pharynx or being swallowed [3].

Breathing Pattern

The rate of breathing and depth of breathing also influence drug deposition in the airways. Rapid, shallow inspiration promotes central deposition of a drug, whereas slow, deep inspiration leads to peripheral airway deposition [4]. Furthermore, the rate of ventilation and tidal volume (volume of air inspired each breath) determines the residence time of the drug in the lungs, that is, the period in which the airways are exposed to drug [1]. Holding one's breath at the end of inspiration of an aerosol promotes deposition through sedimentation (by gravitation) and diffusion.

Airway Geometry

The caliber and tortuosity of the airway influences the flow of air through the segment and, thereby, affects aerosol particle impaction [1]. Disease states that alter airway caliber, such as obstructive airways disease, influence the pattern of aerosolized drug deposition in the airways by influencing airway geometry.

Aerosol particle diameter (μm)	Deposition site
≥ 10	Oropharynx
> 5	Central airways (tracheobronchial)
< 3	Peripheral airways (alveolus)

CENTRAL AIRWAY

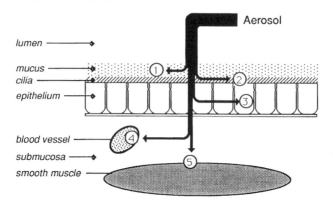

ALVEOLUS

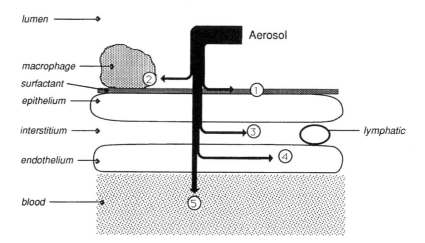

FIGURE 1   Fate of inhaled drugs depositing in the airways. Aerosolized compounds delivered to the lumenal surface of central (i.e., tracheobronchial) and peripheral (i.e., alveolus) airways may be subject to different pharmacokinetic pressures. The sites of loss of a drug in passage from the airway lumen to the site of therapeutic action in the central airways (e.g., smooth muscle) and peripheral airways (e.g., blood in pulmonary circulation) are depicted in upper and lower diagrams, respectively. In the central airways, a drug may (1) interact with the mucus layer, (2) be removed by the mucociliary escalator, (3) have restricted access through the epithelium and be biotransformed or be complexed by epithelium-associated

Pharmacokinetic Factors

Once a drug has been deposited on the lumenal surface of the airway segment, pharmacokinetic processes (viz., absorption, distribution, metabolism or biotransformation, excretion) will govern the amount of drug that reaches its therapeutic site of action. The pharmacokinetic pressures exerted on a drug deposited in the central airways differ from those in the peripheral airways, primarily as a result of the varying constituent cellular populations in each region. For demonstrative purposes, the fates of a bronchodilator drug in the central airways and of a drug destined for systemic absorption in the alveolus are considered in the following sections and are shown in Fig. 1.

Central Airways

The lumenal surface of the epithelium of the central airways (trachea to terminal bronchioles) is covered by a blanket of mucus that is a heterogeneous mixture of water, inorganic salts, glycoproteins, proteoglycans, lipids and other proteins, and peptides [5,6]. Inhaled drug would initially deposit on the mucus layer, in which it may become dissolved or complexed [7]. The mucus of the airways, together with concerted, coordinated beating of cilia on ciliated columnar epithelial cells, constitutes what is known as the *mucociliary escalator*. This system serves to move the mucus toward the pharynx for expulsion from the airways, and, accordingly, a portion of drug present in the mucus will be removed by it (Fig. 1). In addition, it is possible that some of the drug may be effectively lost through complexing with constituent substances in the mucus or degradation by enzymes contained in the mucus. A drug that passes through the mucus layer must then traverse the epithelium to gain access to subepithelial target cells.

The epithelium of the central airways consists primarily of ciliated epithelial cells. Adjacent cells of the epithelium are coupled tightly by junctional processes that normally prevent the passage of macromolecules between cells, i.e., paracellular transport [8–10]. As a result, transport of substances across the epithelium requires passage through, rather than between, epithelial cells, a process called *transcytosis* [10]. Under these conditions, absorption of a drug will be influenced by processes governing passive diffusion through cells, i.e., not saturable, and the rate of diffusion will be directly related to the drug

---

components, and (4) be removed by diffusion into submucosal blood vessels before reaching its target cell, e.g., airway smooth muscle cell. In the peripheral airways, a drug designed for delivery to the blood stream may (1) be diluted and diffuse in the surfactant, (2) be taken up by alveolar macrophages, (3) diffuse through the interstitium and be removed by lymphatic capillaries, and (4) be biotransformed by enzymes associated with pulmonary endothelial cells.

concentration gradient across cell membranes, lipid solubility, and inversely related to molecular size and ionization. It is unclear whether this transport is like the alveolar epithelium in using caveolae or vesicles (vide infra), although the presence of caveolins (structural proteins associated with caveolae) in isolated bronchial epithelial cells [11] would support such a possibility. Carrier-mediated transport systems that are saturable, energy dependent, and selective may also contribute to the passage of drugs, such as cromolyn sodium, across the pulmonary epithelium [12]. Paracellular passage of macromolecules may be enhanced under pathophysiological conditions that influence epithelial permeability, such as those attending application of an irritant or inflammatory stimulus to the airways [9,13]. Fecal pellets of house dust mite, a common allergen, contains a proteinase that disrupts airway epithelial tight junctions and thereby enhances its paracellular penetration of the epithelium [14]. Mechanisms governing tight junction permeability represents an area of active research. (for a review, see Ref. 15.) In passage through the epithelium, the drug or inhaled compounds may be biotransformed or inactivated by enzymes associated with the epithelium and/or may react or bind with cellular or extracellular components of the epithelium [16].

Once a compound has traversed the epithelium and the basement membrane (to which the epithelium is attached), it can diffuse through the loose connective tissue of the submucosa to gain access to target tissues, such as proinflammatory cells (e.g., mast cells), glands, sensory nerves, blood vessels, smooth muscle cells, or autonomic nerves. Submucosal blood flow in an airway segment may also represent a site of loss of drug by "washing out" administered drug from the tissue [17].

Alveolus

In the alveolus, aerosolized drug is deposited in a layer of surfactant, a lipoprotein compound that lines the alveolar surface and reduces alveolar surface tension. Drug deposited in the surfactant may diffuse laterally through the surfactant [18], decreasing focal concentrations. Absorption of compounds presented to the alveolar epithelium is determined by molecular size and lipophilicity or hydrophilicity [16]. Lipophilic drugs (i.e., drugs with a high lipid and water partition coefficient) cross cell membranes rapidly and, thereby, traverse the alveolar epithelial cells, the interstitium, and the endothelium to reach the bloodstream. This process is dependent on blood flow [18] insofar as the drug moves down its concentration gradient from the alveolus to the blood. Hydrophilic compounds are less rapidly absorbed and are thought to be dependent on passage through intracellular pores in the epithelium [10,18]. Caveolae, or vesicles, have been identified in alveolar type 1 cells [19]. Macromolecules can be taken up into caveolae at the lumenal surface of the cell and be shuttled through the cell in a vesicle. The contribution of caveolae to the proposed intracellular pores remains uncertain [11], although it has been proposed that fusion of several vesicles may form discontinuous continuous pathways through the cell [19]. Molecular size of the hydrophilic molecule is thought to be the limiting factor in diffusion, and this process applies primarily to hydrophilic molecules of low molecular weight [16]. Higher-molecular-weight hydrophilic substances deposited in the alveolus may be taken up (subject to endocytosis) and removed by pulmonary alveolar macrophages. Once in the interstitium, a drug may diffuse into lymphatic vessels (an important site of loss for large molecules) or into the bloodstream through the endothelium. In addition, binding to epithelial or interstitial cellular constituents may represent an additional site of loss for compounds [16].

The rate of absorption of a compound from the alveolus is approximately two times faster than that in the central airways of a variety of species [20]. This suggests that the membrane permeability of the alveolus is greater than that of the tracheobronchial region [21]. With respect to enzymatic biotransformation of drugs in passage from the airway lumen to the target cells in the central and peripheral airways, relatively little is known. Using histochemical and biochemical techniques, a variety of enzymes have been identified in the airways, and these are summarized in Table 1. It is important to recognize that the distribution of enzymes in the central airways may differ from those in the peripheral airways [22].

At least insofar as blood-borne substances are concerned, the lung serves as an important organ of metabolism. The primary focus of this activity rests in the pulmonary endothelium, i.e., the cells lining pulmonary blood vessels. Compounds known to be metabolized by the pulmonary endothelium include adenine nucleotides (e.g., AMP, ADP, ATP), bradykinin, 5-hydroxytryptamine (serotonin), norepinephrine, and prostaglandins of the E and F series [27]. In general, these processes result in the formation of biologically inactive products. However, pulmonary biotransformation may result in bioactivation, as is the case for conversion of angiotensin I to angiotensin II by angiotensin-converting enzyme on the endothelium. Furthermore, the processes of metabolism are selective, as exemplified by the pulmonary clearance of 5-hydroxytryptamine and norepinephrine but not of histamine or epinephrine [27]. The importance of enzymatic and degradation on the activity of aerosolized drugs remains the subject of little systematic scientific investigation. Nevertheless, the demonstration that inhibition of pulmonary neutral endopeptidase (EC24.11) uncovers a bronchoconstrictor action of the undecapeptide, substance P [28], underscores the potential importance of metabolic processes in regulating the biological actions of aerosolized compounds. The situation is confounded further by pulmonary diseases wherein activated proinflammatory cells, such as macrophages, mast cells, neutrophils, or eosinophils, release proteolytic enzymes

TABLE 1   Enzymes Identified in Airway Tissue

Acid phosphatase	Glycerol 3 phosphate dehydrogenase
Alcohol dehydrogenase	3-Hydroxybutyrate dehydrogenase
Alkaline phosphatase	Insulysin (insulin degrading enzyme)
Amine oxidase	Isocitrate dehydrogenase
Aminopeptidase P	Lactate dehydrogenase
Angiotensin-converting enzyme	Leucine aminopeptidase
Aniline hydroxylase	Lipase
ATPase	Lipoxygenase
Arylsulfatase	Malate dehydrogenase
Carboxypeptidase M	Metallo-endopeptidase
Cyclooxygenase	N-Methyl transferase
Cytochrome oxidase	Monoamine oxidase
Endothelin-converting enzyme	Mixed-function oxidase
	(cytochrome P450 dependent)
Epoxide hydrase	$NADH_2$ diaphorase
Nonspecific esterase	$NADPH_2$ diaphorase
β-Galactosidase	Neutral endopeptidase 24.11
N-Acetyl β-glucosaminidase	Nitro oxide synthase
Glucose dehydrogenase	Nitro reductase
Glucose 6-phosphatase	5′-Nucleotidase
Glucose 6 phosphatase	Peroxidase
dehydrogenase	
β-Glucuronidase	Phosphatidic acid phosphatase
Glucuronyl transferase	Post proline cleaving enzyme
Glutamate dehydrogenase	Prostaglandin dehydrogenase
Glutathione-s-aryl transferase	Succinate dehydrogenase
Glutathione-S-epoxide transferase	Sulfotransferase
Glyceraldehyde 3 phosphate	
dehydrogenase	

Source: Refs. 22–26.

that can modify the bioavailability of inhaled macromolecules as they are being absorbed from the airways.

THERAPEUTIC USES OF AEROSOLS

Aerosol preparations of drugs are most commonly used for the treatment of diseases involving airway obstruction, namely bronchodilators and anti-inflammatory agents in asthma, bronchitis, and emphysema. Other uses of aerosol therapies include mucolytics (for decreasing the thickness or viscosity of mucus in diseases involving abnormal mucus secretion, e.g., pneumonia, bronchitis, cystic fibrosis) and antibiotics (for treatment of lung infections). In addition, aerosols may be used for clinical investigation and diagnosis, an example of which is delineation of airway reactivity using bronchoconstrictors. In general, current therapeutic uses of aerosols exploit the ability of an aerosol to deliver a high concentration of a drug locally to the airways without eliciting the side effects that otherwise attend administration by alternative routes.

Bronchodilators

Associated with airways extending from the trachea to the terminal bronchioles is a layer of smooth muscle. In the trachea, smooth muscle constitutes a fraction of the circumference and connects the ends of incomplete cartilage rings. The fractional contribution of smooth muscle increases in lower airway segments such that the bronchi and bronchioles are encircled by a layer of smooth muscle. The length of the smooth muscle cells at any particular time determines the circumferential length of the airway and thereby influences airway caliber. Smooth muscle contraction (shortening) reduces airway caliber (causes bronchoconstriction) which increases resistance to airflow and makes breathing or ventilation more difficult. Smooth muscle relaxation (lengthening), on the other hand, decreases the work associated with ventilation by increasing airway caliber (causing bronchodilation) and reducing resistance to airflow.

A variety of agents act on airway smooth muscle to affect its state of contraction (tone), the majority of which act by specific receptors on the smooth muscle cell (Table 2). Bronchodilator drugs may be agonists of receptors subserving airway smooth muscle relaxation (e.g., β_2-adrenoceptor agonists) or antagonists of receptors mediating airway smooth muscle concentration (e.g., muscarinic cholinoceptor antagonists). Other drugs may exert actions on cellular mechanisms that influence the intracellular processes of airway smooth muscle contraction or relaxation (e.g., xanthine derivatives). The sites of action of these drugs are shown in Fig. 2.

β-Adrenoceptor Agonists

Agonists of β-adrenoceptors have been used for many years as bronchodilators in the treatment of asthma, and they remain the most widely used group of bronchodilators in therapy. Epinephrine, an agonist exhibiting relative selectivity for β-adrenoceptors, was the first β agonist used in the treatment of asthma. Through the years, agonists have been developed that are selective for the β-adrenoceptor mediating human airway smooth muscle relaxation, viz. the β_2-adrenoceptor. Examples of drugs of this type include albuterol (salbutamol), fenoterol, terbutaline, and metaproterenol. Further development has led to drugs, such as formoterol and salmeterol, which exhibit longer residence times in the airways and consequent increases in duration of action [29]. Stereoisomers of

TABLE 2   Agents That Influence the Tone of Human Airway Smooth Muscle

Classification	Bronchoconstrictors	Bronchodilators
Neurotransmitters	Acetylcholine	Nonadrenergic noncholinergic inhibitory neurotransmitter Norepinephrine Epinephrine
Endogenous substances (e.g., mediators, hormones)	Histamine Leukotrienes Platelet-activating factor Prostaglandin $F_{2\alpha}$ Prostaglandin D_2 Thromboxane A_2 Adenosine 5-Hydroxytrypt-amine (serotonin) Tachykinins (e.g., substance P) Endothelin	Vasoactive intestinal peptide Prostacyclin Prostaglandin E_2
Exogenous substances (e.g., pharmacological agents)	Methacholine	Methylxanthines (e.g., theophylline) β_2-Adrenoreceptor agonists (e.g., albuterol)
Indirectly acting agents[a]	Antigen (release mediators) Irritants Citric acid Capsaicin Sulfur dioxide	

[a] Substances producing changes in tone through the release of bronchoactive substances.

the β_2-adrenoceptor agonist albuterol demonstrate different biological activities and pharmacokinetics, with the R isomer possessing the beneficial therapeutic effects (i.e., bronchodilation) [30] and a shorter half-life in the body [31].

In the treatment of airway obstruction, as may occur in asthma, bronchitis, or emphysema, β_2-adrenoceptor agonists may be used prophylactically (i.e., to prevent impending bronchoconstriction) or to reverse established bronchoconstriction. They represent the most effective bronchodilator drugs available. The longer-acting drugs, such as salmeterol, are used to prevent bronchoconstriction from occurring and are commonly used in combination with an inhaled

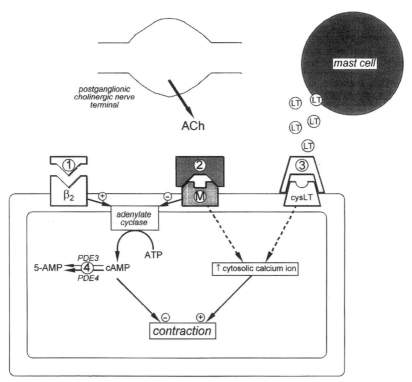

airway smooth muscle cell

FIGURE 2 Mechanisms of action of bronchodilator agents. Bronchodilation may be caused by administering one of the following types of drugs: (1) an agonist of β_2-adrenoceptors (e.g., albuterol), which subserve relaxation of airway smooth muscle, (2) an antagonist (e.g., ipratropium), which blocks the muscarinic cholinoceptor (M)-mediated airway smooth muscle contractile activity of acetylcholine released from cholinergic nerves, (3) an antagonist of cysteinyl leukotriene receptors (cysLT), which blocks airway smooth muscle contractile activity of leukotrienes C_4, D_4, or E_4 (LT) released from activated mast cells, or (4) an inhibitor of phosphodiesterase isozymes 3 (PDE3) and 4 (PDE4), which promotes airway smooth muscle relaxation by increasing intracellular levels of cyclic adenosine 3',5'-monophosphate (cAMP). The interactions between receptor activation, adenylate cyclase, cAMP, intracellular calcium ion concentrations, and the process of contraction are shown. Stimulation is indicated by " + " and inhibition by " − ."

corticosteroid. The shorter-acting agents, such as albuterol, are the drug of choice for reversing established bronchoconstriction. Repetitive or continued activation of β_2-adrenoceptors can lead to tolerance, wherein the extent of bronchodilation or inhibition of bronchoconstriction decreases with increased use of β_2-adrenoceptor agonist. This issue is considered to be more problematic with the longer-acting agents [32].

The evolution of β-adrenoceptor agonists as bronchodilators demonstrates important concepts in drug development. The synthesis of drugs selective for adrenoceptors that mediate airway smooth muscle relaxation served to diminish the side effects associated with their administration. Removal of α-adrenoceptor activity (as exhibited by epinephrine) decreased the incidence of drug-induced increases in blood pressure and removal of β_1-adrenoceptor activity attenuated drug-induced cardiostimulation. Nevertheless, specific β_2-adrenoceptor agonists do induce side effects, including tachycardia (increased heart rate) and muscle tremor, which are physiological manifestations of the actions of these drugs on β_2-adrenoceptors in cardiac and skeletal muscle. For these effects to manifest, the drug must be present in the circulation or blood supply to these tissues. Inhalation of an aerosol of β_2-adrenoceptor agonist serves to deliver a high concentration of drug to the airway smooth muscle while minimizing the amount of drug available to the circulation.

Muscarinic Cholinoceptor Antagonists

Airway smooth muscle cells are innervated (receive nerve supply) by cholinergic nerves. Increased cholinergic nerve activity is associated with irritant stimulation postganglionic cholinergic nerves to result in the release of acetylcholine from postganglionic nerve terminals, thus of sensory nerves in the airways that send impulses to the central nervous system and result in an increase in cholinergic nerve activity to the airways. Electrical impulses (action potentials) emanating from the central nervous system pass down preganglionic cholinergic nerves, traverse a ganglionic synapse (by acetylcholine-dependent neurochemical transmission), and send impulses along postganglionic cholinergic nerves to result in the release of acetycholine from postganglionic nerve terminals. Acetycholine, thus released, acts on muscarinic cholinoceptors that subserve airway smooth muscle contraction and bronchoconstriction (Fig. 3). These actions are prevented by antagonists of muscarinic cholinoceptors or by so-called "atropinelike" drugs. The efficacy of muscarinic cholinoceptor antagonists as bronchodilators is dependent solely on their capacity to reverse airway tone established by acetylcholine or, stated more simply, to terminate bronchoconstriction caused by acetylcholine. Accordingly, the bronchodilator activity of these drugs is dependent on the level of activation of cholinergic nerves, in that the higher the activity of efferent cholinergic nerves, the greater will be the apparent bronchodilator effect of the muscarinic antagonist. This distinguishes muscarinic

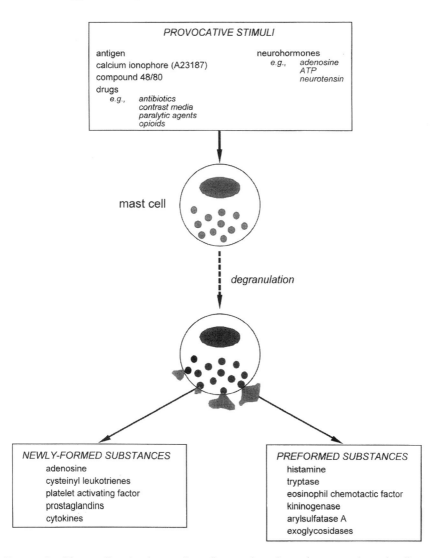

FIGURE 3 Mast cell activation and mediators. A variety of provocative stimuli act on mast cells to cause degranulation and consequent release of stored or preformed substances or mediators and the synthesis of newly formed substances or mediators.

antagonists from β_2-adrenoceptor agonists, in that the latter are nonspecific in reversing bronchoconstriction induced by a variety of stimuli, including acetylcholine and other bronchoconstrictors, such as inflammatory mediators. Increased activity of cholinergic nerves has been implicated in asthma [33]. However, the efficacy of muscarinic cholinoceptor inhibitors, such as ipratropium bromide, in the treatment of this disease appears to be variable and, in general, inferior to β_2-adrenoceptor agonists [34], a situation that may reflect the variable participation of cholinergic nerves in asthmatic bronchoconstriction. In chronic obstructive pulmonary disease, aerosol coadministration of a muscarinic antagonist with a β_2-adrenoceptor agonist induces more profound bronchodilation that either agonist alone [34] and exploits the rapid onset of action of the β_2-adrenoceptor agonist and the long duration of action of the muscarinic antagonist. Studies such as these have fostered the development of combination aerosol therapies, such as ipratropium + albuterol.

In an attempt to reduce the occurrence of side effects associated with absorption into the systemic circulation, quaternary ammonium compounds have been developed as muscarinic cholinoceptor antagonists, for example, ipratropium bromide, glycopyrrolate methylbromide. As a result of their polar nature, these compounds are poorly absorbed across lipid membranes and, therefore, do not easily enter the systemic circulation or the central nervous system (to produce undesirable side effects), but they do induce bronchodilation of long duration [34,35]. The only significant side effect of the quaternary ammonium compounds is dry mouth, an effect perhaps to be expected for a muscarinic cholinoceptor antagonist administered as an aerosol via the mouth.

Three functional subtypes of muscarinic cholinoceptors exist in the airways, designated M_1, M_2, and M_3. In the airways, agonist activation of M_1 and M_2 receptors have been proposed to inhibit autonomic ganglionic transmission and acetylcholine release from postganglionic nerves, respectively. M_3 receptors are the subtype on airway smooth muscle that mediate contraction of airway smooth muscle [36]. The muscarinic cholinoceptor antagonists used initially as bronchodilators in obstructive airways disease were nonselective for the receptor subtypes. Their ostensible lack of efficacy in treatment of airway obstruction was hypothesized to result from their enhancement of acetylcholine release (by blockage of presynaptic M_2 receptors), overwhelming their (postsynaptic M_3 receptor) blockade of the contractile actions of released acetylcholine [37]. This encouraged the development of muscarinic antagonists lacking inhibitory activity at the presynaptic M_2 receptors, an example of which is tiotropium, which inhibits M_1 and M_3 cholinoceptors [38].

Xanthine Derivatives and Phosphodiesterase Inhibitors

Xanthine derivatives, which include theophylline and its salt, aminophylline, are very effective in treating obstructive airways disease. However, the means by which these agents induce airway smooth muscle relaxation remains unclear. The primary mechanisms proposed include: (1) inhibition of phosphodiesterase, the enzyme responsible for metabolism of the intracellular messenger, cyclic adenosine $3',5'$-monophosphate (cAMP) [39] and (2) antagonism of receptors for adenosine, an agent that is proinflammatory and induces airway smooth muscle contraction in asthmatics [40]. It has become clear that several phosphodiesterase (PDE) isozymes (or subtypes) exist in the airways [42]. PDE3 and PDE4 are important in regulating cAMP levels in airway smooth muscle, and theophylline likely induces bronchodilation as a nonselective inhibitor of both isozymes [39]. PDE4 appears to be the primary cAMP-metabolizing enzyme in inflammatory (e.g., mast cells) and immune cells [41]. Consistent with these observations are the documented anti-inflammatory effects of recently developed inhibitors of PDE4 [41]. Xanthine derivatives are administered to the systemic circulation via the intravenous or oral routes of administration. Cardiovascular and central nervous system side effects represent a concern with the use of these agents because of their relatively narrow therapeutic index; i.e., side effects begin to manifest at the upper limits of therapeutic doses. Several pharmaceutical companies are developing isozyme-selective inhibitors with the hope of maintaining anti-inflammatory activity (PDE4 inhibition) to treat airways disease and diminishing side effects associated caused by inhibition of other isozymes, e.g., cardiovascular effects caused by PDE3 inhibition [41,42]. Several PDE4 inhibitors are advancing through early clinical studies [43], with cilomilast demonstrating beneficial effects in patients with chronic obstructive pulmonary disease [44]. Limited studies evaluating the activity of aerosolized xanthines have been conducted and have shown these compounds to induce bronchodilation, albeit less effectively than aerosolized β_2-adrenoceptor agonists [45,46]. Currently in trials, PDE4 inhibitors are administered orally, with nausea and gastrointestinal side effects representing the most common adverse events [41,44]. It remains to be seen whether administration by inhalation could be used to reduce these systemic side effects.

Antiasthma Drugs

Asthma is a disease characterized by reversible airways obstruction and increased responsiveness of the airways to specific and nonspecific bronchoconstrictor stimuli. Indeed, the latter feature may be used in diagnosis of asthma (vide infra). Obstruction to the flow of air in asthma is the product of three factors: smooth muscle contraction, mucosal edema, and augmented mucus secretion. Pathological features, such as infiltration of the airway walls with inflammatory cells (e.g., eosinophils, neutrophils), and the efficacy of anti-inflammatory steroids in treating the disease have pointed to an important role of inflammation in the disease process.

Episodes of airway obstruction or bronchoconstriction may be induced in asthmatics by exposure to stimuli to which they are sensitized, such as inhalation of a specific pollen or house dust mite, or exposure to an occupational stimulus, e.g., red cedar dust [47]. Binding of antigen (e.g., pollen) to specific receptors (antibodies) on the surface of an inflammatory cell (e.g., mast cell) results in the elaboration of prestored mediators, such as histamine, and in the synthesis of newly formed mediators, such as arachidonic acid metabolites (e.g., prostaglandins and leukotrienes). Cellular sources of the various mediators are shown in Table 3. Cytokines and chemokines are proteins that participate in pulmonary immune and inflammatory responses. While important, these have not been subjected to discussion in this chapter because these fields are changing very

TABLE 3 Biologically Active Mediators Derived from Inflammatory Cells

Cell type	Mediator
Eosinophil	Leukotrienes
	Nitric oxide
	Platelet-activating factor
	Reactive oxygen species
	Cotaxin
Macrophage	Nitric oxide
	Platelet-activating factor
	Prostaglandins
	Reactive oxygen species
	Thromboxane A_2
Mast cell	Adenosine
	Histamine
	Leukotrienes
	Platelet-activating factor
	Prostaglandin D_2
	Tryptase
Neutrophil	Elastase
	Leukotriene B_4
	Prostaglandins
	Platelet-activating factor
	Reactive oxygen species
Platelet	5-Hydroxytryptamine
	Lipoxygenase metabolites
	Platelet-activating factor
	Thromboxane A_2

Source: Ref. 78.

rapidly. Readers are directed to excellent review articles [48,49]. Mediators, thus released, exert potent biological actions that include airway smooth muscle contraction, increased capillary permeability (to result in mucosal edema), increased epithelial permeability, mucus secretion, inflammatory cell chemotactic activity, and increased airways responsiveness, i.e., their actions are proinflammatory. Other stimuli in addition to specific antigen may also educe the release of mediators from inflammatory cells, some of these are shown in Fig. 3.

In the treatment of airways diseases involving mediator release, therapeutic interventions have been directed at: (1) inhibition of mediator release or synthesis or (2) inhibition of the biological actions of released mediators. Should mediator release or the resultant inflammatory state be responsible for induction of airway hyperreactivity, it would be expected that these same therapeutic interventions would be beneficial in returning the airway reactivity of asthmatics toward that of nonasthmatic individuals.

Inhibition of Mediator Release or Synthesis

Prevention of the release or synthesis of biologically active mediators from inflammatory cells has represented an important target for drugs in the treatment of asthma. Inhaled drugs, such as cromolyn, β_2-adrenoceptor agonists, and glucocorticoids, have proven to be effective in the prophylactic treatment of asthma, i.e., administered before exposure to a provocative stimulus such as antigen [50]. The mechanisms by which these groups of drugs inhibit mediator release are not well understood. Studies of their mechanisms not only provide valuable leads to new directions for drug development but also serve to elucidate the processes involved in the mediator secretory process.

Cromones. Cromolyn sodium was first available for use as a therapeutic agent in the United States in 1973. Administered as an aerosol, it is widely used for the prophylactic treatment of asthma, with the onset of activity manifesting after several weeks, and it causes few side effects. Nedocromil sodium possesses cromolyn-like activity [51] and is efficacious in the treatment of asthma when administered as an aerosol [52,53]. Despite a concerted research effort, the mechanism by which cromones exert their therapeutic activity remains enigmatic. Inhibition of mediator release from mast cells and a direct suppressive action on other inflammatory cells appear to be features of their clinical actions [54,55].

β-Adrenoceptor Agonists. In addition to possessing potent airway smooth muscle relaxant activities and thereby attenuating bronchospasm induced by released mediators, β_2-adrenoceptor agonists administered prophylactically may inhibit mediator release [50,56]. It has been proposed that the β_2-agonist-induced increase in intracellular cAMP inhibits mediator secretion by altering phospholipid metabolism and cell membrane function [50]. Nevertheless, this is not a primary therapeutic action of this group of drugs.

Corticosteroids. Corticosteroids represent the most valuable therapeutic agents for the prophylactic treatment of asthma [57]. This group of drugs, which include beclomethasone, budesonide, dexamethasone, flunisolide, fluticasone, and triamcinolone, exert a variety of actions on mediator release, including inhibition of mediator secretion from inflammatory cells and of the generation of cyclo-oxygenase (e.g., prostaglandins) and lipoxygenase (e.g., leukotrienes) metabolites of arachidonic acid [58]. Corticosteroids differ from most other drugs in producing a biological effect by diffusing into cells, interacting with a cytoplasmic receptor, and inducing or repressing the synthesis of various proteins that then elicit the biological or therapeutic action [59]. For example, induction of the synthesis of lipomodulin or the macrocortin by the corticosteroids causes the inhibition of phospholipase A_2, the enzyme responsible for releasing arachidonic acid (the substrate for cyclo-oxygenase and lipoxygenase enzymes) from membrane phospholipids [58]. Other important anti-inflammatory actions occur by transrepression of proinflammatory transcription factors NFκ-B and AP-1 [59]. Corticosteroids can also influence other immune system functions and thereby interfere with the inflammatory process at several loci [58,60]. Furthermore, corticosteroids may modify β-adrenoceptor populations [61] and exert a permissive effect on β-adrenoceptor function [62]. Oral corticosteroids are administered as therapy for chronic asthma that cannot be controlled by other therapies [63]. However, severe side effects, including suppression of the hypothalamic–pituitary–adrenal axis, Cushing's syndrome, osteoporosis in the elderly, and growth retardation in children, occur with systemic administration [64], and these limit the maintained use of such therapy. Topical application of corticosteroid as an inhaled aerosol is considered preferable, in that therapeutic concentrations may be delivered locally to the airways, thus minimizing systemic concentrations and the attendant systemic side effects. Principal side effects associated with inhaled corticosteroids reflect steroid deposition in the oropharynx and include oropharyngeal candidiasis, dysphonia, and hoarseness of the voice [64,65]. However, the use of spacers in combination with metered-dose inhalers can reduce these side effects [66], as can rinsing the mouth after aerosol therapy [67]. It is possible that systemic side effects may develop in patients using high-dose inhalation therapy. As a result of the potential for side effects, research efforts are directed toward the development of corticosteroids that possess anti-inflammatory activity but have minimal catabolic side effects [65,68].

Lipoxygenase Inhibitors. The leukotrienes are a series of compounds, generated by 5-lipoxygenase (5-LO) metabolism of arachidonic acid, that possess potent biological actions in the airways, including bronchoconstriction, mucosal edema (leukotrienes C_4, D_4, and E_4), and chemotactic activity (leukotriene B_4)

[69]. As a result of their prolonged and potent bronchoconstrictor actions, a role for the cysteinyl leukotrienes (viz. C_4, D_4, and E_4) in the genesis of asthmatic bronchospasm was suspected and is now well established. Consistent with this, inhibition of 5-LO using zileuton has been shown to relieve mild to moderate asthma [70]. Compared to their cysteinyl leukotriene receptor antagonist brethren (vide infra), 5-LO inhibitors are in their early stages of development. Currently, zileuton is the only 5-LO inhibitor available and is administered as an oral formulation. It is likely that more inhalable 5-LO inhibitors will available in the future.

Inhibition of Mediator Actions

Delineation of the role of a specific mediator in the bronchomotor response to a proinflammatory stimulus is usually obtained by the ability of a specific receptor antagonist to block the response. This process of identification is dependent on the antagonist's being applied in doses sufficient to block the receptor for the endogenously released mediator and selective for the receptor of the mediator at the applied doses. Specific antagonists have been developed or are currently being developed for many of the inflammatory cell-derived mediators possessing bronchoconstrictor or proinflammatory activity.

Histamine Antagonists. The first mediator to be implicated in the pathogenesis of asthma was histamine. Bronchoconstriction induced by histamine is inhibited by histamine H_1-receptor antagonists, or so-called classical antihistamines. Drugs of this group include clemastine, chlorpheniramine, asternizole, and terfenadine. In general, antihistamines are administered orally for the treatment of a variety of allergic disease. However, aerosolized clemastine has been shown to cause bronchodilation in asthmatic subjects [71] and to inhibit antigen-induced bronchoconstriction [72]. Interestingly, the aerosol route of administration of the antihistamines appears to be more effective in eliciting bronchodilation than the oral route [73], an observation related, in part, to the limitation on oral dosage caused by the sedative actions of these drugs. The newer, nonsedating antihistamines (e.g., astemizole, cetirizine, loratadine), while effective in treating some allergic conditions, have proven to be of little benefit in the treatment of asthma when given orally [74]. No studies have been undertaken in which these agents were applied directly to the airways by inhalation.

Leukotriene Antagonists. The leukotrienes are metabolites of arachidonic acid generated de novo after inflammatory cell activation [69,75] and are potent bronchoconstrictors and proinflammatory agents (vide supra). The biological effects of the cysteinyl-leukotrienes (viz. C_4, D_4, and E_4) and of leukotriene B_4 are mediated via $cysLT_1$ and BLT receptors, respectively [69,76]. The development of potent, selective cysLT receptor antagonists, such as montelukast, pranlukast, and zafirlukast, have permitted a clearer understanding of the contribution of the cysteinyl leukotrienes to asthma. The efficacy of these drugs in relieving asthmatic bronchoconstriction is significant (indicating a role of cysteinyl leukotrienes in asthmatic airway obstruction) but inferior to inhaled β_2-adrenoceptor agonists or inhaled corticosteroids [69,76]. As a result, they are often used in combination with other therapies [77]. These drugs are administered orally and exhibit relatively innocuous side effects [69]. This, together with their demonstrated clinical efficacy when administered orally, provides little impetus for the development of an inhalation formulation.

Platelet-Activating Factor Antagonists. Platelet-activating factor (PAF) is generated by a variety of inflammatory cells from membrane phospholipids under the actions of phospholiphase A_2 and acetyl CoA-dependent acetyltransferase [78,79]. Interest in PAF was aroused by the observation that PAF administration mimicked many features characteristic of asthma, including bronchoconstriction, lung inflammation, and airways hyperreponsiveness [79]. The poor clinical efficacy of PAF antagonists, such as apafant (WEB2086) and foropafant (SR27417A), in preventing the symptoms of asthma [80,81] argues against a role for PAF in this disease and makes it unlikely that these agents will be developed for lung delivery.

Mucus Secretion and Clearance

The superficial surface of the tracheobronchial epithelium is covered by a blanket of mucus, a heterogeneous mixture of water, inorganic salts, glycoproteins, proteoglycans, lipids and other proteins, and peptides [5,6]. Airway mucus humidifies inspired air and traps inhaled matter, such as particulates, bacteria, viruses, irritant gases, and aerosols [82]. This latter action of mucus in concert with coordinated ciliary beating (which transports the mucus toward the mouth) or coughing serves an important defensive mechanism in the normal airways for removal of foreign particulates.

The rate of removal of mucus from the airways is determined by such factors as mucus viscosity, the amount of mucus produced, and the degree of ciliary activity. These processes may be influenced by a variety of diseases, including asthma, cystic fibrosis, and chronic bronchitis [82,83]. In patients suffering from cystic fibrosis or chronic bronchitis, mucus hypersecretion is evident and mucociliary function is impaired. The failure to clear mucus from the airways leads to airway obstruction and to chronic colonization of the airways with bacterial organisms (which leads to lung infections and airway inflammation and damage). In asthmatic subjects, airway mucus is more viscous and ciliary transport mechanisms are inhibited [82,83]. In these diseases, the therapeutic objective is to improve mucus clearance from the airways. For example, aerosols of water or saline (especially hypertonic saline) promote clearance of mucus by liquefying secretions [84,85]. Acetylcysteine is a compound that reduces disulfide bonds in mucoproteins and mucopolysaccharides and thereby diminishes mucus viscosity by reducing the size of constituent molecules [86]. Administered as an aerosol, acetylcysteine may irritate the airways and induce bronchospasm in hyperreactive individuals, necessitating the concomitant administration of a β_2-adrenoceptor agonist. A more efficacious mucolytic agent for the treatment of cystic fibrosis is human DNase (dornase), a recombinant human protein. Delivered to the airways as an aerosol, this agent reduces mucus viscosity by degrading extracellular DNA released from neutrophils infiltrating the mucus [87].

Antibiotic and Antiviral Agents

Under pathological conditions involving mucus hypersecretion and diminished mucociliary function (such as cystic fibrosis), bacterial organisms may colonize the airways and produce infection, a process that leads to pulmonary tissue damage. Antibiotics are administered to reverse the lung infection by killing the responsible bacteria, most commonly either *Pseudomonas aeruginosa* or *Staphylococcus aureus*. In general, short-term therapy involves intravenous administration of high doses of antibiotics and oral antibiotics for prophylactic therapy. Aerosol administration has been suggested for the delivery of antibiotics that are not orally active and as an alternative to the oral route of antibiotic administration because, in general, high blood levels of antibiotics (which increase the chance of systemic toxicity) are necessary to attain adequate concentrations in the sputum [88]. Aerosolized antibiotics have the advantage of delivering high concentrations directly to the site of infection and reducing the systemic concentrations of antibiotic. This approach is best illustrated by tobramycin, an aminoglycoside commonly used to treat pulmonary infections associated with cystic fibrosis [89]. High systemic concentrations necessary to be effective against pulmonary *P. aeruginosa* can cause nephrotoxicity and ototoxicity. As a result, tobramycin has been formulated for inhalation as a nebulized solution and proven to be effective in the treatment of *P. aeruginosa* in cystic fibrosis patients [89,90]. Pentamidine is administered as an aerosol for the treatment of and prophylaxis against *Pneumocystis carinii* pneumonia in patients with acquired immunodeficiency syndrome [91]. Like tobramycin, pulmonary delivery minimizes systemic side effects while maintaining a desirable therapeutic effect. The success of these agents portend the development of other antibiotics as inhalation treatment of lung diseases in the future [92].

Ribavirin is a virustatic agent approved for administration as an aerosol for the treatment of lower respiratory tract infections caused by respiratory syncytial virus [93,94]. However, its therapeutic efficacy in this disease has come into question of late [95]. A newer group of antiviral agents have been developed that inhibit neuraminidase, a viral enzyme necessary for the release of viruses from infected cells. Oseltamivir and zanamivir, examples of neuraminidase inhibitors, can be used to treat influenza A and B [96]. Zanamivir, having low oral bio-availability [97], is administered intranasally or by inhalation as a dry powder, whereas oseltamivir is taken orally [98].

Pulmonary Vasodilation

The cyclo-oxygenase metabolite prostacyclin is a potent, short-lived vasodilator and antithrombotic agent. Intravenous administration of the commercially available form of prostacyclin, epoprostenol, relieves the symptoms of primary pulmonary hypertension by dilating the pulmonary vasculature [99]. A stable prostacyclin analogue, iloprost, appears to be similarly effective when administered as an aerosol and obviates the logistical problems associated with maintained intravenous administration [100].

Diagnostic Uses

The airways of asthma subjects are exquisitely sensitive (hyperresponsive) to the bronchoconstrictor actions of specific (e.g., bronchoconstrictor agonist) and nonspecific (e.g., airway irritants) stimuli. Indeed, the degree of airway hyper-responsiveness has been shown to correlate with the severity of asthma [101]. This characteristic is exploited by clinicians in the diagnosis of asthma, particularly in subjects who do not exhibit clinical manifestations of the disease. Pulmonary function tests that assess airway caliber (e.g., forced expiratory volume in one second, FEV_1) are performed before and after administration of incrementally increasing concentrations of bronchoconstrictor aerosol. The concentration producing a specified level of bronchoconstriction (e.g., 20% reduction in FEV_1) permits an assessment of the airway reactivity relative to established figures for normal subjects and mild and severe asthmatics (Fig. 4). In these studies, aerosols of bronchoconstrictor agonists, such as methacholine (a selective agonist of muscarinic cholinoceptors) and histamine, are used [102]. Other stimuli that are not direct bronchoconstrictors, such as exercise and inhaled adenosine monophosphate, have also been proposed for use in bronchial provocation tests [102,103].

Other Possible Uses

The foregoing represent currently accepted therapeutic uses of aerosols. Other uses have been or are being investigated and these exploit the lungs as a site for delivery of a drug to bypass absorption and metabolic processes that limit their use by other routes or to exert a local action in the airways.

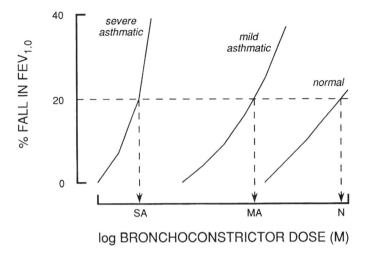

FIGURE 4   Determination of airway reactivity using an aerosolized broncho-constrictor. Incrementally increasing concentrations of bronchoconstrictor agonist aerosol are administered to a subject. The decrease in forced expiratory volume in one second (FEV1.0) is measured after each concentration. The dose of bronchoconstrictor that induces a 20% decrease in $FEV_{1.0}$ is then interpolated from the dose-response curve obtained in the subject. This concentration provides an index of airway sensitivity or reactivity. Severe asthmatics are extremely sensitive to bronchoconstrictor stimuli (i.e., respond to a lower concentration of bronchoconstrictor), more so than mild asthmatics and nonasthmatic subjects.

Insulin

Insulin is a pancreatic hormone that regulates carbohydrate, protein, and fat metabolism. An absolute or relative deficiency of insulin characterizes certain forms of diabetes mellitus, and treatment requires insulin supplementation. Being a protein, insulin is not orally active and is usually administered by subcutaneous injection [104]. As a result of patient compliance concerns, alternative routes of administration for insulin have been sought [105]. Promising results have been reported in a recent phase II clinical trial conducted in type II diabetes patients [106]. Phase III studies in larger populations of patients with diabetes are undoubtedly in progress, as are studies investigating means of delivering insulin more efficiently to the peripheral airways [107]. Other proteins used for therapy are burdened by the same constraints as insulin, viz. orally inactive (due to degradation in the gastrointestinal tract) and paren-teral administration (which diminishes patient compliance). The demonstrated efficacy of inhaled insulin provides proof in concept for the delivery of other proteins to the systemic circulation via the lung. This is particularly important given the increasing number of therapeutic proteins being developed by biotechnology companies.

Anticancer Agents

More so than other therapeutic agents, anticancer drugs exert profound side effects upon systemic administration. Commonly, other therapies need to be applied to treat the side effects of these drugs. Pulmonary delivery, therefore, represents a rational route of administration for the treatment of lung cancers. Relatively few drugs have been investigated, however. In a recent phase I clinical study, inhaled vitamin A was shown to suppress epithelial metaplasia and, therefore, was proposed as a potential agent for the prevention of lung cancer [108]. Other inhaled agents evaluated in phase I human studies for cancer treatment include granulocyte macrophage-colony stimulating factor (GM-CSF) [109], interferon α [110], and interleukin 2 [111]. There are also several other anticancer drugs being examined using pulmonary delivery in animal models of cancer [112]. However, one wonders how effective an inhaled chemotherapeutic agent will be at treating an established tumor that occludes the airway and, consequently, hinders aerosol deposition at the tumor site. It is more likely that inhaled drugs will be used prophylactically for chemoprevention in cancer, i.e., to *prevent* the development of lung tumors in vulnerable patients.

Protease Inhibitors

α_1-Antitrypsin (or α_1-proteinase inhibitor) and secretory leukoprotease inhibitor (SLPI) are proteins generated by the body that protect the connective tissue of the lungs from degradation by neutrophil elastase. A genetic deficiency or defect in α_1-antitrypsin leads to alveolar destruction and emphysema [113], and intravenous administration of exogenous α_1-antitrypsin can be used to halt these pathological processes. Progressive lung damage can similarly occur in patients with cystic fibrosis through the action of elastase released from infiltrating neutrophils. For a given intravenous dose of α_1-antitrypsin, only 2% has been estimated to reach the lungs [114]. As a result, aerosol administration is viewed as a more efficient means of achieving therapeutic repression of elastase-induced lung damage. Inhaled α_1-antitrypsin and recombinant human SLP1 have been shown to be well tolerated [115,116]. Currently, phase II human trials investigating the efficacy of inhaled α_1-antitrypsin are being completed by Bayer®/PPL Therapeutics. With the discovery of the matrix metalloproteinases (MMPs) in the lung and as a clearer understanding of their role in lung disease is made [117], it is possible that we may see MMP inhibitors delivered by inhalation for therapeutic benefit in the future.

Immunization

Vaccination against viruses, such as influenza and measles, commonly involves parenteral (subcutaneous or intramuscular) administration of a live, attenuated virus or a killed virus. The inhalation route is being examined as a means of immunizing patients because it circumvents logistical problems associated with parenteral administration, such as needle sterility issues, patient aversion to needles, and the need for administration by a health care professional. In very young children, maternally derived IgG antibodies may prevent successful immunization [118]. The inhalation route may allow vaccination of these children because the immunological response of the airways is less likely to be influenced by maternal antibodies [118]. Aerosol immunization has been shown to be effective against measles [119] and, in some respects, is more efficacious than parenteral immunization [120].

WHAT LIMITS AEROSOL USE?
Patient Compliance

Although aerosol administration is an extremely effective means of delivering a drug to the airways, the oral route remains the preferred means of drug delivery for a variety of airway diseases. This course of therapeutic action relates primarily to patient preference and compliance. Breathing pattern determines the amount and the pattern of drug deposition in the airways [1]. Indeed, when using patient-actuated metered-dose inhalers (MDIs), coordination of dose release with inspiration constitutes a problem for approximately 50% of patients [121]. It is important, therefore, that the patient be well versed in the correct technique for aerosol inhalation, especially those generated by metered-dose inhalers. Dry powder inhalers, by their design, simplify timing of drug delivery with inspiration. However, dose preparation (e.g., puncturing dosage blister pack) can be more complicated than for an MDI. The advent of spacers and inspiration-activated devices have simplified the maneuvers required to be performed by the patient during aerosol administration, and the resultant subjective improvement in aerosolized drug efficacy may be envisioned to improve patient compliance. Patient perception also affects their use of inhaled medication (and medications in general). For example, the beneficial effects of inhaled corticosteroids develop over a period of weeks. Poor patient compliance with therapy is though to be caused by the failure of these agents to elicit a discernable physiological or beneficial effect with each use, leading the patients cease to using the medication because they perceive no benefit [122].

Breathing Maneuvers

The manner in which a subject breathes has a great bearing on the amount of aerosolized drug deposited in the airways and the pattern of distribution of the drug in the pulmonary tree, i.e., central versus peripheral airways. Minute volume influences the amount of drug delivered to the airway lumen. Ventilatory frequency, tidal volume, and lung volume determine the residence time of an aerosol in the airways [1] and thereby dictate the duration during which the airways are exposed to drug. The distribution of aerosolized agent can be controlled by the pattern of breathing. For example, rapid, shallow breathing results in a deposition in the central airways, whereas slow, deep breathing results in peripheral airway deposition [4]. Under conditions of moderate-to-severe airway obstruction, as might occur during asthmatic bronchospasm, functional residual capacity and ventilation rate tend to increase while tidal volume tends to decrease. As such, the bronchospasm-induced changes in ventilatory parameters are envisaged as modifying the deposition of the aerosol and, therefore, its therapeutic activity. Fortuitously, the rapid, shallow breathing promotes deposition in the central airways that, in general, are the sites of bronchoconstriction. However, the increases in ventilatory rate, airways resistance, and apparent lung stiffness result in an increase in the work of breathing, particularly during inspiration [123] and may lead to fatigue of ventilatory muscles. Under these conditions, the capacity of a severely compromised patient to inhale an aerosol effectively may be limited. These subjects would require more rigorous (e.g., intravenous) therapy.

Irritant Activity

Ramifying within and beneath the epithelium of the central airways are nerves that serve a sensory function and that may be characterized on the basis of their structure, physiology, and susceptibility to stimulation by chemical substances. The two most important (as far as inhaled substances are concerned) are irritant (rapidly adapting receptors) and afferent C-fibers. Impulses received from either nerve type are processed in the central nervous system and results in centrally mediated changes in respiratory rhythm and depth (coughing or sneezing and rapid, shallow breathing), airway smooth muscle tone (bronchoconstriction), and mucus secretion [124]. Airborne substances, such as chemically inert dusts, cigarette smoke, and irritant aerosols (e.g., citric acid, capsaicin, histamine), stimulate sensory nerves to produce an irritant effect, characterized by the previously mentioned physiological changes [124]. This central reflex arc is responsible for the bronchoconstrictor action of nonspecific stimuli (e.g., dust and smoke) and, in addition, may contribute to the bronchoconstrictor action of pharmacological agents, such as histamine. In asthma and other pulmonary diseases, increased sensitivity of sensory nerves to irritants has been proposed as a mechanism by which the airways become hyperresponsive. In the context of aerosol administration, this process has important ramifications, in that a therapeutic agent may actually induce a bronchospastic episode should it prove to stimulate airway sensory nerves, i.e., act as an irritant. Cromolyn administration as an inhalable powder initially induced coughing, wheezing, and, in some instances, bronchospasm, which are actions emanating from an effect on sensory nerve endings. Reformulation as an inhalable solution obviated these problems. Interestingly, a component of therapeutic action of the cromones, such as cromolyn and nedocromil, may rest in their ability to diminish the sensitivity of airway sensory nerves to irritant stimuli [125,126].

Epithelial Permeability

A major factor regulating the pharmacological or biological actions of substances delivered to the lumen of the airways is epithelial permeability. Passage of drug through the epithelium is prerequisite for an action or subepithelial target cells, such as airway smooth muscle.

Studies on changes on epithelial permeability have centered on investigations of mechanisms associated with induction of airway hyperreactivity. In support of an important role for epithelium in regulating the biological activity of inhaled substances, airway reactivity to aerosolized bronchoconstrictors has been correlated inversely with the epithelial thickness [127]. A variety of irritant stimuli, such as antigen and cigarette smoke, increase airway epithelial permeability to small solutes in animal models [128,129]. On the basis of such studies, this process has been suggested to enhance the penetration of irritants or bronchoactive substances to their bronchoconstrictor sites of action (such as sensory nerves, inflammatory cells, or smooth muscle cells) and thereby to contribute to airway hyperreponsiveness [130,131]. The mechanism by which the permeability of the epithelium changes is not well understood, although disruption of intercellular epithelial tight junctions [130] and penetration through disrupted cells [129] have been suggested. In addition to known chemically induced influences on epithelial permeability, disease states, such as asthma, may also be associated with changes in epithelial permeability [132,133]. In addition, regions of epithelium may be absent from the airways of asthmatics [134].

In the same way that epithelial penetration of aerosolized tracer molecules may be enhanced by certain pathological conditions, so too might aerosolized drugs be more efficiently delivered to the airways. Accordingly, it may be hypothesized that, under conditions of augmented epithelial permeability, therapeutic agents delivered into the airway lumen may become more potent because they have readier access to their subepithelial targets.

Metabolism

Enzymatic and nonenzymatic biotransformation of drugs administered to the airways represents an emerging and important area of research. Most is known about of the degradation of select bronchoactive peptides in the airways and a discussion of the findings relating to substance P serves as an example of the nature, efficiency, and regional differences in pulmonary metabolism. Substance P perfused through the pulmonary vasculature is subject to enzymatic metabolism by angiotensin-converting enzyme (presumably associated with vascular endothelium) and neutral endopeptidase [135]. When delivered to the airway lumen, it is principally degraded by neutral endopeptidase and other (as yet to be identified) peptidases [136,137], a result that is consistent with the observed presence of neutral endopeptidase on airway epithelial cells [138]. Enzymatic biotransformation regulates the bronchoconstrictor activity of the tachykinins to the extent that aerosolized substance P, which normally lacks bronchomotor activity, induces significant bronchoconstriction after animal pretreatment with a neutral endopeptidase inhibitor [28]. The expression of neutral endopeptidase has been shown to be influenced by several factors. For example, viral infection, cigarette smoke, and lung tumorigenesis inhibits the expression of neutral endopeptidase [139–141], whereas glucocorticoid treatment increases neutral endopeptidase expression in epithelial cells [142]. Therefore, diseases and therapeutic interventions have the potential to influence the metabolic fate of an inhaled substance.

Metabolic processes in the lung may be exploited in drug design, as is the case for bitolterol. This compound is administered as an inactive ester that must be hydrolyzed by tissue-associated esterases to form the active β_2-adrenoceptor agonist colterol [143]. This process takes several hours and results in a long duration of action of the bronchodilator.

From the foregoing, it is evident that the activity of inhaled drugs can be influenced by metabolic processes in the airways and that various interventions can influence drug activity by modifying metabolic processes. Cellular location of enzymes would be anticipated to have important consequences on the activity of aerosols. For example, enzymes associated with pulmonary endothelium will have little influence on the actions of drugs designed to exert pharmacological activity in the central airways but will be important in regulating the actions of aerosolized therapeutic agents destined for systemic administration via the pulmonary circulation. These considerations notwithstanding, further research into drug biotransformation in the airways is necessary, particularly in the central airways, where aerosol therapy is commonly targeted.

Bronchoconstriction

Airway caliber has a dramatic influence on the pattern of deposition of aerosols in the airways. Deposition increases during bronchoconstriction, primarily as a result of changes in inertial impaction and turbulent flow experienced by aerosol particles after irregular airway obstruction [144]. The presence of excessive mucus may act to enhance further deposition [145]. Indeed, total lung aerosol deposition has been suggested as being a sensitive (perhaps diagnostic) indicator of airways obstruction or lung abnormality [146]. These processes may be envisaged as being advantageous insofar as they would function to deposit aerosolized drug at its site of desired action (i.e., the obstructed airway for a bronchodilator) but disadvantageous under circumstances in which the aerosol is to be delivered to the alveoli, because obstruction would result in a shift in the deposition pattern toward the central airways, that is, the sites of significant bronchoconstriction. In general, aerosolized drug will be deposited in regions of the pulmonary tree where airflow exists, and, accordingly, deposition in occluded airways probably will be diminished as a result of redirection of airflow through patent airways.

FUTURE DIRECTIONS FOR AEROSOL USE

In general, drugs currently administered as aerosols are used principally for the treatment of pulmonary disorders. This line of thinking centers on providing a high local concentration while diminishing systemic absorption and associated side effects. Current research emphasizes this doctrine, examples of which are the development of longer-acting bronchodilator drugs by hindering absorption through molecular modifications (e.g., salmeterol, formoterol) [29] or incorporation into liposomes [147]. What then lies in the future for aerosols in pharmacology, other than the treatment of obstructive airways disease? The potential of aerosols as a means of delivering drugs to the pulmonary and systemic circulations is now starting to be explored and it represents a valuable direction for future research. The rapid onset of action and circumvention of first-pass hepatic metabolism favor the airways as a site of drug disposition for systemic activity. With continuing advancements being made in recombinant DNA technology, therapeutic entities of the future will undoubtedly comprise peptides and proteins. These agents are currently administered via the subcutaneous, intramuscular, or intravenous routes, which lead to poor compliance by patients and necessitate greater health care professional involvement. As a result, alternative routes that are more "patient friendly" are being examined, such as intranasal and aerosol inhalation. The development and success (or failure) of inhaled insulin as a therapeutic entity will serve as an important yardstick for the future of inhaled proteins. The efficiency of delivery and retention in the lung of a significant portion of a total dose of an aerosol are critical for the inhalation route of administration to be useful, particularly when using expensive recombinant products. Introduction of the use of spacer devices with metered-dose inhalers may advance the cause of aerosols by increasing the amount of aerosol introduced into the airways (making the therapy more effective) and decreasing the amount depositing in the mouth (and thereby diminishing side effects associated with oral or gastrointestinal absorption).

These considerations notwithstanding, the extent to which the airways can be used as a site of drug delivery to the systemic circulation remains to be fully defined. Although a considerable amount is known about the manner in which airway caliber and mucus secretion are influenced by pharmacological agents, relatively little is understood about the pharmacokinetic effect of drugs delivered to the lumen of the central and peripheral airways. What happens to a drug in passage from the lumen to its therapeutic target tissue (be it airway, smooth muscle, or blood)? In the development of an aerosolized drug for therapeutic use, the overriding emphasis lies in its capacity to produce a therapeutic or biological response. Perhaps if more were known about the pharmacokinetic processes of the airways, biologically active drugs that are inactive as an aerosol may be structurally modified to resist absorptive or metabolic pressures and thereby establish a therapeutic entity.

REFERENCES

1. Brain JD. In: Hargreave FE, ed. Airway Reactivity: Mechanisms and Clinical Relevance. Ontario, Canada: Astra Pharmaceuticals, 1980:3.
2. Task Group on Lung Dynamics, Health Phys 1966; 12:173.
3. Davies DS. Scand J Respir Dis (Suppl) 1978; 103:44.
4. Valberg DS, Brain JD, Sneddon SL, LeMott SR. J Appl Physiol 1982; 53:824.
5. Jeffery PK. Eur J Respir Dis 1987; 71(suppl 153):34.
6. Finkbeiner WE. Respir Physiol 1999; 118:77.
7. Khanvilkar K, Donovan MD, Flanagan DR. Adv Drug Del Rev 2001; 48:173.
8. Hogg JC, Hulbert W. In: Hargreave FE, ed. Airway Reactivity. Mechanisms and Clinical Relevance. Ontario, Canada: Astra Pharmaceuticals, 1980:35.
9. Godfrey RWA. Microsc Res Tech 1997; 38:488.
10. Patton JS. Adv Drug Del Rev 1996; 19:3.
11. Racine C, Belanger M, Hirabayashi H, Boucher M, Chakir J, Couet J. Biochem Biophys Res Commun 1999; 255:580.
12. Gardiner TH, Schanker LS. Xenobiotica 1974; 4:725.
13. Hogg JC. J Allergy Clin Immunol 1981; 67:421.
14. Wan H, Winton HL, Soeller C, Tovey ER, Gruenert DC, Thompson PJ, Stewart GA, Taylor GW, Garrod DR, Cannell MB, Robinson C. J Clin Investig 1999; 104:123.
15. Mitic LL, Anderson JM. Ann Rev Physiol 1998; 60:121.

16. Oberdorster G. J Aerosol Med 1988; 1:289.
17. Kelly L, Kolbe J, Mitzner W, Spannhake EW, Bromberger-Bamea B, Menkes H. J Appl Physiol 1986; 60:1954.
18. Effros RM, Mason GR. Am Rev Respir Dis 1983; 127(suppl):S59.
19. Gumbleton M. Adv Drug Dev Res 2001; 49:281.
20. Schanker LS, Mitchell EW, Brown RA. Drug Metab Dispos 1986; 14:79.
21. Brown RA, Schanker LS. Drug Metab Dispos 1983; 11:355.
22. Etherton JE, Conning DM. In: Bakhle YS. Vane JR, eds. Lung Biology in Health and Disease. Vol. 4, New York: Marcel Dekker, 1977:233.
23. Battistini B, Dussault P. Pulm Pharmacol 1998; 11:79.
24. Dendorfer A, Vordermark D, Dominiak P. Br J Pharmacol 1997; 120:121.
25. Shen Z, Ziand Q, Weng S, Nagai T. Int J Pharm 1999; 192:115.
26. Philpot RM, Anderson MW, Eling TE. In: Bakhle YS. Vane JR, eds. Lung Biology in Health and Disease. Vol. 4, New York: Marcel Dekker, 1977:123.
27. Gail DB, Lenfant CJM. Am Rev Respir Dis 1983; 127:366.
28. Dusser DJ, Umeno E, Graf PD, Djokic T, Borson DB, Nadel JA. J Appl Physiol 1988; 65:2585.
29. Lotvall J. Respir Med 2001; 95(suppl. B):S7.
30. Page CP, Morley J. J Allergy Clin Immunol 1999; 104:S31.
31. Boulton DW, Fawcett JP. Clin Pharmacokinet 2001; 40:23.
32. Abisheganaden J, Boushey HA. Am J Med 1998; 104:494.
33. Nadel JA, Barnes PJ. Am Rev Med 1984; 35:451.
34. COMBIVENT Inhalation Solution Study Group, Chest 1997; 112:1514.
35. Schroeckenstein DC, Bush RK, Chervinksy P, Busse WW. J Allergy Clin Immunol 1988; 82:115.
36. Barnes PJ. Life Sci 1993; 52:521.
37. Minette PAH, Lammers J-W, Dixon CMS, McCusker MT, Barnes PJ. J Appl Physiol 1989; 67:2461.
38. Barnes PJ. Chest 2000; 117:63S.
39. Rabe KF, Magnussen H, Dent G. Eur Respir J 1995; 8:637.
40. Feoktistov I, Polosa R, Holgate ST, Biaggioni I. Trends Pharmacol Sci 1998; 19:148.
41. Torphy TJ. Am J Respir Crit Care Med 1998; 157:351.
42. Hood WB, Jr. Am J Cardiol 1989; 63:46A.
43. Sturton G, Fitzgerald M. Chest 2002; 121:192S.
44. Compton CH, Gubb J, Nieman R, Edelson J, Amit O, Ayres JG, Creemers JPH, Schultze-Werninghaus G, Brambilla C, Barnes NC. Lancet 2001; 358:265.
45. Bohadana AB, Peslin R, Teculescu D, Polu JM, Belleville F, Massin N. Bull Ear Physiopathol Respir 1980; 16:13.
46. Cushley MJ, Holgate ST. Thorax 1983; 38:223.
47. Newman-Taylor AJ. Thorax 1980; 35:241.
48. Streiter RM, Belperio JA, Keane MP. J Clin Investig 2002; 109:699.
49. Blease K, Lukacs NW, Hogaboam CG, Kunkel SL. Respir Res 2000; 1:54.
50. Wanner A, Ahmed T, Abraham WM. In: Jenne JW, Murphy S, eds. Lung Biology in Health and Disease. Vol. 31. New York: Marcel Dekker, 1987:413.

51. Eady RP. Eur J Respir Dis 1986; 69(suppl. 147):112.

52. Lal S, Malholtra S, Gribben D, Hodder D. Thorax 1984; 39:809.

53. Fairfax AJ, Allbeson M. J Int Med Res 1988; 16:216.

54. Murphy S. In: Jenne JW, Murphy S, eds. Lung Biology in Health and Disease. Vol. 31. New York: Marcel Dekker, 1987:669.

55. Leung KB, Flint KC, Brostoff J, Hudspith BN, Johnson NM, Lau HY, Liu WL, Pearce FL. Thorax 1988; 43:756.

56. Howarth PH, Durham SR, Lee TH, Kay AB, Church MK, Holgate ST. Am Rev Respir Dis 1985; 132:986.

57. Barnes PJ. N Engl J Med 1995; 332:868.

58. Toogood JH. In: Jenne JW, Murphy S, eds. Lung Biology in Health and Disease. Vol. 31. New York: Marcel Dekker, 1987:719.

59. Adcock IM. Pulm Pharmacol Ther 2001; 14:211.

60. Schleimer RP. Am Rev Respir Dis 1990; 141:S59.

61. Fraser CM, Venter JC. Biochem Biophys Res Commun 1980; 94:390.

62. Gebbie T. In: Clark TJH, ed. Steroids in Asthma: A Reappraisal in the Light of Inhalation Therapy. Auckland, New Zealand: ADIS Press, 1983:83.

63. Crompton GK. In: Clark TJH, ed. Steroids in Asthma: A Reappraisal in the Light of Inhalation Therapy. Auckland, New Zealand: ADIS Press, 1983:166.

64. Cochrane GM. In: Clark TJH, ed. Steroids in Asthma: A Reappraisal in the Light of Inhalation Therapy. Auckland, New Zealand: ADIS Press, 1983:103.

65. Williams AJ, Baghat MS, Stableforth DE, Cayton RM, Shenoi PM, Skinner C. Thorax 1983; 38:813.

66. Toogood JH, Baskerville J, Jennings B, Lefcoe NM, Johansson S-A. Am Rev Respir Dis 1984; 129:723.

67. Selroos O, Halme M. Thorax 1991; 46:891.

68. Belvisi MG, Brown TJ, Wicks S, Foster ML. Pulm Pharmacol Ther 2001; 14:221.

69. Leff AR. Ann Rev Med 2001; 52:1.

70. Liu MC, Dube LM, Lancaster J. J Allergy Clin Immunol 1996; 98:859.

71. Nogrady SG, Hartley JPR, Handslip PDJ, Hurst NP. Thorax 1978; 33:479.

72. Phillips MJ, Ollier S, Gould C, Davies RJ. Thorax 1984; 39:345.

73. White MV, Slater JE, Kaliner MA. Am Rev Respir Dis 1987; 135:1165.

74. Mincarini M, Pasquali M, Cosentino C, Fumagalli F, Scordamaglia A, Quaglia R, Canonica GW, Passalacqua G. Pulm Pharmacol Ther 2001; 14:267.

75. Drazen JM, Austen KF. Am Rev Respir Dis 1987; 136:98.

76. Drazen JM. Am Rev Respir Crit Care Med 1998; 158:S193.

77. NIH National Asthma Education and Prevention Program expert panel report, 2002.

78. Barnes PJ, Chung KF, Page CP. Pharmacol Rev 1998; 50:515.

79. Braquet P, Touqui L, Shen TY, Vargaftig BB. Pharmacol Rev 1987; 39:97.

80. Spence DP, Johnston SL, Calverley PM, Dhillon P, Higgins C, Ramhamadany E, Turner S, Winning A, Winter J, Holgate ST. Am J Respir Crit Care Med 1994; 149:1142.

81. Evans DJ, Barnes PJ, Cluzel M, O'Connor BJ. Am J Respir Crit Care Med 1997; 156:11.

82. Phipps RJ. Int Rev Physiol 1981; 23:213.

83. Knowles MR, Boucher RC. J Clin Investig 2002; 109:571.
84. Clark SW. Eur J Respir Dis 1987; 71(suppl. 153):136.
85. Robinson M, Regnis JA, Bailey DL, King M, Bautovich GJ, Bye PT. Am J Respir Crit Care Med 1996; 153:1503.
86. Ziment I. Biomed Pharmacother 1988; 42:513.
87. Shak S. Chest 1995; 107:65S.
88. MacLusky I, Levison H, Gold R, McLaughlin FJ. J Pediatr 1986; 108:861.
89. Moss RB. Chest 2001; 120:107S.
90. Prober CG, Walson PD, Jones J. Pediatrics 2000; 106:E89.
91. Monk JP, Benfield P. Drugs 1990; 39:741.
92. Flume P, Klepser ME. Pharmacotherapy 2002; 22:71S.
93. Eggleston M. Inf Control 1987; 8:215.
94. Knight V, Gilbert B. Eur J Clin Microbiol Infect Dis 1988; 7:721.
95. Vujovic O, Mills J. Curr Opin Pharmacol 2001; 1:497.
96. Ison MG, Hayden FG. Curr Opin Phamacol 2001; 1:482.
97. Cass LM, Efthymiopoulos C, Bye A. Clin Pharmacokinet 1999; 36(suppl. 1):1.
98. McNicholl JR, McNicholl JJ. Ann Pharmacother 2001; 35:57.
99. McLaughlin VV, Genthner DE, Panella MM, Rich S. N Engl J Med 1998; 338:273.
100. Moeper MM, Schwarze M, Ehlerding S, Adler-Schuermeyer A, Spiekerkoetter E, Niedermeyer J, Hamm M, Fabel H. N Engl J Med 2000; 342:1866.
101. Juniper EF, Frith PA, Hargeave FE. Thorax 1981; 36:575.
102. Crapo RO, Casaburi R, Coates AL, Enright PL, Hankinson JL, Irwin CG, MacIntyre NR, MacKay RT, Wanger JS, Anderson SD, Cockcroft DW, Fish JE, Sterk PJ. Am Rev Respir Crit Care Med 2000; 161:309.
103. Cain H. Clin Chest Med 2001; 22:651.
104. Davis SN, Granner DK. In: Hardman JG, Limbird LE, eds. The Pharmaceutical Basis of Therapeutics. 10th ed. New York: Macmillan, 2001:1679.
105. Heinemann L, Pfutzner A, Heise T. Curr Pharm Des 2001; 7:1327.
106. Cefalu WT, Skyler JS, Kourides IA, Landschulz WH, Balagtas CC, Cheng S-L, Gelfand RA. Ann Intern Med 2001; 134:203.
107. Laube BL. Chest 2001; 120(suppl.):99S.
108. Kohlhaufl M, Haussinger K, Stanzel F, Markus A, Tritschler J, Muhlhofer A, Morresi-Hauf A, Golly I, Scheuch G, Jany BH, Biesalski HK. Eur J Med Res 2002; 7:72.
109. Anderson PM, Markovic SN, Sloan JA, Clawson ML, Wylam M, Arndt CAS, Smithson WA, Burch P, Gornet M, Rahman E. Clin Cancer Res 1999; 5:2316.
110. van Zandwijk N, Jassem E, Dubbelmann R, Braat MC, Rumke P. Eur J Cancer 1990; 26:738.
111. Huland E, Heinzer H, Huland H, Yung R. Cancer J Sci Am 2000; 6(suppl. 1):S104.
112. Sharma S, White D, Mondi AR, Placke ME, Vail DM, Kris MG. J Clin Oncol 2001; 6:1839.
113. Hutchinson DCS. Br J Chest 1973; 67:171.
114. Wewers MD, Casolaro MA, Sellers SE, Swayze SC, McPhaul KM, Wittes JT, Crystal RC. N Engl J Med 1987; 316:1055.

115. Vogelmeier C, Kirlath I, Warrington S, Banik N, Ulbrich E, Du Bois RN. Am J Respir Crit Care Med 1997; 155:536.

116. McElvaney NG, Doujaji B, Moan MJ, Burnham MR, Wu MC, Crystal RG. Am Rev Respir Dis 1993; 148:1056.

117. Parks WC, Shapiro SD. Respir Res 2001; 2:10.

118. Barry PW, O'Callaghan C. Thorax 1997; 52(suppl. 2):S78.

109. Cutts FT, Clements CJ, Bennett JV. Biologicals 1997; 25:323.

120. Bellanti JA, Zeligs BJ, Mendez de Inocencio J, Omidvar BM, Omidvar J, Awasum M. Allergy Asthma Proc 2001; 22:173.

121. Crompton GK. Eur J Respir Dis 1982; 63(suppl. 119):101.

122. Bosley CM, Parry DT, Cochrane GM. Eur Respir J 1994; 7:504.

123. Flenley DC, In: Kay AB, Austen KF, Lichenstein LM, eds. Asthma: Physiology, Immunopharmacology and Treatment. New York: Academic Press, 1984:375.

124. Widdicombe JG. Resp Physiol 2001; 125:3.

125. Richards IM, Jackson DM, Altounyan REC. Agents Actions 1983; 13(suppl.):51.

126. Chung KF. J Allergy Clin Immunol 1996; 98:S116.

127. Yanta MA, Snapper JR, Ingram RH, Drazen JM, Coles S, Reid L. Am Rev Respir Dis 1981; 124:337.

128. Boucher RC, Pare PD, Hogg JC. J Allergy Clin Immunol 1979; 64:197.

129. Walker DC, Bums AR. Prog Clin Biol Res 1988; 263:25.

130. Hogg JC, Paré PD, Boucher RC. Fed Proc 1979; 38:197.

131. Boushey A, Holtzman MJ, Sheller JR, Nadel JA. Am Rev Respir Dis 1980; 121:389.

132. Ilowite JS, Bennett WD, Sheetz MS, Groth ML, Nierman DM. Am Rev Respir Dis 1989; 139:1139.

133. Godfrey RWA. Microsc Res Tech 1997; 38:488.

134. Laitinen LA, Heino M, Laitinen A, Kava T, Haahtela T. Am Rev Respir Dis 1985; 131:599.

135. Shore SA, Stimler-Gerard NP, Coats SR, Drazen JM. Am Rev Respir Dis 1988; 137:331.

136. Martins MA, Shore S, Gerard NP, Gerard C, Drazen JM. J Clin Investig 1990; 85:170.

137. Martins MA, Shore S, Drazen JM. Int Arch Allergy Appl Immunol 1991; 94:325.

138. Nadel JA. Prog Clin Biol Res 1988; 263:331.

139. Jacoby DB, Tamaoki J, Borson DB, Nadel JA. J Appl Physiol 1988; 64:2653.

140. Dusser DJ, Djokic TD, Borson DB, Nadel JA. J Clin Investig 1989; 84:900.

141. Cohen AJ, Bunn PA, Franklin W, Magill-Solc C, Hartmann C, Helfrich B, Gilman L, Folkvord J, Helm K, Miller YE. Cancer Res 1996; 56:831.

142. Borson DB, Gruenert DC. Am J Physiol 1991; 260:L83.

143. Orgel HA, Kemp JP, Tinkelman DG, Webb DR. J Allergy Clin Immunol 1985; 75:55.

144. Kim CS, Garcia AL, Sackner MA. Am Rev Respir Dis 1989; 139:422.

145. Kim CS, Abraham WM, Chapman GA, Sackner MA. Am J Respir Dis 1985; 131:618.

146. Kim CS, Lewars GA, Sackner MA. J Appl Physiol 1988; 64:1527.

147. McCalden TA, Abra B, Mihalko P. J Liposome Res 1989; 1:211.

3

Targeting by Deposition

Igor Gonda

Acrux Limited, West Melbourne, Victoria, Australia

INTRODUCTION

The word *targeting* in the context of therapeutics can be interpreted as a desire to achieve distinct concentration–time profiles for a biologically active agent at different sites in the body to maximize therapeutic effects while minimizing or eliminating toxicity. Thus, targeting in general implies a certain degree of specificity of the agent in space and time. If this goal is to be reached by design rather than by chance, the knowledge of the ideal spatial and temporal patterns for each drug is required. As discussed in the following, this information for inhalation therapy of respiratory disease with drug aerosols is incomplete. Nevertheless, some basic guidelines for optimum physical characteristics of these aerosols can be laid down. Exploration of systemic delivery of pharmaceutical drugs has become a major area of academic and industrial research in the last decade. The mechanistic basis for optimum targeting for this purpose is obviously quite different from applications intended for therapies of respiratory disease.

Drug targeting has been primarily the domain of medicinal chemists. The familiar concept of selective toxicity [1] was turned into practical discoveries by design of the molecular properties of drugs that imparted the selective distribution characteristics and pharmacokinetic behavior suitable for therapy. Indeed, it can be argued that one of the most successful types of drugs used in respiratory therapy—the β2 agonists, with their bronchodilating properties—are an excellent example of selective toxicity achieved by the chemical targeting method. However, it should be appreciated that a very significant improvement in the therapeutic efficacy can be achieved when these agents are delivered directly to the site of action in the respiratory tract by inhalation [2–6]. In this way, the local concentration to reach the therapeutic levels is achieved while the systemic levels are kept low. This would be even more important for drugs used in treating respiratory diseases that do have serious systemic side effects when administered by routes other than inhalation [7,8]. Macromolecules are not readily transported from the bloodstream into the airways and alveoli, and the delivery of a variety of biologics for the treatment of respiratory disease is therefore likely to be by inhalation [9].

It is well known that inhalation therapy, especially for asthma and bronchitis, is very successful, even though only a small fraction of the inhaled dose (typically less than 20%) actually reaches the bronchial airways and alveoli of the respiratory tract [10–18]. The rest of it deposits in the mouth and in the upper airways, from where it is eventually swallowed. This swallowed dose may be poorly absorbed, and, in absolute terms, it would still be small compared to the dose that would have to be given systemically to exert the same therapeutic effect. Therefore, inhalation aerosols for the treatment of respiratory disease are an excellent example of site-directed delivery by physical means. In addition to the spatial aspect of targeting by an aerosol, achieving a better temporal pattern of drug activity should be possible: Sometimes extended duration of action is desirable (e.g., to prolong the activity of bronchodilators in the airways). A rapid absorption into the systemic circulation may be preferable, e.g., for the treatment of breakthrough pain by inhalation of analgesics. The commonsense criteria for preference of site directed over systemic administration are listed in Table 1.

The extent to which selectivity of spatial targeting within the respiratory tract is required will depend on the sites of the desired drug receptors and those for the toxic effects, and their concentration–response curves. Other factors that may be important are reduction in acceptance by patients due to, for example, unpleasant taste of the material depositing in the mouth or the cost of inefficiency resulting from having to use a much higher dose than just that actually needed at the site of action. For example, good spatial targeting is needed for inhaled corticosteroids: The portion of the drug that deposits in the upper airways is the cause of fungal infections and dysphonia [19,20]. Similarly, the antibiotic pentamidine used in the prophylaxis and treatment of *Pneumocystis carinii* pneumonia is thought to cause toxicity unless deposited predominantly in the infected regions of the alveoli [21].

TABLE 1 Reasons for Using Direct Inhalation Delivery When the Site of Action is in the Respiratory Tract

Disadvantages of the systemic route
1. Poor or irreproducible delivery. These are problems such as inadequate absorption from the gastrointestinal tract (e.g., the absence of oral absorption of cromolyn sodium or recombinant human proteins) and presystemic and systemic metabolism of the active compound before it reaches the site of action (e.g., proteins, peptides, small molecules such as isoprenaline).
2. Serious systemic side effects (e.g., with oral corticosteroids)
3. Rapid systemic clearance causing a short duration of action

Advantages of the site-directed route
1. Absence of systemic side effects at drug levels adequate to exhibit the desired local therapeutic activity (e.g., antibiotic tobramycin)
2. Slow clearance from the site of action compared to the systemic clearance (e.g., biologics, pentamidine)
3. Activation of a prodrug at the site of action
4. Inactivation of the drug (at the site of action) before its release into the systemic circulation

MECHANISTIC FACTORS AFFECTING THE DEPOSITION OF AEROSOLS

Factors affecting the deposition of aerosols can be divided into two groups: those that are determined primarily by the patient and those that are due essentially to the properties of the aerosol themselves.

Mechanisms

There are five basic physical mechanisms that cause the deposition of aerosols.

Inertial Impaction

Inertial impaction is caused by the tendency of particles and droplets to move in a straight direction instead of following the gas streamlines. Hence, impaction may occur on the obstacle downstream in the trajectory of the particle.

If a particle with mass m is moving with initial velocity v_0, through still air, then it can be shown [22] that, as a result of frictional forces, the particle will stop after traveling the stopping distance, S:

$$S = B \times m \times v_0$$

where B is the mechanical mobility of the particle (i.e., the velocity per unit of force). The stopping distance in an extreme impaction situation is the distance the particle would travel in the original direction of motion from the point where the gas stream, which carries it, turns at a right angle. Clearly, the greater the particle mobility, mass, and initial velocity, the longer it will persist flying in the original direction, and, therefore, its chances of hitting the obstacle placed in front of it are increased.

Sedimentation

Sedimentation [22] of the disperse phase usually takes place under the force of gravity. (It may be caused also by an imposed centrifugal force field). A sphere of diameter D and density d under the influence of gravitational force F_g will have a terminal settling velocity V_{ts} in the laminar region governed by Stoke's law:

$$V_{ts} = \frac{d \times D^2 \times g}{18 \times \eta} = B \times F_g$$

where g is gravitational acceleration and η is the viscosity of air. It follows that the probability of deposition by sedimentation also increases with increasing particle mobility, similar to inertial impaction.

When the particles become very small so that using the Stokes picture of an object moving in a continuous medium is no longer permissible, the so-called slip correction factor, C_c, must be applied [22]. The particle can "slip" through the medium, and, consequently, its velocity is greater than that predicted by the previous equation.

$$V_{ts} \,(\text{with slip}) = V_{ts} \times C_c$$

where

$$C_c = 1 + \left(\frac{s}{D}\right) \times \left(2.514 + 0.800 \times \exp\left[-0.55 \times \frac{D}{s}\right]\right)$$

and where s is the mean free path of the atoms, or molecules, in the air.

In the other extreme, the Stokes regimen ceases to be applicable for particles with high Reynolds numbers, Re:

$$\text{Re} = D \times v \times \frac{d}{\eta}$$

where v is the particle velocity. Correction factors need to be applied to aerosols with particles or droplets in the regimes with Re > 1 [22].

When deposition is governed primarily be impaction and sedimentation, the independent variable that is used to relate to these processes is called the aerodynamic diameter, D_{ae} [22,23]. It is defined as the diameter of a sphere of unit density that has the same terminal sedimentation velocity as the particle in question. Therefore, the sedimentation velocity in terms of the aerodynamic diameter can be rewritten as follows:

$$V_{ts} = \frac{d_0 \times D_{ae}^2 \times g}{18 \times \eta} \times C_c$$

where d_0 is unit density (i.e., 1 g/cm^3 or 1 kg/dm^3). For spherical particles that are sufficiently large compared to the mean free path in the gas so that the slip correction, C_c, does not need to be applied, D_{ae} is simply related to the actual diameter of the sphere D and its density, d:

$$D_{ae} = D \left(\frac{d}{d_0} \right)^{1/2}$$

For nonspherical particles, D_{ae}, in addition to the size and density, depends on particle shape. For relatively simple geometries, D_{ae} can be estimated from a theoretical expression [22,24,25].

One problem with D_{ae} is that it does not provide a unique, one-to-one correspondence to deposition. Impaction for particles with the same D_{ae} will vary depending on the flow rate, Q. A different composite variable, the impaction parameter $d \times D^2 Q$, was found to predict uniquely the deposition in the human mouth and nose. Deposition increases with an increase of this variable, that is, as the particle size, density, and velocity become larger [26].

Diffusion

When the particles become sufficiently small, their deposition by diffusion becomes a significant mechanism. The rate of diffusion is proportional to the diffusion coefficient, Dif, that can be calculated from the Stokes–Einstein equation:

$$\text{Dif} = \frac{kT}{3\pi\eta D}$$

where k is Boltzmann's constant and T is absolute temperature [22]. In contrast to impaction and sedimentation, diffusional deposition increases with decreasing size of the particle and is independent of the particle density. Hence, diffusion coefficient should be a more suitable independent variable to describe the deposition of ultrafine particles than aerodynamic diameters.

Interception

Interception is a mechanism of deposition that denotes the situations in which the center of gravity of the particle is within the streamlines of the gas phase but a distal end of the particle is already touching a solid, or liquid, surface. Deposition in the respiratory tract by this mechanism is important when the dimensions of the anatomical spaces become comparable to the typical dimensions of the particles. As would be expected, this mechanism is particularly pertinent to the deposition of elongated particles on nasal hair, in small airways, and in alveoli [27].

Electrostatic Precipitation

At the generation stage, significant electrostatic charges are often imparted to the droplets and particles of an aerosol. These electric charges are subsequently reduced by partial neutralization with ions from the surrounding gas, until an equilibrium charge distribution is reached. In principle, a charged particle can induce a charge of opposite sign in the walls of airways and then becomes electrostatically attracted to it. This can enhance the deposition of highly charged aerosols by electrostatic precipitation, but, at present, there is very little evidence that such a mechanism can increase significantly the deposition and targeting of therapeutic aerosols in the human respiratory tract.

The Patient Factors

The patient factors enter into play in several ways. The effectiveness of all aerosol delivery systems depends to some extent on the ability of the patients to use them properly. This has been shown for different types of inhalation systems, such as metered-dose inhalers [28,29] and the breath-driven powder generators [15,30]. The second determinant is the state of the patient's airways. These effects are discussed in greater detail in the following section.

REVIEW OF DEPOSITION STUDIES IN THE HUMAN RESPIRATORY TRACT
Methodology

The reader should be aware that the description of the deposition of inhaled materials in the human airways and alveoli is based almost entirely on indirect information and is colored to a large extent by theoretical ideas. For experimental reasons, the respiratory tract is conventionally divided into three regions: the head (or extrathoracic region), tracheobronchial tree (airways, bronchial region), and alveoli (sometimes also referred to as the peripheral region or the "deep lung") [31,32]. The first region is characterized spatially and also by its short mucociliary clearance half-life (of the order of minutes). The last two regions are named after the corresponding anatomical spaces, but, in fact, they are defined experimentally in terms of clearance: the fraction of the dose retained after 24 hours has been thought to be deposited in the nonciliated parts of the lung, that is, the alveoli. The remaining fraction of the dose that is cleared in normal subjects within 24 hours is then the "tracheobronchial deposition."

In several disease states, the mucociliary clearance is impaired, and in such subjects the clearance from the trachcobronchial tree almost certainly exceeds 24 hours [33,34], making the concept of alveolar deposition in terms of retention in excess of 24 hours invalid. The slowly cleared material in normal subjects has been, however, regarded by most investigators as a true reflection of alveolar deposition. More recently, this assumption was seriously questioned [34] as a result of some problems with interpretation of experiments in which attempts were made to deposit materials selectively in the bronchial airways. In these investigations, despite the supposedly exclusive airway deposition that should be subject to mucociliary clearance, a slow phase of clearance was found in normal volunteers. The most plausible explanation of these observations was suggested to be a slow component of clearance from the tracheobronchial tree [35]. Although the classification of the regions in the respiratory tract in terms of clearance rates creates some difficulties with spatial targeting, it is, in fact, the relevant way for the understanding and design of optimal temporal patterns of drug action in the lung [36,37]. Duration of residence in the designated areas can be analyzed and modeled on the basis of this kinetic information, despite the uncertainty of the exact anatomical location of these compartments.

Two-dimensional anterior and posterior images (by gamma scintigraphy), or their geometric averages, of radiolabeled aerosol that are deposited in the respiratory tract should in principle provide an improved understanding of the spatial distribution of the deposited therapeutic and diagnostic aerosols. These studies customarily divide the respiratory tract into the oropharynx (or "extrathoracic deposition," which should include the radiolabeled aerosol swallowed into the stomach) and the pulmonary region. It is not unreasonable to expect that the oropharyngeal deposition should correspond to the head region and that the pulmonary deposition should correspond to the combined tracheobronchial and alveolar fractions as defined in the techniques described previously.

The pulmonary region of the two-dimensional images is sometimes subdivided into the central and peripheral regions. A measure of regional distribution, the penetration index [38,39], is calculated by taking the ratio of the radioactivity in these two regions, with the intention that this reflects the distribution of radioactivity between the central (large) airways and the small airways combined with the alveoli. However, it has been suspected for some time that the radiolabeled material deposited in the latter region is superimposed over the radioactivity residing in the large (central) airways [40]. This was confirmed in a single-photon emission computerized tomography (SPECT) study [39,41]. Therefore, the interpretation of two-dimensional gamma-scintigraphic images, or the use of the clearance data obtained by techniques with poor spatial resolution, requires some care. Morphometric analysis after SPECT studies may facilitate even more detailed spatial interpretations of the tomographic images [42].

Studies with Stable Monodisperse Aerosols

Much of our early understanding of deposition of inhaled particles in the human respiratory tract as a function of aerodynamic diameters and breathing parameters comes from experiments conducted with monodisperse, stable aerosols (i.e., systems with a well-characterized size that does not change between the point of generation and deposition) under carefully controlled breathing conditions [31,32]. Experimental data in normal adults breathing such aerosols by mouth have been obtained by numerous investigators (see reviews in Refs. 8, 26, 32, and 34). In these experiments, the particle velocity is controlled by the subjects' inspiratory flow rate. Steady breathing with moderate inspiratory flow rates and inspired volumes, coupled with a brief respiratory pause, was typically employed in these studies. (This should be contrasted with special breathing maneuvers employed with most therapeutic delivery systems.) There is a general agreement from these studies that particles with aerodynamic diameters greater than about 15 μm deposit entirely in the head region. The maximum tracheobronchial deposition of about 20% occurs for aerodynamic diameters of 5–10 μm. Above ~1 μm, there is a maximum in alveolar deposition of about 60% for aerodynamic diameters of about 3 μm. However, it should be appreciated that at this optimum size for alveolar deposition, a significant amount of material also deposits in the tracheobronchial (~10%) and extrathoracic (~10%) regions, which renders this size range somewhat nonselective if the aerosol cloud is generated and inhaled continuously.

Under normal breathing, submicronic particles are exhaled [unless they are of ultrafine sizes (<0.01 μm), in which case they can deposit sufficiently rapidly by diffusion]. However, breath holding allows more time for small particles to deposit by sedimentation and diffusion [43].

There is a substantial intersubject variation observed in the previously mentioned studies, despite the restrictive selection of the subjects (mostly normal nonsmoking adult males) and the control of breathing conditions. Reduction in the deposition in the head region, which shows large variability, could result in more predictable deposition in the distal parts of the respiratory tract. More information is required on intrasubject and intersubject variability in subjects with respiratory diseases. Experimental studies in patients with airway obstructions indicate that there is more deposition in the central, large airways than in the peripheral regions containing small airways and alveoli [44,45]. There is likely to be more deposition in the vicinity of the obstruction [46]. In an in vitro model, the deposition downstream from a flow-limiting element was shown to increase as the aerodynamic diameter was increased from 1.2 to 4 μm [46].

Several theoretical models exist describing the regional deposition of aerosols [47–50]. These models are in reasonable agreement with experimental data and therefore can be used to understand and design the delivery of therapeutic substances. They can reduce the number of in vivo experiments and enable investigations to be performed that would be difficult or even impossible experimentally. One particularly interesting and important aspect of modeling is the estimation of the effects of age, body size, and sex on deposition [51,52].

There is an important aspect of the deposition patterns that often escapes the unwary reader, who may be getting the impression that the three "compartments" can be treated as homogeneous. In fact, it is expected and observed experimentally that the deposition in the upper respiratory tract and central airways, which is primarily by impaction, tends to take place at the bifurcations. It would be expected, however, that in the lower part of the respiratory tract, where sedimentation and diffusion dominate and the gas flow should be essentially laminar, the deposited material would be evenly spread on the surface. Evidence from studies of experimental animals indicates that this is not so [53,54]. Even material that passes all the way through the small airways tends to deposit at the alveolar duct bifurcations, instead of covering evenly the alveolar spaces.

Indirect evidence indicates that droplets of solutions administered to human volunteers do not spread too rapidly on the surfaces of the respiratory tract, suggesting that even liquids will form deposits of hot spots of material that may never spread uniformly over the surfaces. This affects the clearance rate [55], and it may also modulate the magnitude of the local biological (i.e., both therapeutic and toxic) effects.

Deposition of Therapeutic Aerosols

The early medicinal inhalation products deposited to a large extent in the oropharyngeal cavity (80–95% of the inhaled dose), with the majority of the dose swallowed into the gastrointestinal tract [10–18]. This was true even in normal volunteers, despite the fact that nominally the aerodynamic size was often in the range that, in principle, should deliver at least 60% of the dose to the tracheobronchial and pulmonary regions. The specific reasons for this discrepancy are several, and some need to be discussed with reference to a particular means of aerosol delivery system (i.e., the combination of the formulation and the generation device). However, there are two fundamental differences between the aerosols used in the studies described in the previous section and those administered in clinical practice [56]. Therapeutic aerosols are polydisperse (heterodisperse), and their size usually changes after generation, in contrast to the stable monodisperse aerosol studies reviewed earlier.

Because the therapeutic aerosols frequently have a log-normal type of size distribution, polydispersity usually implies that there is a long tail of particles with large aerodynamic diameters. These big particles contain a significant fraction of the therapeutic dose. Several theoretical calculations indicate that there should be very significant differences in the regional deposition of aerosols with the degree of polydispersity found in conventional therapeutic aerosols compared to the deposition of monodisperse aerosols [50,57–61]. A reduction in alveolar deposition from about 60% of the inhaled dose to less than 30% was calculated for a polydisperse aerosol with a mass median aerodynamic diameter of about 3 μm and a degree of polydispersity characterized by the geometric standard deviation of 3.5 compared to a monodisperse aerosol with the same mass median aerodynamic diameter [59]. These more recent findings are in sharp contrast to an earlier, widely quoted occupational hygiene report [62].

The instability of the particle size of therapeutic aerosols is exhibited in several ways. Perhaps the most thoroughly studied effects are those associated with the generation of drug particles from the propellant-driven metered-dose inhalers. These have usually been formulated as suspensions of drug particles. On release from the metered-dose inhaler, the particles are surrounded by a large volume of propellant and other excipients. The effective aerodynamic size of the drug is, therefore, initially much greater than the intended size (i.e., the size of primary drug particles) [63]. This, together with the high velocity of the aerosol released from the metered-dose inhaler, is predominantly responsible for the high proportion of the dose that deposits at the back of the patient's mouth. If sufficient time is given between generation and entry into the mouth (e.g., by using a holding chamber or a spacer), the propellant may evaporate. It is possible, however, that the resulting particles will be markedly greater than the primary drug particles. This is because they may be associated with involatile excipients and also with other drug particles that were in the same droplet of propellant. Whichever pattern develops with a particular device or formulation, the changing aerodynamic properties of the whole system of the dispersed phase, and not the static properties of the naked drug particles, determine the deposition [64,65]. Recent advances in the design and formulation of metered-dose inhalers using hydrofluoroalkane (HFA) propellants resulted in a product in which a corticosteriod, beclomethasone dipropionate, is dissolved rather than suspended. This metered-dose inhaler (MDI) generates more favorable droplets and evaporation dynamics, leading to significantly smaller particle size and resulting in higher lung deposition and lower loss in the oropharynx than those obtained with the older, chlorofluorocarbon suspensions [66].

The second reason for the difference between the deposition of stable aerosols and many therapeutic aerosols is hygroscopic growth and evaporation. For drugs to be effective, they must show an appreciable aqueous solubility. Solid drug particles may pick up water vapor and dissolve, and droplets of drug solutions can exchange water with the environment to equalize vapor pressure. The relative humidity profile in the respiratory tract depends on the ambient conditions and the breathing pattern [67].

The relative humidity eventually reaches almost 100% in alveoli [67]. The drug particles, or droplets of solution, therefore, will tend to exchange water with the surrounding atmosphere, to equilibrate as isotonic solutions at 37°C. Of course, they may deposit, or be exhaled, before the equilibrium is reached if the rate of water transfer is slow. This instability of particle size has been thought for a long time to be a significant factor causing major differences between the deposition patterns of nonhygroscopic and hygroscopic aerosols (note that at very high relative humidity, almost all reasonably soluble substances become hygroscopic). Hygroscopic growth and evaporation were studied in theoretical and in vitro models [68–72]. The impact of this size instability on the distribution of nonisotonic aqueous aerosols in the human respiratory tract was investigated by gamma scintigraphy [73,74]. A computational model of aerosol deposition that can also deal with aerosol hygroscopicity showed good agreement with the human gamma scintigraphic data [75].

OPPORTUNITIES FOR CONTROL OF DEPOSITION AND TARGETING

Except in situations when an aerosol is deliberately targeted for deposition in the mouth or in the nose, the material landing in these regions has no useful purpose for the therapy of respiratory diseases. Therefore, minimizing the extrathoracic deposition of inhalation aerosols is usually a desirable design feature of these delivery systems. Although there are many studies providing the evidence that inhalation therapy is improved by shifting the deposition from the oropharyngeal to the pulmonary region, data that would show that a more selective targeting within the latter region is desirable are rather scarce. The advantages of delivering pentamidine aerosols selectively to the lung periphery is the clearest case, because the receptors, the infecting microorganisms, reside in the alveolated parts [21]. Bronchodilator drugs contained in particles or droplets with smaller mass median aerodynamic diameters achieve a more potent therapeutic effect than the coarser aerosols [76,77], but how this is affected by changes in the regional deposition is not known. Similar results of improved efficacy with smaller particles were obtained with the prophylactic drug cromolyn sodium [78]; in this case, however, the less effective particles tested had a mass median aerodynamic diameter so large (11 μm) that they would have deposited almost entirely in the oropharynx.

Particle Velocity and Flow Rate

The deposition in the mouth is largely due to impaction (except for ultrafine aerosols). This mode of deposition therefore increases with particle size and velocity. The reduction of oropharyngeal deposition is desirable both to improve the efficiency of lung deposition and to reduce its variability [26]. To accomplish this, the velocity of the particles must be sufficiently low. The lower bound for the particle velocity is dictated by the inspiratory flow carrying the aerosol cloud. But some aerosol generators impart high velocity to the particles in the course of formation of the aerosol cloud.

In particular, the propellant-driven metered-dose inhalers release the aerosol cloud at the very high velocity caused by the pressure of the propellant. The open-mouth technique of inhalation [79] helps to slow down the droplets (and to evaporate the volatile excipients). An even more effective solution is to use spacer devices [4,79–87], in which the aerosol cloud can slowed down, the volatile constituents can evaporate, and any large particles will sediment out. Moreover, the patient can then inhale the remaining aerosol under optimal conditions for pulmonary delivery [4,8,56,79], that is, with a slow inspiratory flow rate.

With breath-driven dry powder inhalers, as with nebulizers, the aerosol cloud is inhaled at the inspiratory flow rate. However, experimental evidence from both in vitro [88] and in vivo studies [15,30] indicates that at least some of these inhalers require high inspiratory flow rates to achieve adequate deaggregation of the drug power. The higher the flow, the more energy is available to emit the dose from the device and disperse the particles; however, this is accompanied by higher inertial impaction. To avoid the dependence on the patient's inspiratory effort and the negative impact of high inspiratory flow rate on lung deposition, "active" dry powder inhalers have evolved that use other forms of energy (e.g., compressed air) to disperse the powder [89].

For aerosols in which the particle velocity is determined by the inspiratory flow rate and the particle size is not sensitive to it, it is expected that the increase in flow rate increases the upper and central airway deposition. For example, Ryan et al. [90] found that fast vital capacity inhalation resulted in a greater proportion of nebulizer aerosol depositing in the central airways than when the aerosol was inhaled slowly. However, the dependence on the inspiratory flow rate becomes more subtle when the particles have intrinsic velocity (such as droplets generated by propellant-driven metered-dose inhalers that need to be entrained into the inhaled air) or the particle size is inspiratory flow dependent (as in the case of passive dry powder inhalers).

Other Inhalation Mode Factors

Timing of the aerosol entry at a particular point in the breathing cycle can have a profound effect on deposition. With the metered-dose inhaler without a spacer, poor synchronization of inspiration with the firing of the valve can result in a substantial loss of the aerosol bolus. For this reason, breath-actuated valves have been developed [91–93].

Stahlhofen's group [94,95] developed the technique of delivering boluses of monodisperse aerosols at predetermined points in the breathing cycle to achieve very selective deposition, especially in the upper and central airways. Early work by Gottschalk et al. [96] indicated that tidal breathing of an aerosol produced by an ultrasonic nebulizer caused less deposition than a deeply inspired aerosol followed by breath holding. Other breathing maneuvers, such as forced expiratory effort that enhances the central deposition of aerosols [97], can be used in principle to control to some extent the sites of deposition. However, it must be remembered that most patients are unable to follow even relatively simple inhalation instructions [28,29]. A complex breathing pattern might be impossible for a patient with compromised respiratory function to exercise, and even in able patients, the breathing patterns should be enforced as much as possible by the aerosol-producing device. A study utilizing an electronic device that managed the patient's breathing was carried out by Farr et al. The device guided the patient with a light prompt into a preprogrammed inspiratory flow rate range, and it automatically actuated the aerosol generation from the MDI at a preprogrammed inspired volume. Using gamma scintigraphy, the authors demonstrated profound differences in lung deposition between the different settings simulating both correct and incorrect use of MDIs [98]. This study also provided evidence that visual prompting using color signals and electronic actuation of aerosol generation at specified inhaled volume was a practicable way to manage the patient's inhalation delivery technique.

An effective and feasible method to enhance deposition in the small airways and alveoli is breath holding; this is important, especially for submicronic particles that would be otherwise exhaled [99].

Size Distribution

To avoid oropharyngeal deposition, the drug-carrying particles should be either generated with low D_{ae} (1–3 μm) or, if bigger particles are present, removed before entry into the patient's mouth. The extent to which the loss in the oropharynx is significant will depend on the acceptable variability of lung delivery and the cost of the drug. Since micron-size particles have poor flow properties, traditionally it has been necessary to include some large particles in the formulation. This could be achieved by mixing the micronized drug powder with a carrier material, such as lactose, which consists of particles so large that they will deposit almost entirely in the mouth. A different solution was found to improve the powder flow of cromolyn sodium without an excipient. Respirable-size particles of the drug were made to aggregate into larger, free-flowing spheres (pellets) that are broken up into the primary particles during the generation of the aerosol cloud in the Spinhaler [15].

Calculations predict that substantial changes in regional deposition would result not only if the median diameter of the size distribution is changed but also if the aerosols have different widths of size distribution [50,57–61]. It would be expected that, at the macroscopic level, a more selective delivery would be obtained with less polydisperse aerosols.

Shape

The shape can have a profound effect on the aerodynamic behavior of particles. Perhaps the best-studied nonspherical shapes are those of elongated particles, because of the toxic effects of mineral fibers such as asbestos. It has been known that the aerodynamic diameters of particles with high axial ratios are almost independent of their length and equal to approximately two to three times the D_{ae} of a sphere of the same density and diameter equal to the short dimension of the particle in question [22,24,25]. It is this peculiar behavior that enables even very long, thin fibers to deposit in alveoli [100, 101]. The deposition of these fibers in the peripheral lungs is enhanced by interception (see the earlier section on Interception as a mechanism of deposition); particles with compact shapes and the same D_{ae} would be more likely to be exhaled under normal breathing conditions. It is possible to prepare drug particles with these types of shapes, for example, by control of the crystallization conditions. If the crystal growth takes place preferentially in the longitudinal direction so that the drug particles have similar thickness, then a powder with a narrow distribution of aerodynamic diameters should be obtained. This was, indeed, observed with two drugs engineered in the manner described previously [25,102,103]. Preparation of drug powders with elongated particles may, therefore, provide the means to achieve a more selective delivery, especially to the lung periphery. The modification of the shape is probably useful only for drugs that have a relatively slow dissolution rate in water. Otherwise, the original shape would change, ultimately into spherical droplets, on entry into the respiratory tract.

Traditionally, nonspherical particles have been avoided because of the potential problems with powder flow. This phenomenon has not been studied in depth, but some published work suggests that the respirable fraction of the drug obtained from a breath-driven dry powder inhaler may not depend very much on the particle shape [104].

Density

Although the dependence of the aerodynamic diameter on particle density is relatively weak, recent advances in particle engineering produced pharmaceutically interesting porous particles [105]. The geometric diameters of these porous particles are several times greater than the aerodynamic diameters, because the density of the porous material is much lower than that of water. Of course, it is expected that the deposition of these particles will be governed by their aerodynamic, rather than geometric, size. These particles are also claimed to be more resistant to phagocytosis by alveolar macrophages and could therefore provide increased duration of action in the alveolar regions ("temporal" or "kinetic" targeting—see later).

Hygroscopic Growth

The ability of drug-containing particles and droplets to exchange water with the atmosphere in the respiratory tract has been discussed so far only in the context of being a factor contributing to the loss in the useful fraction of the drug reaching the lung. However, theoretical models predict that hygroscopic growth may be used to enhance deposition of therapeutic aerosols [106–108]. Once again, theory is somewhat ahead of experimental work in this field. Good predictive models of hygroscopic growth require reliable information about the nature of the environment in the airways. There has been much interest in recent years in investigating the distribution of relative humidity and temperature in the respiratory tract [67,109–115]. If the aerosol is present in sufficient quantity, it can affect the relative humidity in the respiratory tract and hence its own hygroscopic growth. This was demonstrated in human deposition studies in which nonisotonic aqueous aerosols with identical initial particle size distributions and aqueous solution properties were used but the droplet number concentrations were different [73,74]. To be able to predict correctly the rate and extent of hygroscopic growth, it would appear that the rate of dissolution of drugs and their solution properties (without and with excipients) need to be determined, because the nonideal behavior of these solutions is likely to cause significant deviations from the growth dynamics predicted for simple inorganic salts [70,73,116,117].

Control of the hygroscopic growth rate may be achieved, for example, by preparation of drugs in solid forms with reduced aqueous solubility [102,103] or by coating the drug with hydrophobic films [118–120]. These formulation interventions can prevent hygroscopic growth altogether, if desired, because the growth rate will be retarded to the point where no enlargement would take place during the transit of the particle in the respiratory tract.

Kinetic Aspects for Local and Systemic Delivery

Increasing the duration of action of inhaled drugs is an area of great interest for the short-acting substances, because, generally speaking, the less frequent the need for dosing, the better the patient's compliance. Therapeutic efficacy may be improved if the drug levels in the respiratory tract are relatively constant, as shown by the improved therapeutic effects achieved with a corticosteroid inhaled four times a day compared to two times a day [121].

The regional differences in the mucociliary clearance rate provide opportunities to increase the duration of residence of drugs in the respiratory tract by depositing the drug initially in the regions with the slow clearance rates [36,37]. This suggests that deposition in the peripheral regions is desirable. However, the very slow clearance component, presumably representing mainly the material deposited on the nonciliated parts of the peripheral lung, may never get transported to the more central parts, where the receptors could be located. Furthermore, the drug may disappear by absorption. The latter can be prevented by placing the drug in a carrier that either is absorbed slowly or is nonabsorbable. The release rate of the drug from the carrier is critical to achieve adequate levels of the free drug in the lung for therapy, because drug still present in its delivery system is usually incapable of causing the desired therapeutic effect [37]. The sustained-release effect may be achieved in a number of ways. Four methods have been described in the literature: (1) magnesium hydroxide precipitates as a model for sustained release [122], (2) entrapment of drugs in liposomes and other hydrophobic microcarriers [123–131], (3) sparingly soluble drugs [25,132,133], and (4) the use of poorly soluble, porous carrier particles, with the view also to minimize the digestion of the drug-loaded material by phagocytosis [105].

Drug entrapment in liposomes has been most extensively investigated, and evidence has been presented both in experimental animals and in humans that the drug residence time in the lung can be substantially extended [123–129,131].

To increase the residence times of drugs in the conducting airways served by the mucociliary escalator, mucoadhesive formulations were investigated [134]. This approach can be effective, but safety consequences of slowing down this natural clearance mechanism will need to be investigated.

Absorption and Metabolism

It is well established that the deeper in the lung the aerosol deposits, the higher is the proportion of the drug that gets absorbed into the systemic circulation. These observations span different animal species, including humans, and range from small molecules to peptides and proteins [135–140]. A number of factors contribute to this: (1) depositing the drug beyond the mucociliary escalator removes a significant mechanism competing with absorption; (2) although there is no conclusive evidence yet that different parts of the respiratory tract have different permeabilities (for a review, see Ref. 8), it would be expected that the thin alveolar membranes are more permeable than the airway surfaces; (3) the surface area grows rapidly with increasing airway generations. However, as mentioned in the earlier section on Studies with Stable Monodisperse Aerosols, the mixing of liquids on the mucosal surface appears to be incomplete, and, therefore, the rate of absorption will be probably affected by the initial surface area covered by the deposited material [55]. Even though the mechanistic aspects are not entirely understood, for systemic delivery of drugs via the lung, "deep" lung should be targeted.

For activity in the respiratory tract, the absorption should be slowed down. Controlled deposition in the tracheobronchial region to slow down the absorption is likely to be counterproductive because the overall clearance, which includes the mucociliary escalator, has to be taken in account. In other words, even if the conducting airways were less permeable to the substance in question than the lung periphery, mucociliary clearance would remove the drug more rapidly from the more central location. For locally acting drugs, selecting drug molecules with intrinsically long absorption half-life in the lung would be advantageous; pentamidine serves as an example [141]. Other drugs may require controlled-release absorption to prolong their residence time in the respiratory tract, as discussed in the previous section [37].

Studies with homogenized lung tissues show that the alveolated parts generally have higher metabolic rates than the tracheobronchial tissue [142,143]. These studies are not directly relevant, though, to the effect of a drug deposited for local activity on the respiratory lumen. On the other hand, this information is more directly pertinent to drugs intended for systemic effects. Interestingly, the bronchial circulation was shown to have a lower metabolic capacity than the pulmonary circulation [144]. There does not appear to be any clinical evidence, though, that drugs absorbed from the central airways would be metabolized to a lesser extent than following absorption from the lung periphery.

Rate of Delivery

The concentrations of the drug at the desired sites and at the sites of toxicity within the respiratory tract will depend on the balance of the drug supply and clearance rates at these sites [37]. We may speculate that this is one of the reasons for the higher doses required for the delivery of topical medications by nebulizers (typically over 10–25 min) vs. metered-dose inhalers or dry powder inhalers that deliver the medication in one or two breaths. There is little doubt that prolonged inhalation reduces the patient's enthusiasm for the therapy. It is therefore appropriate to evaluate nebulizers in terms of their useful output, that is, the dose of the therapeutic or diagnostic agent delivered in the desired aerodynamic size range per unit time [145].

For systemic administration of readily absorbed molecules, the rate of delivery may be the rate-limiting step. This is evidenced with small molecules, such as morphine, whose absorption rate following deep lung delivery is practically indistinguishable from that after intravenous injection [146].

Airway Caliber

The caliber of airways through which the aerosol has to pass to get to the more distal parts of the lungs is of utmost importance. In functional terms, the forced expiratory volume in one second, FEV_1, is usually taken as a measure of the instantaneous resistance (and, hence, the caliber) of the airways. Therefore, it is customary to attempt to relate FEV_1 to the deposition pattern. Using such functional tools, bronchoconstriction, or low values of FEV_1, were shown to be associated with a hindrance of penetration of aerosols to the distal lungs [73,147–152], and, conversely, bronchodilation enhanced the shift of deposition to the peripheral lungs [151]. This may have important therapeutic consequences. For example, it is known that the bronchodilatory potency can be increased by successive inhalation spaced by 10-min intervals to allow for bronchodilation. This was interpreted by the ability of the aerosol to reach receptors deeper in the lung by successive opening of the airways [153].

CONCLUSIONS

A range of options exists to increase or decrease the fraction of dose deposited in different parts of the respiratory tract and to control the concentration–time profiles of the drug at these sites. New techniques are being developed that enable noninvasive monitoring of the drug [12] or monitoring of a labeled marker compound [16–18,39–41,87] in the respiratory tract in vivo so that the degree of achievement of spatial and temporal selectivity can be investigated. Better spatial resolution is now possible with the greater availability of tomographic technique, such as single-photon emission computerized tomography (SPECT) and positron emission tomography (PET) [154,155].

The primary objective for the development of targeting strategies is to improve the safety and efficacy of therapy. This requires intrasubject reproducibility of delivery within the margins of therapeutic and toxic responses to the drug. In the first instance, the aerosol generators should give adequately reproducible output in terms of drug mass and its aerodynamic size distribution. It is now possible to incorporate features into the aerosol delivery systems that minimize the dependence on patient factors. In particular, the management of the patient's inspiratory flow rate and the volume of air inhaled at the time of actuation of the aerosol delivery reduces the variability of the dose to the lung and its distribution [98]. In aerosol administration to subjects with poor respiratory function, the most frequent dominant source of variability is the state of the patient's airways. For patients with reversible obstructive airway disease, this may be controlled with appropriate therapy. Interestingly, the greatest advances in pulmonary targeting have been obtained in recent years with "deep lung" delivery. Complete pulmonary absorption of small molecules in human volunteer studies has been found with these specially developed aerosol delivery systems, resulting in blood levels that are practically indistinguishable in terms of the pharmacokinetics and variability from intravenous administration [146].

Systems producing fine-particle insulin aerosols have been tested extensively in humans [156]. A clear dose response of glucose reduction and reproducibilities comparable to subcutaneous injections were obtained with an inhaler that combines almost monodisperse insulin particles (MMAD ~ 2–$3\ \mu m$)

with electronic control of inspiratory flow rate and delivery of the aerosol bolus early in the inspiration, followed by a chase volume ("deep breath") [157].

REFERENCES

1. Albert A. Selective Toxicity. 6th ed. London: Chapman and Hall, 1979.
2. Anderson SD, Seale JP, Rozea P, Bandler L, Theobald G, Lindsay DA. Am Rev Respir Dis 1976; 114:493.
3. Neville A, Palmer JBD, Gaddie J, May CS, Palmer KNV, Murchison LE. Br Med J 1977; 1:413.
4. Newman SP, Clarke SW. In: Morén F, Newhouse MT, Dolovich MB, eds. Aerosols in Medicine. Amsterdam. Elsevier, 1985:289.
5. Svedmyr N, Löfdahl G-G. In: Jenne JW, Murphy S, eds. Drug Therapy for Asthma. New York: Marcel Dekker, 1987:177.
6. Taylor RG. In: Ganderton D, Jones T, eds. Drug Delivery to the Respiratory Tract. Chichester, UK: Ellis Horwood, 1978:27.
7. Clark TJH. Lancet 1972; 6:1361.
8. Gonda I. CRC Rev Ther Drug Carrier Syst 1990; 6:273.
9. Cipolla D, Farr S, Gonda I, Otulana B. In: Hansel TT, Barnes PJ, eds. New Drugs for Asthma. Basel, Switzerland: Karger, 2001:20.
10. Laros CD, van Urk P, Rominger KL. Respiration 1997; 34:131.
11. Blackwell EW, Briant RH, Conolly ME, Davies DS, Dollery CT. Br J Pharmacol 1974; 50:587.
12. Spiro SG, Singh CA, Tolfree SEJ, Partridge MR, Short MD. Thorax 1984; 39:432.
13. Moss GF, Jones KM, Ritchie JT, Cox JSG. Toxicol Appl Pharmacol 1971; 20:147.
14. Neale MG, Brown K, Hodder RW, Auty RM. Br J Clin Pharmacol 1986; 22:373.
15. Auty RM, Brown K, Neale MG, Snashall PD. Br J Dis Chest 1987; 81:371.
16. Vidgren MT, Kärkkäinen A, Paronen TP, Karjalainen P. Int J Pharm 1987; 39:101.
17. Davies DS. In: Junod AF, deHaller R, eds. Lung Metabolism. New York: Academic Press, 1975:201.
18. Vidgren M, Kärkkäinen A, Karjalainen P, Paronen P, Nuutinen J. Int J Pharm 1988; 42:211.
19. Milne LJR, Crompton GK. Br Med J 1974; 3:797.
20. Toogood JH. In: Jenne JW, Murphy S, eds. Drug Therapy for Asthma: Research and Clinical Practice. New York: Marcel Dekker, 1987:719.
21. O'Doherty MJ, Thomas S, Page C, Barlow D, Bradbeer C, Nunan TO, Bateman NY. Lancet 1988; 2:1283.
22. Hinds WC. Aerosol Technology. New York: Wiley, 1982.
23. Raabe OG. In: Crapo JD, Smolko ED, Miller FJ, Graham JA, Hayes AW, eds. Extrapolation of Dosimetric Relationships for Inhaled Particles and Gases. San Diego, CA: Academic Press, 1989:81.
24. Stöber W. In: MercerTT, Morrow PE, Stöber W, eds. Assessment of Airborne Particles. Springfield, IL: Charles C Thomas, 1972:249.
25. Gonda I, Khalik AFAE. Ann Occup Hyg 1985; (suppl VI):379.

26. Morrow PE, Yu CP. In: Morén F, Newhouse MT, Dolovich MB, eds. Aerosols in Medicine. Amsterdam: Elsevier, 1985:149.

27. Timbrell V. Ann N Y Acad Sci 1965; 132:255.

28. Epstein SW, Manning CPR, Ashley MJ, Corey PN. Can Med Assoc J 1979; 120:813.

29. Munt P. Can Med Assoc J 1979; 120:781.

30. Richards RS, Simpson SF, Renwick AG, Holgate ST. Eur Respir J 1988; 1:896.

31. Lippmann M, Albert RE. Am Ind Hyg Assoc J 1969; 30:257.

32. Stahlhofen W. In: Smith H, Gerber G, eds. Lung Modeling for Inhalation of Radioactive Materials. Office for Official Publications of the European Communities, 1984:39.

33. Warmer A. Am J Med 1979; 67:477.

34. Agnew JE. In: Clarke SW, Pavia D, eds. Aerosols and the Lung: Clinical and Experimental Aspects. London: Butterworths, 1984:49.

35. Stahlhofen W. Extrapolation of Dosimetric Relationships for Inhaled Particles and Gases. San Diego, CA: Academic Press, 1989:153.

36. Byron PR. J Pharm Sci 1986; 75:433.

37. Gonda I. J Pharm Sci 1988; 77:340.

38. Agnew JE, Pavia D, Clarke SW. Eur J Respir Dis 1981; 62:239.

39. Phipps PR, Gonda I, Bailey DL, Borharn P, Bautovich G, Anderson SD. Am Rev Respir Dis 1989; 139:1561.

40. Logus JW, Trajan M, Hooper HR, Lentle BC, Man SFP. J Can Assoc Radial 1984; 35:133.

41. Phipps PR, Gonda I, Bailey DL, Borham P, Bautovich G, Anderson SD. J Pharm Pharmacol 1987; 39(suppl):78P.

42. Coleman RE, Mercer RR, Jaszczak RJ, Greer KL, Crapo JD. In: Crapo JD, Smolko ED, Miller FJ, Graham JA, Hayes AW, eds. Extrapolation of Dosimetric Relationships for Inhaled Particles and Gases. San Diego, CA: Academic Press, 1989:201.

43. Palmes ED, Altshuler B, Nelson N. In: Davies CN, ed. Inhaled Particles and Vapors II. New York: Pergamon Press, 1976:339.

44. Santolicandro A, Giuntini C. J Nucl Med All Sci 1979; 23:115.

45. Laube BL, Swift DL, Wagner HN, Norman PS, Adams GK. Am Rev Respir Dis 1986; 133:740.

46. Christensen WD, Swift DL. J Appl Physiol 1986; 60:630.

47. Heyder J, Rudolph G. In: Smith H, Gerber G, eds. Lung Modeling for Inhalation of Radioactive Materials. Office for Official Publications of the European Communities, 1984:17.

48. Ferron GA, Hornik S, Kreyling WG, Haider B. J Aerosol Sci 1985; 16:133.

49. Yu CP, Diu CK. Aerosol Sci Technol 1982; 1:355.

50. Gonda I. J Pharm Pharmacol 1981; 3:692.

51. Phalen RF, Oldham MJ, Kleinman MT, Crocker TT. Ann Occup Hyg 1988; (suppl VI): II.

52. Knight V, Yu CP, Gilbert BE, Divine GW. J Infect Dis 1988; 158:443.

53. Lippmann M. In: Lee SD, Schneider T, Grant LD, Verkerk PJ, eds. Aerosols: Research, Risk Assessment and Control Strategies. Chelsea, MI: Lewis, 1986:43.

54. Brody AR, Yu CP. In: Crapo JD, Smolko EE, Miller FJ, Graham JA, Hayes AW, eds. Extrapolation of Dosimetric Relationships for Inhaled Particles and Gases. New York: Academic Press, 1989:91.

55. Groth S, Mortensen J, Lange P, Vest S, Rossing N, Swift D. J Appl Physiol 1989; 66:2750.

56. Gonda I. In: Aulton ME, ed. Pharmaceutics: The Science of Dosage Form Design. Edinburgh, UK: Churchill Livingstone, 1988:341.

57. Persons DD, Hess GD, Muller WJ, Scherer PW. J Appl Physiol 1987; 63:1195.

58. Gonda I. In: Hauck H, ed. Abstracts of the International Symposium on Deposition and Clearance of Aerosols in the Human Respiratory Tract, Bad Gleichenberg. vol. 1. International Society for Aerosols in Medicine.1981:59.

59. Gonda I. J Pharm Pharmacol 1981; 33(suppl):52P.

60. Diu CK, Yu CP. Am Ind Hyg Assoc J 1983; 44:62.

61. Rudolph G, Gebhart J, Heyder J, Scheuch G, Stahlhofen W. Ann Occup Hyg 1988; (suppl VI):119.

62. Task Group on Lung Dynamics, Health Phys 1966; 12:173.

63. Moren F, Andersson J. Int J Pharm 1980; 6:295.

64. Newman SP, Killip M, Pavia D, Moran F, Clarke SW. Int J Pharm 1984; 19:333.

65. Chan H-K, Gonda I. Int J Pharm 1988; 41:147.

66. Leach C. In: Dalby RN, Byron PR, Farr SJ, eds. Respiratory Drug Delivery V. Buffalo Grove, IL: Interpharm Press, 1996:133.

67. Daviskas E, Gonda I, Anderson SD. J Appl Physiol 1990; 69:361.

68. Byron PR, Davis SS, Bubb MD, Cooper P. Pestic Sci 1977; 8:521.

69. Gonda I, Kayes JB, Groom CV, Fildes FJT. In: StanleyWood N, Allen T, eds. Particle Size Analysis 1981: Proceedings of the Fourth Particle Size Analysis Conference. Chichester, UK: Wiley, 1982:31.

70. Smith G, Hiller C, Mazumder M, Bone R. Am Rev Respir Dis 1980; 121:513.

71. Bell K, Ho AT. J Aerosol Sci 1981; 12:247.

72. Martin GP, Bell AE, Marriot C. Int J Pharm 1988; 44:57.

73. Phipps PR, Gonda I, Anderson SD, Bailey D, Bautovich G. Eur Respir J 1994; 7:1474.

74. Chan H-K, Phipps PR, Gonda I, Cook P, Fulton R, Young I, Bautovich G. Eur Respir J 1994; 7:1483.

75. Finlay WH, Stapleton KW, Gonda I, Chan H-K, Zuberhuler P. J Appl Physiol 1996; 81:374.

76. Padfield JM, Winterborn IK, Pover GM, Tattersfield A. J Pharm Pharmacol 1983; 35(suppl):10P.

77. Persson G, Wiren JE. Eur Respir J 1989; 2:253.

78. Godfrey S, Zeidifard E, Brown K, Bell JH. Clin Sci Mol Med 1974; 46:265.

79. Newhouse M, Dolovich M. Respiration 1986; 50(suppl 2):123.

80. Dolovich M, Ruffin R, Corr D, Newhouse MT. Chest 1983; 84:36.

81. Newman SP, Millar AB, Lennard-Jones TR, Moran F, Clarke SW. Thorax 1984; 39:935.

82. Newman SP, Woodman G, Clarke SW, Sackner MA. Am Rev Respir Dis 1985; 131:A96.
83. Vidgren MT, Paronen TP, Kärkkäinen A, Karjalainen P. Int J Pharm 1987; 39:107.
84. Newman SP, Moran F, Pavia D, Little F, Clarke SW. Am Rev Respir Dis 1981; 124:317.
85. Salzman GA, Pyszczynski DR, Allergy J. Clin Immunol 1988; 81:424.
86. Toogood JH, Baskerville J, Jennings B, Lefcoe NM, Johnsson S-A. Am Rev Respir Dis 1984; 129:723.
87. Newman SP, Clark AR, Talaee N, Clarke SW. Thorax 1989; 44:706.
88. Kassem MM, Ho KKL, Ganderton D. J Pharm Pharmacol 1989; 41:14P.
89. Clark AR, Shire SJ. In: McNally EJ, ed. Protein Formulation and Delivery. New York: Marcel Dekker, 2000:201.
90. Ryan G, Dolovich MB, Obminski G, Cockcroft DW, Juniper E, Hargreave FE, Newhouse MT. J Allergy Clin Immunol 1981; 67:156.
91. D'Arcy PF, Kirk WF. Pharm J 1971; 206:306.
92. Armstrong JC. U.S. Patent 3789843, 1974.
93. Baum EA, Bryant AM. J Aerosol Med 1988; 1:219.
94. Scheuch G, Stahlhofen W. J Aerosol Med 1988; 1:29.
95. Scheuch G, Stahlhofen W. J Aerosol Med 1988; 1:210.
96. Gottschalk B, Leupold W, Woller P. Z Erkrank Atm Org 1978; 150:139.
97. Foster WM, Langenback EG, Smaldone GC, Bergofsky EH, Bohning DE. Ann Occup Hyg 1980; (suppl):101.
98. Farr SJ, Rowe AM, Rubsamen R, Taylor G. Thorax 1995; 50:639.
99. Palmes ED, Goldring RM, Wang C-S, Altshuler B. In: Walton WH, ed. Inhaled Particles III. Old Working, UK: Unwin, 1971:123.
100. Harris RL, Jr., Timbrell V. In: Walton WH, ed. Inhaled Particles IV. Part I. Oxford: Pergamon Press, 1977:75.
101. Timbrell V. Ann Occup Hyg 1982; 26(suppl):347.
102. Chan H-K, Gonda I. J Aerosol Sci 1989; 20:157.
103. Chan H-K, Gonda I. J Pharm Sci 1989; 78:176.
104. Wong LW, Kassem NM, Ganderton D. J Pharm Pharmacol 1989; 41(suppl):24P.
105. Edwards DA, Hanes J, Caponetti G, Hrkach J, Ben-Jebria A, Eskew M, Mintzes J, Deaver D, Lotan N, Langer R. Science 1997; 276:1868.
106. Ferron GA, Kreyling WG, Haider B. J Aerosol Sci 1988; 19:611.
107. Persons DD, Hess GD, Scherer P. J Appl Physiol 1987; 63:1205.
108. Martonen TB, Hofmann W, Eisner AD, Menache MG. In: Crapo JD, Smolko ED, Miller FJ, Graham JA, Hayes AW, eds. Extrapolation of Dosimetric Relationships for Inhaled Particles and Gases. New York: Academic Press, 1989:303.
109. Ferron GA, Haider B, Kreyling WG. J Aerosol Sci 1988; 19:343.
110. Hanna LM, Scherer PW. J Biomech Eng 1986; 108:19.
111. Ingenito EP, Solway J, McFadden ER, Pichurko BMI, Cravalho EG, Drazen JM. J Appl Physiol 1986; 61:2252.
112. Ingenito EP, Solway J, McFadden ER, Pichurko BMI, Bowman F, Michaels D, Drazen JM. J Appl Physiol 1987; 63:2075.
113. Saidel GM, Kruse KL, Primiano FP. J Biomech Eng 1983; 105:188.

114. McFadden ER, Denison DM, Waller JF, Assoufi BI, Peacock A, Sopwith T. J Clin Investig 1982; 69:799.

115. McFadden ER, Pichurko BMI, Bowman F, Ingenito EP, Bums S, Dowling N, Solway J. J Appl Physiol 1985; 58:564.

116. Gonda I, Groom CV. J Colloid Interf Sci 1983; 92:289.

117. Groom CV, Gonda I, Fildes FJT. 2nd International Congress on Pharmaceutical Technology, AGPI, Paris, Vol. 5, 1980:124.

118. Hickey AJ. Ph.D. dissertation, University of Aston in Birmingham, UK, 1984.

119. Hickey AJ, Gonda I. In: Gale AE, Wilde W, eds. Abstracts of the 5th Congress of the International Society for Aserosols in Medicine: Medical Aerosols 1984. Adelaide, Australia: South Australian Postgraduate Medical Education Association, 1984:14.

120. Hickey AJ, Gonda I, Irwin WJ, Fildes FJT. J Pharm Sci 1990; 79:1009.

121. Maio JL, Cartier A, Merland N, Ghezzo H, Burek A, Morris J, Jennings BH. Am Rev Respir Dis 1989; 140:624.

122. Hickey AJ, Byron PR. J Pharm Soc 1986; 75:756.

123. Mihalko PJ, Schreier H, Abra RM. In: Gregoriadis G, ed. Liposomes as Drug Carriers. London: Wiley, 1988:679.

124. McCullough HN, Juliano RL. J Natl Cancer Inst 1979; 63:727.

125. Juliano RL, Stamp D, McCullough N. Ann N Y Acad Sci 1979; 308:411.

126. Juliano RL, McCullough HN. J Pharmacol Exp Ther 1980; 214:381.

127. McGurk JG, Ross AR, Dickson CM, Eason CT, Potter CJ. J Pharm Pharmacol 1987; 39(suppl):54P.

128. Woolfrey SG, Taylor G, Kellaway IW. J Control Release 1988; 5:203.

129. Pettenazzo A, Jobe A, Ikegami M, Abra R, Hogue E, Mihalko P. Am Rev Respir Dis 1989; 139:752.

130. Lim JGP, Farr SJ, Kellaway IW. J Pharm Pharmacol 1989; 41(suppl):8P.

131. Taylor KMG, Taylor G, Kellaway IW, Stevens J. Pharm Res 1989; 6:633.

132. Chowhan ZT, Amaro AA. J Pharm Sci 1976; 65:1669.

133. Gonda I, Khalik AFAE, Britten AZ. Int J Pharm 1985; 27:255.

134. Sakagami M, Kinoshita W, Makinon Y, Fujii T. In: Dalby RN, Byron PR, Farr SJ, eds. Respiraroty Drug Delivery VI. Buffalo Grove, IL: Interpharm Press, 1998:193.

135. Johnson M. In: Dalby RN, Byron PR, Farr SJ, eds. Respiratory Drug Delivery. Buffalo Grove, IL: Interpharm Press, 1996:61.

136. Colthorpe P, Farr SJ, Taylor G, Smith IJ, Wyatt D. Pharm Res 1992; 9:764.

137. Colthorpe P, Farr SJ, Smith IJ, Wyatt D, Taylor G. Pharm Res 1995; 12:356.

138. Qui Y, Guptaand PK, Adjei AL. In: Adjei AL, Gupta PR, eds. Inhalation Delivery of Therapeutic Peptides and Proteins. Chap 4. New York: Marcel Dekker, 1997:89–131.

139. Newman SP, Hirst PH, Pitcairn GR, Clark AR. In: Dalby RN, Byron PR, Farr SJ, eds. Respiraroty Drug Delivery VI. Buffalo Grove, IL: Interpharm Press, 1998:9.

140. Sangway S, Agosti JM, Bauer LA, Otulana BA, Morishige RJ, Cipolla DC, Blanchard JD, Smaldone GC. J Aerosol Med 2001; 14:185.

141. Debs RJ, Straubinger RM, Brunette EN, Lin JM, Lin EJ, Montgomery AB, Friend DS, Papahadjopoulous DS. Am Rev Respir Dis 1987; 135:731.

142. Petruzzelli S, de Flora S, Bagnasco M, Hietanen E, Camus A-E, Saracci R, Izzotti A, Bartsch H, Giuntini C. Am Rev Respir Dis 1989; 140:417.

143. Harpur ES, Gonda I. Metabolism of hexamethylmelamine by rodent lung microsomes. Xth Congress of Pharmacology (IUPHAR '87), Sydney, Australia, 1987:1045.

144. Grantham CJ, Jackowski JT, Wannner A, Ryan US. J Appl Physiol 1989; 67:1041.

145. Phipps P, Borham P, Gonda I, Bailey D, Bautovich G, Anderson S. Eur J Nucl Med 1982; 13:183.

146. Farr SJ, Schuster JA, Lloyd P, Lloyd LJ, Okikawa JK, Rubsamen RM. In: Dalby RN, Byron PR, Farr SJ, eds. Respiraroty Drug Delivery V. Buffalo Grove, IL: Interpharm Press, 1996:175.

147. Ilowite JS, Gorvoy JD, Smaldone GC. Am Rev Respir Dis 1987; 136:1445.

148. Sanchis J, Dolovich M, Chalmers R, Newhouse M. J Appl Physiol 1972; 33:757.

149. Garrard CS, Gerrity TR, Schreiner JF, Yeates DB. Arch Environ Health 1981; 47:867.

150. Agnew JE, Bateman JRM, Watts M, Paramanada V, Pavia D, Clarke SW. Chest 1981; 80(suppl):843.

151. Chung KF, Jeyasingh K, Snashall PD. Eur Respir J 1988; 1:890.

152. Richards R, Haas A, Simpson S, Britten A, Renwick A, Holgate ST. Thorax 1988; 43:611.

153. Heitner D, Shim C, Williams MH. J Allergy Clin Immunol 1980; 66:75.

154. Gonda I. Aerosol Sci Technol 1993; 18:250.

155. Dolovich M, Nahmias C, Coates G. In: Dalby RN, Byron PR, Farr SJ, Peart J, eds. Respiratory Drug Delivery VII. Raleigh, NC: Serentec Press, 2000:215.

156. Gonda I. J Pharm Sci 2000; 89:940.

157. Clauson PR, Balent B, Brunner GA, Sendlhofer G, Jendle JH, Hatorp V, Dahl UL, Okikawa J, Pieber TR. In: Dalby RN, Byron PR, Farr SJ, Peart J, eds. Respiratory Drug Delivery VII. Raleigh, NC: Serentec Press, 2000:155.

4

Drug Targeting to the Lung: Chemical and Biochemical Considerations

Peter A. Crooks and Abeer M. Al-Ghananeem
University of Kentucky, Lexington, Kentucky, U.S.A.

INTRODUCTION

This chapter provides an overview of pulmonary drug-targeting strategies that are discussed from a number of different perspectives. An initial section on general considerations discusses the structure of the pulmonary epithelial membrane and considers the various factors affecting drug clearance and absorption through the pulmonary epithelial membrane. There is a section on recent advances in the design of drug molecules, which reviews recent research in the design of drug molecules for pulmonary receptor targeting and addresses new areas of pulmonary drug discovery and development. A section on structural factors governing the uptake of drugs into the lung discusses the structural requirements for the selective uptake and how these data may be used in drug targeting to the respiratory tract. The use of prodrugs for lung targeting and extending drug activity in the lung is addressed in the section on prodrug approaches. A section on the potential utility of cell membrane–bound drug entities deals with the possible usefulness of pulmonary cell membrane–bound enzymes or receptors as targets for drugs covalently linked to respective substrates or agonists and inhibitors or antagonists of these membrane-bound entities. The section on conjugation of drugs focuses on drug conjugation with macromolecules for selective targeting of the lung, which is followed by a section on the use of bioadhesives in drug targeting to pulmonary tissues. A section on the use of drug–monoclonal antibody conjugates for drug targeting to the lung is followed by a concluding section on the future direction of research in this exciting area of pulmonary drug targeting.

GENERAL CONSIDERATIONS

Some years ago, most drugs that were targeted to the respiratory tract were used for their local action, that is, nasal decongestion, bronchodilation, and so on. In recent years, it has become apparent that the lining of the upper respiratory tract (i.e., the nasal mucosa) and the airways may also be used for the absorption of a drug for its systemic effect, particularly if this route of administration avoids the metabolic destruction observed with alternative routes of administration [1,2]. This area has attracted considerable interest, particularly with regard to the delivery of peptides and proteins, which suffer from rapid degradation by peptidases by the oral route. Numerous studies have recently demonstrated that drugs can be administered systemically by application to the respiratory tract, either to the nasal mucosa or to the lungs.

The lung provides substantially greater bioavailability for macromolecules than any other port of entry to the body [3,4]. Large proteins (18–20 kDa), such as human growth hormone, show pulmonary bioavailability approaching or exceeding 50% [5], while bioavailability might approach 100% for small peptides and insulin (<6 kDa) placed in the lung compared to delivery by subcutaneous injection. The lung has several dynamic barriers, the first of which is the lung surfactant layer, which is probably a single molecule thick. Spreading at the air/water interface both in airway and alveolar surface, this surfactant layer may cause large molecules to aggregate, which might enhance engulfment and digestion by air space macophages. Interaction of some drug molecules administered by inhalation may interfere with surfactant function and lead to an increase in local surface tension, which could produce either collapse of the alveoli or edema through altered transpulmonary pressures [6]. Below the molecular layer(s) of lung surfactant lie the epithelial surface fluids. Macromolecules must defuse to get to the epithelial cell layer. It has been shown that the volume and composition of the surface liquids in this layer are regulated by ion transport in pulmonary epithelium [7]. Patton [8] mentioned in his review that in the airway, the thickness of the surface fluid is thought to average about 5–10 μm, gradually decreasing distally until the vast expanse of the alveolar is reached, covered with a very thin layer of fluid that averages about 0.05–0.08 μm thick. This layer may be several microns thick in pooled areas and as thin as 15–20 nm in other areas. The lining fluid of the airway contains various types and amounts of mucus, except on the alveoli, which concentrate on top of the surface. This mucus blanket, which covers the conducting airways and which is moved by ciliated cells in an upward direction to the pharynx, may affect pulmonary drug delivery. Drug transport may be affected as a result of drug binding to mucus compounds; increases in the thickness of the mucus layer may reduce the rate of drug absorption, and a change in the diameter of the airways may also affect the sites of drug deposition.

The ultrastructure of the respiratory membrane is unique by virtue of its function. A diagrammatic representation of the respiratory membrane is shown in Figure 1. The respiratory membrane basically comprises two main layers. The first layer is the alveolar epithelium, which consists of at least three different cell types: alveolar types I, II, and III or brush cells and migratory alveolar macrophages.

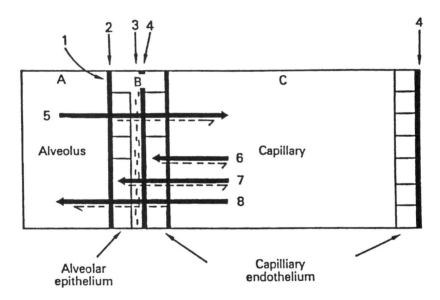

FIGURE 1 Diagrammatic representation of the ultrastructure of the respiratory membrane. Arrows indicate the passage of drugs (horizontal heavy lines) through the respiratory membrane after alveolar or capillary *exposure, or* of metabolites (horizontal broken lines) generated in the epithelial or endothelial layers. Key: (1) monomolecular surfactant layers, (2) thin fluid film, (3) interstitial space, (4) endothelial capillary basement membrane, (5) drug transport from the alveoli, (6) absorption of drug into endothelial cells from the circulation, (7) transport of drug from the circulation to alveolar epithelium, (8) transport of drug from the circulation to the alveoli. (From Ref. 102. Reproduced by permission, CRC Press, Inc.)

The epithelial layer has a thin fluid film that is covered by a monomolecular layer of surfactant. Unlike the endothelium, the epithelial basement membrane is not distinct but is usually observed to be fused into one layer with the epithelial cells. The second layer, the capillary endothelium, with its basement membrane, is separated from the endothelial layer by an interstitial space. The overall thickness of these layers is less than 0.1 μm and in some areas of the respiratory tract is as thin as 0.1 μm. Exposure of the respiratory tract to drugs or xenobiotics can occur by either the airways or the vasculature. Because the venous drainage from the entire body perfuses through the alveolar capillary unit, drugs that are administered at sites other than by direct application to the respiratory tract may still find their way into lung tissue, either by unique lung uptake (endothelial) mechanisms or by designed targeting. In this case of drug delivery by inhalation administration, several factors can affect drug absorption and clearance from the respiratory tract.

The absorption of drug molecules through lung epithelium has received more attention in recent years. The lung is lined by a layer of epithelial cells that extends from the ciliated columnar cells of the conducting airways by an abrupt transition to the flattened cells of the alveolar region. Earlier studies by Schanker et al. [9,10] showed that most xenobiotics are absorbed by passive diffusion at rates that correlate with their apparent partition coefficients at pH. 7.4. Thus, like the gastrointestinal membrane, the endothelial membrane appears to behave like a typical phospholipid membrane. However, poorly lipid-soluble compounds generally diffuse more rapidly than would be expected, suggesting that pulmonary epithelial diffusion may occur through aqueous pores. In addition, certain drugs (e.g., disodium cromoglycate) are known to undergo carrier-mediated transport, which is unique for lung epithelial cells. Pulmonary microvascular endothelial cells form a restrictive barrier to macromolecular flux, even more so than arterial cells. The mechanisms responsible for this intrinsic feature are unknown. However, cAMP improves endothelial barrier function by promoting cell–cell and cell–matrix association [11,12]. Endothelial cells form a semipermeable barrier to fluid and protein transudation in the noninflamed lung that limits accumulation in interstitial spaces [13]. Inflammatory mediators increase pulmonary macrovascular permeability [14,15].

Recently, significant emphasis has been placed on elucidating the cellular and molecular mechanisms governing the pulmonary microvascular endothelial cell response to inflammatory stimuli [16]. Constituent protein flux is greatly attenuated in response to inflammation [17,18]. This enhancement in barrier property is associated with increased expression of focal adhesion complexes that promote cell–cell contact [19–21]. Increases in cAMP may account for enhanced barrier properties of pulmonary endothelial cells, since elevating cAMP may reduce inflammation permeability by promoting cell–cell contact. When an aerosolized drug is administered to the respiratory tract, it must cross the epithelial cell barrier to enter either the lung tissue (topical effect) or the circulation (systemic effect). The pulmonary epithelium has a high resistance to the movement of water and lipid-insoluble compounds, which usually diffuse through the tissue very slowly, either by a vesicular mechanism or by leaks in the intercellular tight junctions. The characteristic feature of this type of junction bestows on the epithelium a 10-fold greater resistance to the permeation by hydrophilic probe molecules than that of the pulmonary vascular endothelium. For the delivery of macromolecules, such as peptides and oligonucleotides, an understanding of these mechanisms of epithelial transport is crucial.

Enhancement of drug uptake by altered junctional (paracellular) or vesicular (transcellular) transport (Fig. 2) is an active area of research [22,23]. The paracellular transport mechanism provides an explanation for the pulmonary absorption of peptides and proteins ≤ 40 kDa.

The pore radius of paracellular channels between epithelial cells is about 1 nm, which is a quarter of the pore radius found between the adjacent endothelial cells. Thus, macromolecules which molecular radii greater than 2 nm are completely excluded from paracellular transport (e.g., horseradish peroxidase, MW 40,000; molecular radius > 3 nm). This implies that the main mechanism of transport of large particles across normal pulmonary epithelium is either by endocytosis by the epithelium itself or by phagocytosis and subsequent penetration of the epithelium. Of note, the epithelial tight junction is characterized by a network of sealing strands made up of a row of protein molecules on each adjacent cell wall; these molecules interlock like a zipper. The greater the number of strands, the more impermeable is the junction. However, it is hypothesized that the intercellular strands can reversibly "unzip" to permit lymphocytes, phagocytic macrophages, and polymorphonuclear leukocytes to enter or leave the airspace. Tight junction structure and function is now a very

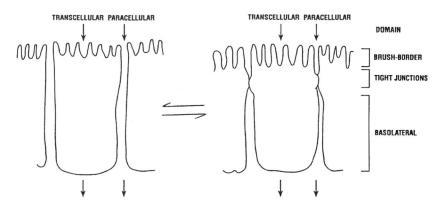

FIGURE 2   Transcellular and paracellular transport pathways across lung epithelial cells.

active area of research. They used to be thought of as simple cell adhesions composed of lipid structures [24]; however, it is now known that these junctions consist of a complex structure of multiple proteins that serves as a dynamic mechanism for the fastening of cells to each other. In fact, there are around 60 miles of cell junction in human airways and over 2000 miles in the alveolar region. The pulmonary endothelial cell barrier is relatively permeable to macromolecules as compared to the epithelium.

Vesicular transport (endocytosis) of drugs may well depend on molecular structure and size. In this respect, the ionic structure of the pulmonary membrane may be an important factor to consider. The predominance of negative charge in the basement membrane structure and the interstitia of the lung [25] will no doubt influence the rate of transport of charged molecules by dipolar interactions. It has been observed that pulmonary absorption of similarly macromolecular fluorophore-labeled poly(hydroxyethylaspartamide) derivatives, either neutral or positively or negatively charged, occurs via both carrier-mediated and diffusive mechanisms. The highest rate of absorption was observed with the polyanionic derivative [26]. A study has also shown that pulmonary absorption of some peptidase-resistant polypeptides [poly-(2-hydroxyethy l)-aspartamides] administered intratracheally to the airways in isolated rat lung is molecular weight dependent [27]. Approximately 70% absorption of a 0.2-mg dose of a 3.98-kDa polymer occurred in 100 minutes, whereas for larger polymers the absorption rates appeared to be slower and suggested a molecular weight cutoff point between 4 and 7 kDa. Nevertheless, according to the investigators, the results strongly suggest that systemic protein and peptide delivery by aerosol is feasible because even the largest polymers (11.65 kDa) were absorbed at finite rates. Intratracheally administered cytochalasin D and calcium ions are known to alter junctional transport by disruption of parts of the cytoskeleton that are attached to tight junctions. Airway epithelium appears to actively secrete chloride ions coupled with sodium ion; the exact organization of these ion pumps remains to be established, but they appear to be dependent on intracellular levels of cyclic adenosine monophosphate (cAMP). In this respect, target receptors on epithelial cell membrane surfaces may be exploitable in the development of bioadhesive carriers conjugated to a drug molecule, resulting in selective binding and rapid internalization. In addition, the observed specific uptake of certain drugs into pulmonary tissue is an intriguing area of study, particularly as it relates to the development of lung-targeting strategies. Both of these approaches to pulmonary targeting of drugs are discussed in later sections of this chapter.

A final, and not insignificant, consideration is the problem of drug metabolism in the respiratory tract. Although a large body of data indicates that pulmonary metabolism is generally relatively lower than hepatic metabolism [28], it is clear that nearly all of the drug metabolism activities found in the liver are present in the respiratory tract [1,25]. In addition, some respiratory tissues contain enzyme activities much higher than corresponding activities found in the liver [29]. Metabolism of drugs in respiratory tract tissue will most likely lead to the formation of more than one metabolite because of the variety of enzymes and their differential location throughout the respiratory tract. The metabolic profile of a particular drug will depend on a number of factors, which include ease of access of the drug to the enzyme active site, availability of cofactors, V_{max} and K_m of the enzyme(s), and possible competition at the active site with other exogenous or possible endogenous substrates and inhibitors, inducers, activators, and so on. Other factors are cell type, age, and health. A recent review addressed the localization of drug-metabolizing enzymes in the respiratory tract [1]. Although pulmonary metabolism may be seen as a disadvantage, particularly in the case of peptides and proteins, because of the wide variety of peptidases and proteinases found in respiratory tract tissues, pulmonary activation of drugs by site-specific metabolism of a prodrug form is a possible way to increase selectivity and duration of action. For example, the bronchodilator bitolterol is converted into its active metabolite by hydrolysis in the respiratory tract (see the section on prodrug approaches), and the antitumor drug hexamethylmelamine owes its activity to pulmonary activation by N-demethylation [30].

Because the main goal of drug delivery is to direct the drug to the target receptors while minimizing interactions with other possible sites of action, the question of receptor specificity is of primary importance in drug design. Although other factors that may affect receptor targeting, such as rate of delivery regional distribution and pharmacodynamics, are of significance, this chapter focuses on structure–activity considerations associated with receptor targeting in the lung.

RECENT ADVANCES IN THE DESIGN OF DRUG MOLECULES FOR PULMONARY RECEPTOR TARGETING

The use of inhalation therapy has been applied mainly to the treatment of asthma and bronchitis. There is an increasing awareness that current treatment is inadequate and that the incidence of asthma is on the rise [31]. Indeed, it has been shown that an apparent increase in the prevalence of asthma at childhood has occurred in recent years [32]. Of particular recent interest is the structure–activity relationships associated with drug residence times in the respiratory tract.

β_2-Adrenoceptor Agonists

Drugs acting at β-adrenoceptors are the most common group of agents used in the treatment of asthma and other related respiratory diseases. Although several drugs in this group, such as isoproterenol and salbutamol, have been used for many years in the symptomatic treatment of bronchospasms, recent research has focused on the use of β_2-adrenergic stimulants as prophylactic drugs because of their ability to inhibit the release of spasmogens and inflammagens from human mast cells; in fact, short-acting β_2-agonists represent an important treatment for the relief of asthma symptoms [33]. Furthermore, asthmatics patients are known to have greater response to bronchodilators than do patients of chronic obstructive pulmonary disease [34].

Early structure–activity studies designed to provide selective β_2-receptor drug–binding clearly established the value of N-substitution for enhancing the β_2 selectivity of norepinephrine analogues [35], and subsequent work also highlighted the importance of uptake mechanisms and biotransformation by catechol-o-methyltransferase (COMT) in the metabolic inactivation of both natural and synthetic catecholamines [36]. These advances have led to the development of potent, β_2 selective bronchodilators, which, when administered by inhalation aerosols, are practically devoid of any major side effects. However, it is generally accepted that aerosol administration of such drugs generally leads to deposition at sites other than the target receptors. In addition, it may be appropriate, for example, in the case of an acute asthmatic attack to attain a rapid, prolonged, and effective concentration of the drug at the desired receptor site. Unfortunately, in this respect, relatively little progress has been made in establishing the regional distribution of β_2-receptors in the lung. Autoradiographic studies in human lung [37] indicated that β_2-receptors are located in smooth muscle from the large and small airways, with a greater population in bronchioli than in bronchi. High densities of receptors were also observed in airway epithelial cells and in bronchial submucosal glands, from the large bronchi to the terminal bronchioli. β_2-receptors appear to be most highly concentrated in the alveolar wall; however, the physiological role of such receptors is not clear.

Recent examples of drugs that exhibit improved affinity for exoreceptor binding in the lung have been reported. The drug salmeterol (**6**) was developed from molecular modification of salbutamol (**4**) [38], and represents a β_2-receptor stimulant with high exoreceptor affinity in order to persist in the vicinity of the β_2-receptors in the respiratory tract. Salmeterol given by inhalation has a markedly prolonged bronchodilatory effect compared to salbutamol, exhibiting sustained bronchodilation over a 12-hour period, with no tachyphylaxis after nine days of treatment [39].

1

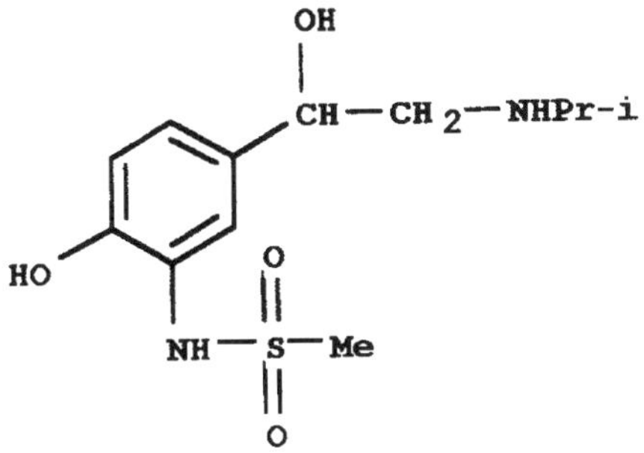

2

Both salmeterol and formoterol (**7**) agonists are structurally related to salbutamol, in that they have an aromatic moiety replacing the catechol group but that is resistant to metabolism by catechol-O-methyl transferase. However, in place of the *N*-isopropyl group, these compounds bear a large lipophilic N-substituent that appears to be responsible for the high affinity in lung and prolonged duration of action of these drugs [40]. Whether this is due to improved receptor-binding characteristics or is the result of a selective uptake mechanism by lung tissue is open to question. This issue is dealt with in detail in the section on structural factors. The drug formoterol, when given by inhalation, is 10 times more potent than salbutamol and produces clinically significant bronchodilation for 8 hours when administered at a dose of 6 µg [41]. In an attempt to obtain optimal control of asthma, a combination therapy of an inhaled long-acting β_2-agonist and an inhaled corticosteroid (i.e., salmeterol/fluticasone and formoterol/budesonide) has been utilized, where the corticosteroids suppresses chronic inflammation of asthma while the β_2-agonist induces bronchodilation and inhibits mast cell mediator release. Furthermore, it has been found that there are more positive interactions between both drug types. Corticosteroids increase the expression of β_2-receptors by increasing gene transcription, while β_2-agonists may potentiate the molecular mechanism associated with corticosteroid action, leading to an additive or sometimes synergistic suppression of inflammatory mediator release [42].

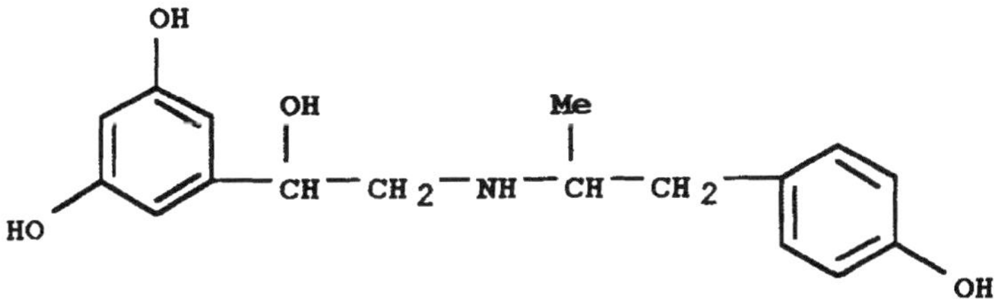

3

Chiarino et al. [43] described some potent and remarkably selective β_2-adrenoceptor agonists in a series of 1-(3-substituted-5-isoxazolyi)-2-alkyl-aminoethanol derivatives in which the isoxazole ring replaces the catechol moiety in the β-adrenergic compounds. From this series, the compound broxaterol (**1**) displayed a marked selectivity toward β_2-receptors of the trachea and was selected for further development as a potential bronchodilatory agent.

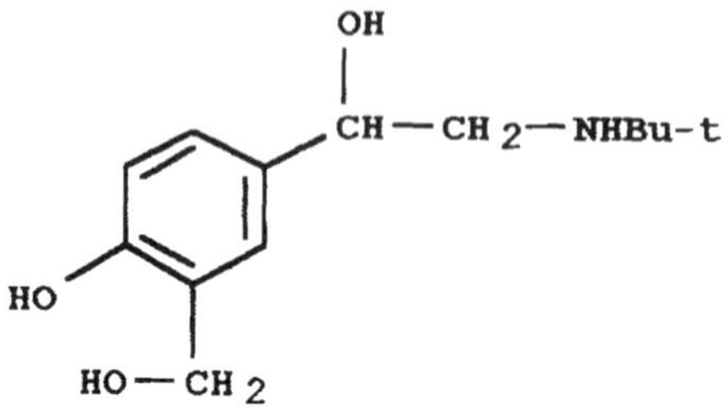

4

It is important to point out that a selective response in vivo does not always reflect selectivity at the receptor level but may depend on organ selectivity. This is particularly true for partial agonists of low intrinsic efficacy, which may exhibit receptor-selective activity in a tissue containing a large receptor pool or may operate the receptor–effector coupling system more efficiently.

β_2-Receptor agonists such as soterenol (**2**), fenoterol (**3**), and salbutamol (**4**) bind with approximately equal affinity to both β_1- and β_2-receptors but apparently owe their selectivity to greater efficacy at the latter receptor [44], whereas other agonists, such as procaterol (**5**), show greater affinity for β_2-receptors [45]. In fact, procaterol is one of the most selective β_2-adrenoceptor drugs known today.

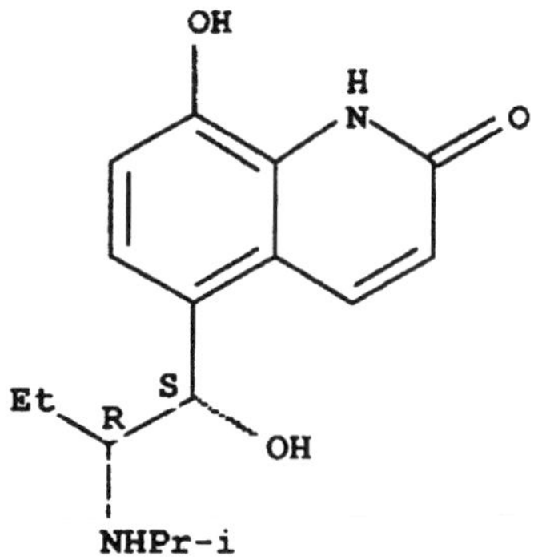

5

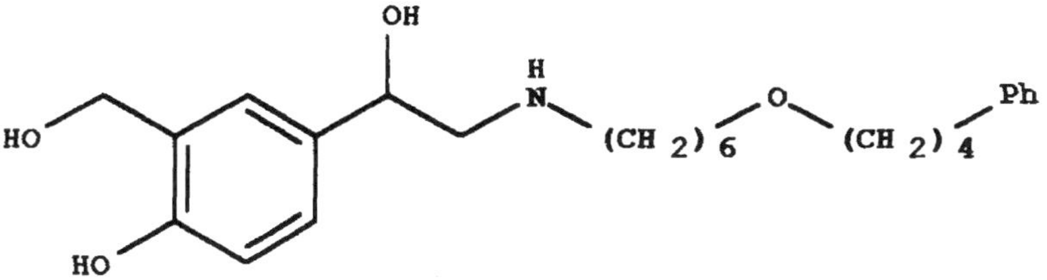

6

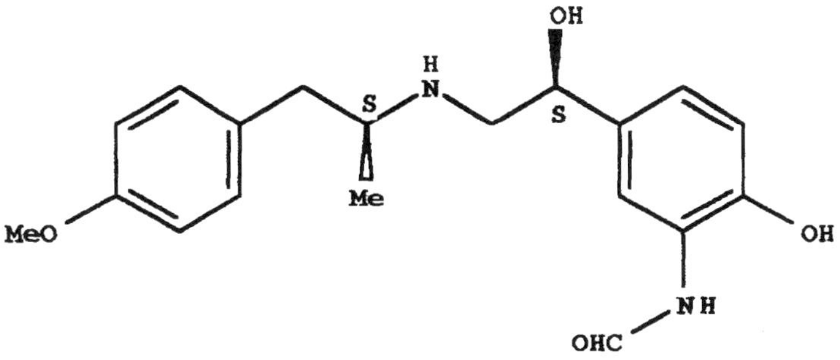

7

There still appears to be a need to further improve the design of β_2-receptor stimulant drugs. Factors such as receptor selectivity, metabolic stability, and structural manipulation to prolong action are actively being investigated. Whether selectivity can ever be achieved is questionable, because skeletal muscle tremor in humans is β_2-receptor mediated [46], and the tachycardia exhibited by bronchodilator drugs appears to be mediated directly and indirectly through β_2-receptors [47]. When given by the inhalation route, the absorption characteristics of β_2-adrenoceptor stimulant drugs may well determine their duration of action; thus, a better understanding of the factors governing drug clearance from the respiratory tract after inhalation delivery is needed.

Another area for improvement is in the relative efficacy of β_2-bronchodilators. Compounds with low efficacy may be effective at low levels of bronchoconstriction. But as the severity of bronchoconstriction increases, such compounds will become partial agonists before those of greater efficacy. Therefore, the relative efficacies of new compounds should be considered in drug development decisions.

Antihistamines

H_1-Receptor agonists are gaining renewed interest as potential antiasthmatic drugs. Such compounds, when given in adequate dosage, not only protect significantly against antigen and exercise-induced asthma but also produce bronchodilation comparable with that seen after inhaled isoproterenol and salbutamol. As in the case of bronchodilator receptors, few attempts have been made to determine the distribution of histamine receptors in the human respiratory tract. It is well known that histamine is used in tests of bronchial reactivity. Histamine receptors are generally thought to reside in the large airways because centrally deposited aerosolized histamine results in significant histamine receptor-mediated responses. However, Ryan et al. [48] have not confirmed this, although it is not known whether adequate differences between peripherally and centrally deposited aerosols was achieved in their studies. Previously, the drawback to using the antihistamines included their marked individual variation in response between patients, specificity of histamine receptor antagonism, and dose and route given. More importantly, the H_1-receptor antagonists were unsuitable for diurnal use because of their marked sedation as a consequence of central nervous system (CNS) uptake. Advances in this drug discovery area [49] have included the development of H_1 antagonists with no H_2-, α-, β-receptor activity, no demonstrable anticholinergic and anti-5-hydroxytryptamine activity, and no ability to cross the blood–brain barrier. The prototype drug terfenadine (**8**) represents the first example of this new class of nonsedating antihistamine possessing the previously mentioned characteristics and exhibits no significant sedation in dosages up to 200 mg three times daily [50]. Terfenadine and the related drug astemizole (**9**) represent the only two drugs of this class marketed in the United States.

8

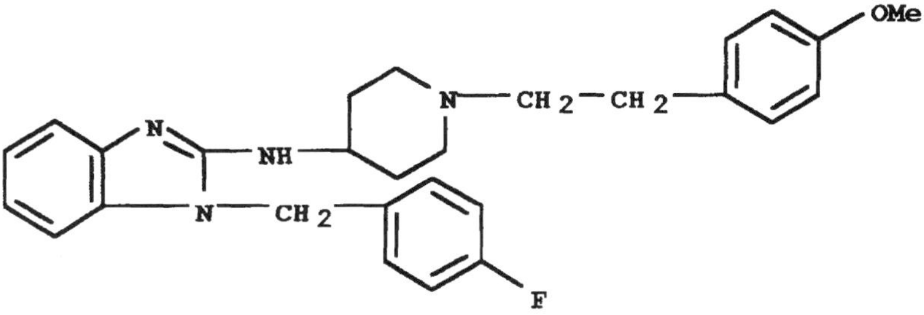

9

Structural modification of the antihistamine azatadine (**10a**) by replacing the N-methyl group with various carbamate groups eliminates CNS activity [51]. Loratidine (**10b**), the most potent compound in this series of carbamates, shows no sedation liability in experimental animals, binds selectively to peripheral histamine receptors [52], and appears likely to be approved by the NDA in the near future. Other nonsedatory H_1 antihistamines that have been reported recently are temelastine (**11**), tazifylline (**12**), cetrizine (**13**), levocabastine (**14**), and epinastine (**15**) [53–57]. Tazifylline is reported to have 10 times the bronchodilator activity exhibited by either asternizole or terfenadine. The recent preclinical pharmacology of AHR-I 1325 (**16**) and PR 1036-654 (**17**) suggests that both these new compounds are potent, nonsedating, long-acting H_1 antagonists [58,59]. Ebastine (**18a**), a structural analogue of terfenadine, has been reported to be a potent, selective, long-lasting antihistamine devoid of sedation at an oral dose of 10 mg [60]. Its mode of action is thought to be due to metabolism to the active form (**18b**) [61].

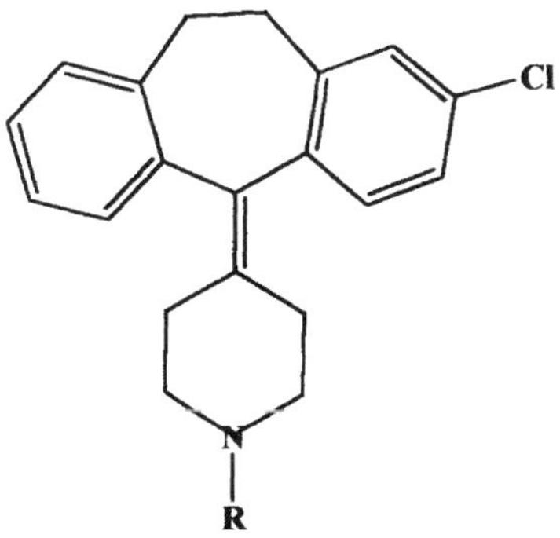

a : R=CH₃
b : R = CO₂CH₂CH₃

10

11

12

13

14

15

16

17

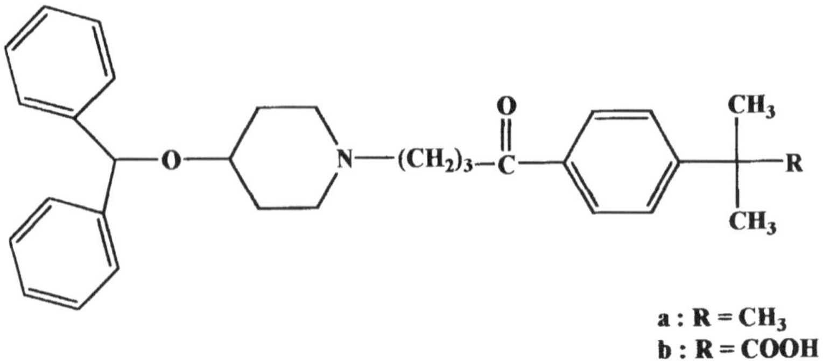

a : R = CH$_3$
b : R = COOH

18

It is clear that these new agents will most likely benefit from being delivered locally into the respiratory tract in therapeutic concentrations that can avoid undesirable systemic side effects.

Anticholinergics

The lung expresses at least three subtypes of muscarinic acetylcholine receptor. M1 receptors are located primarily in the parasympathetic ganglia, where their activation facilitates transmission through the ganglia, whereas M2 receptors are found on presynaptic cholinergic nerve terminals and function to inhibit acetylchdine release, and M3 receptors are present on the smooth muscle and elicit contraction [62]. Although anticholinergic drugs have had a long history of use in the treatment of asthma, the development of a successful antiasthmatic drug in this case has been slow. The major obstacle has been the lack of availability of compounds that produce optimal bronchodilation without accompanying side effects. Two drugs of this class, ipratropium bromide (**19**) and oxitropium bromide (**20**), which are structural analogues of atropine (**21**), have been studied extensively as alternatives to β$_2$ stimulant drugs [63–65]. Although the distribution of cholinergic receptors in the human respiratory tract is not well understood, these quarternary drugs appear to exert their bronchodilatory activity mainly on the large airways, in contrast to β-andrenoceptor agonists, and probably produce bronchodilation by competitive inhibition of cholinergic receptors on bronchial smooth muscle, by antagonizing the action of acetylcholine at its membrane-bound receptor site. Thus, they block the bronchoconstrictor action of vagal efferent impulses; lung irritant receptors provide the chief efferent input for this vagal reflex. Because **19** and **20** are water-soluble quarternary ammonium derivatives, they lack the CNS stimulatory properties of atropine (**21**).

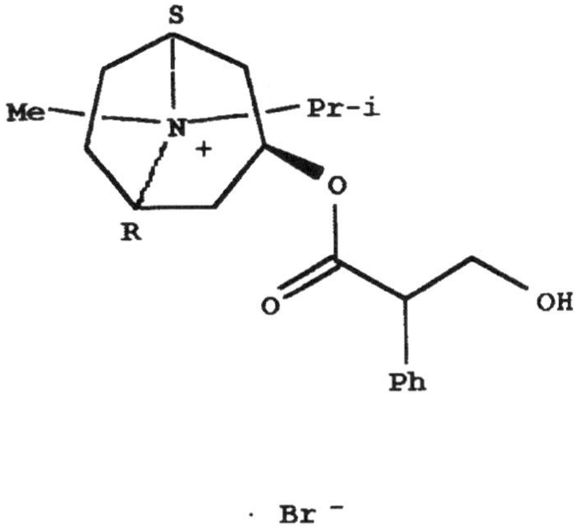

· Br⁻

19

· Br⁻

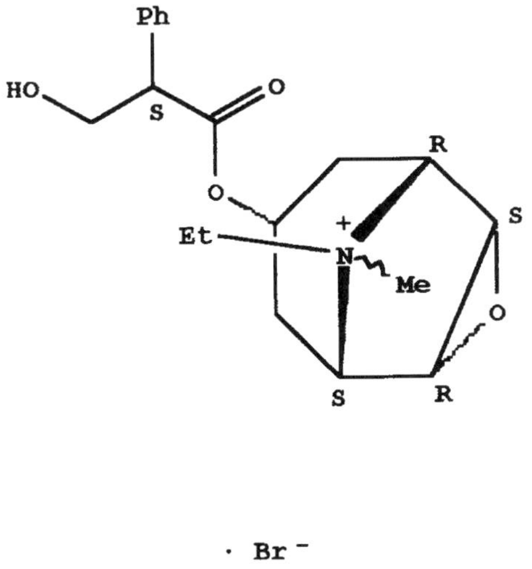

20

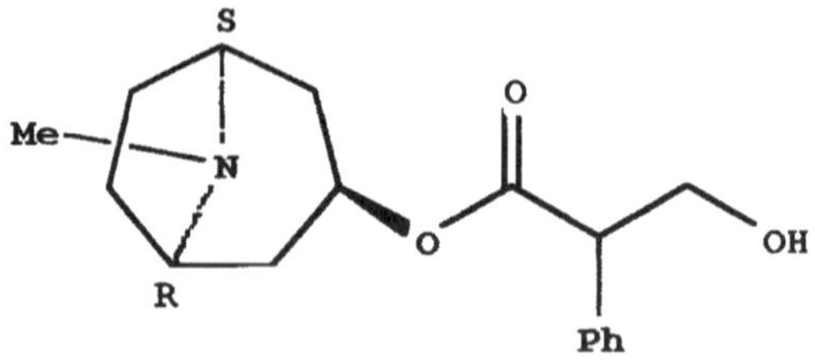

21

When given by inhalation, ipratropium bromide and oxitropium bromide are slower acting than β_2-receptor stimulants but have a longer duration of action [66,67]. Both drugs are considerably more bronchoselective than atropine when given by inhalation and exhibit significantly less systemic anticholinergic side effects.

There is significant interest in identifying and developing either longer-acting, more potent nonselective muscarrinic receptor antagonists than ipratropium, such as tiotropium (**22**) and oxitrope (**23**), or more subtype-selective muscarinic receptor antagonists, such as darifenacin and revatropate (**24**). Revatropate is an M1/M3 receptor-selective muscarininc antagonist with about 50-fold lower potency against M2 receptors. In animal models, revatropate (**24**) inhibited acetylcholine-induced bronchoconstriction but, unlike ipratropium, did not potentiate vagally induced bronchoconstriction [68,69].

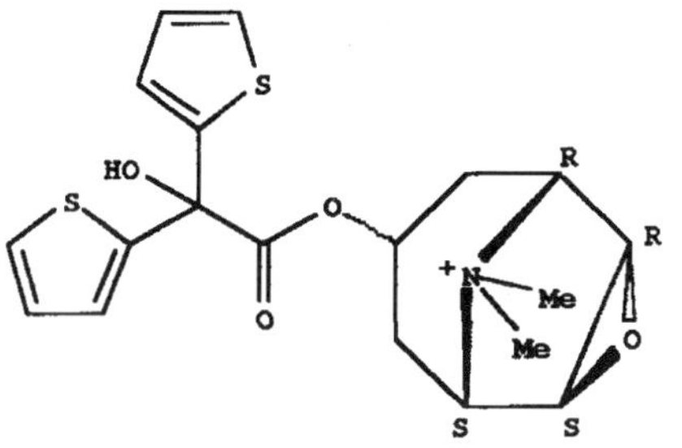

22

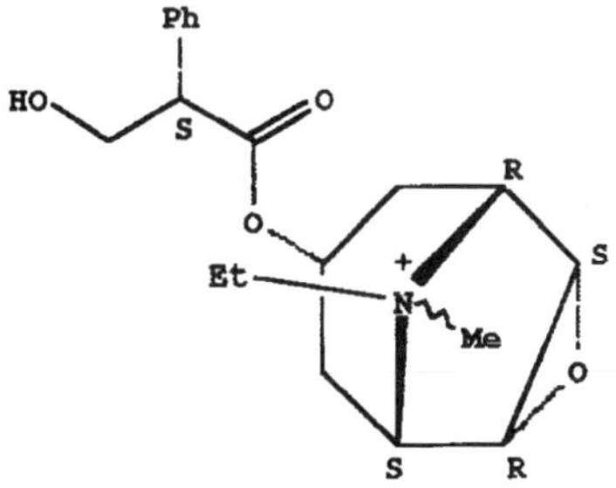

23

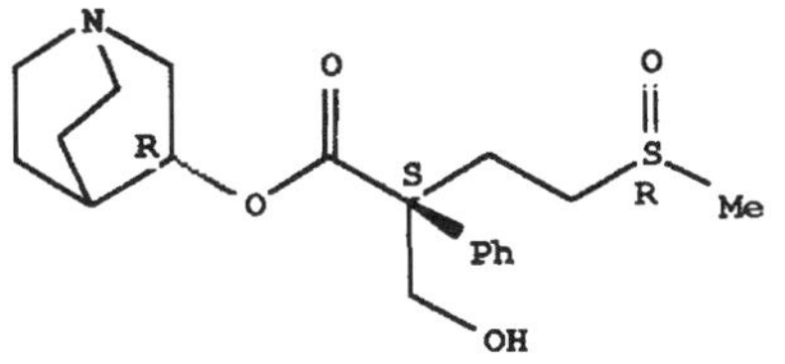

24

Glucocorticoids (GC)

Current effective therapies for asthma have focused on treating the symptoms of the disease. Asthma is characterized by inflammation of the lung; thus, the most prescribed agents to date are the glucocorticoids (GC), due to their widespread anti-inflammatory properties [70–72]. The glucocorticoid drugs budesonide (**25**), beclomethasone dipropionate (**26**), and triamcinolone (**27**) have long been employed for use in treating asthma.

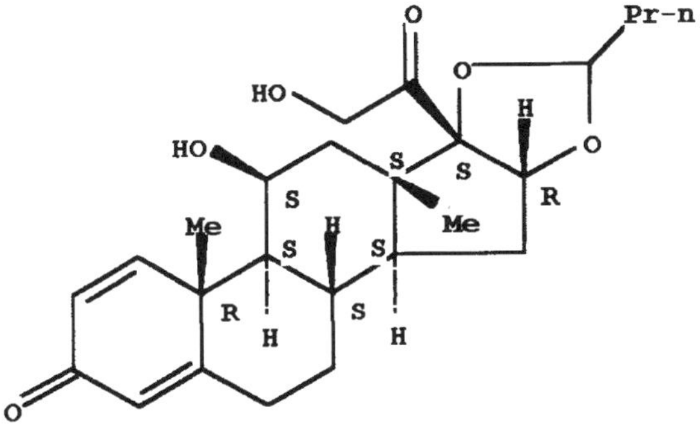

25

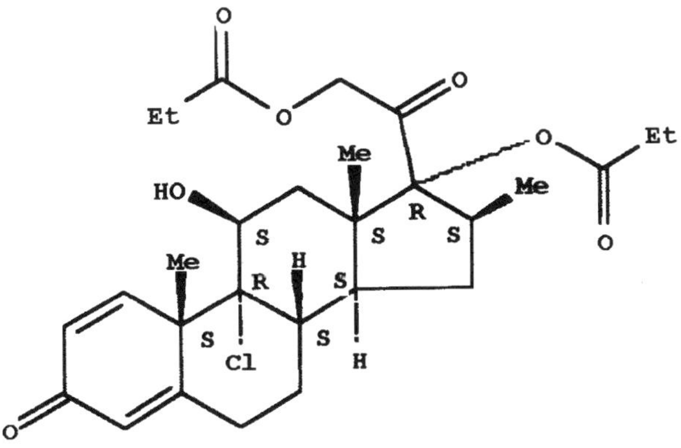

26

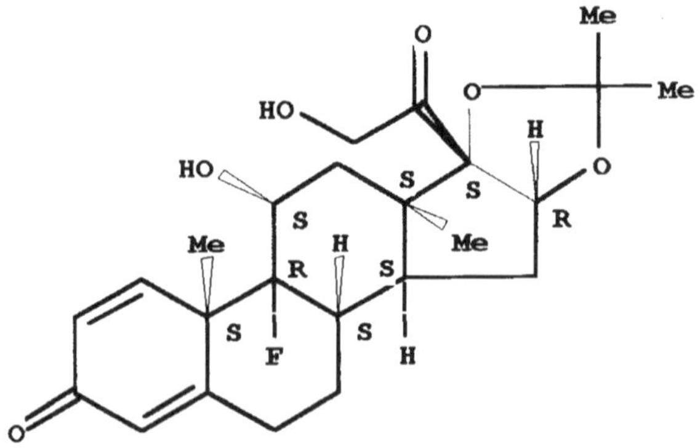

27

Fluticasone propionale (**28**) is a more recent addition, and mometasone furoate (**29**), which is currently under review by regulatory authorities worldwide, has recently been formulated for use in asthma [73]. Many of the adverse effects of elevated systemic glucocorticoid levels have been reduced through the use of inhalation as a method of drug delivery [74]. Inhalation therapy targets the local affected area, where it maximizes local efficacy while reducing systemic bioavailability. Therefore, at therapeutic doses of inhaled glucocorticoids, the risk of systemic effect is considerably reduced when compared to oral glucocorticoid therapy. Mometasone furoate (**29**) is a synthetic glucocorticoid that is structurally similar to the adrenocorticosteroids and prednisolone. The structure was designed to optimize potency; the furoate group at position C17 greatly increases lipid solubility, while the 21-chloromoiety is important for maximum potency and topical activity [75].

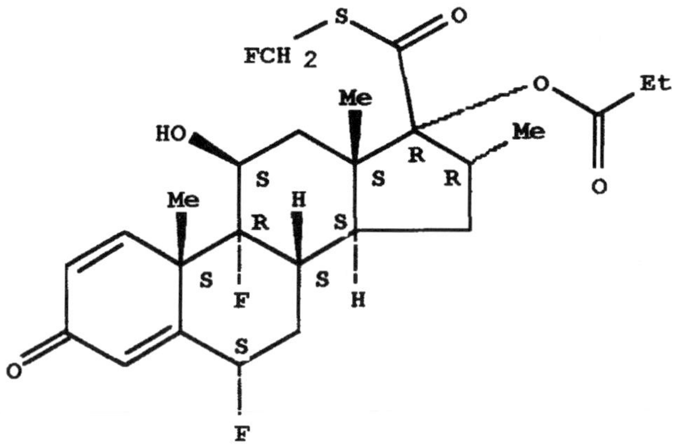

28

29

Recent studies have shown that intact budesonide (**25**) after inhalation binds primarily to available steroid receptors, and mainly excess unbound budesonide is esterified [76,77]. Esterification of budesonide is a rapid process. Thus, in the rat, within 20 minutes of inhalation of radiolabeled budesonide, approximately 80% of the radioactivity within the trachea and main bronchi was associated with budesonide esters, primarily budesonide oleate [78]. The efficacy of topical glucocorticoids in rhinitis and asthma is likely to depend on drug retention in the airway mucosa. With fluticasone propionate (**28**), retention may be achieved exclusively by its inherent lipophilicity, whereas for budesonide an additional possibility may be provided by its ability to form fatty acid esters in the airway mucosa that release the active drug [79]. Recent studies have investigated the role of inhaled corticosteroids in the long-term management of chronic obstructive pulmonary disease (COPD) [80,81]. This disease is characterized by the presence of airflow obstruction due to chronic bronchities or emphysema; in this respect, the airflow obstruction may be partially reversible, in contrast with asthma, which is largely a reversible disease. Although inflammation seems to be present in the airway of patients with COPD, the specific immunopathology is thought to be different from that of asthma [82]. There is conflicting information on the ability of glucocorticoids to modulate the progression of COPD [83]. Short-term treatment with both inhaled and systemic glucocorticoids may have beneficial effects on symptoms and lung function in subgroups of COPD patients, in particular those with partially reversible airways obstruction [84].

Glucocorticoid mimics the action of the endogenous hormones (i.e., Cortisol) that are involved in the regulation of the inflammatory response in the airway. The sequence of events in glucocorticoid action begins when this lipophilic corticosteroid molecule crosses the cell membrane and binds to the intracellular GR receptor that is located in the cytoplasm. Glucocorticoids bind to GR receptor with different affinities, for example, triamcinolone acetonide (**27**), budesonide (**25**), and dexamethasone are 10–90-fold less potent than mometasone furoate in activating transcription [74,85]. Thus, large differences in potency between GC can be observed in in vitro systems.

Combinations of medications has been common practice for the treatment of COPD. There is evidence of increased efficacy of combinations of the β-adrenoceptors agonists and cholinergic receptor antagonists. Such combined therapy has recently been introduced, e.g., Combivent®, which is an aerosol formulation of the β-adrenoceptor agonist, salbutamol, and ipratropium [86].

Regulators of Lipid Mediators
Leukotrienes

This area of drug discovery has seen intense activity, and several orally active leukotriene (LT) antagonists have been clinically evaluated. A number of first-generation LTD_4 antagonists were found to have an activity that was too weak to be effective in asthmatics [87]. Clinical studies showed that ICI 204,219 (**30**) when given orally, could reduce antigen-induced bronchoconstriction in asthmatic patients [88]. ICI 204,219 was reported to be a selective, competitive antagonist of LTD_4-induced contractions of isolated human bronchioli and was effective in reversing LTD_4-induced bronchoconstriction in a dose-dependent manner in guinea pigs by both oral and aerosol routes [89]. The styryl quinoliness (**31a–31c**) are another LTD_4-receptor antagonist with good potential as antiasthmatic [90]. One of these, MK-571, is a recemic compound that has been evaluated as an inhibitor of LTD_4-induced bronchoconstriction following intravenous administration to healthy volunteers and patients [91]. Development of the R-isomer of MK-679, which was selected for clinical evaluation based on preclinical in vitro and in vivo pharmacology, has been terminated due to poor tolerance. Compound RG 12525 (**32**), when dosed orally to mild asthmatics, was found to cause a 7.5-fold shift in the dose response to inhaled LTD_4 [92].

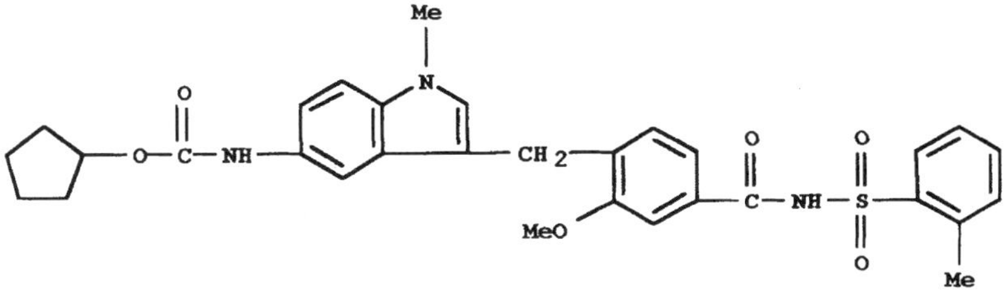

30

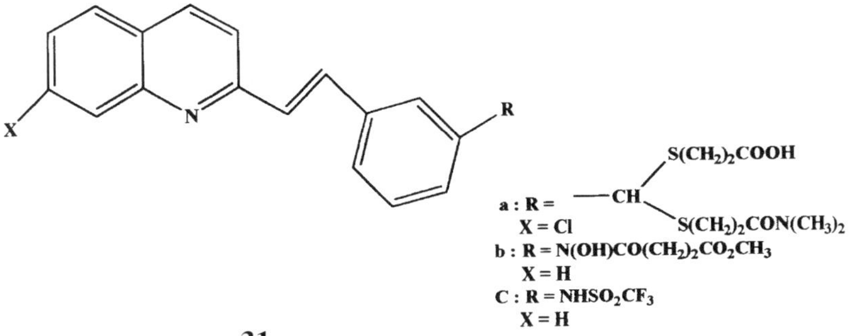

a : R = —CH⟨S(CH₂)₂COOH / S(CH₂)₂CON(CH₃)₂
    X = Cl
b : R = N(OH)CO(CH₂)₂CO₂CH₃
    X = H
C : R = NHSO₂CF₃
    X = H

31

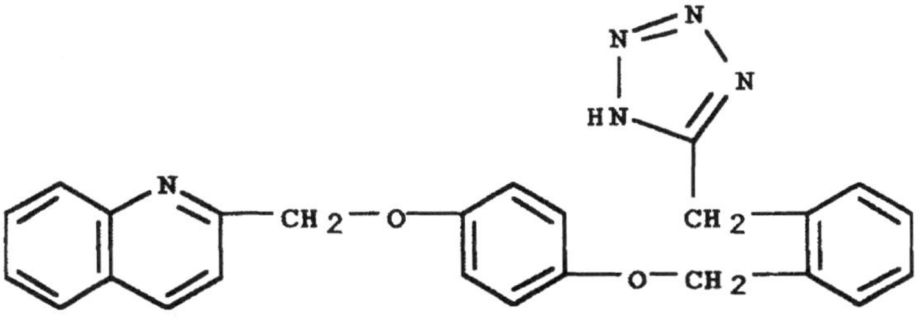

32

The clinical use of LTD$_4$ antagonists is being enthusiastically pursued, although no definitive clinical evidence has been presented that supports a role for the peptide LTs in asthma and allergy. With respect to aerosolized drug studies, SKF 104353-22 (**33**) has been shown to block LTD$_4$- and antigen-induced bronchoconstriction in asthmatics on aerosol administration [93,94]. L-648051 (**34**) represents another aerosol-administered antagonist that has reached the clinic. Relatively large doses ($\sim$ 12 mg) are required to inhibit LTD$_4$ bronchoconstriction [95].

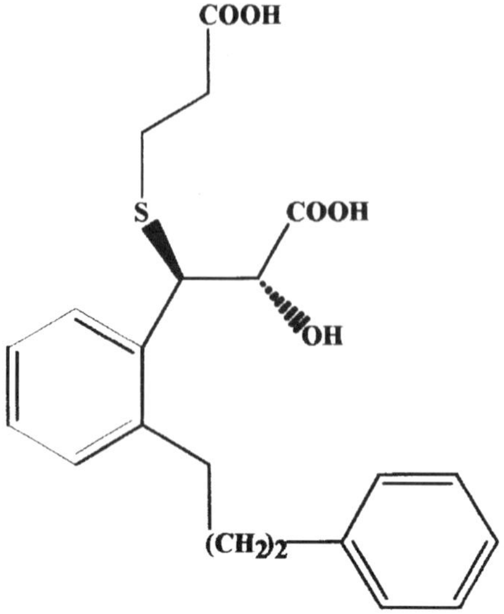

33

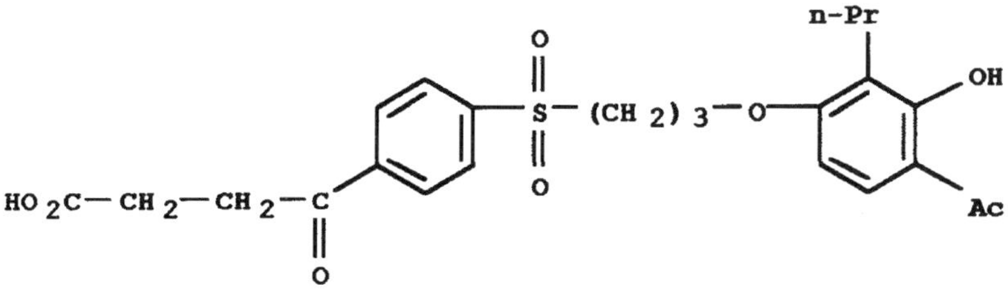

34

5-Lipoxygenase Inhibitors

An interesting correlation between pseudoperoxidase activity and 5-lipoxygenase inhibitory potency has been observed for a series of N-hydroxy ureas, suggesting that the redox properties of this class of drug contribute to their ability to inhibit 5-lipoxygenase [92]. Some compounds has been investigated; the Zileuton (A-64,077) (**35**) shows activity in humans [96]. A series of quinoline-containing inhibitors of LT biosynthesis—WY-49,232 (**36**), L-674,573 (**37**), and REV-5,901 (**38**)—have been found to bind to the 5-lipoxygenose-activating protein (FLAP); their ability to interact with FLAP correlated well with inhibition of LT biosynthesis.

HO
O
N
C
NH 2
CH
Me
S

35

O
CH 2
N
HO 2C
CH
Me

36

N
CH 2
O
CH
(CH 2) 3
Ph
S
CH 2
CO 2 H

37

N
CH 2
O
CH
(CH 2) 4
Me
OH

38

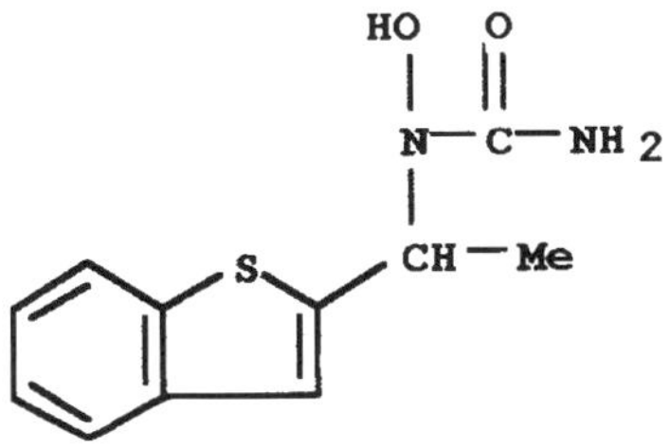

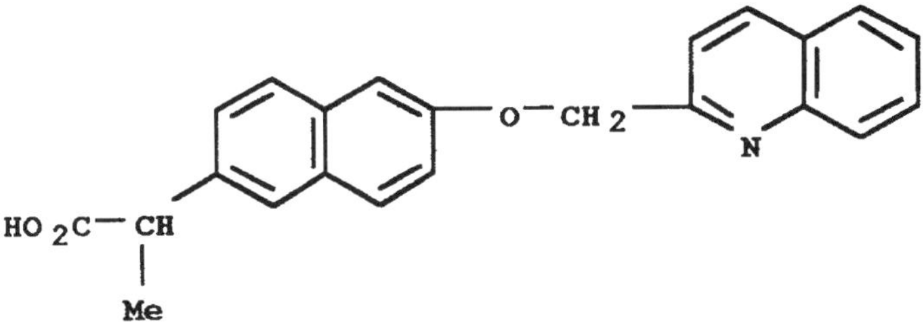

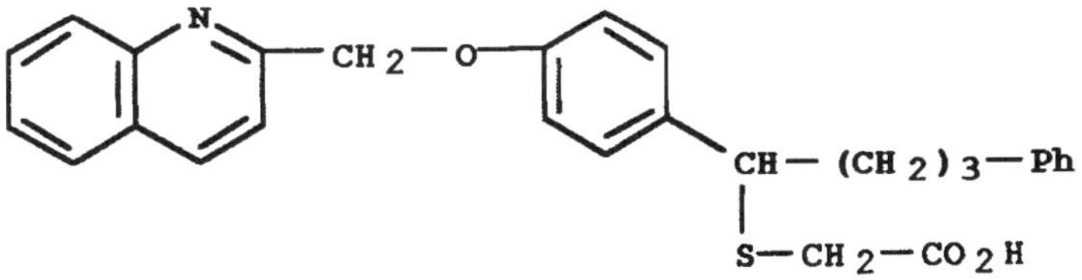

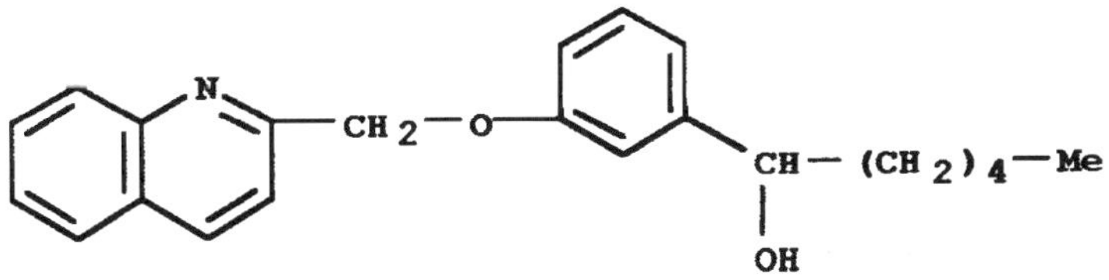

A-69,412 (**39**) was reported to be a potent and selective inhibitor of 5-lipoxygenase with a long duration of action, and 1C1-211,965 (**40**) emerged from a structure–activity relationship study of a (methoxyalkyl) thiazole series designed to inhibit 5-lipoxygenase [97].

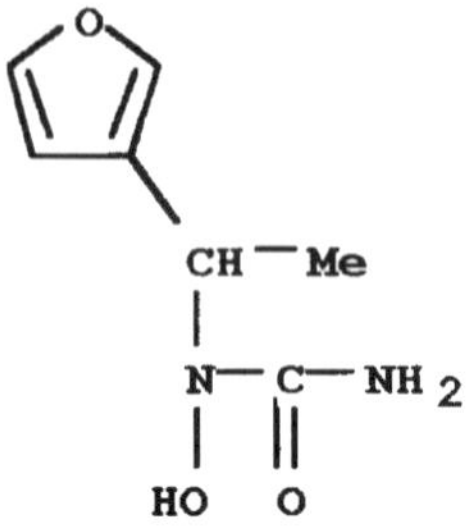

39

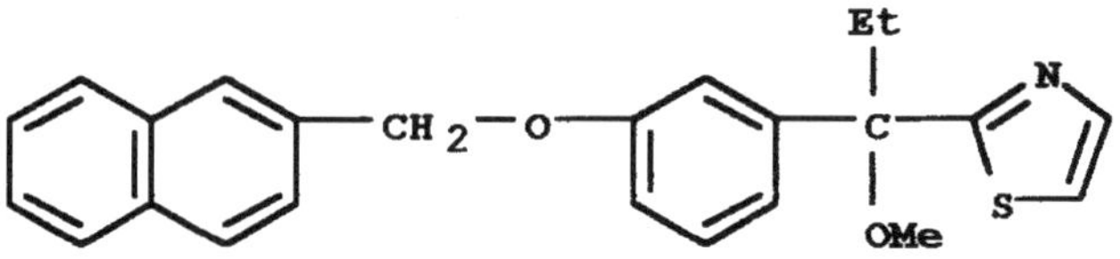

40

Thromboxane-Receptor Antagonists

The role of thermoboxane antagonists is asthma treatment still remains uncertain. AA-2414 (**41**) oral administration to asthmatic subjects favorably attenuated their response to methacholine challenge [98]. Modification of a 7-oxabicyclo heptane of drug candidates by incorporation of a phenylene spacer in the α-chain afforded SQ 35,091 (**42**), which shows longer duration of action ($t_{1/2} = 16\,hr$) [99]. GR 32191 (**43**) shows PGD_2-induced bronchoconstriction in asthmatics at 80 mg PO [100].

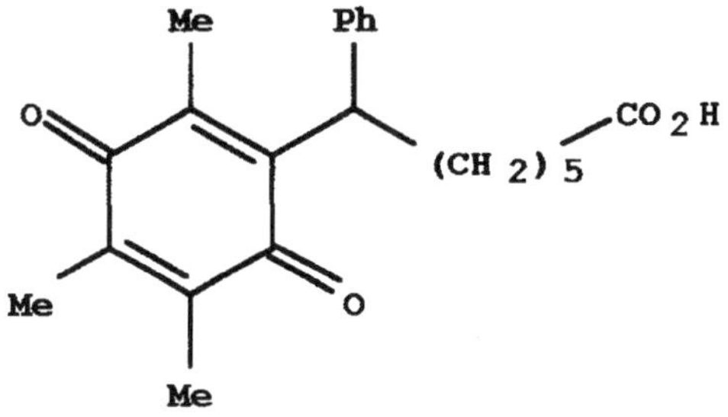

41

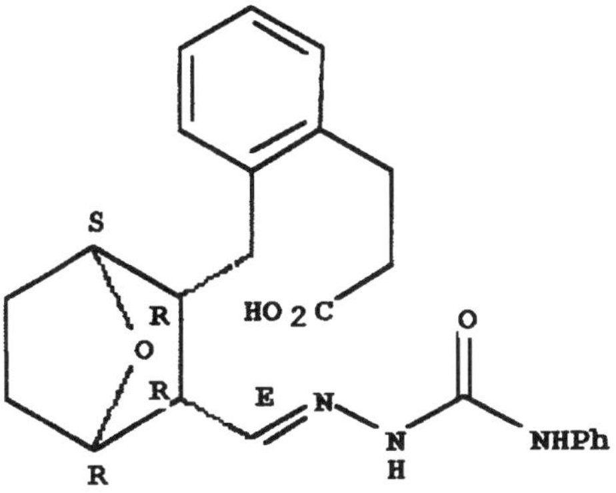

42

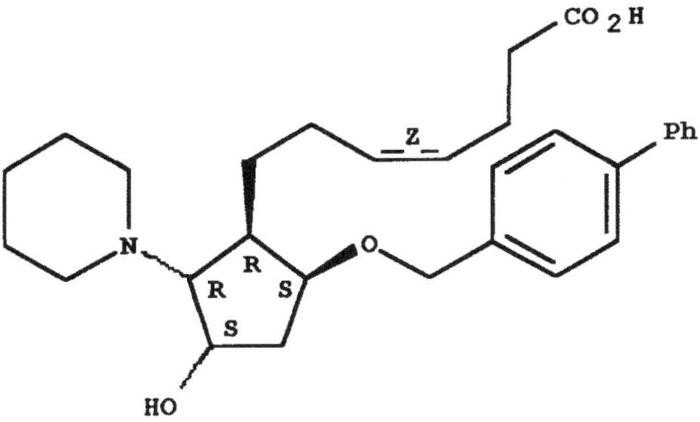

43

Platelet Activating Factor (PAF) Antagonists

These agents may be useful in PAF-induced bronchoconstriction. In the hetrazepine class of PAF antagonist, apafant (WEB-2086) (**44**) has been shown to be rapidly absorbed following oral administration and produced no significant adverse effects [92]. Two other compounds—WEB-2347 (**45**) and E-6123 (**46**)—also from the hetrazepine class, have emerged as orally active derivatives with profiles superior to WEB-2086 (**44**).

44

45

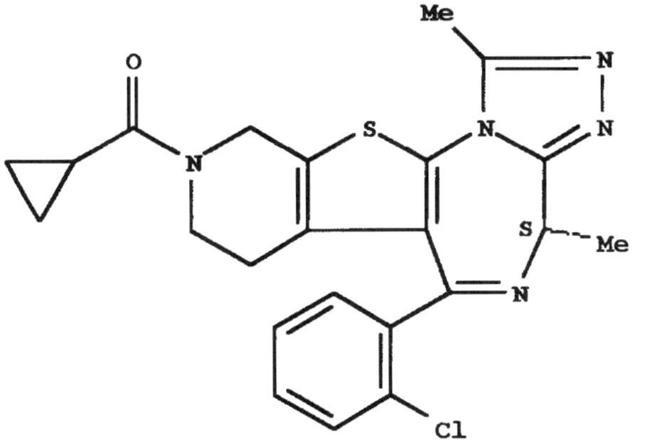

46

Elastase Inhibitors

Strategies for designing inhibitors of human neutrophil elastase (HNE), the enzyme whose unrestrained action may result in the lung damage underlying the development of emphysema, has been under active research. Prolastin, the natural human α_1-antitrypsin that inhibits HNE, was administered by aerosol, with demonstrated effectiveness in restoring the protease–antiprotease balance in genetic emphysema [101,102]. Several other peptide drugs when administered intratrachealy appear to have good residence times in the lung. Intratracheally administered L-6592866 (**47**),

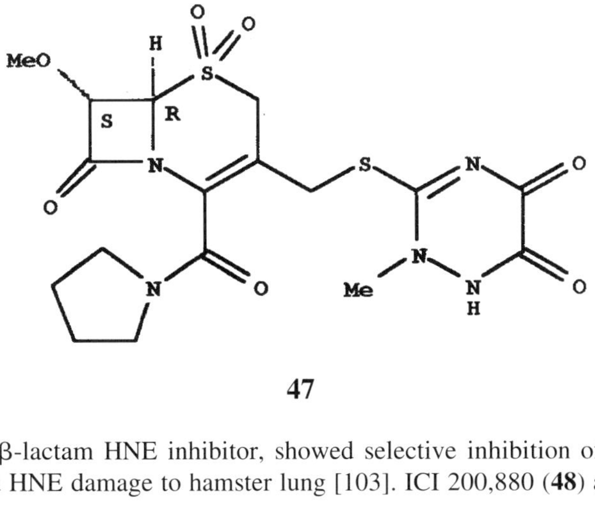

47

a modified β-lactam HNE inhibitor, showed selective inhibition of lung HNE and blocked HNE damage to hamster lung [103]. ICI 200,880 (**48**) also showed a long residency time in the lung and potent HNE inhibition after intratracheal administration [104].

48

SOME STRUCTURAL FACTORS GOVERNING THE UPTAKE OF DRUGS

It has been known for several years that the lung is capable of active uptake of a number of endogenous and exogenous compounds. These include the neurotransmitters norepinephrine and 5-hydroxytryptamine, which are sequestered by lung endothelial cells [105,106], and the lung toxins parquat [107] and 4-ipomeanol [108]. Paraquat is selectively accumulated in type II alveolar cells by an energy-dependent process, whereas the site-specific toxicity of 4-ipomeanol appears to be due to the selective uptake by Clara cells that, because of the presence of cytochrome P-450 PB-B activity, bioactivates the molecule into a toxic species. In the case of the neurotransmitters norepinephrine and 5-hydroxytryptamine, both compounds have been shown to be avidly sequestered by the canine lung; pulmonary extraction percentages after intravenous injection in the nanmolar range into the pulmonary artery amount to 70% and 50%, respectively [106]. Although it is not clear what structure–activity relationships govern the uptake of these compounds into lung endothelia, a possible strategy for lung targeting might be to chemically conjugate a drug molecule with either 5-hydroxytryptamine or norepinephrine or, better still, to conjugate the drug to pharmacologically inactive metabolites or analogues of these neurotransmitters that still retain the selective lung uptake properties. Generally, it is recognized that the lung has a mechanism for the high-affinity uptake of amines that are protonated at physiological PH and that also possess a hydrophilic moiety in their structure. In most cases, such compounds are metabolized by lung tissue and, therefore, do not accumulate. However, a select number of amines of this type that are resistant to lung metabolism have been observed to accumulate in lung tissue for prolonged periods [109–111]. It is important to note that, generally, quarternary ammonium compounds, which are unable to dissociate into an unionized form, are not effectively taken up by lung tissue, although a notable exception is paraquat. Thus, the equilibrium between ionized and unionized drug is important and suggests that the unionized hydrophobic form may be required for transport, whereas the protonated form is necessary for binding to anionic sites in lung tissue. The exact nature of these anionic sites is not known, although they may be negatively charged phospholipid molecules, which are known to exist in high concentrations in lung tissue, Also, the uptake mechanism may involve a mechanism of preferential pH partitioning of the amine species into the lung or the involvement of a lipophilic ion-pair transport process. Several studies showed that lipophilic cationic drugs bound to anionic sites in the lung can be displaced by other lipophilic cationic drugs [112].

The nature of the uptake site, or the involvement of any particular lung cell type in the uptake process, is as yet unknown. It seems possible that drugs conjugated to lipophilic amines of the types described previously can undergo efficient pulmonary targeting. Several amines may be useful in this respect; that is, the compounds chlorphentermine, amiodarone, desethylarniodarone, and desmethylimipramine all exhibit high affinity to lung tissue. Thus, drugs that normally have poor access to the lung may be targeted to this tissue through appropriate chemical combination of an available functional group (i.e., OH or COOH) with the amino function of the carrier molecule (Fig. 3). Of course, the success of this drug design also depends on the ability of lung tissue to release the bound drug from the carrier molecule by some enzymic process; in other words, the approach basically would have to be a targeted prodrug design. Kostenbauder and Sloneker [113] recently investigated the usefulness of chlorphentermine as a carrier for lung targeting by conjugating it to an unspecified pulmonary drug to give a conjugate of general structure **49** (Fig. 4). In this design, the released carrier molecule is anionic and would be predicted to be rapidly washed out of the lung. Isolated, perfused lung experiments indicated that the prodrug was able to displace chlorphentermine from lung-binding sites and that subsequent prodrug hydrolysis occurred with carrier wash out from the lung. However, the in vivo activity of the prodrug could not be evaluated because of its extreme toxicity.

It has been argued that, because many strongly basic lipophilic amines have been found to exhibit high uptake but only very few truly sequester in the lung and exhibit slowly effluxable pools in vivo, prodrug design should focus on simply achieving high concentrations of prodrug in the lung rather than developing conjugates that would establish amine effluxable pools in lung tissue [113]. In this respect, simple alkyl amines, such as octylamine, could be used because these compounds show high affinity for lung tissue, which correlate with their octanol–water partitioning. This approach has the added advantage of keeping conjugate structures as simple as possible to avoid pharmacological problems.

Of interest are the β_2 agonists salmeterol (**1**) and formoterol (**3**), both of which exhibit plasma half-lives similar to that of salbutamol (**2**), although the latter compound has a much shorter duration of action. Thus, in these cases,

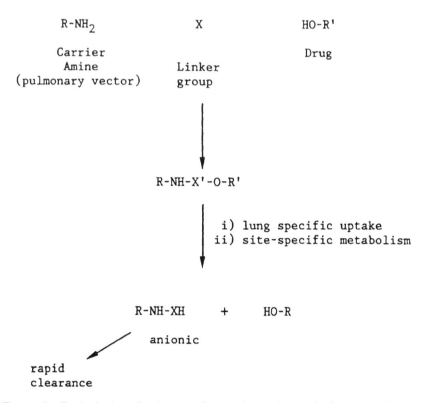

FIGURE 3   Basic design of a drug–amine carrier conjugate for lung targeting.

replacing the *N-t*-butyl group in salbutamol with a highly lipophilic group results in a drug with high affinity for lung tissue and long duration of drug action. It is puzzling, however, that the bronchodilator effects of these drugs are still present even when the drug is no longer detectable or, indeed, even predictable, from elimination half-lives, in plasma [114,115]. This observation may relate to the possible retention in lung of a microfraction of the absorbed dose, presumably in the vicinity of the drug-receptor site.

Salmeterol (**1**) was designed by modifying salbutamol to obtain a drug with much greater affinity for its receptors because of increased "exoreceptor" binding [116] and, consequently, a persistent localization in the vicinity of β_2-receptor. However, there is no evidence for this hypothetical mechanism, and the alternative suggestion that the drug is able to diffuse into the airway epithelium, which then acts as a reservoir for the drug, appears to be a more likely mechanism [117].

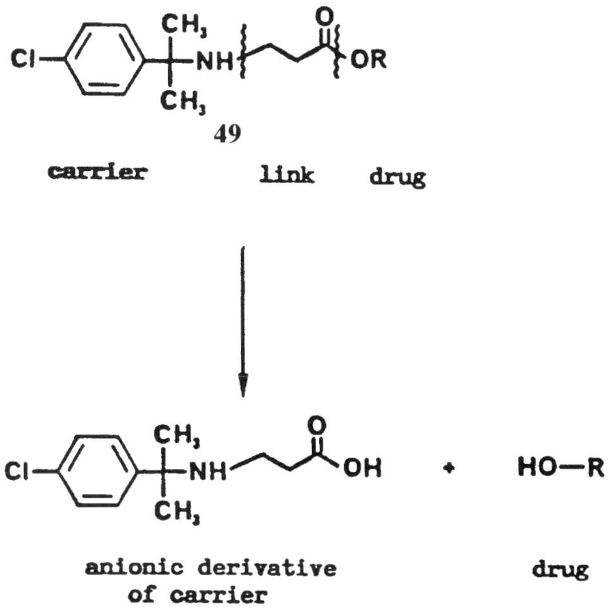

FIGURE 4   Design of chlorphentermine–drug conjugates for lung targeting.

Specific uptake by lung tissue is not restricted to lipophilic amines of the type previously mentioned. Certain antibiotics, such as leucomycin A3, show a high deposition in lung tissue at low concentration of drug [113]. A recent report [118] on erythromycin derivatives, in which the 6, 11, 12 and 4′-hydroxyl groups were totally or partially replaced with O-methyl groups, indicated that these compounds, compared to the parent drug, exhibited a marked increased in lung tissue uptake (four to five times greater) after administration into the external jugular vein of rats (Fig. 5). Of note, erythromycin also has a strongly basic nitrogen. It is interesting that such a significant structural change to the erythromycin molecule does not apparently result in a loss of antimicrobial activity. The tissue levels obtained were in the decreasing order: 6,11,12,4′-OCH$_3$ EM $>$ 6,11,4′-OCH$_3$ EM $>$ 6,4′-OCH$_3$ EM$=$6,11-OCH$_3$ EM$=$6-OCH$_2$CH$_3$EM $>$ 11-OCH$_3$ EM $>$ EM. The most potent antimicrobial derivative was shown to be 6-OCH$_3$ EM. Some derivatives of steroidal drugs also exhibit better uptake in lung tissue than their parent compounds. Budesonide (Fig. 6) is a glucocorticosteroid that has been used in inhalation therapy for several years [119]. It possesses a 16α, 17α acetal group that makes the molecule less polar and confers on the molecule better uptake properties in lung tissue. (Note:

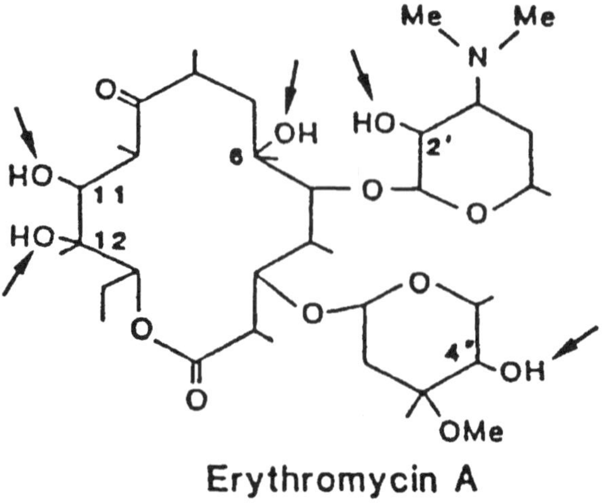

Erythromycin A

FIGURE 5 Erythromycin structure and position of O-methylation for obtaining increased lung uptake.

Budesonide is used as a 1:1 mixture of the 22R- and 22S-epimers.) Budesonide is not metabolized in lung tissue and is slowly released from lung to the systemic circulation. However, it is rapidly metabolized to the 23-hydroxylated 22S-epimer and 16α-hydroxyprednisolone, which is selectively formed from the 22R-epimer. The rapid inactivation of systemic budesonide by the liver minimizes the potential for systemic side effects [120–123]. In isolated lung perfusion studies, a difference in the distribution between lung tissue and perfusion medium for the two epimers of budesonide was found. Interestingly, the pharmacodynamically more potent epimer 22R showed an uptake in lung tissue that was 1.4 times higher than that of epimer 22S. This property may be due to the fact that epimer 22R is less water soluble than epimer 22S [123].

PRODRUG APPROACHES TO EXTENDING DRUG ACTIVITY IN THE LUNG

Most of the research centered on the targeting of drugs by the prodrug approach has been carried out on β_2 stimulants structurally related to isoproterenol and similar drugs. The basic approach has been to esterify the catechol functions of isoproterenot to achieve better uptake in lung tissues of the resulting inactive lipophilic drug, which may then be metabolically cleaved by lung esterases to release the active parent compound [124,125]. In addition, esterification of the catechol function acts to protect the drug from deactivation by metabolic

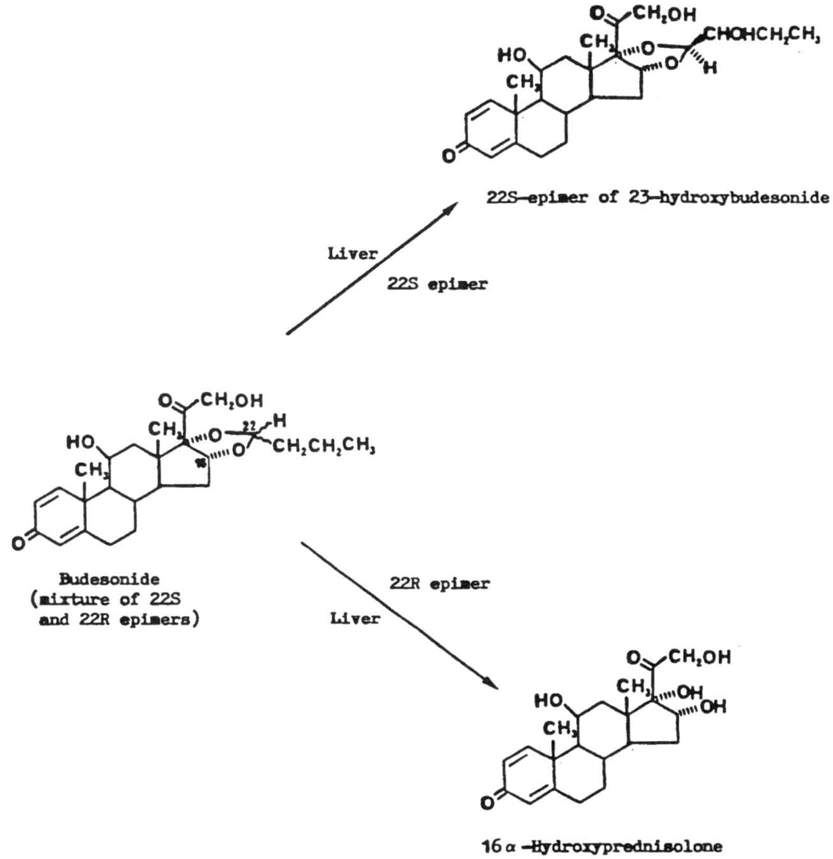

FIGURE 6   Stereoselective metabolism of budesonide.

conjugation. The elimination of cardiovascular side effects using this approach depends on the preferential uptake of the prodrug by the lung and the greater esterase activity in lung tissue relative to heart tissue. However, prolonged therapeutic effect may also be obtained simply by increasing drug residence time in the body through reduced renal clearance. This can be achieved by conjugation of the drug to form a lipophilic prodrug containing a slowly hydrolyzable linker group (e.g., a carbamate) [126].

A few drugs have been investigated that are members of this class (**50–51**). Bitolterol (**50a**) is the di-β-toluolyl ester of *N-t*-butylarterenol (**50b**) and is an effective long-lasting bronchodilator when given by intravenous injection, aerosol, or intraduodenal administration [127]; it is rapidly hydrolyzed after oral administration. Although the improved activity of this compound compared to the parent compound was thought to be due to its avid uptake by the lung followed by slow hydrolytic release of the active drug, recent lung perfusion studies in rabbits have shown that this is not the case [128]. These studies indicate rapid pulmonary hydrolysis of prodrugs such as bitolterol; however, it was pointed out the rabbit lung has greater esterase activity than that of dogs or humans. Nevertheless, it is hard to rationalize that the effect of the drug persists long after any drug remains in the lung. The β_2 drugs ibuterol (**51a**) and bambuterol (**51b**) are further examples of pulmonary prodrugs. Ibuterol (**51a**) is the di-isobutyryl ester of the resorcinol function of terbutaline (**51c**). After inhalation, ibuterol is three times as effective as terbutaline in the inhibition of bronchospasm [129]. Five minutes after inhalation, ibuterol has been shown to exhibit a greater pulmonary pharmacological effect or potency than does terbutaline when administered by this route.

Studies have shown that ibuterol is absorbed more rapidly than terbutaline after administration to the lung but that at all time points both lung and serum terbutaline concentrations were higher after terbutaline administration [130]. Thus, it appears that the prodrug ibuterol exhibits a greater pulmonary pharmacological effect or potency than does terbutaline when administered by inhalation.

Bambuterol (**51b**), the bis-*N*-*N*-dimethylcarbamate of terbutaline, produces a sustained release of terbutaline, a result of the slow, mainly extrapulmonary hydrolysis of the carbamate linkage. Unfortunately, because of its poor metabolism in the lung, it is not effective by the inhalation route. But it has been reported to yield good oral results and can be administered at much less frequent intervals than terbutaline [131]. In fact, bambuterol has been approved for treatment of asthma in almost 28 countries, in oral tablets as the hydrochloride salt. Bambuterol is stable to presystemic elimination and is concentrated by lung tissue after absorption from the gastrointestinal tract. The prodrug is hydrolyzed to terbutaline primarily by butyryl cholinesterase, and lung tissue contains this metabolic enzyme. Bambuterol is also oxidatively metabolized to products that can be hydrolyzed to terbutaline [132]. Bambuterol displays high first-pass hydrolytic stability and is only slowly hydrolyzed to terbutaline; hence, it can be administered orally, as infrequently as once a day. Bambuterol and its metabolites appear to be preferentially distributed to the lung, where an advantageous distribution and metabolism to active drug occurs. Thus, the prodrug is able to generate adequate concentrations of terbutaline levels in the lung. It has been reported that bronchodilator effects at low dosage are greater than can be predicated by plasma concentrations of terbutaline [133]. This may explain the significantly reduced systemic side effects compared to other oral bronchodilators. A study [134] postulated that several explanations can account for the disparity between plasma levels and drug effects as observed for several of the pulmonary products; that is, (a) the prodrug is metabolized in lung to an unknown but potent and long-acting pharmacological agent, (b) the prodrug releases small amounts of the parent drug at sites in lung from which its does not readily efflux, and (c) small amounts of the prodrug not reflected by bulk concentrations of prodrug in lung or plasma may sequester specific sites in the lung.

A related approach to the design of prodrugs of terbutalaine is the cascade ester approach. In this design, the phenolic functions of terbutaline are esterified with 4-0-(2,2-dimethylpropionyloxy)-benzoic acid (**51d**). The cascade effect is postulated initially to involve cleavage of the pivolate ester and 0 conjugation during first-pass metabolism to protect the terbutaline phenolic groups; the subsequent hydrolysis of the hydroxybenzoyl link would, therefore, be delayed. However, data indicate that in dogs and humans this type of prodrug has no advantage over bambuterol, because both compounds are very slowly hydrolyzed in plasma, and significant plasma concentrations of the monoester of these prodrugs are not seen in vivo [134]. Another related approach to the design of prodrugs to target alveolar macrophages has been carried out using microspheres as a primary carrier of the prodrug [135].

The drug isoniazid has been used in this fashion, it was structurally modified into an ionizable form suitable for hydrophobic ion pairing. The charged prodrug, sodium isoniazid methanesulforate, was then ion paired with hydrophobic cations, such as alkyltrimethyl ammonium ion. The drug was then encapsulated into polymeric microspheres to form hydrophobic ion-paired complexes. The ion-pair complex and polymer were coprecipitated using supercritical fluid methodology [136].

POTENTIAL USEFULNESS OF CELL MEMBRANE–BOUND ENZYME SUBSTRATES AND INHIBITORS, AND CELL MEMBRANE–BOUND RECEPTOR AGONISTS AND ANTAGONISTS AS DRUG CARRIERS WITH LUNG SPECIFICITY

Ranney [137,138] postulated that pulmonary clearance of drug molecules from the systemic circulation may be achievable by targeting selective binding sites on the pulmonary endothelial membrane. In this regard, a possible strategy may be to link drug molecules to ligands that have high affinity for these endothelium binding sites. For example, several hydrolytic enzymes, such as peptidases and phosphorylases, are known to be located on the surface membrane of lung epithelium and endothelium [139–142]. Such enzymes may be targetable by designing drug conjugates with appropriate substrates or tight-binding inhibitors (i.e., nonhydrolyzable substrates). Table 1 illustrates the number and types of peptidase enzymes that are known to be bound to pulmonary endothelial or epithelial membranes. The existence of a selection of membrane-bound epithelial enzymes may well be useful in designing appropriate drug conjugates with multiple ligands for these enzyme-active sites as bioadhesive targeting agents. Ranney [137] pointed out that ligands that bind multiple active sites may be more useful as drug carriers on the grounds that populations of some receptors may be significantly decreased or lost entirely in some diseased states, for example, membrane-bound dipeptidyl aminopeptidase (angiotensin-converting enzyme), and phosphodiesterase enzymes (PDEs). The cyclic nucleotide PDEs comprise a family of enzymes whose role is to regulate cellular levels of the second messengers, cAMP and cGMP, by hydrolyzing them to inactive metabolites. PDE IV is the predominant PDE isozyme in inflammatory and immune cells and thus regulates a major pathway of cAMP degradation. Elevation of cAMP levels supresess cell activation in a wide range of inflammatory and immune cells [143]. The attraction of PDE IV inhibition as a therapy for asthma derives from the potential of selectively elevating cAMP levels in the airway smooth muscles and the inflammatory response [144].

TABLE 1   Membrane-Bound Enzymes on Lung Endothelial and Epithelial Cells

Enzyme	Location
Dipeptidyl carboxypeptidase (ACE) (EC 3A.15.1)	Endothelial membrane
Dipeptidyl aminopeptidase IV (EC 3.4.14.5)	Endothelial membrane
Carboxypeptidase N (Arginine carboxypeptidase) (EC 3.4.17.3)	Endothelial membrane
Aminopeptidase M (EC 3.4.11.1)	Endothelial membrane
Aminopeptidase A (Microsomal aminopeptidase) (EC 3.4.11.2)	Endothelial membrane
Aminopeptidase P (aminoacyl-peptide hydrolase) (EC 3.4.11.9)	Endothelial membrane
Neutral metallo endopeptidase (enkephalinase) (EC 3.4.24.11)	Epithelial membrane
5'-Nucleotidase (EC 3.1.3.5)	Endothelial membrane
Adenyl cyclase	Endothelial and epithelial membrane
Carbonic anhydrase	Endothelial membrane
ATPase (EC 3.6.1.8)	Endothelial membrane
ADPase (EC 3.6.1.5)	Endothelial membrane

Source: Ref. 149.

In order to achieve the desired pharmacological effects without unwanted side effects it is likely that selective targeting of specific enzymes will be necessary. Selective inhibition of a specific target enzyme has recently been achieved using Rolipram (**52**) a selective PDE IV inhibitor, which shows reduction in allergen-induced bronchiol hyperreactivity in guinea pigs dosed at 75 µg/kg i.p. [145].

52

In a structure–activity correlation study, a number of N-substituted derivatives of rolipram (**52**) were prepared and evaluated [146]. A carbamate ester of rolipram was found to be approximately 10-fold more potent than rolipram itself at inhibiting human PDE IV. A methyl ketone derivate of rolipram shows more potent inhibition of PDE IV compared to rolipram or its carbamate ester. Based on proton NMR spectroscopy and computer modeling studies, a pharmacophore model of the methyl ketone derivative was proposed [147]. This model showed that the ketone carbonyl oxygen atom is involved in an important interaction within the PDE IV active site. Sodium orthovanadate, a phosphotyrosine phosphate inhibitor, exhibits dose- and time-dependent suppression of Lewis lung carcinoma A11 cells spreading. Protein tyrosine phosphorylation levels in A11 cells was elevated after treatment with orthovanadate; this increase was partially deminished by the tyrosine kinase inhibitor ST 638, concomitantly with restoration of the suppressed cell spreading, as well as invasive and metastatic ability [148]. These results suggest tyrosine phosphorylation influences adhesion of cancer cells to lung surface endothelia and that a valid approach in treating cancer is inhibition of phosphotyrosine phosphatase.

Activity in the lung is known to be reduced by multiple diseases and by exposure to drugs and medical procedures, because of reversible endothelial damage [150]. Thus, the ideal carrier would be a nonpharmacological substrate (or inhibitor) with a broad spectrum affinity substrate for membrane-bound epithelial enzymes.

For such an approach to drug targeting to be effective, it is assumed that the drug and carrier are able to become internalized by transport across the contralumenal membrane and passage into the basement membrane tissues. In this respect, the use of macromolecule carriers such as dextran (see later discussion) that can conjugate both drug and multiple-binding molecules may be an advantage. This approach can also be considered a viable strategy for the transendothelial route in the lung because several different peptidases are known to be bound to the endothelial membrane [151–153] (Table 1).

Another strategy for obtaining an enhancement in pulmonary clearance of drugs is to conjugate the drug molecule to a chemical entity that binds to one or more surface receptors on endothelial or epithelial cells. Examples of the receptor agonists serotonin and norepinephrine have already been mentioned. However, there are examples of lung targeting that have used other pulmonary receptor substrates as targeting vectors.

Human pulmonary carcinomas have been shown to contain high levels of opioid peptides and their corresponding membrane-bound receptors [154]. Rigaudy et al. [154] targeted drugs to these receptors using modified metabolically stable enkephalins linked to cytotoxic drugs. These conjugates were expected to specifically internalize within opiate receptor-baring cells. Cell culture studies with NG 108-15 mouse tumor cells indicated that the peptide–ellipticinium conjugates 53a and 53b were internalized and were intracellularly stable but showed much lower cytotoxicity than their parent drug toward the opioid receptor–bearing cells. Nevertheless, the study did indicate that enkephalin-derived peptides could be used as specific carriers to target cytotoxic agents toward opioid receptor–rich cells. A similar approach for targeting pulmonary epithelial membrane–bound enkephalinase (Table 1) may also be valid, using enkephalin drug or enkephalinase inhibitor–drug conjugates. One potential problem with the drug-targeting strategy is the likelihood that in disease states membrane receptor populations may not be maintained. In this respect, an approach that uses a carrier capable of binding to multiple types of receptors may be more successful.

53

A cell-based drug delivery system for lung targeting has been investigated. Doxorubicin was loaded into B16-F10 murine melanoma cells [a drug-loaded tumor cell (DLTC)]. The amount and rate of drug released from the DLTC mainly depended on the drug loading and carrier cell concentration. After a bolus injection of 30 μg doxorubicin either in the DLTC form or in free solution into the mice tail veins, drug deposit ion in the lung from DLTC was 3.6-fold greater than that achieved by free drug solution. This DLTC system demonstrated a lung-targeting activity that may be due to specific surface characteristics [155,156].

Some recent studies [157] indicate that insulin is efficiently absorbed from the lung when administered either by intratracheal instillation in the rat or by aerosol inhalation in the rabbit. Because insulin is also actively cleared from the systemic circulation [158] and has a lower potential for acute pharmacological effects, the conjugation of appropriate drug molecules to this polypeptide may also be a useful strategy for lung targeting.

CONJUGATION OF DRUGS WITH MACROMOLECULES FOR SELECTIVE TARGETING TO THE LUNG

One approach to the selective targeting of drugs into those cells where their action is required is the conjugation of a pharmacologically active agent to a macromolecular vector that is recognized and actively taken up by the target cell, where bound drug can then be released in its active from. Several examples where macromolecules have been used as carriers in an effort to alter the tissue localization of a carrier-linked drug have been reported [159]. Selectivity of targeting is largely dependent on the properties of the macromolecular vector and usually results in an altered distribution of the free drug compared to the parent drug itself when administered by the same route.

It is clear that macromolecule–drug conjugates or, more accurately, macromolecular prodrugs may well alter the pharmacological and immunological activity of the parent compound. The macromolecular transport vector may vary considerably in size, electrical charges, hydrophobicity and hydrophilicity, and its ability to act as a substrate for transmembrane transport mechanisms.

Desirable properties of the macromolecular vectors are no intrinsic toxicity (e.g., nonantigenic), biodegradability with no accumulation in the body, and presence of functionalized moieties for drug conjugation. In addition, the macromolecule–drug conjugate must not possess the pharmacological activity of

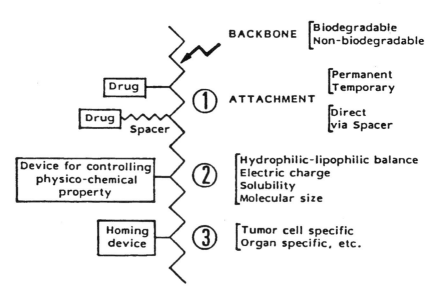

FIGURE 7   Model for macromolecule–drug conjugates. (From Ref. 102. Reproduced by permission, CRC Press, Inc.)

the parent drug, but the conjugate should retain the desirable targeting specificity of the parent macromolecular vector. With regard to the drug molecule, certain properties are also desirable for the formulation of an effective prodrug. For example, the therapeutic effect of the drug must be shown at relatively low doses to afford a reasonably low load of carrier macromolecule, and the macromolecule–drug conjugate structure must be chemically stable before drug release. Not all therapeutic drug molecules are capable of being conjugated to macromolecular vectors, simply because they lack adequate functional groups in their molecular structure for chemical fixation.

A variety of covalent linkages have been used in the design of macromolecule–drug conjugates, that is, esters, amides, hydrazones, imides, and disulfides. These linkages must be designed to be readily formed without chemical destruction of either the macromolecular vector or the drug during synthesis, and they must be readily broken by chemical or enzymatic hydrolysis. Figure 7 illustrates the various components of a macromolecule–drug conjugate.

In Vivo Fate of Macromolecular Prodrugs and Lung Targeting

The fate of macromolecular conjugates when administered by the systemic route is heavily dependent on the distribution and elimination properties of the prodrug. In addition, endothelial and epithelial membrane transport is of primary importance with regard to targeting and drug action. Distribution and elimination profiles are primarily determined by factors such as molecular size, charge, water solubility, and hydrophilic and lipophilic balance. Apart from the incorporation of specific targeting features into the conjugate (i.e., antibodies), such physiochemical factors can play an important role in tissue targeting. The administration of macromolecule–drug conjugates by inhalation has received relatively little attention, although some studies involving anticancer agents are available. If such conjugates are required to access the circulatory system, then initial diffusion or transport across the alveolar capillary membrane must take place. In addition, interaction will occur with other structures, such as the alveolar epithelial cells that face the air spaces, the capillary endothelial cells that are the major constituents of the pulmonary macrocirculation, and the phagocytic pulmonary intravascular macrophages.

The relationship between pulmonary sequestering of macromolecules and molecular weight or particle size is not clear. Hashida et al. [160] showed that distribution of C-dextran-mitomycin C conjugates was dependent on molecular weight when given intravenously in rats, conjugates of MW 10,000–500,000 being sequestered mainly by spleen, liver, and lymph nodes, with no significant accumulation in the lung, heart, or muscle. Interestingly, cationic dextran conjugates of MW 70,000 or less are immediately distributed to the kidney and excreted, indicating that the glomerular capillary membrane is impermeable to polycationic macromolecules in excess of MW 70,000. There have been numerous studies in dogs and rats that indicate that particles exceeding 7 μm are retained in the lung after intravascular administration [161]. However, other studies in ruminants have shown that liposomes, bacteria, and magnetic iron microaggregates are sequestered in the lung, even at particle sizes much smaller than 7 μm [162,163]. Studies [164] have suggested that particulate trapping in the pulmonary circulation may not be solely dependent on size but may also be determined by other factors, for example, the involvement of pulmonary intravascular macrophages (PIMs), because pulmonary sequestration is often associated with pulmonary hypertension and lung injury, conditions that increase the lung burden of pulmonary intravascular macrophages. Other studies [165] have shown that disruption of hepatic bacterial clearance mechanisms may also induce PIM formation in the lung; of importance in this connection, patients with impaired hepatic function often exhibit substantial pulmonary uptake of intravascular colloidal imaging agents that are normally localized in the liver, spleen, and bone marrow of healthy patients.

Targeting of Macromolecule–Drug Conjugates to the Lung

In general, the major problem in targeting macromolecules to the lung after intravascular administration is to overcome the biodistribution of such molecules to phagocytes in the reticuloendothelial organs (liver, spleen, and bone marrow). With a growing body of data on the nature of endothelial and epithelial receptors that enhance pulmonary drug clearance, the morphological factors governing transport of molecules through basement membranes, the effects of disease on endothelial and sequestered tissue receptors, and the availability of receptor-binding substrates that can be used for targeting entities in macromolecule–drug conjugates, the efforts to improve pulmonary targeting of drugs is already under way. Recent developments that have effected this progress have been due to new technologies, leading to an improvement in the design and production of drug-carrier molecules and coatings that afford circulating agents with specific affinity for lung endothelium and epithelium. As previously mentioned in the section on structural factors governing drug uptake, several endogenous compounds are known to be actively taken up from the plasma by the pulmonary endothelium, for example, serotonin and norepinephrine. Drugs conjugated to these agents have been suggested to undergo pulmonary targeting; this has yet to be determined conclusively. A more rational approach is to use pharmacologically inactive analogues of these agents or their inactive metabolites, which would still retain their targeting abilities, in drug–drug or macromolecule–drug conjugates.

It is generally recognized that the use of liposomes, microparticulates, and colloidal carriers to achieve drug targeting has proven to be largely unsuccessful because of the difficulties in gaining access to targeted tissues, penetrating vascular barriers, and evading phagocytic capture by the reticuloendothelium system. However, the coating of microspheres and emulsions with block copolymers may overcome the latter problem. Illum et al. [166,167], for example, coated model polystyrene microspheres with a poloxamine-980 block copolymer, and they observed a much longer circulatory half-life in the vascular compartment after intravenous injection, with little or no uptake by the reticuloendothelium system. Deposition of coated microspheres was observed to be significantly reduced in the liver and spleen, with high levels in the lungs. The conjugation of tissue-targeting vectors (e.g., sugar residues, lectins, monoclonal antibodies, apolipoproteins) to appropriate functionalities on a hydrophilic coating may allow colloidal carriers to be actively targeted to specific sites, either by systemic or intracavity administration (N-2-hydroxyporpyl)-methacrylamide copolymer macromolecules have also been used as targetable drug-carrier systems [168,169]. The advantages of these systems is that they can be tailor-made to include oligopeptide drug linkages that are stable in the circulation but are readily digested intracellularly by the lysosomal thiol-dependent (cysteine-) proteinases. They are readily synthesized and are efficiently internalized by cells via pinocytosis, and cleavage of linkages to drug can be controlled by appropriate structural manipulation. Thus, they provide good opportunities for controlled intracellular delivery of drugs. In addition, they can be synthesized to include potentially useful targeting residues, such as sugars, immunoglobulins, and antibodies.

Soluble macromolecule-drug carriers seem to offer greater potential because they can transverse compartmental barriers more efficiently and, therefore, gain access to a greater number of cell types and, in most cases, are not subject to clearance by the reticuloendothelial cells. Dextrans, human serum albumin, polysomes, and even tumor-specific antibodies (see the section on drug monoclonal–antibody conjugates) have all been evaluated as drug carriers for lung targeting [170,171]. Each system has advantages in terms of specificity or ease of chemical conjugation, but each also presents problems of limited body distribution or immunogenicity. Conjugation of methotrexate of poly-L-lysine has markedly increased the drug's tumoricidal activity in vitro [172], and intermittent administration of methotrexate–albumin conjugates has been shown to be more effective than free drug in reducing the number of lung metastases in mice after receiving subcutaneous inoculation of Lewis lung carcinoma [173].

Mammalian macrophages contain a transport system that binds and internalizes glycoprotcins with exposed mannose residues. It has been shown that small multivalent synthetic glycopeptides with mannose residues covalently linked through a spacer arm to the α- and ε-amino groups of lysine, dilysine, or trilysine are competitive inhibitors of rate alveolar macrophage uptake of the neoglycoprotein-bovine serum albumin with inhibition constants in the low micromolar range [174] (Fig. 8). Various compounds can be covalently attached

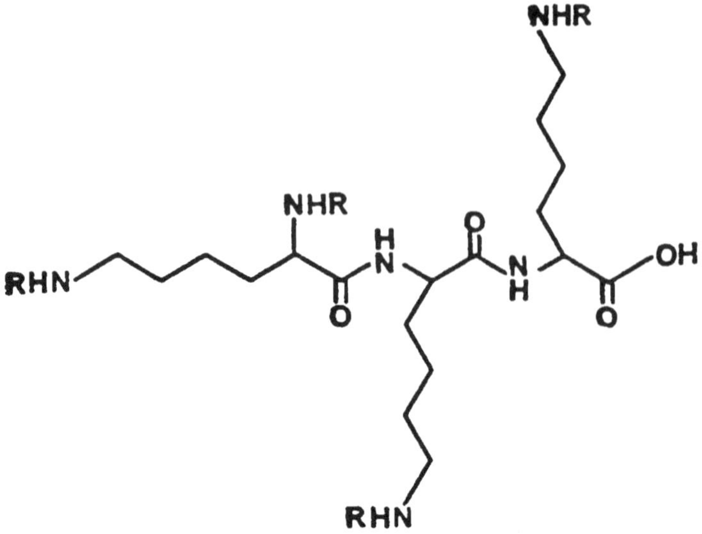

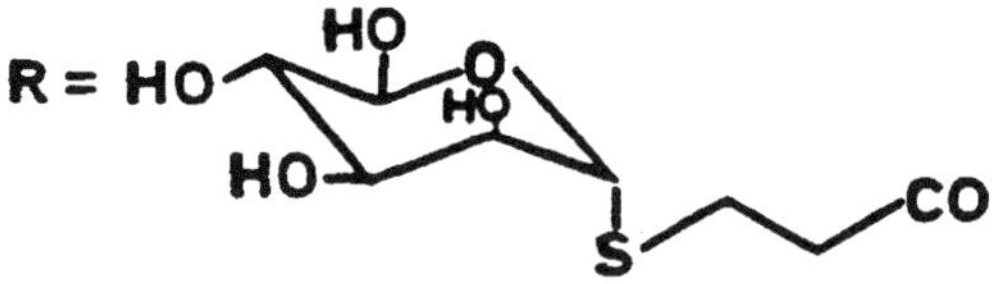

FIGURE 8   Structure of mannosylpeptides.

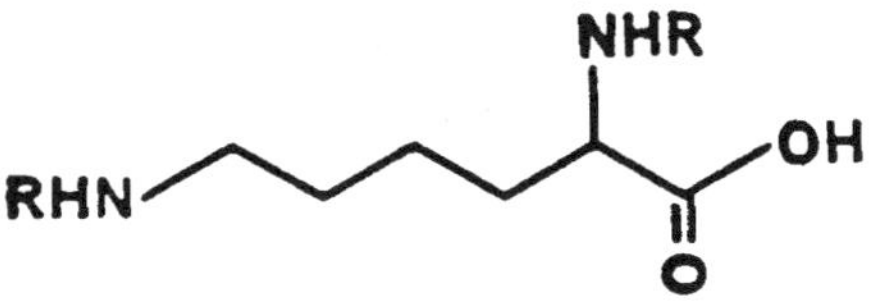

to the α-carboxyl group of these glycopeptides without substantial loss of inhibition.

These synthetic substrates may be useful models for targeting pharmacological agents to alveolar macrophages as well as other cell types. Monsigny et al. [175] have conjugated the immunostimulant muramyldipeptide with neoglycoprotein and have shown that the conjugate was actively endocytosed by murine alveolar macrophages, leading to their dramatic activation, even at very low concentrations of the conjugate. Intravenous and intraperitoneal administration of the conjugate led to maximal activation of alveolar macrophages at 48 hours in mice and 72 hours in rats. This interesting example of drug targeting may have potential usefulness in the design of carrier-mediated anticancer, antiparasitic, or antiviral chemotherapy.

An attempt has been made to target the antitumor drug daunomycin to human squamous lung tumor cell monolayers by conjugating the drug with low-density lipoprotein. Although rapid uptake of the conjugate afforded equilibrium in 3 hours, the in vitro cytotoxicity of the conjugate was no different than that of the parent drug [176]. The high level of expression of high-affinity receptors for EGF on lung tumors may possibly be used as a target for ligand-complexed (conjugated) drugs [177]. Antibodies to EGF have been shown to inhibit tumor growth [178], and ligand-complexed drugs can concentrate in receptor-positive cells by affinity targeting [179].

The correct strategy for accomplishing the successful targeting and delivery of drugs using macromolecule–drug conjugates must be a judicious choice, based on the characteristics of the target tissue or cell type and the drug. Initially, the properties of the cell type, sites of complexation, transport, and internalization mechanisms, as well as the pharmacological and physicochemical properties of the drug molecule, its site of action (i.e., nature of interaction with receptors or enzyme active sites), and chemical stability, must be considered. The conjugation of the drug molecule to the carrier is also an important consideration because the bond must be stable enough to withstand cleavage before reaching the target site but must be designed to release the drug at the site of action.

BIOADHESIVES AND DRUG TARGETING TO THE LUNG

The use of bioadhesive targeting as a means for specific delivery of drugs has gained some impetus since the late 1980s [180]. The term *bioadhesion* refers to interactions involving multiple molecular and usually noncovalent bonds. However, a bioadhesive agent, to be effective as a drug carrier, must initially be trapped or sequestered by endothelial or epithelial cells, followed by multiligand binding of the surface material of the carrier particle to cell surface determinants, which then induces the rapid (10 to 15-minute) envelopment of the carrier by the cell either by transcytosis or migrational overgrowth mechanisms, followed by transfer to the proximal tissues. Bioadhesion targeting is, therefore, a combination of biophysical trapping and biochemical adherence. The carrier is usually a hydrophilic macromolecule or microparticulate, and, for systemic delivery, a particle size between 3 and 5 μm (nonembolizing) is preferable for pulmonary trapping, whereas larger particle sizes between 5 and 250 μm (embolizing) are also usable. Multivalent binding agents may comprise substance such as heparins, lectins, and antibodies to endothelial antigens, epithelial antigens, and glycosylated albumin.

Lectins are naturally occurring glycoproteins of nonimmunological origin. They have the unique ability to recognize and bind to exposed carbohydrate residues on glycoproteins, such as those exposed at the surface of epithelial cells, and therefore have been classified as second-generation bioadhesives. In a recent study [181], lectin-functionalized liposomes, in contrast to lectin-free liposomes, specifically bound to A 549, a tumor-derived cell line. This suggests that lectin-mediated bioadhesion and uptake of liposome-carriers may provide a useful technology for lung cancer treatment. The administration of liposome-encapsulated drugs by aerosols seems to be a feasible way of targeting these delivery systems to the lung. The tolerability and safety of liposome aerosols has been tested in animals as well as human volunteers, and no unwanted effects have been observed [182].

Both transendothelial and transepithelial migration of particles and molecular aggregates larger than about 2 nm in diameter have been shown to be accelerated by application of surface coatings that bind multiply to cell surface receptors or antigens [138]. Such particles conjugate at least two molecules of drug or diagnostic agent and a multivalent binding agent (bioadhesive) that is specific for cell surface determinants. Table 2 lists carrier particles, multivalent binding agents, and endothelial and epithelial cell surface determinants of potential usefulness in bioadhesive targeting to the lung. This list is by no means exhaustive. Carrier particles, preferably having a size between 1 nm and 250 μm, or coatings comprising carbohydrates, oligosaccharides, or monosaccharides, proteins or peptides, and lipids or other biocompatible synthetic polymers are usually used. The chemical structure may be a simple single-chain polymer, a molecular microaggregate (i.e., a molecular carrier or aggregate that acts as both the cell target binding moiety and the backbone for linking prodrug moieties), or a more complex structure incorporating multiple matrix material or serial coating that is able to interact with multiple cell surface determinants, resulting in rapid sequestration and transport of the carrier. Substances from a wide range are known that bind to native endothelium and epithelium and to basement membrane constituents. All are promising candidates with potential usefulness as bioadhesive agents for lung-targeting studies. Laminin is a noncollagenous high-molecular-weight (10^6) protein that interacts with glycosaminoglycans and promotes adhesion of various cell types. Laminin is located in the lamina lucida

TABLE 2 Composition of Bioadhesives

Carrier particles	Multivalent binding agents	Endothelial and epithelial surface determinants
Macromolecules	Heparin and heparin derivatives	Receptors
Microaggregates	Heparin fragments	Enzyme active sites
Microparticles	Lectins	Antigens
Microspheres	Antibodies	Endothelial and epithelial tissue factors
Nanospheres	Dextrans	Subcellular tissue moieties
Liposomes	Peptides	Fibrin D–D dimers
Microemulsions	Enzyme inhibitors Receptor agonists; and antagonists Albumins and glycosylated albumins	Glycoprotein complexes

of a cell's basal surface and the supporting matrix of type IV (basement membrane) collagen [183–185]. Laminin receptors occur on cells that normally interact with basement membranes as well as on cells that extravasate, for example, metastasizing cancer cells, macrophages, and leukocytes [186]. In vitro studies have clearly shown that laminin can mediate the attachment of a wide variety of epithelial and endothelial cells to type IV collagen [183,184], and a cell surface receptor protein for laminin has been isolated from murine fibrosarcoma cells that may mediate the interaction of the cell with its extracellular matrix [187].

Fibronectin, another constituent of basement membrane, may also be an effective constituent for promoting extravascular migration of particulate matter [188,189], and glycosylated serum albumins appear to undergo greater vesicular endothelial micropinocytosis by rat microvessels as compared to unmodified albumin, which may indicate a useful role for nonenzymatic glycosylated serum albumin in drug targeting [190].

Heparin sulfates, the side-chain moieties of cell surface proteoglycans, are important factors in cell recognition phenomena. The proteoheparan sulfates are ubiquitous cell surface proteglycan components of the cell coat or glycocalyx. They undergo chain–chain self-association in a structure-specific manner. Studies show that such compounds are useful bioadhesives [191]. Lipoprotein lipase also attaches to endothelial cells through heparin sulfate interaction on the cell surface and is released by heparin through a detachment from this binding site [192]. Factor VIII antigen has been widely used as a marker for endothelial cells [193], and studies have shown that *Ulex europaeus* 1 agglutinin (UEA-1), a lectin that is specific for α-L-fucose-containing glycocompounds, is also a marker for vascular endothelium in human tissues [193]. UEA-1 appears to be a more sensitive marker than factor VIII antigen for the factor VIII binding site and has a particularly high affinity for alveolar capillary endothelium and bronchial epithelium [194]. In vivo studies indicate that intravenously injected fucose-blocked UEA-1-coated microspheres in CBA mice allowed approximately 90% of the injected dose to be concentrated in the lung after 20 minutes, with 80% of this amount being in extravascular locations [138]. The use of UEA-1 lectin as a diagnostic agent for tumors derived from human endothelial cells was recently described [195].

Anionic sites on the lumenal surface of pulmonary microvascular endothelium have been shown to bind cationic ferritin in isolated, perfused rat lung studies [196]. The cationic ferritin is taken up by vesicles and discharged into the capillary membrane. Similar anionic sites are also present on alveolar epithelial surfaces [25].

In some cases, cell surface expression of certain species can be induced; for example, interleukin-1 has been shown to induce the biosynthesis and cell surface expression of procoagulant activity in human vascular endothelial cells [197]. Such materials may also be exploitable as candidates for bioadhesion studies. Millions of lives of patients with diabetes have been saved since the introduction of insulin therapy. However, several daily injections of insulin are required to maximize glucose control in diabetic patients. Insulin is administered by subcutaneous injection, but this route of administration has a slow onset and subsequent prolonged duration of action. These limitations show up more when higher doses of insulin are injected, which results in a long duration of action and forces the patients to consume additional amounts of food to limit the risk of hypoglycemia [198].

This limitation has been reduced by the availability of newer, short-acting insulin analogues (Lipro and Aspart). However, this form of insulin must be injected subcutaneously. Technosphere™ insulin is a formulation of regular human and Technosphere™, a new drug-delivery system for pulmonary administration. The formulation is designed for efficient transport of insulin across the intact respiratory epithelium into the systemic circulation [199]; its duration of action is more than 3 hours, and maximal serum insulin levels can be reached within 13 minutes after inhalation [200], which is considerably shorter than those observed with rapid-acting insulin analogues administered subcutaneously or other insulin inhalations [201].

Other molecules have been suggested as being useful lung-specific bioadhesive agents [137,138], for example, insulin, transferrin, prostaglandins, hirudin-inhibited thrombin (which binds thrombomodulin), anionic polysaccharides, oligosaccharides (such as dextran sulfate, dermatan sulfate, chondroitin sulfate, hyaluronic acid), peptides (such as benzoyl-phe-ala-pro [BPAPI] that bind angiotensin-converting enzyme, $5'$-nucleotidies that bind $5'$ nucleases, and inactive analogues of biogenic amines (such as 5-hydroxytryptamine) that interact with surface neuroreceptors. Such a list of compounds also includes antibodies directed against cell surface targets, such as factor VIII antigen and type IV collagen of the basement membrane, glycoproteins, and other antigens (see the later section on monoclonal antibody conjugates).

Bioadhesive agents have been hypothesized to interact with endothelial or epithelial cell surface determinants, inducing the cell to undergo transient separation or opening, thereby exposing subcellular determinants for which the agent may also have binding affinity. The interaction results in an acceleration of transport across at least one of the associated endothelial and epithelial structures or subcellular structures into a proximal tissue compartment. The basic premise is that this phenomenon will result in an improvement in the therapeutic index so that a reduced total dose of drug (or diagnostic agent) is required to obtain pharmacological effects comparable to significantly higher doses of free drug (or diagnostic agent).

Ranney [138] showed that intravenously administered heparin-amphotericin Pluronic B-F108 nanospheres and microspheres in adult male CBA/J mice are specifically targeted to lung, endothelium uptake being complete within 15 minutes after injection (i.e., zero blood levels) (Table 3). The results indicate that preferential and rapid uptake in the lung occurs with both subernbolizing

TABLE 3 Organ Localization of Heparin–Amphotericin B Formulations After Intravenous Injection into Adult Male CBA/J Mice

	Organ concentration (μg amphotericin/g tissue) (%) 1 hr after injection		
Tissue	Amphotericin B[a] (unbound)	Heparin (nonembolizing) (nanospheres[b])	Heparin (marginally embolizing) (microspheres[c])
Lung	4.0 (14)[d]	15.0 (52)[d]	25.7 (94)[d]
Liver	6.7 (24)	8.3 (29)	5.0 (18[d])
Kidney	2.5 (9.2)	1.1 (3.8)	0.4 (1.4)[d]
Spleen	11.0 (38.3)	6.2 (21)	2.2 (8.2)
Heart	0.3 (1.3)	0.2 (0.7)	0.3 (0.4)
Brain	0.0 (0)	1.4 (4.8)	0.2 (0.5)

[a] Biodistribution of fungizone (amphotericin β-deoxycholate nanoemulsion).
[b] Total body drug recovered, 70%.
[c] Total body drug recovered, 55%.
[d] Percent of injected dose localized per gram of tissue (wet weight).

and embolizing particle diameters. Such a rapid and efficient uptake was not observed for dextran and agarose placebo particles that lack the heparin surface coat.

Histochemical analysis of lung deposition showed the amphotericin B to be distributed in the alveoli, pulmonary interstitium, respiratory epithelium, and bronchial and tracheal lymph nodes, thus indicating extensive tissue percolation of the drug carrier; no significant kidney deposition was observed. (Note: This is a major site of amphotericin toxicity.) The results establish that it is possible to achieve high-efficiency endothelial bioadhesion, selective drug uptake, and retention in the lung using this approach.

In the same study, intravenous injection of *Ulex europaeus* 1 lectin microspheres were shown to be specifically taken up by lung endothelial cells and rapidly underwent migration into the extravascular tissues and into the airspace within 5–10 minutes after injection, with 90% of the injected dose being identified in the lung. Intratracheal administration of heparin nanospheres of 200 to 800-nm diameter containing iron oxide (Fe_3O_4) and ionic iron (Fe^{3+}) to pentobarbital-anesthetized adult male CBA/J mice indicated a very similar deposition profile to that observed after intravenous injection of amphotericin B–containing nanospheres (Table 3) [138].

Liver and kidney deposition was negligible to very low, showing that stabilized heparin nanosphere carriers with heparin surfaces are taken up by epithelial transport and that a high proportion of the dose becomes localized in lungs relative to other organs when administered by the airways. This novel example of epithelial uptake may provide the rationale for administering drug–bioadhesive carrier conjugates by the inhalation route and may be particularly useful for the topical or systemic delivery of highly toxic drugs (e.g., antitumor drugs, antifungals, antivirals, antibiotics), drugs that are very labile (e.g., peptides, proteins, oligonucleotides), or drugs that for one reason or another exhibit poor access by conventional formulations to pulmonary tissues.

DRUG–MONOCLONAL ANTIBODY CONJUGATES FOR TARGETING TO THE LUNG

Another drug-carrier system that has been investigated as a means of achieving specific tissue targeting is the use of an antibody directed against the tissue that is the proposed site of action of the drug. Although this approach is not new, because pioneering work in this area was carried out as early as 1958 [202]. Recently, it has become evident that monoclonal antibody (mAb) biotechnology is effective in a wide range of disease. The current estimated market for these agents is about $25 billion each year. The application of antibodies is broad ranging and includes therapeutics, diagnostic tools, and research tools. The first therapeutic antibodies were mouse monoclonal antibodies that were selected against cytokines and cell surface proteins of proinflammatory, immunologic, or cancer cells [203]. The development of monoclonal antibodies to human tumor–associated antigens has been achieved, and this has led to a renewed interest in the use of drug–antibody conjugates for cancer therapy [204,205].

There are several questions that need to be addressed before considering the use of drug–monoclonal antibody conjugates.

1. Are sufficiently lung-specific antibodies available?
2. Is there evidence that such antibodies will localize only in lung tissues and not in other tissues in vivo?
3. Do the antibodies contain appropriate functionalities to enable covalent linkage of drug molecules, and, if so, will the conjugated antibody exhibit targeting characteristics similar to those of the parent antibody?
4. Will the formation of an antibody–drug conjugate result in an immunologically active entity on repeated administration?

With regard to these considerations, it is important to determine whether, after either regional or systemic administration, a drug–antibody conjugate can deliver potentially therapeutic doses of the drug. This may depend on the loading of drug at multiple sites of conjugation on the antibody surface. In this respect, the greater the number of drug molecules conjugated to each antibody molecule, the more ineffective the resultant molecule might be, because attachment of drug molecules near or around the antibody–antigen binding site or at locations that compromise the three-dimensional integrity of the antibody will lead to decreased tissue specificity or increased immunological activity, respectively. Thus, an evaluation of the therapeutic index of the conjugate must be undertaken to determine whether it is superior to the free drug.

When considering the targeting of therapeutic agents to lung tissue by this approach, the choice of cell surface antigens would appear to be most appropriate, although there is evidence that antibodies that can recognize in vivo antigens that are expressed extracellularly [206] can also be used for specific tissue targeting. A recombinant humanized mAb to human IgE has been found to inhibit mast-cell-dependent airway narrowing and other components of the asthmatic inflammatory response [207]. Currently, omalizumab is undergoing clinical testing for a number of indications, including asthma. Omalizumab is a mAb that specifically recognizes human IgE [208].

The most commonly used route of administration of antibody–drug conjugates has been the intravenous route, but intracavity administration has also been investigated; and, generally, localization of antibody conjugates in the targeted tissue by this latter route appears to be superior to the intravenous route [209]. The mechanism of antibody-drug delivery at the cellular level is believed to involve initial binding to the specific cell surface antigen. This binding is followed by internalization and endocytosis into lysosomes, where digestion of the conjugate by lysosomal proteinases would release free drug from where it would diffuse to the site of action [210].

As mentioned previously, a significant reduction in antibody reactivity is often observed after multiple sites of conjugation of drug with antibody. This has led to the development of carriers that, when covalently linked to antibody, are able in turn to covalently bind many drug molecules to appropriate carrier functionalities. Examples of carrier molecules that have been used include dextran [211–213], human serum albumin [214], and poly-L-glutamate [215]. Obviously, such a gross molecular modification of the parent antibody may well affect its overall properties, and this often leads to significant differences in biodistribution of an antibody–carrier-drug complex relative to the parent antibody. In addition, for reasons stated previously, such a structural derivitization may also result in lower tissue specificity and increased toxicity.

More innovative approaches to the targeting of drugs by antibody–drug complexes involve the use of hybrid–hybrid antibodies [216–218]. This approach uses hybrid antibodies with dual specificity, one site binding with, say, a cell surface antigen and the other with drug or cytotoxic agent. Such bispecific antibodies are prepared by reassociation of enzyme-prepared fragments of two antibodies or by hybridization of two existing hybridomas, one producing antibody to cell antigen and the other producing antibody to drug. The application of this strategy to the development of therapeutic agents could be twofold: Bispecific antibody would be initially administered, resulting in specific tissue localization (i.e., pretargeting), followed by drug, some of which would be taken up by the localized antibody; alternatively, binary complexes of both drug and antibody could be preformed in vitro and then administered, or drug and antibody could be given simultaneously. The concept of pretargeting is not new and has been investigated for diagnostic tumor imaging with the high-affinity avidin–biotin system [219]. In this system, antibody conjugated to avidin was evaluated for localization in tumors followed by administration of radiolabeled biotin. It is conceivable that such a system may be useful for the pretargeting of drugs to the lung, by using a biotin–drug conjugate in place of biotin.

The use of drug-antibody fragments has been examined as a means for tissue targeting [220,221]. Generally, fragments appear to be poorer targeting agents than intact antibody, although they do exhibit relatively faster overall clearance and catabolism, which may result in less systemic toxicity. However, studies indicate that the increased clearance and kidney metabolism of antibody fragments may lead to renal toxicity [222]. The use of antibody fragments lacking a more immunogenic portion of the intact antibody molecule has generally not resulted in a decrease in immunogenic properties.

Some recent reports involving monoclonal antibodies directed against epithelial and endothelial cell surface components suggest that this approach to drug targeting in the lung may have good potential. For example, monoclonal antibodies to a glycoprotein involved in fibronectin-mediated adhesion mechanisms has been reported for fibroblasts [223], and the injection of rabbit antisera or purified antibodies against basement membrane proteins type IV collagen and laminin into inbred mice results in cellular infiltration of mainly lung and kidney tissue. Antibody location was shown to be on the basement membranes of glomeruli, alveoli (pronounced), choroids plexus, liver, and blood vessels and in epidermal junctions [224].

Developments in the cancer area are also worthy of mention. An immunotoxin consisting of a murine monoclonal antibody (B4G7) that recognizes EGF receptor conjugated with gelonin, a ribose-inactivating protein, was specifically cytotoxic to EGF receptor-hyperproducing cells in mice and was nontoxic at $250 \mu m$ conjugate per mouse [225]. The results suggest that this conjugate may be useful for target therapy to epidermal growth factor receptor-hyperproducing squamous carcinoma. Also, a ^{125}I-labeled monoclonal antibody directed against MW 48,000 human lung cancer–associated antigen may be useful in the diagnosis and treatment of lung cancer [226]. Chan et al. [227] reported that a set of mouse monoclonal antibodies directed against the c-myc oncogene product, a 62,000-d nuclear binding protein involved in cell cycle control, was constructed by immunization with synthetic peptide fragments. After intravenous adminis-tration, these monoclonal antibodies exhibited good tumor localization with primary bronchial carcinoma patients, thus indicating that monoclonal antibodies directed against oncogene products may provide novel selective tools for diagnosis and targeted therapy of cancer. Utilization of mAb to prevent cancer cell metastasis has been examined too. Studies have been done to utilize mAb such as the inhibitor of lung endothelial cell adhesion molecule (anti-lu-ECAM-1) to inhibit colonization of the lung by lung metastatic murine B16 melanoma cells [228]. Lung endothelial cell adhesion molecule (Lu-ECAM-1) has been isolated and characterized [229]; this molecule selectively binds lung-metastatic melanoma cells [230]. In a similar manner mAb 6A3 selectively binds a membrane glycoprotein of rat lung capillary endothelia and has been shown to inhibit specific adhesion of lung endothelial vesicles to lung metastatic breast cancer cells.

Because most monoclonal antibodies that have been studied for tissue targeting are from mouse or, occasionally, from rat, the problem of antibody production to such foreign proteins always exists. While murine-derived mAbs are well tolerated for acute therapy, their use in chronic therapy is limited, due to severe human anti–mouse antibody response (HAMA) [231]. The HAMA response is elicited due to the foreign nature of the antibody itself. Molecular engineering is being utilized to replace the foreign components of the murine antibody with human antibody sequences to overcome their immunogenicity [232].

Recently, successful attempts have been made to develop fully human monoclonal antibodies. Takacs et al. [102] mentioned in their review that, to date, greater than 12 fully human antibodies are currently being profiled in clinical studies.

Future directions for the more effective utilization of monoclonal antibodies as drug targeting agents must focus on a more rational design of the antibody–drug conjugate. Currently, attempts are under way to develop bispecific antibodies combining the VH and VL of two different antibodies into one molecule to ensure cellular targeting constitutes an effective disease treatment [233]. In particular, the chemistry of the linker groups in relation to release mechanisms at the site of action must be carefully evaluated. In addition, chemical entities that could be incorporated into the conjugate structure that may influence its biodistribution should also be investigated. Also, more emphasis should be placed on determining the precise mechanism of action to avoid misinterpretation of in vivo data. In instances where a therapeutic effect has been observed, little attempt has been made to determine whether site specificity has been achieved by the proposed mechanism. Finally, with the increasing availability of human monoclonal antibodies, it is clear that drug–antibody conjugates have even greater potential for clinical therapy, although the cost of manufacturing and purifying monoclonal antibodies still limits their clinical utility.

CONCLUSIONS AND FUTURE DIRECTIONS

The continuing development of targetable drugs to the respiratory tract looks promising. Much emphasis will probably be focused on the respiratory tract as a suitable entry point for proteins and peptides for delivery into the systemic circulation. The use of macromolecule– and monoclonal antibody–drug conjugates will almost certainly increase with the advent of new polymer technology and the availability of human monoclonal antibodies. However, these advances may well be tempered unless parallel progress is made in other important areas. One area that has received relatively little attention is establishing the distribution of metabolizing enzymes throughout the respiratory tract. An in-depth study of the distribution of pulmonary metabolizing enzymes is necessary to achieve a greater cellular selectivity by the activation of appropriately designed prodrugs or drug conjugates in the vicinity of the target cell or a more efficient inactivation to minimize the systemic absorption of the drug.

A greater emphasis will also need to be placed on elucidating epithelial membrane transport mechanisms, especially with regard to improving the epithelial transport of macromolecules. Studies are presently focusing on the microstructural aspects of macromolecular transport across pulmonary epithelia; the results of these investigations will certainly be of value in pulmonary drug-targeting strategies. The discovery of new epithelial and endothelium membrane receptors and of selective materials for binding or adhering to these receptors will also aid in the targeting of drugs to the respiratory tract.

Specific targeting of drugs to other pulmonary targets, such as the alveolar macrophages, which lie in contact with the surfactant lining of the alveoli [234] and which have well-defined surface membrane receptors for initiating particle attachment and phagocytosis [235], may also be exploitable for improving selectivity. If one considers the inhalation route as a means for delivery of drugs to the systemic circulation, then inhaled drugs must enter the circulatory system principally by diffusion or transport across the alveolar capillary membrane. Drug molecules will, therefore, come into contact with the alveolar membrane, the alveolar epithelial cells, the capillary endothelial cells, and other "residents" of the pulmonary circulation, such as the pulmonary intravascular macrophages (PIMs).

These PIMs have been considered a cellular target of potential utility for inhaled drugs [164]. These cells reside in "thick" portions of the pulmonary capillaries and are attached to the capillary endothelium by an electron-dense membrane–adhesive complex. It is likely that such cells would be exposed to high concentrations of inhaled drugs. The PIM cell density appears to increase with pathological stimuli; thus, acute lung injury or lung infection augments the lung burden of PIMs and raises the question of the role of this cell type in the development of lung injury.

Gillespie et al. [164] suggested that microparticulate delivery systems given by intravascular administration might be targeted to PIMs. This suggestion is based on these investigators' observation that particles exceeding 7 μm are often retained in the lung, while smaller particles localize in the liver and spleen. The sequestering in the lung is associated with pulmonary hypertension and lung injury, and, in some cases, it is not related to particle size. Thus, lung sequestering of particles was speculated to be a result of phagocytosis by PIMs and that this could be sued as a means of targeting conventional drug entities, synthetic genes, or antisense oligonucleotides that could perturb PIM function. Any PIMs that have sequestered particulate drug-delivery systems may serve as depots for the release of drug entities into the circulation.

Thus, the future of pulmonary drug targeting is promising, and although drug discovery efforts will no doubt lead to the development of agents with greater selectivity for pulmonary receptors, a greater emphasis will be placed on cell targeting and the development of new macromolecular vectors and cellular targets for this purpose.

REFERENCES

1. Crooks PA, Damani LA. Drug application to the respiratory tract: metabolic and pharmacokinetic considerations. In: Byron PR, ed. Respiratory Drug Delivery. Boca Raton, FL: CRC Press, 1989:61.
2. Brown DT, Marriott C, Beeson MF. J Pharm Pharmacol 1983; 35(suppl):83P.
3. Byron PR, Patton JS. J Aerosol Med 1994; 7:49.
4. Patton JS, Platz RM. Adv Drug Deliv Rev 1992; 8:179.
5. Colthorpe PF, Smith SJ, Wyatt IJ, Taylor D. Pharm Res 1995; 12:356.
6. Possmayer F, Yu S, Weber JM, Harding PGR. Can J Cell Biol 1984; 62:1121.
7. Boucher RC. Human airway ion transport—part one. Am J Respir Crit Care 1994; 150:271.
8. Patton JS. Mechanism of macromolecule absorption by the lung. Adv Drug Deliv 1996; 19:3.
9. Schanker LS. Biochem Pharmacol 1978; 27:381.
10. Schanker LS, Mitchell EW, Brown RA. Drug Metab Dispos 1986; 4:79.
11. Adamson RH, Liu B, Fry GN, Rubin LL, Curry FE. Microvascular permeability and number of tight junctions are modulated by cAMP. Am J Physiol 1998; 274:H1885.
12. Walter U, Geiger J, Haffner C, Market T, Nehls C, Silber RE, Schanzenbacher P. Platelet–vessel wall interactions, focal adhesions, and the mechanism of action of endothelial factors. Agents Action 1995; 45(suppl):255.
13. Taylor A, Khimenko P, Moore T, Adkins W. Fluid Balance. Philadelphia: Lippincott-Raven, 1997.
14. Chetham PM, Babal P, Bridges J, Moore T, Stevens T. Segmental regulation of pulmonary vascular permeability by store operated Ca^{2+} entry. Am J Physiol 1999; 276:L41.
15. Townsley M, Parker J, Longenecker G, Perry M, Pitt R, Taylor A. Pulmonary embolism: analysis of endothelial pore sizes in canine lung. Am J Physiol 1988; 255:H1075.
16. Moore T, Chetham PM, Kelly JJ, Stevens T. Signal transduction and regulation of lung endothelial cell permeability: interaction between calcium and camp. Am J Physiol 1998; 275:L203.
17. Del Vecchio P, Siflinger-Birnboim A, Belloni PN, Holleran LA, Lum H, Malik AB. Culture and characterization of pulmonary microvascular endothelial cells. In Vitro Cell Dev Biol 1992; 28A:711.
18. Schaeffer R Jr, Bitrick M Jr. Effects of human a-thrombin and 8-bromo-cAMP on large and microvessel endothelial monolayer equivalent "pore" radii. Microvasc Res 1995; 49:364.
19. Schnitzer J, Siflinger-Birnboim A, Del Vecchio PJ, Malik AB. Segmental differentiation of permeability, protein glycosylation, and morphology of cultured bovine lung vascular endothelium. Biochem Biophys Res Commun 1994; 199:11.
20. Seibert AF, Thompson WJ, Taylor A, Wilborn WH, Bernard J, Haynes J. Reversal of increased microvascular permeability associated with ischemia-reperfusion: role of cAMP. J Appl Physiol 1992; 72:389.

21. Stevens T, Creighton J, Thompson J. Control of cAMP in lung endothelial cell phenotype. Implications for control of barrier function. Am J Physiol 1999; 277:L119.

22. Wangensteen D. Microstructural aspects of macromolecular transport across pulmonary epithelia. In: Proceedings of the Second International Symposium on Respiratory Drug Delivery (in press).

23. Burton PS. The influence of peptide structure on transport across epithelial cells. In: Proceedings of the Second International Symposium on Respiratory Drug Delivery (in press).

24. Schnee EE, Lynch RD. Am J Physiol 1992; 262:L647.

25. Vaccaro CA, Brody JS. J Cell Biol 1981; 91:427.

26. Sun, JZ, Byron PR, Rypacek F. Pharm Res 1999; 16(7):1104.

27. Niven RW, Rypacek F, Byron PR. Pharm Res 1990; 7:990.

28. Benford DJ, Bridges JW. Prog Drug Metab 1986; 9:53.

29. Sabourin PJ, Dahl AR. Distribution of the FAD-containing monooxygenase in respiratory tract tissues. Annual Report LMF-114. In: Medinsky MA, Muggenburg BA, eds. National Technical Information Service. Springfield, VA, 1985:156.

30. Gonda I, Harpur ES. Metabolism of hexamethylmelamine by rodent lung microsomes. In: Proceedings of 10th International Congress of Pharmacology (IUPHAR), 1987; 1045.

31. Sly RM. J Allergy Clin Immunol 1989; 84:421; Buiet AS. J Allergy Clin Immunol 1989; 84:275.

32. Lenny W, Wells N, O'Neal BA. Eur Respir Rev 1994; 4:49.

33. Barnes NC. J Pharm Pharmacol 1997; 49:13.

34. Chhabra SK, Bhatnager S. Indian J Chest Allied Sci 2002; 44(2):91.

35. Lands AM, Ludena FP, Buzzo HJ. Life Sci 1967; 6:2241; Collier JG, Dornhurst AC. Nature 1969; 223:1283.

36. Iversen LL. Br J Pharmacol 1971; 41:571.

37. Carstairs JR, Nimmo AJ, Barnes PJ. Am Rev Respir Dis 1985; 132:541.

38. Ullman A, Svedmyr N. Thorax 1988; 43:674.

39. Bradshaw J, Brittain RT, Coleman RA, Jack D, Kennedy I, Lunts LHC, Skidmore IF. Br J Pharmacol 1987; 92:590.

40. Ullman A, Svedmyr N. Am Rev Respir Dis 1988; 137(suppl):32A.

41. Lofdahl CG, Svedmyr N. Am Rev Respir Dis 1988; 137(suppl):330A.

42. Barnes PJ. Eur Respir J 2002; 19(1):182.

43. Chiarino D, Fantucci M, Della Bella D, Frigeni V, Sala R. Farmaco Ed Sci 1986; 41:4401.

44. Minneman KP, Hegstrand LR, Molinoff PB. Mol Pharmacol 1979; 16:21; Minneman KP, Hedberg KP, Molinoff PB. J Pharm Exp 1979, 211:502.

45. Rugg EL, Barnett DB, Nahorski SR. Mol Pharmacol 1978; 14:996.

46. Levy GP, Apperley GH. In: Szabadi E, Bradshaw CM, Bevan P, eds. Recent Advances in the Pharmacology of Adrenoceptors. Amsterdam: Elsevier/North Holland, 1978:201.

47. Gibson DJ, Coltart DJ. Postgrad Med J 1971; 45(S):40.

48. Ryan G, Dolovich MB, Obminski G, Cockcroft DW, Juniper E, Hargreave FE, Newhouse MT. J Allergy Clin Immunol 1981; 67:156.
49. Shaw A. Annu Rep Med Chem 1989; 25:61.
50. Cheng HC, Woodward JK. Drug Dev Res 1982; 2:11.
51. Villani FJ, Magatti CV, Vashi DB, Wong J, Popper TL. Arzneim Forschd/Drug Res 1986; 36:1311.
52. Ahn HS, Barnett A. Eur J Pharmacol 1986; 127:153.
53. Brown EA, Griffiths R, Harvey CA, Owen DAA. Rev J Pharmacol 1986; 87:569.
54. Nicholson AN, Stone BM. Br J Clin Pharmacol 1995; 19:127P.
55. deVos C, Rihoux JP, Juhlin L. In: Proceedings of the Congress of the European Academy of Allergology and Clinical Immunology. Budapest, 1986.
56. Stokbroekx RA, Luyckx MGM, Willems JJM, Janssen M, Bracke JOMM, Joosen RLP, Van Wauwe IP. Drug Dev Res 1986; 8:87.
57. Fugner A, Bechtel WD, Kuhn FJ, Mierau J. Arzneim-Forschd/Drug Res 1988; 32:1445.
58. Nolan JC, Stephens DJ, Proakis AG, Leonard CA, Johnson DN, Kilpatrick BF, Foxwell MH, Yanni JJ. Agents Actions 1989; 28:53.
59. Palmer GC, Radov LA, Napier JJ, Griffiths RC, Stagnitto ML, Garske GE. FASEB J 1989; 3:A639.
60. Vincent J, Liminana R, Meredith PA, Reid JL. Br J Clin Pharmacol 1988; 26:497.
61. Vincent J, Summer DJ, Reid JL. Br J Clin Pharmacol 1988; 26:503.
62. Zaagsma J, Roffel AF, Meurs H. Life Sci 1997; 60:1061.
63. Buckle DR, Smith H. Development of Anti-asthma Drugs. London: Butterworths, 1984:159–183.
64. Rominger KL. Chemistry and pharmacokinetics of ipratropium bromide. Scand J Respir Dis 1978; 103(suppl):116–129.
65. Frith PA, Ruffin RE, Cockcroft DW, Hargreave FE. J Allergy Clin Immunol 1978; 61:175.
66. Storms WW, DePico OA, Reed CE. Am Rev Respir Dis 1975; 111:419.
67. Schlueter DP, Neuman JL. Chest 1978; 73(suppl):982.
68. Tamoaki J, Chiyotani A, Tagaya E, Sakai N, Konno K. Thorax 1994; 49:545.
69. Alabaster VA. Life Sci 1997; 60:1053.
70. Kelly HW. J Allergy Clin Immunol 1998; 102:S36.
71. Pedersen S, O'Byrne P. Allergy 1997; 52:1.
72. Allen DB. Acta Paediatr 1998; 87(2):123.
73. Bernstein DI, Berkowitz RB, Chervinsky P, Dvorin DJ, Finn AF, Gross GN, Karetsky M, Kerap JP, Laforce C, Lumry W, Mendelson LM, Nelson H, Pearlman D, Rachelefsky G, Ratner P, Repsher L, Segal AT, Selner JC, Settipare GA, Wanderer A, Guss FM, Nolop KB, Harrison JE. Respir Med 1999; 93:603.
74. Barnes PJ, Pedersen S, Busse WW. Am J Respir Crit Care Med 1998; 157:S1.
75. Onrust SV, Lamb HM. Drugs 1998; 56(4):725.
76. Petersen H, Kullberg A, Edsbacker S, Greiff L. Br J Clin Pharmacol 2001; 51(2):159.
77. Miller-Larson A, Mattsson H, Hjertberg E, Dahlback M, Tunek A, Brattsand R. Drug Metab Dispos 1998; 26(7):623.

78. Sorkness CA. J Allergy Clin Immunol 1998; 102:S52.
79. Petersen H, Kulbery A, Edsbacker S, Creiff L. Br J Clin Pharm 2001; 51(2):159.
80. Van Grunsen PM, Van Schaych CP, Derenne JP, Kerstjens HA, Renkema TE, Postma DS, Similowski T, Akkermans RP, Pasker PC, Jong D, Dekhuijzen PN, Van Herwaarden CL, Van Weel C. Thorax 1999; 54:7.
81. Douglas WP, Barnette HS, Barnette MS. Annu Rep Med Chem 1999; 34(11):111.
82. Lacoste JY, Bousquet J, Chanez P, et al. J Allergy Clin Immunol 1993; 92:537.
83. Ziment I. Clin Chest Med 1990; 11:461.
84. Van Schaych CP, Van Grunsven PM, Dekhuijzen PNR. Eur Respir J 1996; 9:1969.
85. Wilson JD, Serby CW, Menjoge SS, Witek TJ Jr. Eur Respir J 1996; 6:286.
86. Barnes PJ. J Allergy Clin Immunol 1996; 97:159.
87. Britton JR, Hanley SP, Tattersfield AE. J Allergy Clin Immunol 1987; 79:811; Fleisch JH, Cloud ML, Marshall WS. Ann NY Acad Sci 1988; 524:356; Barnes N, Evans J, Zakrzewski J, Piper P, Costello J. Ann NY Acad Sci 1988; 524:369.
88. Smith L, Geller S, Ebright, L, Glass M, Thyrum PT. Am Rev Respir Dis 1990; 141(4):988.
89. Krell RD, Buckner CK, Keith RA, Snyder DW, Brown FJ, Bernstein PR, Matussa V, Yee YK, Hesp B, Giles RE. J Allergy Clin Immunol 1988; 81:276.
90. Jones TR, Zamboni R, Belley M, Champion E, Charette L, Ford-Hutchinson AW, Frenette R, Gauthier J-Y, Leger S, Masson P, McFarlane CS, Piechuta H, Rokach J, Williams H, Young RN, Dehaven R, Pong SS. Can J Physiol Pharmacol 1989; 67:17.
91. Depre M, Margolskee DJ, Van Hecken A, Hsieh JSY, Buntinx A, De Schepper PJ, Rogers JD. Eur J Clin Pharmacol 1992; 43(4):431.
92. Jacob RT, Veale CA, Wolanin DJ. Annu Rep Med Chem 1992; 27(12):109.
93. Joos GF, Kips JC, Puttemans M, Pauwels RA, Van Der Straeten ME. J Allergy Clin Immunol 1989; 83:187.
94. Creticos PS, Bodenheimer S, Albright A, Lichtenstein LM, Norman PB. J Allergy Clin Immunol 1989; 83:187.
95. Evans JM, Barnes NC, Zakzewski JT, Sciberras DG, Stahl EG, Piper J, Costello JF. Br J Clin Pharmacol 1989; 28:125.
96. Brooks DM, Summers JB, Gunn BP, Martin JC, Martin MB, Mazdiyasni H, Holms JH, Stewart AO, Moore JL, Young PR, Albert DH, Bouska JB, Dyer RD, Bell RL, Carter GW. 197th ACS Annual Meeting (abstr) (MEDI 69 1989).
97. Bruneau BJ, Crawley GC, Edwards MP, Foster SJ, Girodeau JM, Kingston JF, McMillan RM. UK J Med Chem 1991; 34(7):2176.
98. Hoshino M, Sim JJ, Shimizu K, Nakayama H, Koya A. J Allergy Clin Immunol 1999; 103(6):1054.
99. Misra RN, Brown BR, Han WC, Harris DN, Hedberg A, Webb ML, Hall SE. J Med Chem 1991; 34(9):2882.
100. Beasly RCW, Featherstone RL, Church MK, Rafferty P, Varley JG, Harris A, Robinson C, Holgate ST. J Appl Physiol 1989; 66:1685.
101. Hubbard RC, Casolaro MA, Mitchell M, Sellers SE, Arabia F, Matthay MA, Crystal RG. Proc Natl Acad Sci 1989; 86:680.
102. FDC Reports, May 22, 1989.

103. Bonney RJ, Ashe B, Maycock A, Dellea P, Hand K, Osinga D, Fletcher D, Mumford R, Davies P, Frankenfield D, Nolan T, Schaeffer L, Hagman W, Finke F, Shah S, Dom C, Doherty J. J Cell Biochem 1989; 39:47.

104. Williams JC, Stein RL, Knee C, Egan J, Falcone R, Trainor D, Edwards P, Wolanin D, Wildonger R, Schwartz J, Heap B, Giles RE, Krell RD. Am Rev Respir Dis 1988; 137:206.

105. Iwasaw Y, Gillis CN, Aghajanian G. J Pharmacol Exp Ther 1973; 186:498.

106. Pitt BR, Hammond GL, Gillis CN. J Appl Physiol 1982; 52:1545.

107. Baron J, Bruke JP, Guengerich FP, Jakoby WB, Voigt JM. Toxicol Appl Pharmacol 1988; 93:493.

108. Forman HJ, Aldrich TK, Posner MA, Fisher AB. J Pharmacol Exp Ther 1982; 221:428.

109. Wilson AGE, Pickett RD, Eling TE, Anderson MW. Drug Metab Dispos 1979; 7:420.

110. Lullmann H, Rossen E, Seiler KU. J Pharm Pharmacol 1973; 25:239.

111. Minchin RF, Barber HE, Ilett KF. Drug Metab Dispos 1982; 10:356.

112. Fowler JS, Gallagher BM, MacGregor RR, Wolf AP. J Pharmacol Exp Ther 1976; 198:133.

113. Kostenbauder HB, Sloneker S. Prodrugs for pulmonary drug targeting. In: Byron PR, ed. Respiratory Drug Delivery. Boca Raton, FL: CRC Press, 1990:91–106.

114. Kostenbauder HB. Extending duration of drug activity in the lung. In: Proceedings of the Second International Conference on Respiratory Drug Delivery (in press).

115. Lofdahl CG, Svedmyr N. Acta Pharmacol Toxicol 1986; 5(suppl):229.

116. Brittain RT, Dean CM, Jack D. Int Encycl Pharmacol Ther 1981; 104:613.

117. Ullman A, Svednyr N. Thorax 1988; 423:674.

118. Suwa T, Kohno Y, Yoshida H, Morimoto S, Suga T. J Pharm Sci 1989; 79:783.

119. Clissold SP, Heel RC. Drugs 1984; 28:485.

120. Edsbacker S. Studies on the Metabolic Fate and Human Pharmacokinetics of Budenoside. Ph.D. dissertation, University of Lund, Sweden, 1986.

121. Andersson P, Lihne M, Thalen A, Ryrfeldt A. Xenobiotica 1987; 17:35.

122. Ryrfeldt A, Edsbacker S. Clin Pharmacol Ther 1984; 35:525.

123. Ryrfeldt A, Persson G, Nilsson E. Biochem Pharmacol 1989; 38:17.

124. Hussain AA, Truelove JE. U.S. Patent 3,868,461, 1975.

125. Shargel L, Dorrbecker SA. Drug Metab Dispos 1976; 4:72.

126. Olsson AT, Svensson L-A. Pharm Res 1984; 1:19.

127. Friedel HA, Brogden RN. Drugs 1988; 35:22.

128. Small D, Kostenbauder HB. Unpublished data, 1985.

129. Andersoon P. Acta Pharmacol Toxicol 1976; 39:225.

130. Ryrfeldt A, Bodin N-O. Xenobiotica 1975; 5:521.

131. Holstein-Rathlou N-H, Laursen LC, Madsen F, Svendsen UG, Grosspelius Y, Weeke B. Eur J Clin Pharmacol 1986; 30:7.

132. Sitar DS. Clinical pharmacokinetics of Bambuterol. Clin Pharmacokinet 1996; 31(4):246.

133. Svensson LA. Acta Pharm Suec 1987; 24:333.

134. Svensson LA. Pharm Res 1985; 2:156.

135. Sharma R, Saxena D, Dwivedi AK, Misra A. Pharm Res 2001; 18:1405.
136. Zhou H, Lengsfeld C, Claffey DJ, Ruth JA, bertson B, Rondolph TW, Ng K, Manning M. J Pharm Sci 2002; 91(6):1502.
137. Ranney DF. Biochem Pharmacol 1986; 35:1063.
138. Ranney DF. International Patent, WO 88/07365, 1988.
139. Krepela E, Vicar J, Zizkova L, Dazafirek E, Kolar Z, Lichnovsky V. Lung 1985; 163:33.
140. Catravas JD, White RE. J Appl Physiol 1981; 50:1161.
141. Ryan US, Ryan JW, Whitaker C, Chiu A. Tissue Cell 1976; 8:125.
142. Ryan JW. Am J Physiol 1989; 257(2):L53.
143. Dent G, Giembycz MA, Rabe KF, Barnes PJ. Br J Pharmacol 1991; 103:1339.
144. Staford JA, Feldman PL. Annu Rep Med Chem 1996; 34(8):71.
145. Santing RE, Olymunder CG, Molen KV, Meurs H, Zaagsma J. Eur J Pharmacol 1995; 275:75.
146. Tanaka T, Yamamoto A, Amenomori A. European Patent Applications. EPO671389.
147. Stafford JA, Veal JM, Feldman PL, Valvano NL, Baer PG, Brackeen MF, Brawley ES, Cornolly KM, Domanico PL, Han B, Rose DA, Rutkowske RD, Sekut L, Strickland AB, Verghese MW. J Med Chem 1995; 38:4972.
148. Takenag AK. Invasion Metastasis 1997; 16(2):97.
149. Crooks PA. Lung peptidases and their activities. In: Proceedings of the Second International Conference on Respiratory Drug Delivery (in press).
150. Catravas JD, Lazo JS, Dobuler KJ, Mills LR, Gillis CN. Am Rev Respir Dis 1983; 128:740.
151. Ryan US, Ryan JW. Clin Lab Med 1983; 3:577.
152. Ryan US. Endothelial cell activation response. In: Ryan US, ed. Pulmonary Endothelium in Health and Disease. New York: Marcel Dekker, 1987:3.
153. Ryan JW. Assay of pulmonary endothelial surface enzymes in vivo. In: Ryan US, ed. Pulmonary Endothelium in Health and Disease. New York: Marcel Dekker, 1987:161.
154. Rigaudy R, Charcosset J-Y, Garbay-Jaureguiberry C, Jacquemin-Sablon A, Roques BP. Cancer Res 1989; 49:1836.
155. Shao J, Dettaven J, Laman D, Weissman DN, Ruyan K, Malanga C, Rojanasakul Y, Ma J. Drug Deliv 2001; 8(2):61.
156. Shao J, Dettaven J, Laman D, Weissman DN, Malanga C, Rojanasakul Y, Ma J. Drug Deliv 2001; 8(2):71.
157. Jones AL, Kellaway IW, Taylor G. J Pharm Pharmacol 1989; 41:92P.
158. King GL, Johnson SM. Science 1985; 227:1583.
159. Sezaki H, Hashida M. CRC Crit Rev Ther Drug Carrier Syst 1984–1985; 1:1.
160. Hashida M, Kato A, TakaBura Y, Sezaki H. Drug Metab Dispos 1984; 12.
161. Tomlinson E. Site-specific drug deliver using particulate systems. In: Bunker G, Rhodes CT, eds. Modern Pharmaceutics. 40:673–693.
162. Miyamoto K, Shultz E, Heath T, Mitchell MD, Albertine KH, Staul NC. J Appl Physiol 1988; 64:1143.
163. Warner AE, Molilna RM, Brain JD. Am Rev Respir Dis 1987; 136:683.

164. Gillespie MN, Aziz SM, Pauly TH. Pulmonary intravascular macrophages: cellular targets of opportunity for inhaled drugs. In: Proceeds of the Second International Conference on Respiratory Drug Delivery (in press).

165. Brain JD, Warner AE, Molina RM, DeCamp MM. Am Rev Respir Dis 1988; 137:A147.

166. Illum L, Davis SS, Muller RH, Mak E, West P. Life Sci 1987; 40:367.

167. Illum L, Davis SS. FEPS Lett 1984; 107:79.

168. Kopecak J, Duncan R. Poly N-(2-hydroxypropyl) methacrylamide macromolecules as drug carrier systems. In: Ilium L, Davies SS, eds. Controlled Release of Drugs from Polymeric Particles and Macromolecules. Bristol, UK: Adam Hilger, 1988.

169. Kopecek J. Synthesis of tailor-made soluble polymeric drug carriers. In: Kim SW, Anderson J, eds. Recent Advances in Drug Delivery Systems. New York: Plenum Press, 1984:41.

170. Kojima T, Hashida M, Muranishi S, Sezaki H. J Pharm Pharmacol 1980; 32:30.

171. Fimm MV. CRC Crit Rev Ther Drug Carrier Syst 1988; 5:189.

172. Ryser HJP, Shen WC. Proc Natl Acad Sci USA 1978; 75:3867.

173. Chu BCF, Whiteley JM. Mol Pharmacol 1980; 17:382.

174. Robbins JC, Lam MH, Tripp CS, Bugianesi RL, Ponpipom MM, Shen TY. Proc Natl Acad Sci USA 1981; 78:7924.

175. Monsigny M, Roche A-C, Bailey P. Biochem Biophys Res Commun 1984; 121:579.

176. Kerr DJ, Hynds SA, Shepherd J, Packard CJ, Kaye SB. Biochem Pharmacol 1988; 37:3981.

177. Veale D, Kerr N, Gibson GJ, Harris AL. Cancer Res 1989; 49:1313.

178. Masui H, Kawamoto T, Sato JD, Wolf B, Sato G, Mendelsohn J. Cancer Res 1984; 44:1002.

179. Vollmar AM, Banker DE, Mendelsohn J, Herschman HR. J Cell Physiol 1987; 131:418.

180. Gu J-M, Robinson JR, Leung S-HS. CRC Crit Rev Ther Drug Carrier Syst 1988–1989; 5:21.

181. Bruck A, Abu-Dahab R, Borchard G, Schafer UF, Lehr CM. Drug Targeting 2001; 9(4):241.

182. Waldrep JC, Gilbert BE, Knight CM, Black MB, Scherer PW, Knight V, Eschenbacher W. Chest 1997; 111:316.

183. Terranova V, Rohrbach D, Martin GR. Cell 1980; 22:719.

184. Vlodavsky D. Gospodarowicz. Nature (London) 1980; 289:304.

185. Rennard SI, Gullino M, Martin JR, Katz SI. Lab Investig 1980; 42:336.

186. Lopes JD, dos Reis M, Brentani RR. Science 1985; 229:275.

187. Malinoff HL, Wicha MS. J Cell Biol 1983; 96:1475.

188. Newman SA, Frenz DA, Tomasek JJ, Rabuzzi DD. Science 1985; 228:885.

189. Brown PJ, Juliano RL. Science 1985; 228:1448.

190. Williams SK, Devenny JJ, Bitensky MM. Proc Natl Acad Sci USA 1981; 78:2393.

191. Fransson L-A. Eur J Biochem 1981; 120:251.

192. Shimada K, Gill PJ, Silbert JE, Douglas WH. J Clin Investig 1981; 68:995.

193. Ordonez NG, Batsakis JG. Arch Pathol Lab Med 1984; 108:129.

194. Holthofer H, Virtanen I, Kariniemi A-L, Hormia M, Linder E, Miettinen A. Lab Investig 1982; 47:60.
195. Miettinen M, Holthofer H, Lehto V-P, Miettinen A, Virtanen I. Am J Clin Pathol 1983; 79:32.
196. Pietra GG, Sampson P, Lanken PN, Hansen-Flaschen J, Fishman AP. Lab Investig 1983; 49:54.
197. Bevilacqua MP, Pober JS, Majeau GR, Cotran RS, Gimbrone MA. J Exp Med 1984; 160:618.
198. Anderson JH, Koivisto VA. Drugs Today 1998; 34:37.
199. Owens D. Nat Res Drug Discov 2002; 1(17):529.
200. Steiner S, Pfutzner A, Wilson BR, Harzer O, Heinemann L, Rave K. Exp Clin Endocrinol Diabetes 2002.
201. Skyler JS, Cetalu WT, Kourides IA, Landschulz WH, Balagtas CC, Cheng SL, Gelfand RA. Lancet 2001; 357(9253):331.
202. Mathe G, Tran BL, Bernard J. Compt Rend 1958; 246:1626.
203. Takacs L, Vazquez-Abad MD, Elliott EA. Annu Rep Med Chem 2001; 36(23):237.
204. Stephens S, Emtage S, Vetterlein O, Chaplin L, Bebbington C, Nesbitt A, Sopwith M, Thwal DA, Novak C, Bodmer M. Immunology 1995; 85:668.
205. Pimm MV. CRC Crit Rev Ther Drug Carrier Syst 1988–1989; 5:189.
206. Chan YT, Evans GI, Ritson A, Watson J, Wraight P, Sikora K. Br J Cancer 1986; 54:761.
207. Milgrom H, Fick RB Jr., Su JQ, Reimann JD, Bush RK, Watrous ML, Metzger WJ. N Engl J Med 1999; 341:1966.
208. Easthope S, Jarvis B. Drugs 2001; 61(2):253.
209. Colcher D, Esterban J, Carrasquillo JA, Sugarbaker P, Reynolds JC, Bryant G, Larson SM, Schlom J. Cancer Res 1987; 47:4218.
210. De Duve C, De Barsy T, Poole B, Trouet A, Tuckens P, Van Hoof F. Biochem Pharmacol 1975; 23:2495.
211. Pimm MV, Jones JA, Price MR, Middle JG, Embleton JM, Baldwin RW. Cancer Immunol Immunother 1982; 12:125.
212. Hurwitz E, Schechter B, Arnon R, Sela M. Int J Cancer 1979; 24:461.
213. Tsukada Y, Ohkawa K, Hibi N. Cancer Res 1997; 47:4293.
214. Garnett MC, Embleton MJ, Jacobs E, Baldwin RW. Int J Cancer 1983; 31:661.
215. Tsukada Y, Kato Y, Takeda Y, Hara T, Hirai H. J Natl Cancer Inst 1984; 73:721.
216. Corvalan JRF, Smith W, Gore VA, Brandon DR. Cancer Immunol Immunother 1987; 24:133.
217. Corvalan JRF, Smith W. Cancer Immunol Immunother 1987; 24:127.
218. Corvalan JRF, Smith W, Gore VA, Brandon DR, Ryde PJ. Cancer Immunol Immunother 1997; 24:138.
219. Ilnatowich DJ, Virzi F, Rusckowski M. J Nucl Med 1987; 28:1294.
220. Andrew SM, Perkins AC, Pimm MV, Baldwin RW. Eur J Nucl Med 1988; 13:598.
221. Buchegger F, Haskell CM, Schreyer M, Scazziga BR, Randin S, Carrel S, Mach I-P. J Exp Med 1983; 158:413.
222. Rowland GF, Simmonds RG, Gore VA, Marsden CH, Smith W. Cancer Immunol Immunother 1986; 21:183.

223. Brown PJ, Juliano RL. Science 1985; 228:1448.
224. Wick G, Muller PU, Timpl R. Clin Immunol Immunother 1982; 23:656.
225. Hirota N, Ueda M, Ozawa S, Abe O, Shimizu N. Cancer Res 1989; 49:7106.
226. Endo K, Kamma H, Ogata T. Cancer Res 1987; 47:5427.
227. Chan SYT, Evan GI, Ritson A, Watson J, Wraight P, Sikora K. Br J Cancer 1986; 54:761.
228. Zhu D, Cheng CF, Pauli BU. J Clin Investig 1992; 89:1718.
229. Elble RC, Widom J, Levine R, Goodwin A, Cheng HC, Pauli BU. J Biol Chem 1997; 272:27853.
230. Zhu D, Pauli BU. Int J Cancer 1993; 53:628.
231. Schroff RW. Cancer Res 1985; 45:879.
232. Birch JR, Lennox ES, eds. Monoclonal Antibodies. New York: Wiley-Liss, 1995.
233. Van Spriel AB, Van Ojik HH, Van De Winkel JGJ. Immunol Today 2000; 21:391.
234. Weibel ER, Gil J. Respir Physiol 1969; 4:42.
235. Rowlands DT, Daniele RP. N Engl J Med 1975; 293:26.

5

Lung Deposition Simulation

W. H. Finlay
University of Alberta, Edmonton, Alberta, Canada

INTRODUCTION

Inhaled pharmaceutical aerosols cannot act unless they deposit in the respiratory tract. However, the amount and location of such deposition is strongly affected by several factors, including aerosol properties, breath pattern, and lung geometry. Since some control over aerosol properties and breath pattern is possible when designing an inhaled aerosol formulation, access to tools that permit parametric exploration of lung deposition is useful in order to optimize these parameters and guide preclinical development. It is for this reason that methods allowing simulation of deposition in the lung have become increasingly common in the respiratory drug delivery arena.

An example of the kind of information that can be obtained with lung deposition models is given in Fig. 1, where a one-dimensional Lagrangian dynamical model (see later in this chapter for an explanation of this term) is combined with a model of the mucous and periciliary layers to give estimates of drug concentration in the liquid lining the airways when a novel liposomal antimicrobial peptide is delivered as an inhaled aerosol [1]. A similar approach was used by Finlay et al. [2] to guide the development of an inhaled aerosol

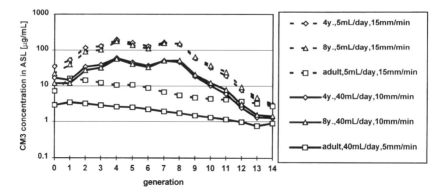

FIGURE 1 Estimated concentrations of liposomally encapsulated peptide (CM3) in the airway surface liquid (ASL) immediately after completion of nebulization for various simulated subject ages, mucus production rates, and tracheal mucous velocities. Generation 0 corresponds to the trachea, while the terminal bronchioles are generation 14. (From Ref. 1, with permission.)

therapy for the treatment of pulmonary infection and mucous clearance in cystic fibrosis.

Information like that in Fig. 1, and the respiratory tract deposition information that lies behind this data, is increasingly becoming part of the preclinical development process with inhaled pharmaceutical aerosols. The purpose of the present chapter is to briefly outline some of the deposition models that have been used with inhaled pharmaceutical aerosols and their basis. The reader is referred to Finlay [3] for a detailed treatment of the underlying mechanics.

It should be noted that throughout this chapter, the words *model* and *simulation* are used to mean a procedure that solves mathematical equations to represent reality. This may be a less common definition of the word *model* for some readers. However, since the equations governing aerosol and fluid motion are well established and represent reality exactly, such models have the ability to represent reality exactly, at least in principle.

It should be also be mentioned that little attention has been paid to modeling deposition in lungs altered by disease, largely because the geometry of diseased lung airways has not been well characterized and is different for each disease as well as being dependent on the progression of the disease. Application of the approaches discussed in this chapter to diseased lungs is thus largely a topic for future research.

THE NEED FOR SIMPLIFICATION

Most readers would probably intuitively agree that simulating the behavior of an aerosol as it is inhaled and dispersed throughout the entire respiratory tract is a difficult task. In fact, at the present time it is impossible to precisely simulate this behavior because the geometry of the lung, including the time-dependent shape of all several hundred million alveoli, is not known. However, let us say that some dramatic breakthrough in imaging technology allowed us to determine the detailed three-dimensional geometry of all airspaces in the lung throughout an entire breath. Would it then be feasible to precisely simulate what happens to an inhaled aerosol in the respiratory tract?

To answer this question, let us take the simplest case of a dilute aerosol consisting of spherical, stable (i.e., nonevaporating, noncondensing) particles. To determine the fate of this aerosol, we must solve the governing equations, which are based simply on mass conservation and Newton's second law, both for the air that carries the aerosol and the aerosol itself. It is not possible to solve these equations at the infinite number of spatial locations in the respiratory tract, so instead we solve these equations on a computer at a finite number of "grid points" and interpolate the solution at all other points. To achieve reasonable accuracy, each individual airway (with associated alveoli) in each generation in the lung needs to be divided into approximately 10^5 grid points. With 23 lung generations, there are

$$\sum_{i=0}^{23} 2^i = 16,777,215$$

individual airways in the lung, resulting in the need for more than 10^{12} grid points in total. At each grid point we need to store the air and aerosol conditions, so we will require several terabytes (i.e., several thousand gigabytes) of RAM on any computer on which we hope to solve these equations. This is a major limitation, since only a handful of computers in the world have this kind of memory capacity, and access to these computers is severely restricted, usually to military applications.

Assuming we did manage to find a computer with terabytes of RAM, how long would it take for such a computer to solve the governing equations at our 10^{12} grid points? A reasonable estimate can be made by assuming 10^3 floating point operations are needed to solve for the air and aerosol conditions at a grid point, with these operations being needed at each of approximately 100 steps in time throughout a breath (since the lung geometry varies with time as the alveoli fill), yielding a total of 10^{17} floating point operations. Typical desktop computers can perform less than 10^9 floating point operations per second (flops), so we would need to wait over 10^8 seconds, which is more than three years!

Even the latest ASCI (Advanced Strategic Computing Initiative) computer developed by the U.S. Department of Defense, costing $200 million, occupying 21,000 square feet, and running at 30×10^{12} flops, would take an hour to solve this problem.

From these simple estimates, it is seen that while a three-dimensional full lung simulation (hereafter abbreviated as FLS, with "three-dimensional" always implied) of the air and aerosol flow in the entire respiratory is not beyond the realm of possibility if the detailed geometry of the lung was known, such a large calculation is impractical at present. Assuming that, according to "Moore's law," computers double in speed every 18 months, it will be less than 20 years before FLS takes less than 20 minutes on a good desktop computer, which may make it a more attractive approach at that time. However, deposition of aerosol particles in the respiratory tract is merely the first step in a series of relatively poorly understood steps (at least from a mechanistically predictive point of view) that lead to the onset of action of a drug. Simulation of the subsequent disposition of drug, including its dissolution, pharmacokinetics, and finally pharmacodynamics, requires an understanding at a cellular and molecular level that remains incomplete. As a result, although FLS may be useful in developing and refining simpler deposition models, at present it is not feasible from the perspective of aiding preclinical development. Instead, simplifications are used, to which we now turn.

EMPIRICAL MODELS

At the other end of the spectrum from FLS in terms of computational requirements lie the simplest models that can be considered, which are the empirical models. These models are usually based on parametric curve fits to in vivo data of aerosol deposition in humans or to data from more complicated lung deposition models. The simplest of all such models is the rule of thumb that inhaled pharmaceutical aerosol should have particle diameters in some "fine particle" range of, e.g., 1–5 μm, which is based on observations that lung deposition during tidal breathing (of monodisperse aerosols from tubes inserted partway into the mouth) decreases for particles with diameters on either side of this range (see, e.g., Ref. 4).

Several popular empirical models adopted for respiratory pharmaceutical use owe their existence to the need for radiological dose estimation of inhaled particulates, beginning with the ICRP Task Group on Lung Dynamics [5], now superseded by ICRP [6] or alternatively NCRP [7]. Yeh et al. [8] compare the ICRP [6] and NCRP [7] models, with the largest differences between these models occurring for particles that are smaller than those used in respiratory drug delivery (i.e, <0.1 μm diameters). Other empirical models include Yu et al. [9] and Davies [10].

For inhaled pharmaceutical aerosols, the principal attractions of empirical models are the ease with which they can be programmed (requiring little more than entering a handful of algebraic equations into a spreadsheet) and the small amount of computation time they require (typically taking less than a second on a PC). Compared to simply using some rule of thumb specifying that particle size must be in some range, empirical models give considerable additional information. In particular, they can provide predictions of doses depositing in various morphological regions (e.g., alveolar, tracheobronchial, and extrathoracic regions), and these predictions depend on the particle size distribution and inhalation parameters (e.g., flow rate and inhaled volume), which the user supplies as input. Thus, these models allow a degree of parametric optimization that a particle size rule of thumb does not allow.

However, empirical models must be used with caution, for several reasons. First, the mouth–throat (oropharyngeal) deposition predictions of existing empirical models usually differ considerably from reality when inhaling from existing dry powder inhalers and metered-dose inhalers [11,12]. DeHaan and Finlay [13] and Finlay et al. [14] show that these models predict mouth–throat deposition well for devices with mouthpieces and exit fluid flow that resemble a straight tube exit (which these models are based on), such as nebulizers, but do not perform well for devices that differ from this, such as dry powder inhalers. For metered-dose inhalers, additional errors occur due to the high speed of the aerosol relative to the inhaled air, an effect not present in the experimental in vivo data on which these models are based. These concerns are not minor, since correct prediction of lung deposition is entirely dependent on correct prediction of mouth–throat deposition. This is because with single-breath inhalation devices there is negligible exhaled aerosol, especially with breath holding, so any aerosol not depositing in the mouth–throat deposits in the lung. As a result, underestimation of mouth–throat deposition by 50% of the inhaled dose, which is not uncommon with these empirical models [13], results in overestimation of the lung dose by the same amount.

A partial solution to this failing of existing empirical models is to use them only to predict deposition distal to the mouth–throat, relying instead on benchtop measurements in mouth–throat replicas to give the particle size and dose delivered distal to the oropharynx [15,16]. Such a procedure is not without its drawbacks though, since mouth–throat deposition varies dramatically between different individuals (see Ref. 4), so care must be taken to ensure the mouth–throat replica is an "average" one in its particle size vs. flow rate filtering properties (e.g., Ref. 14). In addition, inhaler aerosols (and their deposition) are often flow rate dependent, so care must be taken to ensure that the flow rates used in the benchtop testing are similar to those used during delivery in vivo. This will depend on the device, but if a constant-flow-rate sizing apparatus is used, this may mean using flow rates from the early part of the breath, not the average of peak inhalation flow rates, since aerosol delivery may occur during the flow acceleration phase of the breath, when flow rates are below their average or peak values [17,18]. Alternatively, breath simulation can be done to avoid this issue [19], although this complicates particle sizing by cascade impaction and may not be necessary if appropriate constant flow rates are used [20].

A second drawback of empirical models lies in the danger of extrapolating to parameter values outside the range of the experimental data on which they are based. In particular, these models have been developed for tidal breathing of aerosols in healthy subjects. Using them for subjects with lung disease involves extrapolation, with largely unknown error. In addition, except for nebulizers, inhaled pharmaceutical aerosols are not delivered with tidal breathing but instead with a single large breath, often with a breath hold. This is a very different breathing pattern than tidal breathing, and it can be argued that deposition in the alveolar region may then be different because chaotic mixing due to periodic stretching and folding as the alveoli repeatedly expand and contract, which may play a significant role in alveolar deposition during tidal breathing [21], is not present during a single-breath maneuver. However, whether this causes significant errors in empirical models applied to single-breath inhalation devices remains to be determined, since it is necessary first to correct these models for their errors in mouth–throat deposition filtering and then to compare to measurements of alveolar deposition in vivo with single-breath devices. Unfortunately, such a task is complicated by the lack of methods for determining alveolar deposition in vivo (unknown amounts of slow clearance from the tracheobronchial region hamper the ability of standard 24-hour clearance methods to give these measurements; see, e.g., Ref. 6). Although comparisons to in vivo total lung deposition with single-breath devices have been made (e.g., Ref. 22), such comparisons only assess the ability of the mouth–throat deposition model since, as mentioned earlier, total lung dose with single-breath devices is essentially the inhaled dose minus mouth–throat deposition. The ability of empirical models to predict regional deposition within the lung with single-breath inhaled pharmaceutical devices remains to be examined. However, even if such data are obtained, it must be realized that to avoid extrapolation with empirical models it is necessary to produce new data for every new situation not covered by existing data, a limitation that will always hamper the generality of empirical models.

One final point to bear in mind with existing empirical models is that they cannot be used when droplet size changes occur in moderately dense aqueous aerosols, an increasingly important area with the development of single-breath devices such as the AERx® (Aradigm), AeroDose® (AeroGen), Eflow® (Pari), and Respimat® (Boehringer) and Battelle's electrohydrodynamic inhaler. Droplet size changes in these devices, which can be important in determining respiratory tract deposition, usually involve two-way coupled hygroscopic effects [3,23] which are beyond the capabilities of existing empirical models.

LAGRANGIAN DYNAMICAL MODELS (LDMs)

To overcome some of the limitations just mentioned that are associated with purely empirical models, simulations that include various aspects of the inhaled aerosol dynamics have been developed. The simplest of these belong to a class of models we refer to as *Lagrangian dynamical models* (LDMs), meaning that the model simulates some of the dynamical behavior of the aerosol in a frame of reference that travels with the aerosol (i.e., a "Lagrangian viewpoint").

A complete Lagrangian dynamical model would be ridiculously difficult, since it would follow all individual particles and air parcels as they travel through the entire lung and would require computation times of the same order as FLS mentioned earlier. Instead, existing one-dimensional LDMs make the major simplifying assumption that the aerosol and air travel together at the same velocity, and this velocity is obtained by treating the lung as a sequence of branching circular pipes whose diameter is given by some idealized lung geometry. For example, if the inhalation flow rate is Q, then the flow rate in each airway in the 10th lung generation is $Q/2^{10}$ and the average velocity in these airways is

$$v = \frac{\dfrac{Q}{2^{10}}}{\pi R^2}$$

where R is the radius of the airways in the 10th generation of the idealized lung geometry being used. With the velocity in each airway known, the amount of time the aerosol spends traveling through each airway generation can be obtained by dividing the length of each airway in the idealized lung geometry by this velocity. With this information, then by treating each airway generation as an inclined circular tube, it is possible to predict how much aerosol will deposit due to gravitational sedimentation and by Brownian diffusion in each airway generation (by using exact solutions of the dynamical equations for sedimentation and diffusion in inclined circular tubes—see Ref. 3 for these equations). Deposition in each airway by inertial impaction is dealt with empirically in one-dimensional LDMs (since simulation of the equations governing impaction requires full simulation of at least several lung branches at a time, which dramatically increases computation times). Many different empirical equations for impaction have been suggested, largely based on data from in vitro experiments in branched tubes, although those obtained using several generations probably represent reality more closely [3], since it is known that typically three or more generations of branches are needed before sensitivity to artificial inlet conditions is reduced [24]. Although most LDMs assume each bifurcation is symmetric, this assumption can be removed using a stochastic Monte Carlo approach [25].

A major advantage of LDMs over empirical models is the ease with which they can capture droplet size changes (e.g., due to evaporation) and the effect on respiratory tract deposition. It is for this reason that LDMs have been applied mainly to drug delivery with nebulized aqueous aerosols (e.g., Ref. 26). It should be noted that many aqueous inhaled pharmaceutical aerosols that undergo hygroscopic size changes require two-way coupled heat and mass transfer modeling [23], in which the air properties are affected by the droplets, vice versa. This is unfortunate, since two-way coupled hygroscopic effects complicate the model considerably as well as increasing the computation times (on a typical PC taking seconds without such effects to minutes with two-way coupled effects included). Various hygroscopic models (e.g. Refs. 6,27–29) do not include such two-way coupled effects and are therefore limited to those cases where the inhaled air can be considered as an infinite source of water vapor, otherwise giving varying degrees of inaccuracy, depending on the relevant parameters [30].

A second advantage of one-dimensional LDMs over empirical models is that their inclusion of some of the aerosol dynamics (albeit semiempirically) reduces the dangers of extrapolation, allowing, for example, prediction of deposition with breathing patterns that are quite different from normal tidal breathing. Indeed, Anderson et al. [31] use a one-dimensional LDM to examine extremely slow inhalations consisting of inhalation flow rates of < 2 L/min with a single inhalation duration of 10–20 seconds, which allows much larger particles to deposit in the small airways compared to normal tidal breathing.

The ability of different one-dimensional LDMs to predict the regional deposition of aerosols inhaled from pharmaceutical devices has been examined by several authors without inclusion of particle size changes due to evaporation [32,33] as well as with inclusion of two-way coupled hygroscopic effects [34]. These comparisons show that LDMs are sensitive to the dimensions of the idealized lung geometry being used, with the division of deposition between the alveolar and tracheobronchial regions matching in vivo data with some idealized lung geometries but not others [35]. Such sensitivity of LDMs to the dimensions of the idealized geometry is a concern if a model remains untested in comparison to in vivo data, particularly since the commonly used Weibel A model is known to have narrower tracheobronchial airways than more recent models [35].

Because one-dimensional LDMs include the aerosol dynamics by using solutions of the dynamical equations in simplified versions of parts of the lung geometry and by including empirical data from experiments on inertial impaction, they remain semiempirical in nature. As a result, they share some of the drawbacks of purely empirical models mentioned earlier. In particular, one-dimensional LDMs use the same mouth–throat deposition models used with the purely empirical models and so suffer from the same inability to predict mouth–throat deposition with dry powder inhalers and metered-dose inhalers discussed earlier.

A second drawback with one-dimensional LDMs is associated with the major simplifying assumption that the air and aerosol travel together as a single plug that does not distort (other than splitting in half at each bifurcation). Although this assumption makes LDMs computationally inexpensive, it causes an inhaled aerosol to proceed through the lung without axial dispersion (i.e., stretching and distortion of the aerosol front). Sarangapani and Wexler [36] present a model for axial dispersion suitable for one-dimensional LDMs that allows incorporation of irreversibility of dispersion between inhalation and exhalation. However, the effect of axial dispersion on aerosol deposition remains poorly characterized [3], so it is difficult to assess the magnitude of the errors associated with the lack of its presence. The reasonable agreement of one-dimensional LDMs with in vivo data would suggest that this effect may be minor for inhaled pharmaceutical aerosol deposition, but further research addressing this issue is needed.

A final drawback with one-dimensional LDMs is the difficulty they have in treating the time dependence of inhalation flow rates and aerosol properties (a situation that commonly occurs with single-breath inhalers) as well as the time dependence of the lung geometry. This difficulty is due to their Lagrangian nature, in which a single parcel of air and aerosol is tracked as it moves through an idealized lung geometry. In one-dimensional LDMs, once this parcel has left the mouth–throat, no further regard is paid to the conditions at the mouth, so the only way to capture time dependence of the air and aerosol properties (e.g. MMAD, GSD, inhalation flow rate) is with a quasisteady procedure whereby parcels released at different times in the breath are each tracked separately. However, such an approach increases computation times significantly and, to the author's knowledge, has not been pursued with inhaled pharmaceutical LDMs. To further complicate matters, the partial inclusion of axial diffusivity, as in Sarangapani and Wexler [36], would require some degree of coupling between consecutive parcels in the case of two-way coupled hygroscopic simulations and would also need modifying to include dispersion in both distal and proximal directions.

EULERIAN DYNAMICAL MODELS (EDMs)

To remove some of the limitations associated with one-dimensional LDMs, particularly their clumsiness with axial dispersion and time-varying breathing, more complex models can be considered. The next level of complexity beyond one-dimensional LDMs are what we refer to as the one-dimensional Eulerian dynamical models (EDMs). With these models, the dynamical behavior of the aerosol is viewed not by an observer moving with the inhaled particles, but instead by a stationary observer watching the aerosol's behavior in the entire respiratory tract at once (a so-called "Eulerian" viewpoint). To solve the equations governing the aerosol dynamics without simplification would mean doing FLS, which is not practical as discussed earlier. Instead, the fluid flow is assumed known (e.g., parabolic or plug flow in an idealized lung geometry), and the equation governing the aerosol number density (i.e., number of aerosol particles/ unit volume) is reduced to one dimension by integrating over cross-sectional planes at each axial location in the respiratory tract (see Ref. 3 for a detailed development of the basis of these models). The result is a single, partial differential equation for the aerosol density as a function of depth x into the respiratory tract and time t. This equation is solved numerically, giving the aerosol number density at a number of discrete depths, x, and times, t.

Particle deposition in one-dimensional EDMs is dealt with in the same manner as in LDMs, by using exact solutions of the dynamical equations for sedimentation and diffusion in inclined circular tubes and using empirical equations for inertial impaction from experiments in branched-airway replicas.

Because one-dimensional EDMs require the numerical solution of a partial differential equation (as opposed to simple algebraic equations with empirical models and one-dimensional LDMs, or ordinary differential equations with hygroscopic LDMs), EDMs are more difficult to program, require somewhat more computational resources (typically many minutes on a PC), and have only recently been modified to include two-way coupled hygroscopic effects [37]. For these reasons, only a few examples exist of one-dimensional EDMs being used with inhaled pharmaceutical aerosols (e.g., Ref. 11), although they have been used to aid in the development of purely empirical models (e.g., the ICRP 1994 [6] model is partly a curve fit to data from the one-dimensional EDM of Ref. 38).

The principal attractions of one-dimensional EDMs are their ability to implement time dependence of the aerosol properties at the respiratory tract entrance (e.g., variations in aerosol concentration and size associated with a burst, or "bolus," of inhaled particles), the ease with which simple models of axial dispersion can be incorporated, as well as their ability to include time dependence of the lung geometry associated with lung inflation during inhalation [39–41]. When any of these effects are deemed important, then one-dimensional EDMs are advantageous over the other simpler approaches we have considered thus far.

Of course, one-dimensional EDMs are not without their drawbacks. Indeed, they suffer from several of the same problems that plague empirical and one-dimensional LDMs. In particular, their use of empirical mouth–throat deposition models is a serious drawback to modeling of dry powder and metered-dose inhalers, as discussed earlier with purely empirical models. As with one-dimensional LDMs, the use of simplified lung geometries and empirical impaction data for predicting deposition within each airway gives an element of empiricism to one-dimensional EDMs that limits their generality.

A final drawback with one-dimensional EDMs lies in the information that is lost when the flow and aerosol properties are averaged over cross sections at each depth in the lung in deriving these models. This missing information is crucial in determining axial dispersion [3], so existing one-dimensional EDMs instead model axial dispersion using simple analogies with molecular diffusional transport. This is one of the least scrutinized aspects of one-dimensional EDMs, and although recent work has begun to examine this (e.g., Ref. 42), it remains to be seen how accurate axial dispersion models in one-dimensional EDMs must be for deposition of inhaled pharmaceutical aerosols. It should be noted though that comparisons of regional deposition predictions of a one-dimensional EDM [38] to in vivo data of aerosols inhaled with tidal breathing from tubes show good agreement with in vivo data [6], so such axial dispersion models may be adequate under these circumstances. Whether this is true for single-breath inhaled pharmaceutical aerosols remains for future research.

THREE-DIMENSIONAL PARTIAL LUNG SIMULATION

Some of the major limitations of existing one-dimensional LDMs and EDMs are caused by their use of only one dimension in space. By removing this one-dimensional restriction, these limitations can be removed. This is normally done by simulating the airways instead in three spatial dimensions and performing numerical simulation of the fluid and aerosol equations on a three-dimensional grid placed in each lung airway. Since, as discussed earlier, simulation of the whole respiratory tract in this manner (i.e., FLS) is prohibitively demanding of computational resources, work to date in this direction has limited itself to simulations of small parts of the respiratory tract, which we refer to as *three-dimensional partial lung simulations* (abbreviated as PLS, with "three-dimensional" implied). Since it is easier to solve the fluid flow equations in a Eulerian framework [using standard computational fluid dynamics (CFD) methods] while particle deposition is more naturally dealt with in a Lagrangian framework, most PLS researchers have used a mixed approach, with Eulerian equations for the fluid and Lagrangian equations for the aerosol.

A host of authors since the early 1990s (e.g., Refs. 24,42–47, 52, see Ref. 3 for more of these many references) have performed PLS in various idealized replicas of single-, double-, and triple-bifurcation segments of the lung as well as parts of simplified alveolar ducts. Deposition in the particular respiratory tract segment being simulated can be predicted more accurately with this approach than with the simplified, one-dimensional LDMs or EDMs.

However, PLS is not without its drawbacks, some of which are discussed in Finlay et al. [48]. Perhaps the largest drawback is the inability of such an approach to correctly predict mouth–throat deposition with inhaled pharmaceutical aerosols [49] when a standard semiempirical treatment of turbulence and its effect on particles is used (to avoid having to do direct numerical simulation to resolve all the turbulent motion in this region). A second drawback is the demand on computing time. Although not nearly as demanding as an FLS of the entire respiratory tract, PLS of even just a few lung generations can require many hours on the fastest desktop computers, so patching together simulations done in small parts of the lung in order to make up an entire lung remains impractical for preclinical design purposes.

A major limiting factor with PLS is our lack of knowledge of the three-dimensional geometry of the respiratory tract airways, particularly distal to the first few lung generations. Current imaging technology has been used to give this information only for the mouth–throat and proximal tracheobronchial airways (e.g., Refs. 50,51), so at present PLS in regions distal to the first few airway generations requires speculation as to the actual geometry of these airspaces. This is unfortunate, since the alveolar region has become increasingly important because of its ability to give systemic delivery. Imaging of the alveolar airspaces requires improvement in spatial resolution by at least a factor of 10 over present medical imaging technology. Since the alveoli change shape significantly during inhalation, temporal resolution well below one second is also required in these images. Such imaging demands are likely to remain beyond our technological capabilities for some time to come, so PLS is not yet ready to supplant one-dimensional LDMs and EDMs in inhaled pharmaceutical aerosol design. Its main use at present is to allow research aimed at improving one-dimensional LDMs and EDMs.

SUMMARY

Respiratory drug delivery has matured in recent years to the extent that those working in formulation and device design of inhaled aerosols often desire tools that allow more sophisticated preclinical design optimization than has been the case in past years. As an increasingly useful tool in this regard, lung deposition models allow preclinical estimation of doses delivered to different regions of the respiratory tract with different inhalation and aerosol properties. Empirical models that are essentially curve fits to more accurately obtained data are readily used for this purpose but must be used with caution due to their inability to extrapolate outside the parameter range for which they were developed, the most severe such restriction being their inability to capture mouth–throat deposition accurately with dry powder and metered-dose inhalers. Empirical models are also unable to incorporate two-way coupled hygroscopic size changes, which are common with the new generation of aqueous delivery devices. Dynamical models that incorporate some of the aerosol dynamics have the potential to eliminate these issues. At present, dynamical models that reduce an idealized lung geometry to one dimension in space are most commonly used. The simplest of such models are the one-dimensional Lagrangian dynamical models (LDMs), which assume that the aerosol travels at the same velocity as a nondistorting plug of air traveling through an idealized lung geometry. More complex are the one-dimensional Eulerian dynamical models (EDMs), which instead solve for the aerosol behavior at a series of depths, x, into the lung at each point in time, t, during inhalation. Both types of dynamical models allow more confidence in estimating deposition with single-breath inhalation devices than do the empirical models, since the latter are based on deposition data with tidal breathing rather than single-breath inhalations. In addition, it is possible to capture two-way coupled hygroscopic effects with dynamical models.

At present both one-dimensional EDMs and LDMs use empirical models for mouth–throat deposition, so the aforementioned difficulty with correct prediction of mouth–throat deposition remains a concern for existing one-dimensional EDMs and LDMs.

More accurate predictions of localized deposition within airways can be obtained using computational fluid dynamics (CFD) methods to perform numerical simulation of the equations governing the aerosol and air motion in three-dimensional replicas of the air spaces in the lung. However, such an approach is currently hampered by the large computation times required to simulate a reasonable section of the respiratory tract and our present lack of knowledge of the three-dimensional geometry of the lung airspaces. As a result, such simulations are likely destined to remain solely a research tool for some time yet, being used largely to improve the abilities of simpler models, such as one-dimensional LDMs and EDMs. Future work in this direction may include the use of partial lung simulation (PLS) in the development of LDMs and EDMs for diseased lungs. In vivo validation of such improved deposition models is in itself a daunting task, requiring careful experimental design if meaningful results are to be obtained [35].

Estimating the doses depositing in different regions of the respiratory tract with a lung deposition model is only the first, and probably the most well-characterized, step in predicting the fate of an inhaled therapeutic agent. However, models that allow prediction of the subsequent steps are being developed, an example being airway surface liquid thickness models that allow estimation of drug concentrations in the mucus and periciliary liquid layers that line the tracheobronchial airways [1]. Combination of present-day lung deposition models with increasingly sophisticated models for predicting the behavior of aerosol particles subsequent to their deposition will occupy future research for some time to come.

REFERENCES

1. Lange CF, Hancock REW, Samuel J, Finlay WH. In vitro aerosol delivery and regional airway surface liquid concentration of a liposomal cationic peptide. J Pharm Sci 2001; 40:1647–1657.
2. Finlay WH, Lange CF, King M, Speert D. Lung delivery of aerosolized dextran. Am J Resp Crit Care Med 2000; 161:91–97.
3. Finlay WH. The Mechanics of Inhaled Pharmaceutical Aerosols: An Introduction. London: Academic Press, 2001.
4. Stahlhofen W, Rudolf G, James AC. Intercomparison of experimental regional aerosol deposition data. J Aerosol Med 1989; 2:285–308.
5. ICRP Task Group on Lung Dynamics. Deposition and retention models for internal dosimetry of the human respiratory tract. Health Phys 1966; 12:173–207.
6. ICRP. Human respiratory tract model for radiological protection. Annals of the ICRP, ICRP publication 66, New York: Elsevier, 1994.
7. NCRP. Deposition, retention and dosimetry of inhaled radioactive substances. Report No. 125, National Council on Radiation Protection and Measurement, Bethesda, MD, 1997.
8. Yeh H-C, Cuddihy RG, Phalen RF, Chang IY. Comparisons of calculated respiratory tract deposition of particles based on the proposed NCRP model and the new ICRP66 Model. Aerosol Sci Techn 1996; 25:134–140.
9. Yu CP, Zhang L, Becquemin MH, Roy M, Bouchikhi A. Algebraic modeling of total and regional deposition of inhaled particles in the human lung of various ages. J Aerosol Sci 1992; 23:73–79.
10. Davies CN. Deposition of particles in the human lung as a function of particle size and breathing pattern: an empirical model. Ann Occup Hyg 1982; 26:119–135.
11. Clark AR, Egan M. Modelling the deposition of inhaled powdered drug aerosols. J Aerosol Sci 1994; 25:175–186.
12. Clark AR, Newman SP, Dasovich N. Mouth and oropharyngeal deposition of pharmaceutical aerosols. J Aerosol Med 1998; 11(suppl. 1):116–121.
13. DeHaan WH, Finlay WH. In vitro monodisperse aerosol deposition in a mouth and throat with six different inhalation devices. J Aerosol Med 2001; 14:361–367.
14. Finlay WH, DeHaan W, Grigic B, Heenan EA, Matida EA, Hoskinson M, Pollard A, Lange CF. Fluid mechanics and particle deposition in the oropharynx: the factors that really matter. In: Dalby RN, Byron PR, Farr SJ, eds. Respiratory Drug Delivery 8, Tucson, AZ, May 13–16, 2002. Raleigh, NC: Serentec Press, 171–177.
15. Pritchard JN. Generation and interpretation of in vitro data from dry powder and metered dose inhalers. J Aerosol Med 1997; 10:241.
16. Thiel CG. Can in vitro particle size measurements be used to predict pulmonary deposition of aerosol from inhalers? J Aerosol Med 1998; 11(suppl. 1):S43–S52.
17. Clark AR, Bailey R. Inspiratory flow profiles in disease and their effects on the delivery characteristics of dry powder inhalers. In: Dalby RN, Byron PR, Farr, SJ, eds. Respiratory Drug Delivery V, Buffalo Grove, IL: Interpharm Press, 1996:221–230.
18. Burnell PKP, Grant AC, Haywood PA, Prime D, Sumby BS. Powder inhalers— exploring the limits of performance. In: Dalby RN, Byron PR, Farr SJ, eds. Respiratory Drug Delivery VI, Buffalo Grove, IL: Interpharm Press, 1998:259–266.

19. Burnell PKP, Malton A, Reavill K, Ball MHE. Design, validation and initial testing of the electronic lung™ device. J Aerosol Sci 1998; 29:1011–1025.
20. Finlay WH, Gehmlich MG. Inertial sizing of aerosol inhaled from two dry powder inhalers with realistic breath patterns vs. constant flow rates. Int J Pharm 2000; 210:83–95.
21. Butler JP, Tsuda A. Effect of convective stretching and folding on aerosol mixing deep in the lung, assessed by approximate entropy. J Appl Physiol 1997; 83:800–809.
22. Price AC. Validation of aerosol deposition models for pharmaceutical purposes: the way forward. In: Dalby RN, Byron PR, Farr SJ, Peart J, eds. Respiratory Drug Delivery VII, Raleigh NC: Serentec Press, 2000:197–208.
23. Finlay WH. Estimating the type of hygroscopic behaviour exhibited by aqueous droplets. J Aerosol Med 1998; 11:221–229.
24. Comer JK, Kleinstreuer C, Zhang Z. Aerosol transport and deposition in sequentially bifurcating airways. ASME J Biomech Eng 2000; 122:152–158.
25. Koblinger L, Hofmann W. Monte Carlo modelling of aerosol deposition in human lungs. Part I. Simulation of particle transport in a stochastic lung structure. J Aerosol Sci 1990; 21:661–674.
26. Finlay WH, Stapleton KW, Zuberbuhler P. Variations in predicted regional lung deposition of salbutamol sulphate between 19 nebulizer models.fs J Aerosol Med 1998; 11:65–80.
27. Persons DD, Hess GD, Muller WJ, Scherer PW. Airway deposition of hygroscopic heterodispersed aerosols: results of a computer calculation. J Appl Physiol 1987; 63:1195–1204.
28. Ferron GA, Kreyling WG, Haider B. Inhalation of salt aerosol particles—II. Growth and deposition due to hygroscopic growth. J Aerosol Sci 1988; 19:611–631.
29. Martonen TB. Analytical model of hygroscopic particle behavior in human airways. Bull Math Biol 1982; 44:425–442.
30. Finlay WH, Stapleton KW, Zuberbuhler P. Errors in regional lung deposition predictions of nebulized salbutamol sulphate due to neglect or partial inclusion of hygroscopic effects. Int J Pharm 1997; 149:63–72.
31. Anderson M, Svartengren M, Canmer P. Human tracheobronchial deposition and effect of a cholinergic aerosol inhaled by extremely slow inhalations. Exp Lung Res 1999; 25:335–352.
32. Finlay WH, Hoskinson M, Stapleton KW. Can models be trusted to subdivide lung deposition into alveolar and tracheobronchial fractions? In: Dalby RN, Byron PR, Farr SJ, eds. Respiratory Drug Delivery VI, Hilton Head Island. SC, May 3–7, 1998. Buffalo Grove, IL: Interpharm Press, 1998:235–242.
33. Hashish AH, Fleming JS, Conway J, Halson P, Moore E, Williams TJ, Bailey AG, Nassim MN, Holgate ST. Lung deposition of particles by airway generation in healthy subjects: three-dimensional radionuclide imaging and numerical model prediction. J Aerosol Sci 1998; 29:205–215.
34. Finlay WH, Stapleton KW, Chan HK, Zuberbuhler P, Gonda I. Regional deposition of inhaled hygroscopic aerosols: in vivo SPECT compared with mathematical deposition modeling. J Appl Physiol 1996; 81:374–383.

35. Finlay WH, Lange CF, Li W-I, Hoskinson M. Validating deposition models in disease: what is needed? J Aerosol Med 2000; 13:381–385.

36. Sarangapani R, Wexler AS. The role of dispersion in particle deposition in human airways. Toxicol Sci 2000; 54:229–236.

37. Lange CF, Finlay WH. A fully Eulerian approach to the simulation of volatile hygroscopic aerosols. In: Schneider GE, ed. Proceedings of the Ninth Annual Conference of the CFD Society of Canada, CFD Society of Canada, Waterloo, ON, May 27–29, 2001:279–283.

38. Egan MJ, Nixon W, Robinson NI, James AC, Phalen RT. Inhaled aerosol transport and deposition calculations for the ICRP Task Group. J Aerosol Sci 1989; 20:1305–1308.

39. Taulbee DB, Yu CP, Heyder J. Aerosol transport in the human lung from analysis of single breaths. J Appl Physiol 1978; 44:803–812.

40. Egan MJ, Nixon W. A model of aerosol deposition in the lung for use in inhalation dose assessments. Rad Prot Dos 1985; 11:5–17.

41. Edwards D. The macrotransport of aerosol particles in the lung: aerosol deposition phenomena. J Aerosol Sci 1995; 26:293–317.

42. Lee JW, Lee DY, Kim WS. Dispersion of an aerosol bolus in a double bifurcation. J Aerosol Sci 2000; 31:491–505.

43. Oldham MJ, Phalen RF, Heistracher T. Computational fluid dynamics predictions and experimental results for particle deposition in an airway model. Aerosol Sci Technol 2000; 32:61–71.

44. Balásházy I, Hofman W, Heistracher T. Computation of local enhancement factors for the quantification of particle deposition patterns in airway bifurcations. J Aerosol Sci 1999; 30:185–203.

45. Zhao Y, Brunskill CT, Lieber BB. Inspiratory and expiratory steady-flow analysis in a model symmetrically bifurcating airway. Trans ASME 1997; 199:52–58.

46. Darquenne C, Pavia M. Two- and three-dimensional simulations of aerosol transport and deposition in alveolar zone of human lung. J Appl Physiol 1996; 80:1401–1414.

47. Martonen TB, Yang Y, Xue ZQ, Zhang Z. Motion of air within the human tracheobronchial tree. Part Sci Tech 1994; 12:175–188.

48. Finlay WH, Stapleton KW, Yokota J. On the use of computational fluid dynamics for simulating flow and particle deposition in the human respiratory tract. J Aerosol Med 1996; 9:329–342.

49. Stapleton KW, Guentsch E, Hoskinson MK, Finlay WH. On the suitability of k-ε turbulence modelling for aerosol deposition in the mouth and throat: a comparison with experiment. J Aerosol Sci 2000; 31:739–749.

50. Perzl MA, Schulz H, Paretzke HG, Englmeier KH, Heyder J. Reconstruction of the lung geometry for the simulation of aerosol transport. J Aerosol Med 1996; 9:409–418.

51. Sauret V, Goatman KA, Fleming JS, Bailey AG. Semiautomated tabulation of the 3D topology and morphology of branching networks using CT: application to the airway tree. Phys Med Biol 1999; 44:1625–1638.

52. Gradon L, Orlicki D. Deposition of inhaled aerosol particles in a generation of the tracheobronchial tree. J Aerosol Sci 1990; 21:3–19.

6

Practical Aspects of Imaging Techniques Employed to Study Aerosol Deposition and Clearance

Myrna B. Dolovich
McMaster University, Hamilton, Ontario, Canada

INTRODUCTION

The measurement of lung deposition of inhaled therapeutics and its interpretation has been debated within the field of inhaled drug delivery science for many years. Historically, two-dimensional gamma scintigraphy (planar imaging) has been used to demonstrate total and regional lung deposition of drugs inhaled from selected aerosol delivery systems [1–4]. Efforts have been made to link total lung deposition with the clinical parameters of efficacy and safety, though with limited success. Acquisition of 2D scintigraphic data can be confounded by several factors, such as poor radiolabeling of the study drug, use of inaccurate tissue attenuation factors applied when calculating absolute amounts of radioactivity in the lung, oropharynx, and gut, and poor delineation of the edge of the lung, leading to incorrectly defined lung regions. In addition, factors influencing the inhalation of the radiolabeled aerosols may not be well controlled, producing variability in deposition patterns. Intraindividual variability in data outcomes may result from a lack of adherence to inclusion/exclusion criteria for study subjects or the enrollment of subjects with too broad a range of disease severities. Furthermore, for deposition protocols with concurrent pharmacokinetic measurements, acquisition of imaging data may be constrained by the need to image immediately following inhalation of the labeled drug and to precisely measure plasma drug levels at the same time and, therefore, possibly requiring correction factors to be applied to the data for any discrepancy in time between the two sets of measurements.

The response to a therapeutic aerosol is considered to be a function of the dose deposited at the target site in the lung [5–10]. The dose, in turn, is dependent upon the system producing the aerosol, the particle size characteristics of the inhaled aerosol, the mode of inhalation, and the caliber of the airways [11–16]. The influence of the pattern of deposition of the inhaled dose, that is, selective delivery to the central versus small, peripheral airways, on the response is not as well defined [17–19]. Direct measurements of deposition and distribution of therapeutic aerosols in the lung, mucociliary clearance (MCC), and lung epithelial permeability (LEP) have been made using a variety of tracer methods employing external imaging [4,20,21]. These diagnostic tests (Table 1) [20,21,24] measure the surface transport of secretions (mucociliary clearance) [22–24], transepithelial transport of fluid and hydrophilic solutes (respiratory clearance or epithelial permeability) related to the integrity of the lung epithelium [25–27], and the distribution of inhaled gases or extrafine ($\sim 1\,\mu m$) aerosols in the lung (ventilation) [28–33]; correlations with clinical response have been obtained in a limited number of these same studies. When properly conducted, the procedures are convenient and involve minimal radiation and risk. It should be understood that these tests are dependent on the production, characterization, and inhalation of aerosols within a particular size range [32–35].

While 2D imaging is easy to implement in practice, the blurring caused by structures overlying and underlying the structures of interest limits its usefulness for quantitation of the distribution of an inhaled dose within the lung [36]. However, over the last approximately 30 years, advances in imaging technology have enabled more sophisticated three-dimensional techniques to be utilized to image and provide greater detail about the regional deposition of drugs in the lung, e.g., single-photon-emission computed tomography (SPECT) [28,37–42] and positron-emission tomography (PET) [40,43–46]. Both PET and SPECT provide accurate and highly specific information about the dose and distribution within the body of inhaled or injected tracers, and both are widely used as diagnostic tools in nuclear medicine. Of the two imaging techniques, PET provides greater resolution, with the advantage of utilizing radiolabeled molecular markers to obtain functional imaging of biologic processes in vivo [47–51].

TABLE 1 Aerosols Used in Clinical Investigations

Technique	Application	Aerosol size	Disease or condition
Mucociliary clearance (MCC)	Ciliary dysfunction, airway caliber, mucus production	$>2\,\mu m$	Primary ciliary dyskinesia, bronchial disorders, lung transplantation
Inhalation challenge	Airway responsiveness, allergen challenge, sputum induction	$1-6\,\mu m$	Asthma, COPD
Respiratory solute absorption	Epithelial permeability	$<2\,\mu m$	Interstitial lung disease, lung injury, *Pneumocystis carinii* pneumonia, adult respiratory distress syndrome
Ventilation/ perfusion	Vascular occlusion, presurgery evaluation	$<1\,\mu m$	Pulmonary embolism, localized airway disease
Dosimetry	Drug dose and distribution/response to therapy	$1-5\,\mu m$	Asthma, cystic fibrosis, COPD, bronchopulmonary dysplasia, respiratory syncytial virus, diabetes, adult respiratory distress syndrome

Supporting these measurements are analytical methodologies that have allowed a more precise measure of the pharmacokinetic profiles of many inhaled drugs, enhancing understanding of their absorption, distribution, and clearance kinetics from the respiratory tract [52,53].

This chapter will discuss some of the practical issues to be aware of when performing radiolabeled deposition and clearance studies (Table 2). The considerations apply to both in vivo studies in man and, in animal models and, to some extent, in in vitro models. Nasal deposition and clearance studies and tracheal transport measurements will not be discussed in detail, although it should be understood that the importance of a valid radiolabeled test aerosol is key to the successful interpretation of the deposition data for both nasal and lung studies [54,55].

TABLE 2   Issues in Imaging with Radioaerosols

Characteristics of aerosol system (particle size, drug output)
    Standard curves (impactor plates, filter, inlet, collection tube)
Radiolabeling of drug
    Types of tracers
    Validation of radioaerosol
    Particle size characterization: drug vs. radioactivity
Measurement of emitted dose from inhaler
    Drug vs. radioactivity
Scanner selection
    Scanner resolution and sensitivity
    Type of collimator for gamma camera
Controls during administration and imaging of radioaerosol
    Breathing technique
    Mouthpiece seal
    Gas flow rate
    Subject movement during imaging
Subject characteristics
    Age
    Sex
    Severity of disease
    Stability of baseline pulmonary function
Data analysis
    Defining the lung edge
    Defining regions of interest within the lung
    Correction for tissue attenuation of radioactivity
    Calculation of dose deposited
    Expression of results

ISSUES IN USING RADIOLABELED AEROSOLS TO DETERMINE DRUG DELIVERY TO THE LUNG
Characterization of the Aerosol from the Delivery System

Systems used to provide unit doses of therapeutic aerosols are the pressurized metered-dose inhaler (pMDI), containing drug in a propellant formulation, the dry powder inhaler (DPI), and nebulizers for aqueous and ethanolic formulations [56,57]. Many inhaler systems now available to patients and dispensing a variety of therapies have been tested in vivo with radiolabeled drugs to measure their efficiency of delivery to the lung. These measurements of lung deposition have yielded values on the order of 5–30%, even under optimal inhalation conditions. Newer nebulizer technologies, such as the metered-dose liquid inhalers currently in development, have much greater efficiencies, on the order of 70% or more of the drug dose deposited in the lung [58]. It is widely accepted that knowledge of the lung dose and distribution of inhaled aerosols from these various systems is critical for optimal development of the delivery system technology and for the assessment of the performance of these inhalers in vivo. The information provided is of interest not only to the pharmaceutical industry [30,59,60], but also to physicians prescribing inhalant therapy for a variety of diseases. If deposition from a particular aerosol dispensed from a delivery system is poor, it is likely that the response to therapy given from that aerosol will be suboptimal. The deposition measurements provide the physician with data on which to base the selection of an inhaler or mode of therapy for that particular patient.

Radiolabeling Methods for Aerosols

The first step when embarking on a series of experiments to measure lung deposition for an inhaled pharmaceutic is to produce the radioactive aerosol that mirrors the therapy dispensed from the inhaler being tested [61–63]. This may be a fairly straightforward radiopharmaceutical procedure, in particular for nebulizer and pMDI solution formulations, but it may also take months to produce and validate the tracer. Suspension formulations labeled with a tracer for 2D and SPECT imaging and drugs synthesized with a positron emitter can fall into the latter category. For 2D imaging and SPECT deposition studies, most labeled drugs produced are "association" products; that is, the label is associated with the drug but is not firmly bound. Without firm binding, images must be acquired quickly before the dissociation of the label from the drug leads to a circulating level of absorbed radioactivity that would introduce an unacceptable error in the measurement of radioactivity in the lung. Knowing the effective half-life $(1/t_{effective}^{1/2} = 1/t_{physical}^{1/2} + 1/t_{biological}^{1/2})$ of the tracer in the lung may allow a correction for the uptake, but this is not a desirable solution. Deposition studies using SPECT with these types of absorbable labeled drugs as the test agents are less accurate because the time required for imaging is often greater than the $t_{effective}^{1/2}$, although acquisition times with newer SPECT cameras are much shorter [64].

There are several protocols designed to measure mucociliary clearance. Which protocols are used are dependant upon the question being asked. To measure the acute effect of a pharmaceutic on clearance, the unlabeled drug is inhaled, followed by the nonabsorbable tracer aerosol [65,66]. In other protocols, designed to determine the effect of an intervention on MCC, the tracer aerosol is inhaled and clearance is measured for 30–60 min to establish the control curve. The treatment or intervention is then administered for a fixed length of time while continuing to measure clearance. This period is usually followed by another series of clearance measurements to define changes from the control period postintervention [67,68]. Thus, it is important that there be little or no uptake of the inhaled tracer, more or less guaranteed, i.e., the $t_{1/2 \, effective}$ of the tracer similar to the physical half-life of the isotope.

Production of Radiolabel

A number of methods have been developed to produce radioactive products for inhalation and use in lung deposition measurements. When imaging with 2D planar or 3D SPECT, the tracer most commonly used for diagnostic and research studies in humans is 99m-technetium, i.e., pertechnetate ($^{99m}TcO_4^-$). The short physical half-life of ^{99m}Tc (6.0 hr) and effective half-life of 0.16–6.0 hr, dependent on the compound labeled, coupled with a low gamma emission energy (140 KeV) minimizes the radiation exposure and risk to the subject as well as to personnel handling or preparing the radioactive drugs for inhalation. With the exception of PET tracers, very few radiolabeled studies involve direct labeling of the drug [69]. As already mentioned for inhalation products used for imaging with either planar or SPECT, the tracer is associated with, but not part of, the drug formulation, whether the formulation is a drug in suspension, a drug in solution, or a drug powder. As stated earlier, unless firmly bound, the label and drug rapidly dissociate following deposition on the airway surface; the label then no longer provides a marker for the drug. For $^{99m}TcO_4$, a soluble tracer, the effective half-life in the lung, once separated from the drug, is of the order of 11–15 minutes, while that in the oropharynx is approximately 25 minutes. Thus imaging must be done quickly and over a short period of time, with possible correction of the data for the loss of radioactivity due to absorption through the lungs, seen if the kidneys become obvious within minutes of administering the radioactive aerosol. Accumulation of pertechnetate in tissue may be detected by simultaneously imaging the thigh, although the sensitivity of this measurement will depend on the activity of the dose inhaled and the rates of absorption and excretion from the lungs and other compartments in the body. Measuring radioactivity in the blood by defining a region over the heart is possible with PET but not with planar imaging.

Dose calibrators are standard equipment in all nuclear medicine facilities. They are used to measure the dose of radioactivity of all drugs administered. Because quantitative outcomes based on administered dose are dependent on the exactness of the dose measurement, the accuracy of the dose calibrator must be ensured with routine measurements using reference standards. Quality control and calibration of the scanners must also be scheduled on a regular basis to maintain proper performance. Because a variety of 2D and 3D scanners is used, variability in performance can be a major issue [70].

Deposited doses in the lung and oropharynx vary among infants, children, adults, geriatric patients, and patients being mechanically ventilated, the differences being mainly a function of breathing pattern and oropharyngeal and airway geometry [71–76]. Adjustments to the nominal dose of radioactivity must be made to avoid excessive radiation exposure, in particular when imaging is used to measure deposited dose in children [77]. For research deposition measurements of pMDI drugs in adults, we load approximately 200 mCi into the canister to obtain 150–200 μCi per actuation, for an effective radiation dose of less than 1 mSv [78]. When imaging children and small animals, approximately one-fourth of the adult dose is given. While these administered doses of radioactivity are much less than those used for nuclear medicine diagnostic procedures, counting statistics for the acquired images are well within acceptable limits.

pMDIs. Procedures for labeling some pMDI formulations are described in the literature [74,79–83]. The method varies with the category of drug and the excipients present in the formulation.

The first step in the preparation of a labeled canister is to extract the pertechnetate, using methylethylketone (MEK), into an empty canister. When the MEK has evaporated, the finishing steps must be carried out fairly quickly, aiming for 90 seconds or less to complete the cutting open of the frozen drug canister, the transfer of its contents to the fresh canister containing the radioactivity, and the crimping of a new metering valve onto the radioactive canister. If this procedure takes longer, there is a risk that a significant amount of propellant will evaporate, changing the vapor pressure of the newly sealed canister and subsequently the unit dose and particle size characteristics of the dispensed tracer aerosol.

When the radioactive canister reaches room temperature, 15-unit (emitted or exactuator) doses should be dispensed. The first five doses are considered priming doses and are to be discarded, along with the actuator mouthpiece. The remaining 10 doses are each collected into individual dose collection tubes (Fig. 1) [84] using a fresh actuator mouthpiece. The radioactivity from the single sprays can be measured directly in the dose calibrator and the drug content

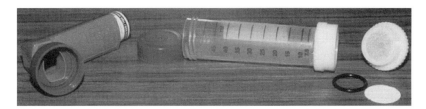

FIGURE 1 Unit Dose Collection Apparatus (UDA) for aerosol emitted from an aerosol delivery device. The setup is shown with a pMDI interface, but similar connecting pieces have been made in our laboratory for nebulizers. The sample is collected in the tube and solvent added to absorb the drug collected on the filter. (From Ref. 91.)

assayed chemically afterwards. However, if the doses are inconsistent, another 10 must be dispensed. The canister should be discarded if the unit doses fall outside of the allowable FDA limits [85]. It is not possible to accurately measure the dispensed dose for each individual subject inhaling a single puff from the pMDI by counting the canister before and after the subject has inhaled his/her dose. The total radioactivity in the labeled canister is much higher than the radioactivity contained in a single actuated dose, and the sensitivity of most dose calibrators is such that the detection of the difference of one dose from the total load tends to be unreliable. One should also not divide the total amount of radioactivity in the pMDI by the number of doses in the canister, for several reasons. The radioactivity that is adsorbed onto the walls of the canister and metering valve, and hence not available for inhalation, is counted as part of the total canister dose. In addition, the number of doses cannot be accurately known because there is usually overfill by the drug company and the evaporation of propellant when the can is opened during the radiolabeling procedure may result in loss of doses. Because the mean of the 10 doses of radioactivity is used in the calculation of lung deposition when expressing the results as a percentage of the inhaled or emitted dose from the delivery system, the introduction of variability in the emitted dose of radioactivity should be minimized, aiming for a coefficient of variation of the measured single unit doses of less than 15%. Good labeling technique, reproducible dose-collection procedures, and correction of dose measurements for decay of isotope all contribute to minimization of error.

Suspension pMDIs are more difficult to label than solution pMDIs, but for both types of pMDIs the label is soluble in the propellant and associated only with the drug or other excipients in the canister. Thus, 2D imaging must begin immediately after inhaling the dose. Radiolabeled pMDI suspensions should be shaken prior to use, particularly if they were prepared several hours earlier and at least three priming doses wasted before the subject inhales the radioactive dose.

Nebulizers.   With nebulizer solution formulations, the labeling process to produce an aerosol for planar and SPECT imaging is fairly straightforward, in that the radioactivity, nonabsorbable tracers such as ^{99m}Tc-HSA or ^{99m}Tc-SC or ^{99m}Tc-DTPA, are mixed into the drug product. These compounds, made either from commercial kits or by implementing approved radiopharmacy protocols, are also used as diagnostic agents in nuclear medicine. Each droplet will contain amounts of drug, carrier, and radioactivity in proportion to the original concentrations. However, the radiolabel is not bound to the drug but is associated with it, within the droplet. With the exception of DTPA in smokers and patients with interstitial lung disease, they all have effective $t^{1/2}$ comparable to the physical half-life of ^{99m}Tc, thus allowing imaging to occur over time and without loss of the tracer, other than from natural decay of the isotope and via mucociliary clearance from the lung. The drug particles in nebulizer suspensions cannot be labeled in this way; mixing the radioactivity into the nebulizer suspension means that only the carrier is labeled and not the drug. While it is the droplet size that determines the deposition distribution of the aerosol in the lung, one cannot infer deposited drug dose from these measurements without a parallel measurement of the drug content within the droplets.

Powders. Techniques for labeling drug powders are more complex than those used for pMDIs. As with pressurized aerosols, pertechnetate must first be extracted from saline. It is possible to apply a nonabsorbable ^{99m}Tc label onto the powder particles, but this technique is dependent on the category of drug being labeled [86]. Lactose, if a part of the formulation, is blended into the powder after the labeling and prior to loading of the labeled powder into capsules or blisters or to placing it in the DPI reservoir. A method devised by Newman et al. mixed radioactivity, following extraction and evaporation of solvent, into the dry powder [87]. While successful, the technique assumes an even mixing of the components and may explain why deposition values for budesonide in the Turbuhaler vary between laboratories [62]. The radioactivity is associated with the drug and is not a firm chemical or physical bond with the drug molecule.

With breath-actuated inhalers such as DPIs, the variability in dispensing the dose between individuals places added importance on knowing the absolute amount of radioactivity actually inhaled. For DPIs designed to dispense multi- or single units doses rather than dispensing from a reservoir, the amount can be obtained if the radioactivity in the inhaler is assayed in a dose calibrator pre- and then postinhalation for *each* study subject to give, respectively, the nominal or metered dose and the dose remaining in the DPI. The difference between these two measurements is the dose of drug emitted from the inhaler or inhaled at the mouth. Fig. 2 shows a reasonable correlation between the deposited lung dose, measured with the gamma camera and expressed as a percentage of the nominal dose, and that portion of the nominal dose containing drug in particles of less than 5 μm (fine particle dose), measured by the dose calibrator [88]. The variability in the fine particle dose for both inspiratory flow rates tested contributed to differences in deposition between subjects, adding to other influencing factors, such as airway caliber. Therefore, it is important to account for dose differences by normalizing the data so as not to introduce additional error in the calculations. Accurate calculations of deposited dose, either as a percentage of the nominal or emitted dose or in absolute terms, i.e., as microcuries of radioactivity or micrograms of drug, cannot be made without the measurement of inhaled dose. When this is done, the fine particle dose of the inhaled aerosol can provide a good estimate for dose deposited below the larynx, as seen in mean data obtained for several other DPIs [89].

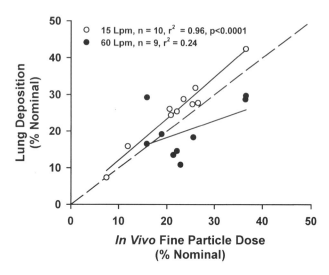

FIGURE 2   Relationship between deposition of a radiolabeled DPI aerosol and the measured fine particle dose of the labeled powder inhaled for each subject. Both variables are expressed as the percent of nominal dose. The correlation is higher for the lower flow rate used to inhale the powder, possibly due to the more consistent amount of drug deposited in the oropharynx. (From Ref. 88.)

For deposition studies to be an accurate representation of the behavior of the drug inhaled, the aerosol produced from the tracer powder must be similar to the unlabeled aerosol, and validation of its performance characteristics must be demonstrated prior to use. This involves the same sizing and dosing measurements described earlier.

Validation of a Radiolabeled Aerosol Formulation: Particle Size and Unit Dose

Deposition is a function of the particle size characteristics of the aerosol and the in vivo response is influenced by the dose of drug inhaled per actuation from the inhaler. Thus, prior to using a labeled aerosol product to measure lung deposition and response, confirmation that the aerosol characteristics have not been altered by the labeling procedure must be obtained, as well as demonstrating that the dose of active substance in the aerosol formulation is dispensed consistently, similar to the original nonlabeled formulation, and that the drug is viable. The latter is particularly important when using imaging and simultaneous pharmacokinetic measurements to assess the response to the radiolabeled drug postinhalation [90].

Particle Size Measurements for Validation. The validity of the radiolabeling process is confirmed by a three-way comparison of drug particle size distributions before and after labeling and to the size distribution of radioactivity in the drug product after labeling [61,63]. The characterization of the aerosols is typically performed using cascade impaction, counting the radioactivity deposited on the impactor stages (Fig. 3) and then assaying the drug chemically. The unit spray content and consistency (drug, radioactivity) of the emitted doses from the aerosol inhaler, that is, a pMDI, DPI, or nebulizer, are assessed by comparing the amount and variability of drug (micrograms) and radioactivity (microcuries) emitted per actuation pre- and postlabeling as well as the coefficient of variation for the unit doses in terms of drug and radioactivity. Limits for acceptability are specified in the U.S. FDA Guidance for Industry— Metered-Dose Inhalers (MDI) and Dry Powder Inhaler (DPI) Drug Products— Chemistry, Manufacturing and Controls Documentation, issued in 1998 [85]. For synthesis of drugs with positron emitters, the structure and purity of the radiotracer must be verified, using HPLC, in comparison to an authentic standard prior to administration to human subjects.

When validating whether a radiolabeled aerosol has the same properties as the original aerosol, one needs to use a sizing system that gives both the measurement of the drug substance and the radioactivity. While there are a number of instruments used for sampling and classifying aerosols, multistage cascade impactors are used for validation work because radioactivity can be

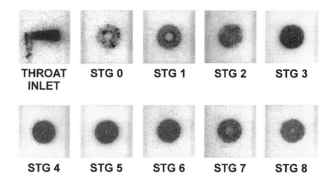

FIGURE 3 Individual stage plates and inlet from the Anderson Cascade Impactor showing the pattern of radioactivity on the plates following sizing of a radiolabeled pMDI formulation. The plates and inlet were placed on the planar gamma camera face and imaged to measure the amount of deposited radioactivity. The plates were subsequently washed with solvent and assayed using UV spectroscopy to obtain the amount of drug deposited.

measured on the individual stage plates and then the drug can be dissolved off the plates and assayed chemically by UV spectroscopy or HPLC. The latter is particularly useful for single doses or small quantities of drug. Using these data allows the frequency distributions for particle diameter in terms of radioactivity and mass of drug to be plotted in parallel.

Fig. 4a and b give examples of graphs plotted from sizing data obtained for a radiolabeled formulation in comparison to the unlabeled or control formulation. The graphs plotted are the frequency and cumulative mass distributions for drug mass and radioactivity [86]. Fig. 4c gives the Line of Identity (LOI) between drug mass and radioactivity in this particular formulation. All the data from all the impactor stages from 19 sizing runs have been plotted. The deviation from the line of identity allows one to see the extent of the variability of the "match" within the aerosol. Statistically, the radiolabel was considered to be a match and reliable surrogate for the drug, and it was subsequently used in a deposition study in asthmatic subjects.

Measurement of Dose of Radioactivity and Drug to be Administered. As described earlier, unit doses of dispensed aerosol—pressurized, powder, or liquid—can be collected in the apparatus shown in Fig. 1 [84,91]. The single doses are dispensed into the tube, using a suction airflow matching that for the impactor sizings and the inspiratory flowrate to be used by the study subjects. The radioactivity in the tube can be counted and the drug content assayed chemically by UV spectroscopy or HPLC to provide the emitted dose. For pMDIs, mean actuator mouthpiece content of radioactivity and drug can be determined from the total of 10 doses by counting the actuator in the dose calibrator; the drug is measured by dropping the actuator into a fixed volume of solvent and assaying the drug content chemically.

Fig. 5 [86] shows an example of the mean unit spray content for drug and radioactivity for several study days using this labeled powder. Each bar of the graph represents a mean ± standard deviation of 10 unit doses. While the CV of the daily measurements for both drug and radioactivity must be within specified limits, it should be understood that the mean daily level of radioactivity in the formulation or nominal dose of radioactivity varies as a function of the level of the specific activity available from the generator on the day of the study. This variability in the amount of radioactivity affects only the absolute dose of radioactivity inhaled and not the measured deposition distribution. Deposition results should be normalized to account for these differences, even for the small, day-to-day variability in the supply of radioactivity.

Because radiolabeling techniques are not precise and specific activities of the isotopes can vary, validation and calibration should be done for each radiolabeled aerosol produced. In particular, the measurement of emitted doses

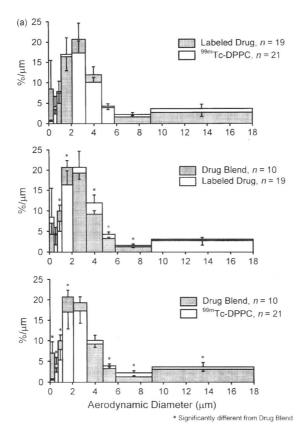

FIGURE 4 (a) Frequency distribution of drug mass and radioactivity for a radiolabeled powder and the drug in the original (control) powder versus aerodynamic particle diameter, obtained to validate the radiolabeled powder for deposition experiments. Measurements were obtained using the Anderson Cascade Impactor operated at 28 lpm. While the statistical comparisons showed significant differences between some of the amounts of drug and radioactivity on several of the stages, the differences were small and not sufficient to preclude the aerosol from being used in deposition studies. The drug was unchanged by the labeling process. (b) Cumulative distribution plotted from the sizing data for drug and radioactivity in the radiolabeled formulation and the drug in the original powder. A mean difference of approximately 3.0% was obtained between the radioactivity and drug on the lowest stage of the impactor. This resulted in a small but significant difference in the FPF (% < 5.8 μm) between the three distributions ($p = 0.01$, ANOVA). The FPF for the control powder and the drug in the labeled powder were the same. (c) Identity plot for the drug and radioactivity on all impactor plates from 19 sizings of a labeled powder formulation. The correlation is high, indicating that the radioactivity mirrors the drug. (From Ref. 86.)

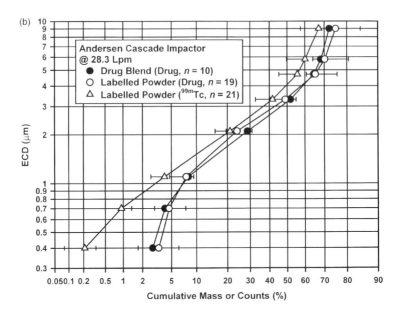

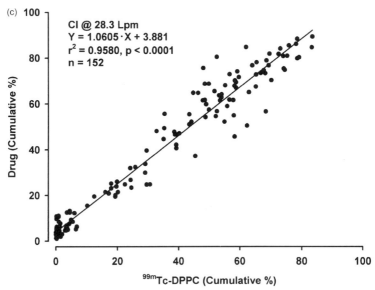

FIGURE 4   Continued.

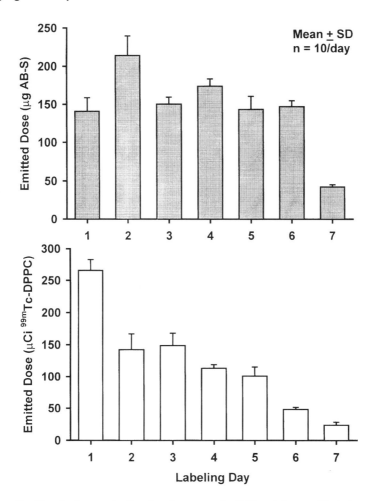

FIGURE 5 Graph demonstrating in vitro reproducibility of the emitted dose for a radiolabeled drug powder inhaled at two different inspiratory flowrates. Although the mean dose of drug and radioactivity varied between study days, the coefficient of variation for the emitted doses of drug or radioactivity on each study day was low. The amount of radioactivity used in the labeling of the powder varied with the specific activity of the $^{99m}TcO_4{}^-$ supply on each labeling day [86].

provides the mean value for the dose of radioactivity administered, which must be further corrected for decay between the time of production and the time of use. This value is critical if calculating absolute doses inhaled rather than percentages of radioactivity distributed within the respiratory tract.

Provided that the radiolabeling process does not alter the particle size distribution of the emitted drug and that the size distribution of the radiotracer is similar, the radiolabeled formulation may be used to measure total lung deposition and distribution of the inhaled drug. If clinical response measurements are performed following inhalation of the radiolabeled pMDI aerosol, the particle size characteristics and dose of drug per actuation in the radiolabeled formulation must match those of the drug in the unlabeled or original formulation. A successful match is indicated by an equivalent in vivo clinical response to the labeled and unlabeled formulations. Useful information from these studies will be obtained only if the label accurately follows the drug during inhalation.

Other Factors.   Additional factors that should be standardized for the in vitro characterization of the aerosol size distribution are:

- The ambient temperature and humidity
- The inlet stage or entry port for the sizing system (Fig. 6 [92])
- The coupling of the inhaler to the inlet stage
- The number of priming doses to be "wasted" from the inhaler prior to sampling the aerosol
- The number of doses sampled

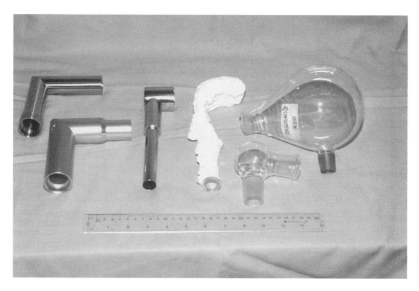

FIGURE 6   Different inlets used to couple a cascade impactor to an aerosol delivery system. The inlets range in volume from 66 to 1080 mL [92] and collect varying amounts of drug, depending on their volume. This in turn affects the amount of aerosol sampled by the impactor.

- The time between actuations
- Whether a pMDI is shaken between doses
- The type of pMDI actuator mouthpiece used
- The expression of the results

With a sensitive balance, it is possible to measure the actual weight of drug deposited on the various stages of the impactor. The weight, however, would include the weight of any excipients in the formulation as well as the drug. For any impactor sizing system used and where drug assays are required for analysis, reproducible standard curves must be produced for each drug tested. Standard curves for the drug on impactor plates, filters, impactor inlets, and the unit dose collection apparatus should be obtained to correct for the possibility of interference from extractibles.

CONTROL DURING INHALATION OF A RADIOLABELED AEROSOL AND SUBJECT VARIABLES

Lung deposition varies with the drug and the formulation. In addition, many of the 2D deposition studies have been performed in normal, healthy volunteers rather than in the patient groups intended for the therapy. This option of using normals is chosen for several reasons. The subject with normal pulmonary function provides the best possible outcome or the "envelope" for the deposition value obtained. Patients with lung disease may have greater or lesser deposition compared to normals, depending upon the particle size characteristics of the test aerosol and the inspiratory volumes and flow rates used during aerosol inhalation. The regional distribution of the inhaled therapy within the lung would, however, be abnormal [11,93–96]. It is often easier to solicit normal healthy volunteers for deposition studies, and certainly there is not the inevitable rescheduling due to variability in baseline lung function or exacerbations of the disease that occurs when doing studies in patients. However, the drugs being tested are to be prescribed for the treatment of respiratory and other diseases. Therefore, knowing the lung deposition and distribution in the various patient groups is more relevant to the assessment of the drug and the delivery device.

When designing protocols to measure deposition, a number of clinical factors need to be considered and incorporated into the study design: subjects' age, sex, smoking history, and current drug regimens, presence of a viral infection, severity of disease, stability of pulmonary function, and other outcome measures that could affect the inhalation of the radioaerosol, the measurement of deposition, and the results. Some of these also apply when using healthy volunteers as subjects for deposition studies. For example, we allow a 4- to 6-week recovery period between repeat studies for subjects who have suffered an exacerbation of their asthma or developed a chest cold or infection after enrollment.

The particle size of therapeutic aerosols range from < 1-μm mass median aerodynamic diameter (MMAD) to 8 μm MMAD. However, the "effect" of particle size, once the inspiratory flowrate is taken into account, can be much greater, shifting the deposition pattern to more proximal airways, as does airway narrowing due to the presence of lung disease, effects demonstrated in a number of published deposition studies. Thus the inhalation variables—inspiratory flowrate, inspiratory volume, and time of breath hold—are important to control during the inhalation of the tracer aerosol [11,97,98]. This can be accomplished by either training the subject prior to the inhalation maneuver or using a monitoring system with or without visual feedback. While this level of control is rarely present during actual patient use of the inhaler, nonetheless it is important to the interpretation of deposition results if the objective is to determine delivery efficiency under optimal conditions of use. Small changes in particle size and/or inspiratory flowrate can influence the deposition measurement (Fig. 7, [99]). Control of these variables may contribute to a reduction in intersubject variability in deposition and, perhaps,

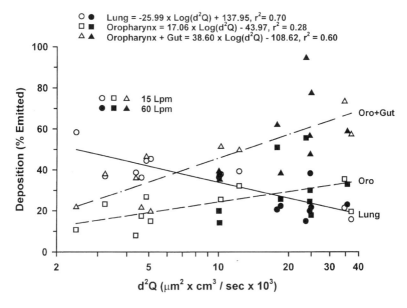

FIGURE 7 Deposition in the lung, the oropharynx, and the sum of the oropharynx and gut, expressed as the percent of nominal dose, plotted against the impaction parameter, d^2Q, where d is particle size and Q is inspiratory flow rate [99]. With this particular inhaler, a fourfold difference in Q caused a marked shift in the distribution of drug between lung and oropharynx + gut. Variability in deposition seen between subjects may be reduced by controlling the particle size of the inhaled drug and the inspiratory flowrate during the inhalation maneuver.

response to the therapy. Similarly, when measuring deposition in patients, clinical classification of their disease must be documented, and an attempt should be made to study patients with similar severities or extent of airway narrowing.

Other technical factors influencing the delivery and measurement of the radioactivity must be well controlled. Some of these are

- Use of the same collimator for all studies.
- Position of the subject in front of the gamma camera and restriction of movement of the subject during imaging [100].
- Careful notation of image acquisition times and times of the in vitro emitted dose measurements prior to administration of the radiolabeled formulation in order that all data can be corrected for decay to a common time (time 0).
- Normalization of acquired counts for time to account for different imaging times between subjects. Images presented should have the same acquisition time because the scans can then be compared visually for differences in deposited radioactivity. This can be done, however, only if the nominal dose is similar between subjects. The use of color palettes can be misleading when presenting images of different subjects within a study, unless the scale relating count levels to color is kept the same for all images.
- Accurate measurement of the various calibration factors to be applied to both the in vivo data and any gamma camera images taken of inhalers and tubing. These latter calibration factors are different from those for the subject and need to be measured using sources or phantoms with known quantities of the same radioactivity as being inhaled.
- Ensuring a tight mouthpiece seal between the subject and the delivery system to avoid loss of aerosol inhaled and contamination of the room [101]. The use of a facemask is not recommended, except for infants.

DATA ANALYSIS

When imaging a subject after inhalation of a radiolabeled formulation, it is the radioactivity that is detected and measured; absolute amounts of deposited drug are inferred from the counts of radioactivity in the lung and other regions, based on the assumption that there is a 1:1 relationship between the two components. This relationship holds true for direct-labeled PET products or for those formulations where a firm bond can be demonstrated between the drug and radioactivity for the time taken to acquire all the images.

Determination of Deposited Dose

A number of investigators have addressed the issue of how to determine the absolute dose of radioactivity deposited in the lung and measured by either 2D or 3D imaging. Radioactivity counted over the lung field (counts/time) can be converted to megabequerels (MBq) or microcuries (μCi) detected in the lung by applying various calibration factors. These factors are measured using several techniques that utilize either external phantoms containing calibrated sources of radioactivity or the injection of a known amount of radioactivity and external detection [102–107]. The main source of reduction in the level of radioactivity detected is the chest wall, and this decrease can be as high as 50%, depending upon the subject [107]. The sensitivity of the imaging detector/collimator affects the detection of radioactivity and should be factored into the measurements [108,109]. Tissue attenuation factors vary between individuals with normal lungs and between those with diseased lungs [110–112], with greater variability in the latter group. Hence, these factors need to be determined for each individual studied to accurately calculate the deposited lung dose.

It should be recognized that the deposited dose is a fraction of the dose inhaled and that the inhaled dose is, in turn, a fraction of the nominal, or label claim, dose of the inhaler. Estimates of inhaled doses correlate with the fine particle dose, calculated from the fine particle fraction (% particles $<4.7\,\mu$m or $<5.8\,\mu$m in diameter) of the aerosol and the emitted ex-actuator or ex-device dose from the aerosol inhaler. The latter are measured in terms of radioactivity and drug prior to delivering the aerosol for deposition measurements. Drug deposition in the lung will further be reduced due to losses occurring in the inhaler device and in the oropharynx. This is particularly true for spacers attached to pMDIs, where upwards of 60% of the metered dose remains in the spacer. Fig. 7 illustrates the losses on the actuator mouthpiece and in the spacer, showing how the emitted dose of radioactivity is calculated. When possible, the device should be assayed for radioactivity postinhalation, either using a dose calibrator to measure the absolute amount of radioactivity or imaging the inhaler using the gamma camera and applying the appropriate calibration factors to obtain an absolute dose of radioactivity in the device. If possible, the inhaler can then be assayed for drug. These measurements will allow an estimation of the dose of tracer and drug delivered to the mouth.

Defining Lung Borders and Regions of Interest

Defining the edge of the lung is critical to determining both total and regional deposited doses. Several methods used for delineating the outer lung boundary are described in the literature. The options are:

- A transmission scan with an external source of radioactivity
- Inhalation of a radioactive gas, i.e., ^{133}xenon (^{133}Xe) or ^{81m}krypton (^{81m}Kr)
- Inhalation of an extrafine aerosol ($<1\,\mu$m MMAD) of Technegas, ^{99m}technetium (^{99m}Tc) sulfide colloid or albumin
- Measuring lung perfusion using an injection of ^{99m}Tc macroaggregated albumin

Fig. 8 illustrates examples of images for all of these procedures, acquired using planar imaging and, with the exception of the transmission scan, obtainable with SPECT imaging. The assessment of ventilation, which usually tracks the edge of the lung, has traditionally been measured with radioactive gases, but the inhalation of extrafine aerosols has been shown to give comparable information both in normals and in patients with airways disease [34,113,114]. While perfusion scanning is considered the "gold" standard [104], all these methods provide an acceptable outline of the lung.

Tissue Attenuation of Radioactivity

Using planar imaging, expressing the dose deposited in the lung in absolute terms requires the measurement of global lung tissue attenuation factors

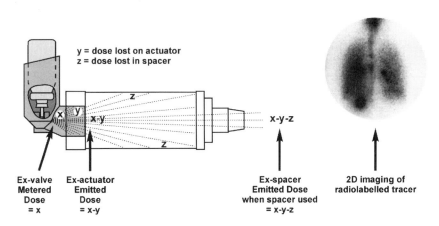

FIGURE 8 Schematic illustrating losses of radioactivity and drug in a pMDI + spacer delivery system. The emitted dose calculated when a spacer is used is reduced compared to when the spacer is not used, reflecting the loss of drug in the spacer. The radioactivity deposited in the oropharynx and stomach, shown in the 2D image, is from the coarse aerosol not collected by the spacer but inhaled.

(TAF) to correct for the reduction of activity due to chest wall absorption. These can be determined from a perfusion scan or a transmission scan or by measuring the thickness of the chest with calipers and calculating the factor from derived equations. The perfusion scan uses a known internal source of injected radioactivity, namely, ^{99m}Tc-microaggregated albumin (MAA) particles. Anterior and posterior images of the lung (Fig. 9) are obtained, the lung edge defined, followed by the calculation of the geometric mean count for the delineated lung. This last step is done to correct the acquired counts for the distance factor, i.e., the decrease in sensitivity of detection of activity emanating from the anterior lung when acquiring a posterior image. An error in the calculation of deposited dose of approximately 15% will be introduced if only the posterior image is acquired (M Dolovich, laboratory data). As the actual dose of injected radioactivity is known, a simple calculation can be made relating counts per minute per microcurie (or megabequeral) of activity in the whole lung as follows:

Tissue attenuation factor (cpm/μCi) from the perfusion scan (Q):

$$\mathrm{TAF}_Q = (N_A \times N_P)_Q^{1/2} \times \left(\frac{1}{A_{\text{injected}}}\right) \text{cpm/μCi} \tag{1}$$

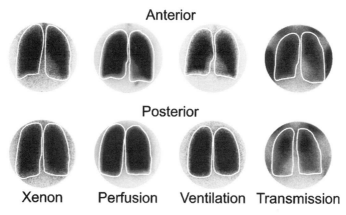

Anterior

Posterior

Xenon   Perfusion   Ventilation   Transmission

FIGURE 9   Methods for outlining the whole lung used in planar or 2D imaging. The area defined by the transmission scan appears to be approximately 10% smaller than with the other techniques. Scatter of low-energy gamma rays into the chest wall area is the most likely explanation for the larger lung seen with inhalation of xenon-133 gas. (From Ref. 114a.)

where

N_A = anterior perfusion cpm = sum of right and left lung cpm

N_P = posterior perfusion cpm = sum of right and left lung cpm

and $(N_A \times N_P)^{\frac{1}{2}}$ is the geometric mean count for the lung, cpm

A_{injected} = amount of ^{99m}Tc−MAA injected, μCi

Factors for the right and left lung and other regions of interest (ROIs) within the lung can be calculated separately by apportioning the amount injected to the area of interest, although this step is not without assumptions, possibly introducing error into the calculations. The factors can then be applied to the emission data for that particular area.

For planar imaging, transmission scans are performed with external pancake sources of ^{58}Co or ^{99m}TcO$_4{}^-$ [109]. To obtain an image, the source is held against the subject's chest and back for a fixed period of time. Both anterior and posterior images are acquired for the calculation of the attenuation factor. In addition, it is necessary to know precisely the dose of radioactivity in the source imaged by the gamma camera and the sensitivity of the gamma camera/collimator system for counting the particular isotope being used.

TAF from the transmission scan (TR):

$$\text{TAF}_{\text{TR}} = (N_O/N_T)^{1/2} \times 1/E \ \text{cpm}/\mu\text{Ci} \tag{2}$$

where

N_O = geometric mean of flood source count rate with regions

   defined from the transmission scan

N_T = geometric mean of count rate from transmission scan for the

   same regions = $(N_A \times N_P)_{\text{TR}}^{1/2}$

E = gamma camera sensitivity, cpm/μCi

This procedure can also be applied to the oropharyngeal region using lateral scans of the head and outlining the oropharynx in the images.

Defining Regions of Interest in the Lung

Defining regions of the lung for determining deposition of an inhaled therapy to the small peripheral (P) vs. large central (C) airways needs to accurately reflect lung geometry. This is especially true with 2D imaging. Because of the overlapping of airway structures, it is not possible to differentiate radioactivity emanating from small versus large airways [36,115], particularly when imaging immediately following inhalation of the tracer aerosol. Repeat imaging at 24 hours allows MCC to remove aerosol deposited on airway surfaces, leaving the remaining activity "representing" aerosol retained on peripheral airways. Aside from the need to align the subject in the same position in front of the scanner, this measurement is not always convenient to obtain. With 2D imaging, the peripheral region should be a narrow region, defined from the outer edge of the lung. Otherwise, the data are confounded by the detection of radioactivity from larger airways. As illustrated in Fig. 10, a number of methods have been applied to planar images to define central and peripheral regions within the lung [114]; a comparison between planar imaging and SPECT, using similar definitions for the lung regions demonstrated greater discrimination between aerosol deposited in central vs peripheral regions for SPECT [116]. As described above, the outer boundary of the lungs must be defined in the gamma camera

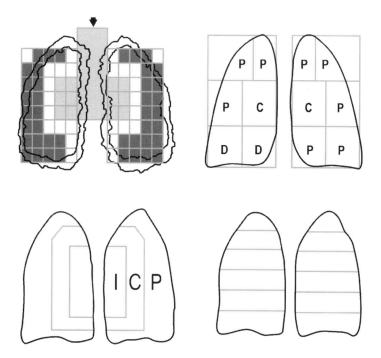

FIGURE 10 Various methods for defining regions of interest within the lung for images obtained with planar (2D) scanning. (From Ref. 114.)

images—this is the first step in mapping regions within the lung. The whole lung (right and left lungs) region is then further divided into regions of interest (ROIs), which correspond to the large (central), medium, and small (peripheral) airways.

Two methods that have been used extensively for defining three ROIs in planar lung images are the 5×8 grid [117] and "onionskin" (OS) contours [113,118] (Fig. 11). The former divides the lung into rectangular areas of variable size around the hilus, while for the latter, concentric rings are drawn from the lung edge to the hilus of approximately 1/4, 1/4, and 1/2 the lung width.

Contour Regions   5 x 8 Grid

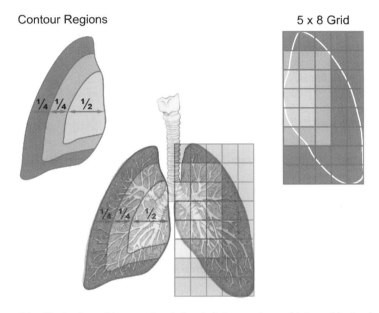

FIGURE 11   Illustration of two methods for defining regions of interest in the lung to calculate the distribution to the central and peripheral areas. For the 5×8 grid technique, rectangular grids, five sections wide by eight sections high, are placed over the right and left gas-filled lungs so that the perimeter of the grids enclose the lungs. The ROIs, containing different numbers of sections, are then drawn as nested rectangles, centered about the hilus, of varying height and width: outer border of $C = 2 \times 3$, $I = 3 \times 5$, and $P = 5 \times 8$ sections. For regions defined by the onionskin contour method, right and left lung areas are drawn by following the outer contours of the gas-filled lungs. The C, I, and P regions are drawn as three concentric regions from the outer edge to the hilus of the lung, with P and I regions each representing one-fourth the width of the lung and C representing one-half the width of each lung. Significant differences were seen between the central and peripheral regions for the two methods affecting the calculation of the P/C ratio. (From Ref. 113.)

A comparison of these two methods [113] for defining central (C), mid-, and peripheral (P) lung showed that the cross-sectional areas for the total lung and the peripheral ROIs were significantly greater for the 5×8 grid than for the OS contours, while the central lung ROI was significantly smaller, as defined by the grid. When the respective areas were applied to a deposition data set, the values for peripheral lung deposition were significantly greater and the central area deposition significantly less applying the grid as compared to the OS ROIs. This resulted in a P/C deposition ratio significantly greater for the 5×8 template, with the conclusion that there was greater drug deposited in the peripheral lung. The comparison points out the need for consensus among investigators imaging the lung for the purposes of assessing drug deposition as to the most appropriate geometry on which to base deposition calculations.

For the other two imaging modalities, SPECT and PET, multiple (up to 10) concentric regions of interest or shells are used to define the geometry for the purpose of calculating regional drug distribution (Fig. 12). The methods used for SPECT images have been developed by Fleming and colleagues and are described extensively in the literature [40,41,43,107,119,120]. For PET images, the shells are generated from the transmission scans for each transverse slice and applied to the specific emission slice (Fig. 13). Because of the way PET data are acquired, absolute quantitation of drug dose is possible for discrete areas within the lung.

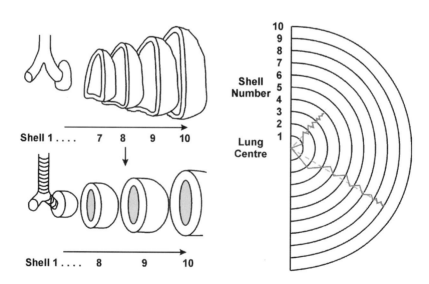

FIGURE 12 Illustration of shells constructed for a SPECT analysis. (From Ref. 132.)

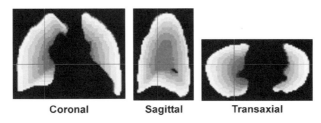

| Coronal | Sagittal | Transaxial |

FIGURE 13 Applying the PET shell analysis program to the lung images. One transmission slice from each of the coronal, transaxial, and sagittal planes is illustrated. The number of shells will vary with the geometry (cross-sectional area) of the slice. The shell configurations, obtained for the transmission scan slices, are then superimposed on the emission scans, slice by slice, providing volume and activity information related to the distribution of drug within the lung.

DIFFERENCES BETWEEN IMAGING MODALITIES FOR THE DETECTION AND MEASUREMENT OF DEPOSITED RADIOACTIVITY

A number of steps need to be implemented when using two- and three-dimensional imaging to measure lung deposition. Protocols should be in place to define the edge of the lung and the regions of interest, the measurement of tissue attenuation correction factors that are applied to the scanner data, and the calculation and expression of the deposition results. If possible, the correlation of dose and distribution data with clinical outcome measurements obtained at the time of imaging should be undertaken. There is still no consensus regarding the methods and protocols that should be used for these, but there is general agreement that the steps outlined are necessary to obtain meaningful deposition data.

Planar (2D) Scintigraphy

Planar (or projection) imaging using a gamma scintillation camera is the conventional technique for imaging the lung, providing two-dimensional analogue/digital information on the inhaled radiotracer. It is widely used to measure the dose and distribution of inhaled drugs. Each pixel (picture element) does not provide information on depth but represents the sum of the radioactivity along the axis perpendicular to the face of the camera. The collective images provide a good sense of total dose, but they are limited in offering information about dose deposited within the lung.

When measuring deposition, anterior and posterior images are obtained (Fig. 14) and the determination of radioactivity deposited is made by calculating

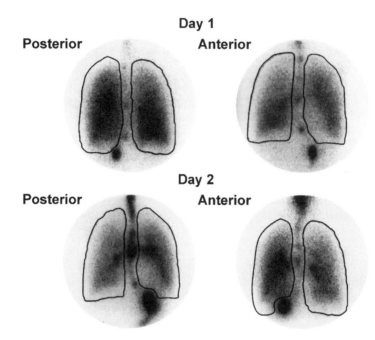

FIGURE 14 Planar anterior and posterior images obtained following inhalation of two different-size pMDI aerosols, with the outline of the lung drawn from the anterior and posterior perfusion scans. The difference in geometry and distribution of deposited radioactivity between the anterior and posterior images reflects the proximity of that area of the lung to the gamma camera face.

the geometric mean count rate of these two images. The result can then be expressed as a percentage of the total counts detected, or alternatively can be converted, using, as discussed earlier, tissue attenuation factors specific for the individual being imaged, to a deposited dose of radioactivity (μCi) or microgram quantities of drug. This value can be used to calculate inhaler deposition efficiency as a percentage of the emitted or inhaled dose of radioactivity or drug from the delivery system.

For example, when using a perfusion scan to outline the lung and to correct for tissue attenuation of radioactivity, the total lung dose deposited (TLD$_d$) is calculated as follows:

$$\text{TLD}_d = (N_A \times N_P)^{1/2} / \text{TAF}_Q, \quad \mu\text{Ci} \tag{3}$$

where

N_A = anterior cpm for the lung following radioaerosol inhalation

N_P = posterior cpm for the lung following radioaerosol inhalation

TAF_Q = tissue attenuation factor using perfusion method, cpm/μCi

The dose deposited in the lung (L) as a percentage of the emitted dose or metered dose is calculated as follows:

$$\%ED_L = dose\ deposited_{ED} = TLD_d/ED \times 100,\ \% \tag{4i}$$

or

$$\%MD_L = dose\ deposited_{MD} = TLD_d/MD \times 100,\ \% \tag{4ii}$$

where ED is the emitted dose or dose available at the mouth, in μCi, and MD is the metered dose from the inhaler, in μCi.

Similar calculations can be done for the different regions of interest in the lung or for the oropharynx and gut. The radioactivity deposited in specified regions of the lung is typically expressed as a percentage of the total lung dose of radioactivity or as a ratio of one region to another, such as the central to peripheral airways. To account for all the activity administered, mouthpieces, actuators, filters, etc. need to be imaged and/or measured in the dose calibrator. In the preceding calculations, the %ED will always be greater than the %MD, but the absolute values calculated for the dose in micrograms will be the same. There is merit in expressing the deposited dose in absolute terms. However, it is essential to measure the emitted dose also in micrograms, particularly when testing subjects with the same inhaler on different days, each day with varying amounts of loaded radioactivity, or when comparing different inhalers in the same subject. As shown in Fig. 15, while the deposition percentages for the lung were vastly different, the absolute amounts of drug delivered were not, a function of different nominal doses.

Single-Photon-Emission Computed Tomography (SPECT)

SPECT imaging is more complex than planar imaging, in that rather than obtaining single anterior and posterior cumulative two-dimensional images of the thorax, the gamma camera rotates through a full 360° obtaining multiple images from different angles [121]. Subsequent manipulation of the data using computers permits tomographic images to be constructed. This approach has potential advantages in that it improves the accuracy of assessing the pattern of deposition within the lungs. However, it has the associated disadvantages of longer acquisition times and requiring relatively high doses to be administered to

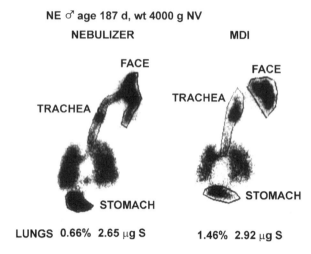

NE ♂ age 187 d, wt 4000 g NV

FIGURE 15 Deposition images obtained on two separate days for a 4-kg nonventilated neonate following inhalation of a pMDI radioaerosol, $^{99m}TcO_4^-$ salbutamol and a 99mTc-sulfide colloid plus salbutamol nebulizer solution. The lung deposition, expressed as percentages of the emitted dose, showed a twofold difference between the inhalers, favoring the pMDI. However, a similar lung dose of drug was received from both inhalers when the percentages were converted to absolute doses of salbutamol by using the nominal dose for each delivery system. (From Ref. 73.)

improve the counting efficiency per slice. Newer, dual- and triple-headed cameras are now available with reduced acquisition times, and they have become the "work horse" camera in many nuclear medicine departments. The per-pixel resolution (8–10 mm) is similar to or better than that of the gamma camera (10–14 mm). To interpret the scans and obtain accurate data, a CT scan or MRI is required to correct for attenuation and define the edge of the lung [122]. Protocols must be in place to coregister the data from the two machines or, alternatively, density factors are calculated for defined regions and applied to the SPECT emission data on a global basis. Calculation of deposited dose is then made from these data.

Positron-Emission Tomography (PET)

PET imaging provides a series of transaxial slices through the lungs, comparable to a CT scan. The transaxial information is used to reconstruct, postimaging, the lung activity for the other two planes, enabling coronal and sagittal images of the lungs to be viewed. PET resolution is approximately 4–6 mm/slice, enabling up to 120 slices per plane to be obtained. Because of the nature of the emissions and the use of coincidence counting, scatter is minimal and location of the pixels or voxels (volume unit) containing the radioactivity is precise. The ability of PET to examine and quantitate regional or local deposition from the coronal, sagittal, or transaxial views has clear advantages over 2D planar imaging (Fig. 16 [10]).

Correction for the natural decay of the PET isotope used is incorporated into the software protocols; correction for tissue attenuation of the radioactivity is made directly using PET and following each procedure by acquiring a transmission (density) scan with an external source of radioactivity. The advantages are that the geometry is constant, because the patient remains in the same position under the scanner as for the original investigation, and that the corrections are applied to each voxel in each slice of each plane. Applying attenuation correction to deposition data from the emission scans allows absolute amounts of radioactivity to be measured per cubic millimeter of lung tissue, giving the actual topographic distribution of drug throughout the lung. The transmission image also defines the lung borders for each slice, providing landmarks from which to delineate regions of interest in the emission scan (Fig. 17). When the lungs are imaged over time, the kinetics of the drug can be described for the whole lung as well as for specific regions. As with SPECT, multiple regions of interest or shells (Fig. 13), concentric about the hilus, can be defined and the deposition data per region of interest, reconstructed in all three planes. Both volume and dose information are obtained from the PET images. The information for deposited dose is obtained by summing the voxel data from the emission scan for designated regions (slices/shells) and applying the appropriate calibration factors; absolute volumes are obtained by summing

Projection View   Projection View Rotated

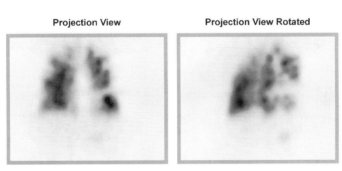

1.5 μm ¹⁸FDG aerosol, CF Subject

FIGURE 16 Projection view from a PET scan for one subject with cystic fibrosis. Rotation of the projection view, shown on the right, indicates that the location of aerosol deposited in both the right lung and left lung is posterior and basal, with some impaction of aerosol in the anterior of the left lung. This information is not apparent in the "head-on" view shown on the left. (From Ref. 10.)

Transmission Scans

Coronal   Transaxial   Sagittal

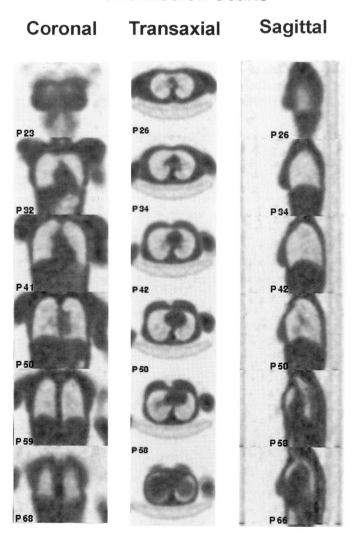

FIGURE 17 PET transmission scans for several slices of lung in the three planes showing the difference in geometry of the lung. During the reconstruction of the data, the tissue attenuation factors obtained from the transmission scan are applied to the absolute counts from the emission scan on a voxel-by-voxel basis. In the slice-by-slice analysis of the images, the emission scan of each slice is superimposed on its own transmission slice, allowing a more accurate location of the lung edge for the drawing of the shell regions, a distinct advantage over 2D imaging.

the number of voxels in the particular regions and applying volume factors. Data can be expressed in a number of ways, including the dose per unit lung volume.

PET techniques offer the important advantage in that the drug under study can be firmly labeled with the appropriate positron emitting isotope, usually ^{11}C or [18]F. Thus, deposition reflects the pharmaceutical itself, without interference from free isotope. Fluticasone dipropionate, triamcinolone acetonide, and zanamivir have all been labeled and their dose and distribution in the respiratory tract and/or the nasal cavity assessed with PET [48,50,123].

AEROSOLS USED IN CLINICAL INVESTIGATIONS OF DISEASE

Several diagnostic tests utilizing specific-size nonradioactive aerosols and also radioactive aerosols with standard nuclear medicine technology are practiced in respiratory medicine (Table 2). For example, inhalation of aerosols of methacholine and histamine is widely used to assess nonspecific bronchial responsiveness in asthma; the concentration of the challenge aerosol that provokes a specific fall in FEV1 gives an indication of the severity of the disease. Changes in the disease with treatment or with exposure to sensitizing agents can be monitored over time with repeated measurements. These measurements are coupled with clinical outcomes such as spirometry and pharmacokinetic and pharmacodynamic measurements in the same group of subjects. In the research laboratory, measurements using radioactive aerosols of these challenge agents have determined the change in distribution effected with changes in airway caliber [124,125] as well as compared techniques and outcomes in inhalation challenge testing [126–128].

Mucociliary clearance (MCC), a measure of the surface transport properties of the lung, and lung epithelial permeability (LEP), a measure of the integrity of the alveolar–capillary membrane, can be assessed using radiotracers and imaging. MCC is determined from the rate of removal (from ciliated airways) of an inhaled tracer aerosol, while LEP is determined from the rate of removal of an inhaled tracer resulting from absorption across the alveolated surface of the lung and into the circulation. Table 3 lists the factors affecting these measurements, some of which need to be controlled when performing these studies [31].

MCC is measured by imaging the lung over time to obtain the retention of an inhaled radioaerosol. Planar imaging is used mainly, and serial measurements are required. Because aerosol size and ventilatory parameters affect where aerosol is initially deposited in the lung and because the rate of transport is more rapid from proximal airways than peripheral airways, changes to the initial deposition pattern as a result of treatment or the factors listed in Table 3 will

TABLE 3   Factors Affecting the Measurement of Lung Mucociliary
Clearance (MCC) and Lung Epithelial Permeability (LEP)

MCC	LEP
Site of deposition of tracer aerosol	Molecular weight of solute probe
Particle size of aerosol	Site of deposition of labeled solute
Pattern of inhalation	Recirculation of labeled solute
Airway caliber	Stability of labeled solute in vivo
Lung capacity	Ventilation
Mucus/cilia interaction	Posture
Mucosal surface damage	Apex–base gradient in LEP
Spontaneous cough	Inspiratory volume
Exercise	PEEP
Disease	CPAP
Drugs	Exercise
	Smoking

have a marked effect on MCC. In addition, inter- and intrasubject variability in deposition makes it difficult to do repeated measurements of MCC and to group subjects. The differences between subjects can be partly attributed to airway geometry and lung size [129]; therefore, measurements of lung volumes and expiratory flowrates should be obtained for each subject studied.

Submicronic aerosols of low molecular weight solutes are used to measure epithelial permeability [25,26]; the site of deposition of these tracers must be distal to the ciliated airway surfaces. LEP is measured by dynamic planar imaging of the lung for 15–30 minutes. Parallel blood samples can be obtained at the same time points to measure plasma radioactivity, but this is not critical to the determination of the rate of absorption of the radiotracer. MCC of the submicronic aerosol is extremely slow, with $t^{1/2}$ in excess of 24 hours. Because LEP is measured over 30 min, the error due to MCC is negligible. Peripheral lung regions of interest are usually chosen for analysis of uptake to avoid the contribution from any radioactivity deposited in the hilar regions [130].

Inhalation of hypertonic saline is a noninvasive diagnostic test using nonradioactive aerosols and results in expectoration of sputum. The cellular content of the sputum, related to the degree of inflammation present in the lung in asthma, is then measured using specific laboratory techniques and provides an objective means of monitoring the disease and the effectiveness of anti-inflammatory therapy. Scheduling of these tests, either pre- or postinhalation of the tracer aerosol, would be determined by the clinical question or the research objective.

SUMMARY

The total and regional dose deposited in the lung, obtained using two- or three-dimensional scintigraphic imaging is a useful measurement of topical drug delivery, made doubly useful when correlated with pharmacodynamic and/or and pharmacokinetic data and preferably in the same subjects that undergo imaging. While the accuracy, sensitivity, and resolution of current 2D detectors is high, the use of 3D imaging is to be encouraged [28,45,52]. Further support for the deposition data must be provided by efficacy and safety studies of the test aerosol in various types of patients that would be prescribed the test medications. Knowledge of the lung dose and distribution of inhaled aerosols from delivery systems is critical for the assessment of their performance in vivo and can provide a rationale for adjusting the therapeutic dose for different categories of patients. Arguments for using imaging as a means of predicting clinical response have been raised [120,131]; however, improved accuracy of both in vitro and in vivo data must be demonstrated before this approach is accepted by the medical community as a suitable substitution for biological data.

REFERENCES

1. O'Doherty MJ, Miller RF. Aerosols for therapy and diagnosis. Eur J Nucl Med 1993; 20(12):1201–1213.
2. Newman SP, Pitcairn GR, Hirst PH. A brief history of gamma scintigraphy. J Aerosol Med 2001; 14(2):139–145.
3. Gonda I. Scintigraphic techniques for measuring in vivo deposition. J Aerosol Med 1996; 9(suppl 1):S59–S67.
4. Newman SP. Scintigraphic assessment of therapeutic aerosols. Crit Rev Ther Drug Carrier Syst 1993; 10(1):65–109.
5. Kunka R, Andrews S, Pimazzoni M, Callejas S, Ziviani L, Squassante L, et al.. From hydrofluoroalkane pressurized metered-dose inhalers (pMDIs) and comparability with chlorofluorocarbon pMDIs. Respir Med 2000; 94(suppl B):S10–S16.
6. Selroos O, Pietinallo A, Riska H. Delivery devices for inhaled asthma medication. Clin Immunother 1996; 6(4):273–299.
7. Edsbacker S. Pharmacological factors that influence the choice of inhaled corticosteroids. Drugs 1999; 58(suppl 4):7–16.
8. Wilson A, Demsey O, Couties W, Sims E, Lipworth B. Importance of drug–device interaction in determining systemic effects of inhaled corticosteroids. Lancet 1999; 353:2128.
9. Taylor I, Hill A, Hayes M, Rhodes CG, O'Shaughnessy K, O'Connor BJ. Imaging allergen-invoked airway inflammation in atopic asthma with [18F]-fluorodeoxyglucose and positron emission tomography. Lancet 1996; 347:937–940.
10. Dolovich M. Aerosol delivery devices and airways/lung deposition. In: Schleimer R, O'Byrne P, Szefler SJ, Brattsand R, eds. Inhaled Steroids in Asthma: Optimizing Effects in the Airways. New York: Marcel Dekker, 2002:169–211.

11. Dolovich MB. Influence of inspiratory flow rate, particle size, and airway caliber on aerosolized drug delivery to the lung. Respir Care 2000; 45(6):597–608.

12. Zanen P, Go LT, Lammers JW. Optimal particle size for beta 2 agonist and anticholinergic aerosols in patients with severe airflow obstruction [see comments]. Thorax 1996; 51(10):977–980.

13. Martin R, Szefler SJ, Chinchilli V, Kraft M, Dolovich M, Boushey HCR, et al. Systemic effect comparisons of six inhaled corticosteroid preparations. Am J Respir Crit Care Med 2002; 165:1377–1383.

14. Byron PR, ed. Pathophysiological and Disease Constraints on Aerosol Delivery. Boca Raton, FL: CRC Press, 1990.

15. Heyder J, Gebbart J, Rudolf G, Stahlhofen W. Physical factors determining particle deposition in the human respiratory tract. J Aerosol Sci 1980; 11:505–515.

16. Everard ML, Dolovich M. In vivo measurements of lung dose. In: Bisgaard H, O'Callaghan C, , Smaldone GC, eds. Drug Delivery to the Lung. New York: Marcel Dekker, 2001:173–209.

17. Bennett WD, Brown JS, Zeman KL, Hu SC, Scheuch G, Sommerer K. Targeting delivery of aerosols to different lung regions. J Aerosol Med 2002; 15(2):179–188.

18. Laube BL, Jashnani R, Dalby RN, Zeitlin PL. Targeting aerosol deposition in patients with cystic fibrosis: effects of alterations in particle size and inspiratory flow rate. Chest 2000; 118(4):1069–1076.

19. Smaldone GC, Fuhrer J, Steigbigel RT, McPeck M. Factors determining pulmonary deposition of aerosolized pentamidine in patients with human immunodeficiency virus infection. Am Rev Respir Dis 1991; 143(4 Pt 1):727–737.

20. Anderson PJ, Dolovich MB. Aerosols as diagnostic tools. J Aerosol Med 1994; 7(1):77–88.

21. Dolovich M, Cockcroft D, Coates G. Aerosols in diagnosis: ventilation, airway penetrance, airway reactivity, epithelial permeability and mucociliary transport. In: Moren F, Dolovich M, Newhouse M, Newman S, eds. Aerosols in Medicine: Principles, Diagnosis and Therapy. Amsterdam: Elsevier Science, 1993:195–234.

22. Robinson M, Eberl S, Tomlinson C, Daviskas E, Regnis JA, Bailey DL, et al. Regional mucociliary clearance in patients with cystic fibrosis. J Aerosol Med 2000; 13(2):73–86.

23. Robinson M, Bye PT. Mucociliary clearance in cystic fibrosis. Pediatr Pulmonol 2002; 33(4):293–306.

24. Knowles MR, Boucher RC. Mucus clearance as a primary innate defense mechanism for mammalian airways. J Clin Investig 2002; 109(5):571–577.

25. Coates G, O'Brodovich H, Dolovich M. Lung clearance of 99mTc-DTPA in patients with acute lung injury and pulmonary edema. J Thorac Imaging 1988; 3(3):21–27.

26. Diot P, Galinier E, Grimbert D, Bugeon S, Valat C, Lemarie E, et al. Characterization of 99mTc-DTPA aerosols for lung permeability studies. Respiration 2001; 68(3):313–317.

27. Effros R. Epithelial permeability. In: Moren F, Dolovich M, Newhouse M, Newman S, eds. Aerosols in Medicine: Principles, Diagnosis and Therapy. Amsterdam: Elsevier Science, 1993:235–246.

28. Reinartz P, Schirp U, Zimny M, Sabri O, Nowak B, Schafer W, et al. Optimizing ventilation-perfusion lung scintigraphy: parting with planar imaging. Nuklearmedizin 2001; 40(2):38–43.

29. Tagil K, Evander E, Wollmer P, Palmer J, Jonson B. Efficient lung scintigraphy. Clin Physiol 2000; 20(2):95–100.

30. Davis SS, Hardy JG, Newman SP, Wilding IR. Gamma scintigraphy in the evaluation of pharmaceutical dosage forms. Eur J Nucl Med 1992; 19(11):971–986.

31. Dolovich MB, Jordana M, Newhouse MT. Methodologic considerations in mucociliary clearance and lung epithelial absorption measurements. Eur J Nucl Med 1987; 13(suppl):S45–S52.

32. Calmanovici G, Boccio J, Goldman C, Hager A, De Paoli T, Alak M, et al. 99mTc-ENS ventilation scintigraphy: preliminary study in human volunteers. Nucl Med Biol 2000; 27(2):215–218.

33. Walker PS, Conway JH, Fleming JS, Bondesson E, Borgstrom L. Pulmonary clearance rate of two chemically different forms of inhaled pertechnetate. J Aerosol Med 2001; 14(2):209–215.

34. Coghe J, Votion D, Lekeux P. Comparison between radioactive aerosol, technegas and krypton for ventilation imaging in healthy calves. Vet J 2000; 160(1):25–32.

35. Suarez S, Hickey AJ. Drug properties affecting aerosol behavior. Respir Care 2000; 45(6):652–666.

36. Martonen TB, Yang Y, Dolovich M. Definition of airway composition within gamma camera images. J Thorac Imaging 1994; 9(3):188–197.

37. Jaszczak R, Coleman RE, Lim C. SPECT: single photon emission computed tomography. IEEE Trans Nucl Sci 1980; 27:1137–1153.

38. Fleming JS, Sauret V, Conway JH, Holgate ST, Bailey AG, Martonen TB. Evaluation of the accuracy and precision of lung aerosol deposition measurements from single-photon emission computed tomography using simulation. J Aerosol Med 2000; 13(3):187–198.

39. Fleming JS, Hashish AH, Conway JH, Nassim MA, Holgate ST, Halson P, et al. Assessment of deposition of inhaled aerosol in the respiratory tract of man using three-dimensional multimodality imaging and mathematical modeling. J Aerosol Med 1996; 9(3):317–327.

40. Fleming JS, Conway JH. Three-dimensional imaging of aerosol deposition. J Aerosol Med 2001; 14(2):147–153.

41. Eberl S, Chan HK, Daviskas E, Constable C, Young I. Aerosol deposition and clearance measurement: a novel technique using dynamic SPET. Eur J Nucl Med 2001; 28(9):1365–1372.

42. Chan HK, Eberl S, Daviskas E, Constable C, Young IH. Dynamic SPECT of aerosol deposition and mucociliary clearance in healthy subjects (abstr). J Aerosol Med 1999; 12:135.

43. Rhodes CG, Hughes JM. Pulmonary studies using positron emission tomography. Eur Respir J 1995; 8:1011–1017.

44. Dolovich MB. Measuring total and regional lung deposition using inhaled radiotracers. J Aerosol Med 2001; 14(suppl 1):S35–S44.

45. Musch G, Layfield JD, Harris RS, Melo MF, Winkler T, Callahan RJ, et al. Topographical distribution of pulmonary perfusion and ventilation, assessed by PET in supine and prone humans. J Appl Physiol 2002; 93(5):1841–1851.

46. Dolovich M, Nahmias C, Coates G. Unleashing the PET: 3D imaging of the lung. In: Byron PR, Dalby R, Farr SJ, eds. Respiratory Drug Delivery VII. North Carolina: Serentec Press, 2000:215–230.

47. Czernin J, Phelps M. Positron emission tomography scanning: current and future applications. Annu Rev Med 2002; 53:89–112.

48. Bergstrom M, Cass LM, Valind S, Westerberg G, Lundberg EL, Gray S, et al. Deposition and disposition of [11C]zanamivir following administration as an intranasal spray. Evaluation with positron emission tomography. Clin Pharmacokinet 1999; 36(suppl 1):33–39.

49. Bailey AG, Gilardi MC, Grootoonk S, Kinahan P, Nahmias C, Ollinger J, et al. Quantitative procedures in 3D PET. In: Bendriem B, Townsend DW, eds. The Theory and Practice of PET. Dordrecht, Netherlands: Kluwer Academic, 1998.

50. Lee Z, Berridge MS, Finlay WH, Heald DL. Mapping PET-measured triamcinolone acetonide (TAA) aerosol distribution into deposition by airway generation. Int J Pharm 2000; 199(1):7–16.

51. Berridge MS, Lee Z, Heald DL. Regional distribution and kinetics of inhaled pharmaceuticals. Curr Pharm Des 2000; 6(16):1631–1651.

52. Aboagye EO, Price PM, Jones T. In vivo pharmacokinetics and pharmacodynamics in drug development using positron-emission tomography. Drug Discov Today 2001; 6(6):293–302.

53. Derendorf H, Lesko LJ, Chaikin P, Colburn WA, Lee P, Miller R, et al. Pharmacokinetic/pharmacodynamic modeling in drug research and development. J Clin Pharmacol 2000; 40(12 Pt 2):1399–1418.

54. Cheng YS, Holmes TD, Gao J, Guilmette RA, Li S, Surakitbanharn Y, et al. Characterization of nasal spray pumps and deposition pattern in a replica of the human nasal airway. J Aerosol Med 2001; 14(2):267–280.

55. Boek WM, Graamans K, Natzijl H, van Rijk PP, Huizing EH. Nasal mucociliary transport: new evidence for a key role of ciliary beat frequency. Laryngoscope 2002; 112(3):570–573.

56. Dolovich MB. Aerosols. In: Barnes P, Grunstein M, Leff A, Woolcock A, eds. Asthma. Philadelphia: Lippincott-Raven, 1997:1349–1366.

57. Fink JB. Metered-dose inhalers, dry powder inhalers, and transitions. Respir Care 2000; 45(6):623–635.

58. Dolovich M. New delivery systems and propellants. Can Respir J 1999; 6(3):290–295.

59. Chan HK, Daviskas E, Eberl S, Robinson M, Bautovich G, Young I. Deposition of aqueous aerosol of technetium-99m diethylene triamine penta-acetic acid generated and delivered by a novel system (AERx) in healthy subjects. Eur J Nucl Med 1999; 26(4):320–327.

60. Cass LM, Brown J, Pickford M, Fayinka S, Newman SP, Johansson CJ, et al. Pharmacoscintigraphic evaluation of lung deposition of inhaled zanamivir in healthy volunteers. Clin Pharmacokinet 1999; 36(suppl 1):21–31.

61. Newman SP. Characteristics of radiolabeled versus unlabeled inhaler formulations. J Aerosol Med 1996; 9(suppl 1):S37–S47.

62. Warren S, Taylor G, Smith J, Buck H, Parry-Billings M. Gamma scintigraphic evaluation of a novel budesonide dry powder inhaler using a validated radiolabeling technique. J Aerosol Med 2002; 15(1):15–25.

63. Dolovich M. In vitro measurements of delivery of medications from MDIs and spacer devices. J Aerosol Med 1996; 9(suppl 1):S49–S58.

64. Chan HK, Eberl S, Daviskas E, Constable C, Young I. Changes in lung deposition of aerosols due to hygroscopic growth: a fast SPECT study. J Aerosol Med 2002; 15(3):307–311.

65. Bennett WD. Effect of beta-adrenergic agonists on mucociliary clearance. J Allergy Clin Immunol 2002; 110(suppl 6):S291–S297.

66. Sabater JR, Wanner A, Abraham WM. Montelukast prevents antigen-induced mucociliary dysfunction in sheep. Am J Respir Crit Care Med 2002; 166(11):1457–1460.

67. Oldenburg FA Jr, Dolovich MB, Montgomery JM, Newhouse MT. Effects of postural drainage, exercise, and cough on mucus clearance in chronic bronchitis. Am Rev Respir Dis 1979; 120(4):739–745.

68. Robinson M, Regnis JA, Bailey DL, King M, Bautovich GJ, Bye PT. Effect of hypertonic saline, amiloride, and cough on mucociliary clearance in patients with cystic fibrosis. Am J Respir Crit Care Med 1996; 153(5):1503–1509.

69. Spiro SG, Singh CA, Tolfree SE, Partridge MR, Short MD. Direct labeling of ipratropium bromide aerosol and its deposition pattern in normal subjects and patients with chronic bronchitis. Thorax 1984; 39(6):432–435.

70. Geworski L, Knoop BO, de Wit M, Ivancevic V, Bares R, Munz DL. Multicenter comparison of calibration and cross-calibration of PET scanners. J Nucl Med 2002; 43(5):635–639.

71. Mallol J, Rattray S, Walker G, Cook D, Robertson CF. Aerosol deposition in infants with cystic fibrosis. Pediatr Pulmonol 1996; 21(5):276–281.

72. Devadason SG, Everard ML, MacEarlan C, Roller C, Summers QA, Swift P, et al. Lung deposition from the Turbuhaler in children with cystic fibrosis. Eur Respir J 1997; 10(9):2023–2028.

73. Fok TF, Monkman S, Dolovich M, Gray S, Coates G, Paes B, et al. Efficiency of aerosol medication delivery from a metered-dose inhaler versus jet nebulizer in infants with bronchopulmonary dysplasia. Pediatr Pulmonol 1996; 21(5):301–309.

74. Fuller HD, Dolovich MB, Posmituck G, Pack WW, Newhouse MT. Pressurized aerosol versus jet aerosol delivery to mechanically ventilated patients. Comparison of dose to the lungs. Am Rev Respir Dis 1990; 141(2):440–444.

75. Anhoj J, Thorsson L, Bisgaard H. Lung deposition of inhaled drugs increases with age. Am J Respir Crit Care Med 2000; 162(5):1819–1822.

76. Salmon B, Wilson N, Silverman M. How much aerosol reaches the lungs of wheezy infants and toddlers? Arch Dis Child 1990; 98:401–404.

77. Everard ML. The use of radiolabeled aerosols for research purposes in paediatric patients: ethical and practical aspects. Thorax 1994; 49(12):1259–1266.

78. Radiation dose to patients from radiopharmaceuticals. A Report of a Task Group of Committees 2 and 3 of the International Commission on Radiological Protection (ICRP). Oxford, UK: Pergamon Press, 1994.

79. Aug C, Perry RJ, Smaldone GC. Technetium 99m radiolabeling of aerosolized drug particles from metered dose inhalers. J Aerosol Med 1991; 4(2):127–138.

80. Farr SJ. The physicochemical basis of radiolabeling metered-dose inhalers with 99mTc. J Aerosol Med 1996; 9(suppl 1):S27–S36.

81. Fok TF, al Essa M, Monkman S, Dolovich M, Girard L, Coates G, et al. Pulmonary deposition of salbutamol aerosol delivered by metered-dose inhaler, jet nebulizer, and ultrasonic nebulizer in mechanically ventilated rabbits. Pediatr Res 1997; 42(5):721–727.

82. Koehler D, Fleischer W, Matthys H. New method for easy labelling of β-agonists in metered-dose inhalers with technetium 99m. Respiration 1988; 53:65–73.

83. Summers QA, Clark AR, Hollingworth A, Fleming JS, Holgate ST. The preparation of a radiolabeled aerosol of nedocromil sodium for administration by metered-dose inhaler that accurately preserves particle size distribution of the drug. Drug Investig 1990; 2:90–98.

84. Byron PR, et al. Recommendations of the USP advisory panel on aerosols on the USP general chapters on aerosols [601] and uniformity of dosage units [905]. Pharm Forum 1994; 7:7477–7503. http://www.fda.gov/cder/guidance/index.htm.

85. Guidance for Industry Metered-Dose Inhaler (MDI) and Dry Powder Inhaler (DPI) Drug Products Chemistry, Manufacturing, and Controls Documentation. Center for Drug Evaluation and Research (CDER), 1998.

86. Dolovich M, Rhem R, Rashid F, Coates G, Hill M, Bowen B. Measurement of the particle size and dosing characteristics of a radiolabeled albuterol–sulphate lactose blend used in the SPIROS[7] dry powder inhaler. In: Byron PR, Dalby R, Farr SJ, eds. Respiratory Drug Delivery V. Buffalo Grove, FL, Interpharm Press: 1996:332–335.

87. Newman SP, Moren F, Trofast E, Talaee N, Clarke SW. Deposition and clinical efficacy of terbutaline sulphate from Turbuhaler, a new multidose powder inhaler. Eur Respir J 1989; 2(3):247–252.

88. Dolovich M, Rhem R, Rashid F, Bowen B. Lung deposition of albuterol sulphate from the Dura Dryhaler in normal adults. Am J Respir Crit Care Med 1996; 153(4(Part 2)):A62.

89. Olsson B, Asking L, Borgstrom L, Bondesson E. Effect of inlet throat on the correlation between measured fine particle dose and lung deposition. In: Dalby RN, Byron PR, Farr SJ, eds. Respiratory Drug Delivery V. Buffalo Grove, IL: Interpharm Press, 1996:273–281.

90. Laube BL. In vivo measurements of aerosol dose and distribution: clinical relevance. J Aerosol Med 1996; 9(suppl 1):S77–S91.

91. Dolovich MB. Assessing nebulizer performance. Respir Care 2002; 47(11):1–15.

92. Dolovich M, Rhem R. Impact of oropharyngeal deposition on inhaled dose. J Aerosol Med 1998; 11(suppl 1):S112–S115.

93. Laube BL, Links JM, LaFrance ND, Wagner HN Jr, Rosenstein BJ. Homogeneity of bronchopulmonary distribution of 99mTc aerosol in normal subjects and in cystic fibrosis patients. Chest 1989; 95(4):822–830.

94. Kim CS, Lewars GA, Sackner MA. Measurement of total lung aerosol deposition as an index of lung abnormality. J Appl Physiol 1988; 64(4):1527–1536.

95. Kim CS, Abraham WM, Garcia L, Sackner MA. Enhanced aerosol deposition in the lung with mild airways obstruction. Am Rev Respir Dis 1989; 139(2):422–426.

96. Kim CS, Kang TC. Comparative measurement of lung deposition of inhaled fine particles in normal subjects and patients with obstructive airway disease. Am J Respir Crit Care Med 1997; 155(3):899–905.

97. Farr SJ, Rowe AM, Rubsamen R, Taylor G. Aerosol deposition in the human lung following administration from a microprocessor-controlled pressurized metered-dose inhaler. Thorax 1995; 50(6):639–644.

98. Smaldone GC. Deposition and clearance: unique problems in the proximal airways and oral cavity in the young and elderly. Respir Physiol 2001; 128(1):33–38.

99. Dolovich M, Rhem R. Small differences in inspiratory flow rate (IFR) and aerosol particle size can influence upper and lower respiratory tract deposition. J Aerosol Med 1997; 10(3):238.

100. Mijailovich SM, Treppo S, Venegas JG. Effects of lung motion and tracer kinetics corrections on PET imaging of pulmonary function. J Appl Physiol 1997; 82(4):1154–1162.

101. Braga FJ, Souza JF, Trad CS, Santos AC, Ghillardi NT, Elias J Jr, et al. An improved mouthpiece to prevent environmental contamination during radioaerosol inhalation procedures. Health Phys 1998; 75(4):424–427.

102. Bailey DL, Jones T, Spinks TJ. A method for measuring the absolute sensitivity of positron-emission tomographic scanners. Eur J Nucl Med 1991; 18(6):374–379.

103. Fok TF, al Essa M, Kirpalani H, Monkman S, Bowen B, Coates G, et al. Estimation of pulmonary deposition of aerosol using gamma scintigraphy. J Aerosol Med 1999; 12(1):9–15.

104. Forge NI, Mountford PJ, O'Doherty MJ. Quantification of technetium-99m lung radioactivity from planar images [published erratum appears in Eur J Nucl Med 1993; 20(4):367]. Eur J Nucl Med 1993; 20(1):10–15.

105. Fleming JS. A technique for using CT images in attenuation correction and quantification in SPECT. Nucl Med Commun 1989; 10(2):83–97.

106. Ruffin R, Kenworthy M, Newhouse M. Response of patients to fenoterol inhalation: a method for quantifying the airway bronchodilator dose. Clin Pharmacol Ther 1978; 23:338–342.

107. Messina MS, Smaldone GC. Evaluation of quantitative aerosol techniques for use in bronchoprovocation studies. J Allergy Clin Immunol 1985; 75(2):252–257.

108. Fleming JS, Alaamer AS. Influence of collimator characteristics on quantification in SPECT. J Nucl Med 1996; 37(11):1832–1836.

109. Macey M, Marshall R. Absolute quantitation of radiotracer uptake in the lungs using a gamma camera. J Nucl Med 1982; 23:39–45.

110. Pitcairn G. Tissue attenuation corrections in gamma scintigraphy. J Aerosol Med 1997; 3:187–198.

111. Langenback EG, Foster WM, Bergofsky EH. Calculating concentration of inhaled radiolabeled particles from external gamma counting: external counting efficiency and attenuation coefficient of thorax. J Toxicol Environ Health 1989; 26:139–152.

112. Itoh H, Smaldone GC, Swift DL, Wagner HN Jr. Quantitative measurements of aerosol deposition: evaluation of different techniques. J Aerosol Sci 1985; 16:367–371.

113. Dolovich M, Rhem R, Kish S, Saab C. Defining lung regions for the purpose of calculating deposition to the small airways. Am J Respir Crit Care Med 2002; 165:A190.

114. Kim CS. Methods of calculating lung delivery and deposition of aerosol particles. Respir Care 2000; 45(6):695–711.

114a. Dolovich MB, Rhem R, Coates G. Defining and quantitating peripheral lung deposition using radiolabeled tracers and 2D imaging. Eur Resp J 2000; 16 (suppl 31):625–P560.

115. Martonen TB, Yang Y, Dolovich M, Guan X. Computer simulations of lung morphologies within planar gamma camera images. Nucl Med Commun 1997; 18(9):861–869.

116. Phipps PR, Gonda I, Bailey DL, Borham P, Bautovich G, Anderson SD. Comparisons of planar and tomographic gamma scintigraphy to measure the penetration index of inhaled aerosols. Am Rev Respir Dis 1989; 139(6):1516–1523.

117. Newman SP, Hirst PH, Pitcairn GR, Clark AR. Understanding regional lung deposition in gamma scintigraphy. In: Dalby RN, Byron PR, Farr SJ, eds. Respiratory Drug Delivery VI. Buffalo Grove, IL: Interpharm Press, 1998:9–15.

118. Sanchis J, Dolovich M, Chalmers R, Newhouse M. Quantitation of regional aerosol clearance in the normal human lung. J Appl Physiol 1972; 33(6):757–762.

119. Fleming JS, Halson P, Conway J, Moore E, Nassim MA, Hashish AH, et al.. Three-dimensional description of pulmonary deposition of inhaled aerosol using data from multimodality imaging. J Nucl Med 1996; 37(5):873–877.

120. Newman SP. Can lung deposition data act as a surrogate for the clinical response to inhaled asthma drugs? Br J Clin Pharmacol 2000; 49(6):529–537.

121. Fahey FH. Positron-emission tomography instrumentation. Radiol Clin N Am 2001; 39(5):919–929.

122. Bailey DL. Transmission scanning in emission tomography. Eur J Nucl Med 1998; 25(7):774–787.

123. Rahman S, Rhodes CG, Constantinou M, Waters S, Aigbirho FOS, et al.. Lung deposition of 18-F-fluticasone propionate in normal subjects using positron emission tomography. Am J Respir Crit Care Med 2000; 161(Part 2):A177.

124. Ruffin RE, Dolovich MB, Wolff RK, Newhouse MT. The effects of preferential deposition of histamine in the human airway. Am Rev Respir Dis 1978; 117(3):485–492.

125. Ruffin RE, Dolovich MB, Oldenburg FA Jr, Newhouse MT. The preferential deposition of inhaled isoproterenol and propranolol in asthmatic patients. Chest 1981; 80(suppl 6):904–907.

126. Ryan G, Dolovich MB, Roberts RS, Frith PA, Juniper EF, Hargreave FE, et al. Standardization of inhalation provocation tests: two techniques of aerosol generation and inhalation compared. Am Rev Respir Dis 1981; 123(2):195–199.

127. Schmekel B, Hedenstrom H, Kampe M, Lagerstrand L, Stalenheim G, Wollmer P, et al. The bronchial response, but not the pulmonary response, to inhaled methacholine is dependent on the aerosol deposition pattern. Chest 1994; 106(6):1781–1787.

128. O'Riordan TG, Walser L, Smaldone GC. Changing patterns of aerosol deposition during methacholine bronchoprovocation. Chest 1993; 103(5):1385–1389.

129. Garrard CS, Gerrity TR, Yeates DB. The relationships of aerosol deposition, lung size, and the rate of mucociliary clearance. Arch Environ Health 1986; 41(1):11–15.

130. O'Doherty MJ, Page CJ, Croft DN, Bateman NT. Lung 99Tcm-DTPA transfer: a method for background correction. Nucl Med Commun 1985; 6(4):209–215.

131. Snell NJ, Ganderton D. Assessing lung deposition of inhaled medications. Consensus statement from a workshop of the British Association for Lung Research, held at the Institute of Biology, London, on 17 April 1998. Respir Med 1999; 93(2):123–133.

132. Fleming JS, Nassim MA, Hashish AH, Bailey AG, Conway J, Holgate ST, et al. Description of pulmonary deposition of radiolabeled aerosol by airway generation using a conceptual three-dimensional model of lung morphology. J Aerosol Med 1995; 8:341–356.

7

Pharmacokinetics and Pharmacodynamics of Drugs Delivered to the Lungs

Manish Issar, Cary Mobley, Patricia Khan, and Günther Hochhaus
University of Florida, Gainesville, Florida, U.S.A.

INTRODUCTION

The focus of this chapter is on the pharmacokinetic and pharmacodynamic aspects of inhalation drugs for topical delivery. For the last 30 years, pulmonary drug delivery has been successfully employed for topical therapy of pulmonary diseases, with the goal of achieving pronounced pulmonary effect while reducing systemic side effects. The degree of pulmonary targeting is determined by a number of pharmacokinetic (PK) and pharmacodynamic (PD) factors. This chapter will discuss these relationships and will review the pharmacokinetic and pharmacodynamic tools suitable for characterizing inhalation drugs.

FACTORS IMPORTANT FOR PULMONARY TARGETING
Pulmonary Targeting—as Seen by a Pharmacokineticist's Eye

Figure 1 illustrates the sequence of events relevant to pulmonary drug administration. Once released from the device, a fraction of the delivered dose (respirable fraction) will be deposited in the lung, while larger particles will be

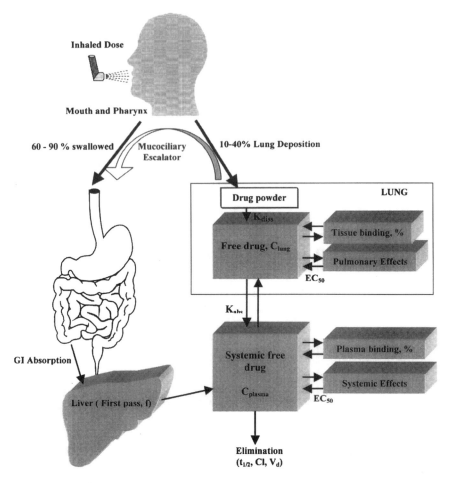

FIGURE 1   PK/PD model describing the fate of an inhaled drug. For a more detailed description, see Sec. 2.1.

deposited in the oropharynx. Drug deposited in the oropharynx will be swallowed and become subject to oral absorption. How much drug will be absorbed through the gastrointestinal (GI) tract will depend on how much drug is reaching the GI tract and the oral bioavailability of the drug. The fate of drug particles deposited in the lung is determined by two competing processes: (1) dissolution of the drug particles in the lung-lining fluid (if deposited as a particle) and subsequent uptake into pulmonary cells, followed by absorption, and (2) removal of solid drug particles from the upper part of the lung by mucociliary transport or in the alveolar region by macrophage uptake. Drug that has been removed from the lung is not available for inducing pulmonary effects; therefore pharmacologically relevant pulmonary drug levels (free drug levels are able to interact with the responsible receptors) will be determined by the complex equilibria between the mucociliary transport rate, dissolution rate of solid particles (if applicable), pulmonary tissue binding (only free drug levels are pharmacologically active), and absorption into the systemic circulation. One needs to realize that once the drug is dissolved in the lung the majority will be absorbed into the systemic circulation and that systemic spillover will occur, even for drugs exhibiting negligible oral bioavailability. The degree of systemic exposure (and the degree of systemic side effects) will depend on how much drug is reaching the systemic circulation through absorption from the lung and the GI tract and the efficiency of the drug removal system (metabolic or other clearance mechanisms). This scheme indicates that pulmonary selectivity or the degree of targeting is determined by an array of pharmacokinetic and pharmacodynamic factors, which are summarized in Table 1 and will be discussed here by using the PK/PD model for simulation purposes.

TABLE 1 Factors Affecting Pulmonary Targeting

Pulmonary components	Systemic components
• How much drug is deposited in the lung?	• How much drug is swallowed?
• Where is the drug deposited in the lung?[a]	• What is the oral bioavailability?
• How long does the drug remain in the lung (dissolution rate, mucociliary transport rate, rates of cellular entrapment)?	• What is the systemic clearance?
• What is the pulmonary tissue binding?	• What is the tissue binding?
• If a prodrug, how efficient is the pulmonary activation?	• What is the plasma protein binding?
• How does the free pulmonary drug concentration relate to the pulmonary effect?	• If a prodrug, how efficient is the systemic activation?
	• How does the free systemic drug level relate to the systemic "side" effects?

[a] Not discussed in simulations.

This PK/PD model essentially represents a mathematical translation of the scheme shown in Fig. 1 and is based on pharmacokinetic models for evaluating the pulmonary fate of inhaled drugs, developed independently by Byron and by Gonda [1–3]. In order to evaluate pulmonary selectivity, descriptors of the fate of the drug in the systemic circulation were incorporated. In addition, drug concentrations in the lung and in the systemic circulation were converted into the pharmacodynamic endpoints (degree of desired pulmonary effects and undesired systemic side effects) by linking free drug concentrations at the site of action (pulmonary or systemic organs) and the pharmacological response by a simple E_{max} model. This allows quantifying the degree of pulmonary targeting as the difference between local pulmonary effects and systemic side effects. In the case of glucocorticoids and a number of other inhalation drugs, a direct correlation between receptor occupancy and the degree of the pharmacological effects has been demonstrated; thus, receptor occupancy was used in the model as a surrogate marker of pulmonary effects and systemic side effects [4]. Differences in the receptor occupancy-time profiles for pulmonary effects and systemic side effects were then used to quantify pulmonary targeting. A typical result of such simulations is shown in Fig. 2. In accordance with previously published work [4–7], this model will be applied in the following paragraphs to visualize how pharmacokinetic and pharmacodynamic factors (Table 1) affect pulmonary targeting. Therefore, two or more hypothetical drug situations will be compared by simulations in subsequent sections of this chapter. Generally, these simulations will differ in only one property (e.g., clearance) while the rest of the PK and PD parameters remain the same.

Pharmacodynamic Factors Important for Pulmonary Targeting

The effects and side effects of a majority of inhalation drugs are mediated through membrane or cytosolic receptors. For glucocorticoids, the activity at the site of action is related to the receptor-binding affinity of the drug [8–10]. In the case of beta-2-adrenergic drugs, very good correlations were observed between in vitro indicators of drug activity in cell culture and the pharmacological activity in vivo [11,12]. Therefore, receptor-binding affinities or other in vitro parameters are often used in discussions describing the pharmacological properties of inhalation drugs at the site of action (e.g., in the lung). To evaluate the importance of the receptor potency of a drug on pulmonary targeting, two cases need to be differentiated. In the first case, such as for glucocorticoids, pulmonary effects and systemic "side" effects are mediated through the identical receptors in pulmonary and systemic tissues. In the second case, such as for beta-adrenergic drugs, two receptor sub-types (β_1/β_2 adrenergic receptors) are involved in the pulmonary and systemic side effects.

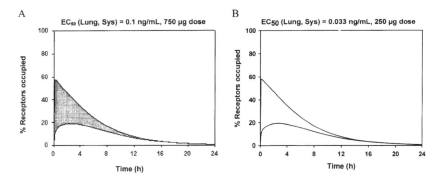

FIGURE 2 Effect of receptor affinity on pulmonary (upper line) and systemic (lower line) receptor occupancies. The simulations try to illustrate pulmonary selectivity of an inhaled drug by utilizing PK/PD relationships and selecting receptor occupancy as a surrogate marker to predict the pulmonary and systemic effects. The difference (shaded area) between the area under the curve (AUC) for pulmonary and systemic receptor occupancy-time profiles indicates the degree of pulmonary targeting. Simulations A and B depict two hypothetical drugs with different receptor-binding affinities; however, by adjusting their dose, the differences in their receptor-binding affinities can be compensated. Both the drugs display the pulmonary and systemic side effects by interacting with the same subtype of receptors. From the figure it is clear that by adjusting the dose of the drug displaying lower receptor-binding affinity, identical pulmonary selectivity can be achieved. The EC_{50} value and the dose were modulated to obtain identical pulmonary selectivities, whereas other parameters (such as clearance, volume of distribution) were fixed during the simulation.

If the "same" receptors are mediating pulmonary and systemic effects, simulations (Fig. 2) show that pulmonary targeting (the difference between lung and systemic receptor occupancy) is not affected by different receptor-binding affinities, as long as these differences are being considered by adjusting the dose (double the dose for a drug with half of the receptor affinity). This means that a low receptor-binding affinity can be compensated by an increase in the dose. Thus, the importance of a high receptor-binding affinity for promoting pulmonary selectivity, often used by marketing publications, should be questioned.

In the second case (Fig. 3), where pulmonary and systemic effects are mediated through different receptors (e.g., beta-2-adrenergic drugs), a high binding selectivity (high affinity to the β_2 receptors, low affinity to the β_1 receptor) is important for the pulmonary selectivity, and drug candidates with the highest degree of selectivity should be selected.

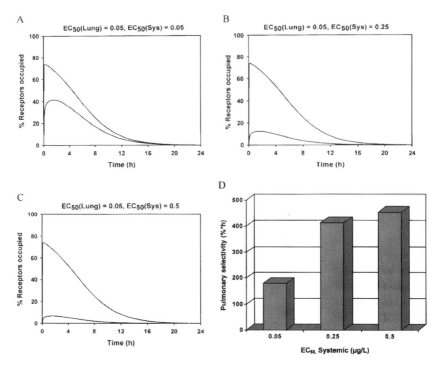

FIGURE 3 Simulations (A, B, and C) showing pulmonary (upper line) and systemic (lower line) receptor occupancies for a hypothetical beta-2-adrenergic drug that display the desired (pulmonary) and undesired (systemic) effect by occupying two different types of receptors. Cases A, B, and C show the occupancy profiles for pulmonary and systemic effects when the receptor affinity of the drug in the lung (for beta-2 receptors) remains unchanged but decreases (for beta-1 receptors) at the systemic organs (compare with A). Thus pulmonary selectivity is achieved at the pharmacodynamic level. Pulmonary selectivities [area between pulmonary (upper line) and systemic (lower line) receptor occupancies] observed in A–C are summarized in D.

Pharmacokinetic and Biopharmaceutical Factors Important for Pulmonary Targeting

Oral Bioavailability

A significant portion of drug delivered by metered-dose inhaler (MDI) or dry powder inhalation (50–90%) reaches the GI tract. The overall amount depends on how much drug is deposited in the oropharynx and swallowed and how much pulmonary deposited drug is removed from the lung by mucociliary clearance, ultimately reaching the GI tract. The oral bioavailability of the drug (F), determined quite often by the hepatic or prehepatic first-pass effect, serves as the final gatekeeper in determining how much drug enters the systemic circulation. Figure 4 shows that the drug with the lower oral bioavailability is more effective in promoting pulmonary targeting. Fluticasone propionate (FP) has been reported to have the lowest bioavailability ($< 1\%$) [13,14]. Bioavailabilities of currently used inhaled glucocorticoids range from 0% to 40% [15–19]. Similarly, oral bioavailabilities of short-acting beta-2-adrenergic drugs vary significantly, from 1.5% to about 50% [11]. These differences are likely to have an impact on the degree of pulmonary selectivity. According to Rohatagi et al., oral bioavailabilities of 25% or less should not induce clinically relevant systemic side effects

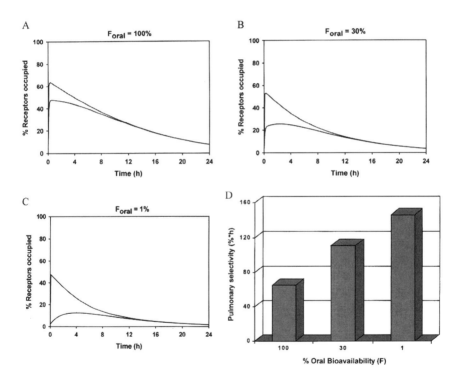

FIGURE 4 Effect of oral bioavailability (*F*-value) on pulmonary (upper line) and systemic (lower line) receptor occupancies. The *F*-value mainly determines the input of the swallowed drug (G.I.) into the systemic circulation. Simulations (A–C) are shown for 100, 30, and 1% oral bioavailability, whereas the other parameters, such as clearance, volume of distribution, and dose, remain unchanged. With a decrease in the oral bioavailability, there was a significant increase in the degree of pulmonary targeting (see D).

as long as a large pulmonary deposition is responsible for a limited amount of drug being swallowed [20].

Systemic Clearance

Systemic clearance is the pharmacokinetic factor describing the efficiency of the body to eliminate systemically absorbed drug. The cumulative systemic exposure, as indicated by the area under the drug plasma concentration time profile, is determined by the amount of drug entering the systemic circulation and the systemic clearance. Thus, if an inhaled drug shows pronounced systemic clearance, systemic exposure will be reduced. This is reflected in simulations shown in Fig. 5 that indicate increased pulmonary targeting with increasing

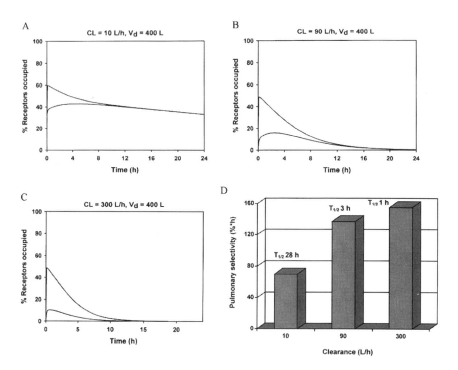

FIGURE 5 Effect of systemic clearance (CL) on pulmonary (upper line) and systemic (lower line) receptor occupancies. Simulations A, B, and C are shown for an increasing CL values of 10, 90, and 300 L/hr, respectively, whereas the other parameters, such as volume of distribution and dose, remain unchanged. An increase in CL (10−300 L/hr) produces a significant increase in the difference (AUC pulmonary−AUC systemic) between pulmonary and systemic receptor occupancies, thus indicating that CL is very beneficial in achieving pulmonary selectivity for an inhaled drug.

systemic clearance. Most inhaled glucocorticoids are predominantly cleared by hepatic metabolism so efficiently that their clearance values are close to the liver blood flow [16,21–23]. For new drug developments in this field this means that further improvements (increases) in the systemic clearance can be achieved only by incorporating extrahepatic clearance mechanisms, for example, by identifying glucocorticoids that are metabolized in the blood [24]. The challenging aspect of such an endeavor is to find enzymatic systems that are present in the blood at sufficient concentrations but that are not expressed in the pulmonary cells, because rapid pulmonary inactivation would result in very low pulmonary drug levels and insufficient pulmonary effects. It is therefore essential that such drugs be stable enough in the lung tissue to show sufficient pulmonary presence.

Volume of Distribution/Plasma Binding

Quite often, the half-life of a drug is used as an indicator of systemic exposure. It is determined by clearance and volume of distribution. While clearance describes the ability of the body to eliminate the drug, volume of distribution (V_d) is the pharmacokinetic parameter that provides an estimate of the extent of distribution of the drug into the tissue compartments.

For lipophilic drugs, which are able to cross membranes and enter most of the tissue compartments (volume of the tissue compartment, V_t), the volume of distribution (V_d) can be calculated by knowing the volume of the plasma (V_p) and the fraction of drug unbound in the plasma (f_u) and in the tissue (f_{uT}):

$$V_d = V_p + V_t \frac{f_u}{f_{uT}}$$

The more pronounced the tissue binding is over plasma protein binding, the larger will be the value of V_d and thus the more drug will be in the peripheral compartment. While this induces a longer half-life of the drug, the degree of pulmonary selectivity is not significantly affected (Fig. 6). Therefore, drugs with a long half-life are not necessarily bad inhalation drugs, if the long half-life is due to a pronounced tissue binding.

Another aspect of tissue and plasma protein binding should be discussed. More lipophilic drugs are currently in development that show both increased tissue and plasma protein binding and, as a consequence, small f_u and f_{uT} values. Yet there are no dramatic increases in the estimates of volume of distribution, because both f_u and f_{uT} are increased. With a decrease in the overall fraction of free drug, the effects (local and systemic) will be smaller than those of an equivalent drug with equivalent volume of distribution but lower tissue and plasma protein binding. In this case, the drug with the higher degree of binding but otherwise identical properties will show reduced systemic side effects and reduced pulmonary effects

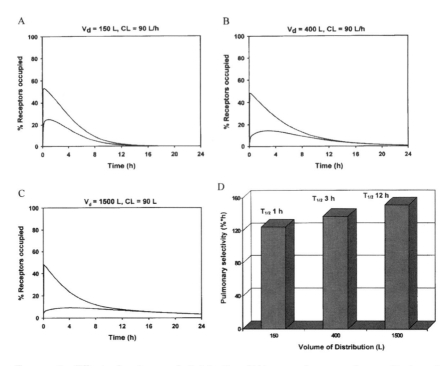

Figure 6 Effect of volume of distribution (V_d) on pulmonary (upper line) and systemic (lower line) receptor occupancies. Simulations, A, B, and C are shown for increasing V_d values of 150, 400, and 1500 L, respectively, whereas the other parameters, such as clearance and dose, remain unchanged. An increase in V_d (100–1500 L) produces only a slight increase in the difference (AUC pulmonary−AUC systemic) between pulmonary and systemic receptor occupancies, thus indicating that V_d does not seem to be that significant in modulating pulmonary selectivity. As a result, drugs with similar clearance but different half-lives due to differences in V_d will produce approximately equivalent degrees of pulmonary and systemic effects.

at a given concentration. Systemic side effects are "hard" parameters in clinical studies, for concentration–response relationships can easily be detected, whereas pulmonary effects are generally "soft" parameters (concentration–effect relationships are difficult to detect). Such high-binding drugs given at identical doses might show very high safety profiles (low systemic effects) while antiasthmatic effects are not statistically significantly different, because of the soft pulmonary surrogate markers. In this case the drug with a high plasma/tissue binding will suggest a higher safety profile.

Pulmonary Deposition Efficiency

Drug deposition to the lungs varies significantly with the type of delivery device. It seems obvious that a pulmonary delivery device with higher pulmonary deposition will be more suitable for achieving pulmonary targeting. This is because the more efficient devices not only increase the amount of drug in the lung but also reduce the amount of drug that is available for absorption from the GI tract. In recent years, improvements in the design of delivery devices have increased pulmonary deposition from 10–20% to up to 40% [25,26]. Simulation studies confirm the obvious, that high pulmonary deposition is beneficial for the degree of pulmonary targeting. However, it is especially beneficial for a drug with high oral bioavailability, because an increase in pulmonary deposition will lead to a reduction in the fraction of the dose available for oral absorption [4]. A high pulmonary deposition is not important at all for a drug with negligible oral bioavailability, because under these conditions, drug entering the GI tract will not be able to induce systemic side effects. However, in this case, using a device with higher pulmonary deposition would permit dose adjustments by reducing the emitted dose.

Daily Dose

Inhaled drugs are often used within a rather broad dose range, with low doses used in patients with light asthma and higher doses prescribed in patients with severe asthma. It might therefore be of interest to evaluate whether pulmonary targeting depends on the prescribed dose. At very low doses of an inhaled drug, most of the pulmonary and systemic receptors are not occupied; thus relatively smaller pulmonary and systemic effects are observed (Fig. 7). As the dose increases, the differences between pulmonary and systemic effects become more pronounced. Finally, at the higher doses, almost all the receptors are occupied both systemically and in the lung, thus leading to loss of targeting. The simulation suggests that there exists an optimal dose that would provide maximal lung selectivity. If a patient needs higher doses to manage the asthma, targeting is lost, and physicians should consider switching the patient from inhalation to oral drug treatment, because the cost/benefit ratio is improved.

Frequency of Dosing

Currently, there is a tendency to maintain patients on once-daily doses of inhaled drugs. While the feasibility of the once-daily dosing depends on a number of drug-specific factors and the disease state itself, one might ask what general relationships exist between dosing frequency and selectivity. As shown in Fig. 8, pulmonary selectivity is improved if the same daily dose is administered in multiple smaller doses throughout the day, for this will extend the time for which

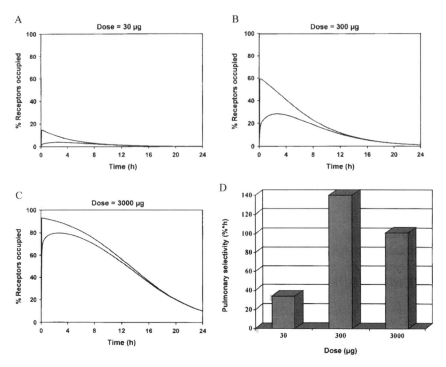

FIGURE 7 Effect of inhaled dose on pulmonary selectivity. Pulmonary selectivities [area between pulmonary (upper line) and systemic (lower line) receptor occupancies] observed in A–C are summarized in D. Simulations are shown for increasing dose values of 30, 300, and 3000 µg. At very low doses, relatively smaller pulmonary and systemic effects are observed, because most of the systemic and pulmonary receptors are unoccupied. With a subsequent increase in the dose, both the pulmonary and systemic effects increase, and so does the difference between them (greater pulmonary selectivity). However, with a further decrease in the dose there is a loss in pulmonary targeting due to the saturation of both pulmonary and systemic receptors.

higher pulmonary levels are present (prolonging the pulmonary drug exposure time). Thus, increasing the frequency of dosing will have a beneficial effect, especially for drugs that are absorbed relatively fast from the lung. This was also demonstrated in a clinical study, which showed that repeated dosing was beneficial in enhancing antiasthmatic efficacy of budesonide [27]. However, increasing the frequency of dosing has its limitations because of problems with patient compliance; therefore other ways of prolonging the contact time of the drug within the lung should be evaluated.

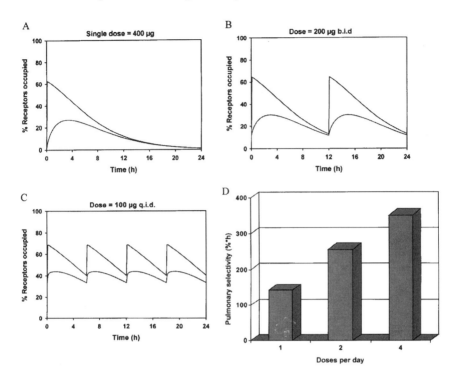

FIGURE 8 Effect of dosing regimen at steady state on pulmonary selectivity. Pulmonary selectivities [area between pulmonary (upper line) and systemic (lower line) receptor occupancies] observed in A–C are summarized in D. Additional doses are shown in D. A daily dose of 400 μg was administered as one single dose (A), 200 μg b.i.d (B), or 100 μg q.i.d. (C). Simulations show that a higher frequency of dosing results in greater pulmonary selectivity.

Pulmonary Residence Time

It seems obvious that the pulmonary fate of an inhaled drug particle is vital for its targeting. Generally, deposited drug particles will dissolve in the pulmonary lining fluid or will be released from delivery systems, such as microspheres and liposomes, and diffuse to the site of action, where they will induce the desired effect and subsequently be absorbed into the systemic circulation. In addition, solid drug particles or macromolecular compounds can be removed from the lung by the mucociliary transporter (predominantly in the upper respiratory tract) or by macrophage uptake and lymphatic removal.

Pulmonary absorption from the lung into the systemic circulation occurs for lipophilic drugs, generally by diffusion across lipophilic membranes [28–32], while hydrophilic drugs are absorbed through water-filled channels [30,33–35]. In addition, active or facilitated transport can be involved in drug absorption [31,36,37]. Because of the physiology of the lung (thin membranes, high number of pores) and the distinct sink conditions realized in the lung due to the high pulmonary blood flow, absorption of inhaled drugs across the pulmonary membranes is often relatively fast (unless it is a drug with very high molecular weight), and inhaled drug in solution will consequently leave the lung in a very short period of time. Thus, the pulmonary residence time of inhaled drugs given as a solution is generally very short. This also indicates that other factors (e.g., the dissolution rate of the inhaled drug particle or the release rate from the drug delivery system) might represent the rate-limiting steps for how long the drug resides in the lung.

Figure 9 shows the relationship between the dissolution rate of inhaled drug particles and pulmonary selectivity, with the assumption that once drug is dissolved, it will be absorbed relatively fast into the systemic circulation. If the drug particle dissolves quickly (or the drug was given as a solution), it will be absorbed rapidly into the systemic circulation and thus reside in the lung for only a short period of time (Fig. 9, short pulmonary residence time). As a result, lung selectivity (higher free drug levels in the lung than in the systemic organs) will last for only a very short period of time, and the free unbound drug in the lung and the systemic circulation will be identical shortly after inhalation, leading to loss in targeting. This does not imply a lack of pulmonary effect, but the beneficial effects could be accompanied by significant systemic side effects. If the pulmonary dissolution rate is slowed down, drug concentrations in the lung will be greater over an extended period of time, compared to the levels in the systemic circulation. Thus, a sustained pulmonary drug release is very beneficial for lung targeting (Fig. 9). However, when the drug is delivered to the upper part of the lung, mucociliary transport needs to be considered, because it will remove undissolved drug particles, resulting in loss of efficacy and pulmonary targeting. As a result, there is an optimal dissolution rate for which maximum targeting will be observed (Fig. 9). It further needs to be stated that the situation is somewhat different in the alveolar region of the lung, because mucociliary clearance is not that pronounced, and an optimum release rate might not easily be defined.

As mentioned earlier, the absorption rate of a number of drugs is often too fast to express maximum targeting. Thus, a significant body of work has concentrated on the design of drug delivery systems that slow down this process and provide the drug with an increased pulmonary residence time. There have been several different approaches to improve the pulmonary residence time of inhaled drugs [38]. These include the use of liposomes [39–41], microspheres [42–45], ultrathin coatings around drug dry powders [46], the use of new excipients such as oligolactic acid [47] and trehalose derivatives [38], or simply

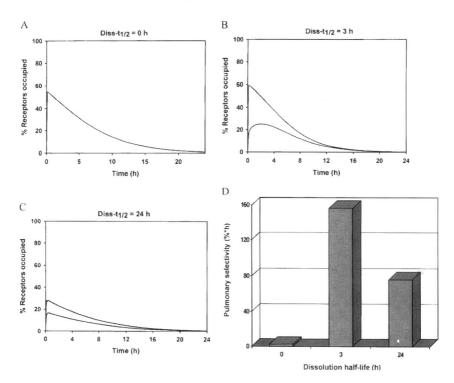

FIGURE 9 Effect of pulmonary dissolution rate on pulmonary selectivity. The dose of 300 μg was allowed to dissolve immediately (A), with a half-life of 3 hr (B), or with a half-life of 24 hr (C). Pulmonary selectivity [area between pulmonary (upper line) and systemic (lower line) receptor occupancies] observed in A–C are summarized in D. The dose was given once a day at steady state. A slower release/dissolution of the drug in the lung does significantly increase pulmonary selectivity; however, very slow dissolution rates further decrease pulmonary selectivity as the undissolved drug particles are removed from the lung by the mucociliary transport system.

the use of slow-dissolving lipophilic drugs. There are also biological approaches to prolong the time the drug stays in the lung. For example, long-acting beta-2-adrenergic drugs bind tightly to pulmonary cell membranes [48], and this fraction of drug provides a reservoir that feeds drug slowly to the receptor. Similarly, reversible formation of fatty acid esters has been described for glucocorticoids. Glucocorticoids will enter the cell, and a fraction of the drug is converted into highly lipophilic inactive ester derivatives that are unable to leave the cell. The trapped ester can also act as depot for the active corticosteroid in the lung because it can be slowly be reactivated into the active glucocorticoid [49–52]. Such systems may serve as alternative mechanisms for enhancing pulmonary residence, if a significant fraction of the drug deposited in the lung will be captured.

Prodrugs

A few inhalation drugs, such as beclomethasone dipropionate, are prodrugs, which are not able to interact with the receptor themselves but need to be metabolized (activated) into an active metabolite before they can induce their desired effects. This activation can happen in the lung or after absorption from the lung or the GI tract. Prodrugs that are absorbed into the systemic circulation without prior activation and that are activated in the systemic circulation can induce pulmonary effects only after redistribution into the lung. Thus free drug levels in the systemic circulation and in the lung will be similar and no targeting will be observed. Therefore in order to obtain optimal pulmonary selectivity, these drugs need to be activated predominantly in the lung. It is not trivial in clinical pharmacological studies to show the degree of pulmonary activation of such prodrugs, because such studies need to include the intravenous administration of drug and active metabolite.

METHODS TO ASSESS PHARMACOKINETIC AND DYNAMIC PROPERTIES OF INHALATION DRUGS

Earlier we described how pharmacokinetic and dynamic properties of inhaled drugs are relevant for pulmonary selectivity. The assessment of pharmacokinetic and dynamic properties is consequently relevant for drug development and clinical practice. This section reviews some of the relevant techniques for assessing such properties. The available tools range from cell culture or isolated lung perfusion models to mucociliary clearance analysis, imaging techniques, and in vivo pharmacokinetic and dynamic analysis of the inhaled drug.

Cell Culture Methods to Assess Drug Transport

Cell culture models to evaluate the pulmonary fate of inhaled drugs have not been used extensively for characterizing inhalation drugs. However, this technique is promising and will be briefly discussed. This section focuses on airway and alveolar epithelial models using cell lines and primary cell culture methods.

Airway Epithelial Cell Cultures

Primary cultures of airway epithelium have been described for many animal species, including humans [53]. These primary epithelial cell cultures have been demonstrated to be useful in investigating the influence of lipophilicity and molecular size on epithelial permeability as well as for investigating mechanisms of absorption. Three of the most promising human bronchial cell lines used as absorption models are 16HBE14o, Calu-3, and BEAS-2B [54].

Alveolar Epithelial Cell Cultures

The primary alveolar epithelial cell cultures [55,56] arises from the alveolar type II cells. The advantage of these cell cultures is that they differentiate into monolayers of cells with morphology similar to Type I cells. Transepithelial delivery of protein, peptides, and macromolecules such as dextran has been evaluated using A549 cells, a lung carcinoma cell line, as a model of the alveolar epithelium. Although these cell culture models are associated with several drawbacks [55], such as being unable to mimic in vivo clearance mechanisms, they do serve as a valuable tool for assessment of drug transport.

Isolated Lung Perfusion Models

Isolated lung perfusion models have been instrumental in assessing the pulmonary fate of inhaled drugs by employing lungs of rabbits, rats, and guinea pigs [57–60]. These models permit investigation of pulmonary dissolution, absorption, lung tissue binding, transport phenomena, and metabolism while maintaining the physiological properties of the lung. The drug is delivered into the ventilated lung either by intratracheal injection or via a modified MDI. These experiments result in typical absorption profiles (drug absorbed as a function of time) of drug and its metabolites (if applicable; see Fig. 10). The isolated perfused lung was one of the models that indicated that a fraction of budesonide is captured in the lung. In addition, estimates of the mucociliary clearance (see next section) can be obtained.

Assessment of the Mucociliary Clearance of a Drug

Pulmonary clearance through the mucociliary transport is relevant for inhalation therapy, mainly for the upper portion of the lung. With more lipophilic drugs being used for inhalation therapy, incorporating the mucociliary clearance in the pharmacokinetic assessment of an inhalation drug is becoming more relevant, because the slow dissolution rate of these drugs makes them more vulnerable for mucociliary removal. As a matter of fact, some of the reported low systemic bioavailabilities of new inhaled steroids might be related to their high lipophilicity and slow dissolution rates, because this provides enough time for the undissolved particles to be removed by the mucociliary transporter.

Mucociliary clearance has been routinely assessed using radioactive-labeling techniques [61]. This technique often involves monitoring mucociliary clearance of inhaled monodisperse 5-μm particles of polystyrene or particles generated from ^{99m}Tc-labeled iron oxide [62]. However, these well-established techniques do not permit direct monitoring of drug particles. Recently, Byron and

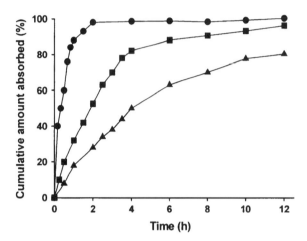

FIGURE 10   Possible absorption profiles obtained from experiments with isolated perfused lung or absorption profiles obtained after proper deconvolution from inhalation studies. Lines present drugs with different absorption rates. Circles = fast, squares = intermediate, and hexagons = slow absorption rates.

coworkers [63] employed an in vitro approach using the isolated perfused lung as a tool for a detailed assessment of the pulmonary fate of fluorescent-labeled analytes, absorbed by carrier-mediated or passive absorption, or removed by the mucociliary escalator. The method was able to generate data on the rate of mucociliary transport of the formulation. Applying this method to other drugs might allow a detailed assessment of the pulmonary pharmacokinetics, including mucociliary removal.

Pharmacokinetic and/or Pharmacodynamic Assessment of Pulmonary Drug Delivery Systems

A variety of pharmacokinetic and pharmacodynamic approaches can be used in preclinical and Phase I–III development to evaluate pulmonary drug delivery. These include studies that evaluate the pulmonary pharmacokinetics directly in the lung (e.g., direct assay of lung tissue), imaging studies, and traditional pharmacokinetic and pharmacodynamic approaches. The most important approaches are discussed next.

Drug Content in Lung Tissue

Determinations of drug levels in the lung and comparison with plasma levels have been used for the pharmacokinetic assessment of inhalation drugs. In such a scenario, drug is typically delivered to the lung of animals or patients, who have to undergo lung resection; subsequently, the lung or lung sections are removed at different time points and the drug concentration-time profile is compared with that in the plasma.

Studies were performed in patients undergoing lung resection surgery [64,65], where lung cancer patients were dosed preoperatively. The drug concentration was determined in the peripheral and central lung tissues and was compared to the blood samples taken during surgery. This enabled calculations of drug ratios between lung and plasma and of the pulmonary half-life of drug. In general, this pharmacokinetic approach is able to evaluate the time profile of disappearance of drug from the lung. However, it needs to be taken into consideration that drug levels in the lung reflect undissolved drug, drug bound to pulmonary tissue components, and pharmacodynamically relevant free drug concentrations. In addition, higher drug levels in the lung than in the plasma are not per se indicative of pulmonary targeting, because even after intravenous administration due to the high volume of distribution (high tissue binding), tissue levels are often higher than plasma levels. Thus, a careful study design [administration of the drug via the lung and after intravenous (IV) administration] needs to be applied if one wishes to use this approach for making selectivity statements.

Imaging Studies

In vivo radiographic imaging techniques are proving to be extremely useful in assessing drug deposition [66,67]. These methods include gamma scinitigraphy (e.g., gamma-emitting nuclide ^{99m}Tc), single-photon emission tomography (SPECT), positron emission tomography (PET), and, for limited applications, magnetic resonance imaging, which does not require radioactive labeling. These techniques, as discussed in more detail in other chapters of this book, are able to provide detailed information on the degree and location of pulmonary deposition. In addition, pulmonary pharmacokinetics can be assessed if the drug particles are labeled and can be followed over an extended period of time [68].

Classical Pharmacokinetic Methods

For a long time classical pharmacokinetic approaches could not be used, because the available analytical techniques were not sensitive enough to measure the low plasma levels in the picogram/mL range often observed after inhalation. However, with the availability of HPLC/MS techniques and their high sensitivity, pharmacokinetic analysis can now be performed for most inhalation drugs.

Influence of Disease-State on Pharmacokinetic Studies. It is important to realize that pharmacokinetics might differ in asthmatics and healthy volunteers. Falcoz et al. and Daley-Yates reported a 2–3 times reduced systemic availability for inhaled fluticasone propionate in asthmatics [69,70], while there was no significant difference in the kinetic parameters after intravenous administration between healthy volunteers and asthmatic patients. This indicates that differences after inhalation between healthy volunteers and asthmatics are due to differences in the pulmonary fate of the drug. These differences are likely to be related to decreased inhalation efficiency in asthmatics or to an increased removal of inhaled drug by increased mucociliary clearance [70]. This decreased systemic availability in asthmatics seems to depend on the severity of the disease. Moderate-to-severe asthmatics exhibited marked PK differences when compared to healthy volunteers, while PK properties were similar in healthy volunteers and mild asthmatics [71]. These findings suggest that pharmacokinetic studies should be performed in the patient population of interest. This would also include children, because differences in the pharmacokinetics between adults and children have also been found [72–74].

Other Important Considerations for Pharmacokinetic Studies. When using systemic (plasma, serum, or urine) drug levels for the evaluation of inhalation drugs, one must take into consideration that these levels are made up of drug absorbed via the lung and the GI tract. Thus, these studies cannot be used a priori for characterization of the pulmonary fate of inhalation drugs (see Table 2).

However, in the case of drugs that show negligible oral bioavailability (e.g., fluticasone propionate), systemic concentration–time profiles mirror what is happening in the lung. In this case, pharmacokinetic parameters (See Table 2) will directly reflect and describe the pulmonary fate of the drug.

TABLE 2 Information Extractable from PK Studies for Inhalation Drugs Showing ($F \gg 0$) or Lacking ($F = 0$) Oral Bioavailability

	Oral bioavailability $F = 0$	Oral bioavailability $F \gg 0$
% Pulmonary deposition	Yes	Not without blocking[a] oral absorption
Systemic exposure (AUC)	Yes	Yes
Pulmonary residence time	Yes	Not without blocking oral absorption
Pulmonary absorption rate	Yes	Only if oral absorption can be blocked or deconvolution is able to differentiate
Absorption through GI Tract	Not applicable	Yes, if PK is assessed with or without blocking

[a] Or other methods able to differentiate between absorption through the lung and GI tract.

For drugs that show significant oral bioavailability (e.g., salbutamol [75]), terbutaline sulfate [76], budesonide [77]), different approaches, such as the charcoal-block technique, or the knowledge of differences in the pulmonary and GI absorption lag times can be utilized to determine the pulmonary fate of the inhaled drug.

The rationale for the charcoal-block design is that for a number of drugs, oral absorption of swallowed drug can be blocked by coadministered charcoal. Typically, using this technique, the subject ingests charcoal slurry both at the time of drug administration and 1 and 2 hours after drug administration. Thus, accurate delineation of pulmonary absorption can be achieved because the absorption of the orally swallowed fraction of the inhaled product is blocked by charcoal. Comparison of drug levels with and without charcoal administration allows one to assess the degree of orally absorbed drug [77]. Such approaches have been described for terbutaline [76], triamcinolone acetonide [78], budesonide [77], and other glucocorticoids [79]. It is, however, vital for this approach to ensure the efficacy of the charcoal treatment by assessing the charcoal block after oral administration of drug [77].

Another approach for drugs with significant oral bioavailability is based on the finding that the absorption rates from the lung and the GI tract differ for a number of drugs, with the pulmonary absorption being much faster. Thus, drug reaching the systemic circulation rapidly after the inhalation represents drug absorbed from the lung. Such differences in the absorption lag times from the lung and the GI tract have been utilized to determine the pulmonary deposition of salbutamol [80]. Hindle et al. showed that under these conditions one does not need to collect blood samples but that the collection of urine is sufficient. Furthermore, negligible amounts of unchanged salbutamol were excreted in the urine within the first 30 min when given orally [80]. In contrast, salbutamol can be detected in the urine within the first half hour when given as inhalation, indicating that the pulmonary absorption is faster. This method was validated in clinical trials, indicating that 30-min urinary excretion of salbutamol following a variety of inhalation maneuvers reflects the pulmonary-absorbed fraction of the dose [81]. Monitoring the urine levels over long time periods can then be used as a marker for the total systemic drug exposure. The time lag between the oral and pulmonary absorption has been utilized for other drugs, such as nedocromil [82], sodium cromoglycate [83], and gentamicin [84]. One needs, however, to consider that this approach is drug specific and cannot be applied to all classes of drugs and that the time resolution is limited when urine is collected, especially if only done once.

It is clear that pharmacokinetic studies in humans provide significant information for inhalation drugs. Relevant key parameters obtained from PK studies include the pulmonary deposition efficiency, parameters assessing the pulmonary absorption, and the overall degree of systemic exposure (Table 2). Some approaches suitable for assessing these and other pharmacokinetic properties are discussed next.

Pharmacokinetics After Oral and Intravenous Administration.   For proper characterization of an inhalation drug, information on the systemic pharmacokinetic properties needs to be provided. One of the major challenges for such studies is to provide a suitable formulation for injection, especially because new drug candidates are often very lipophilic. The resulting parameters of such studies (systemic clearance, volume of distribution, half-life, mean residence time) can then easily be extracted from concentration–time profiles after IV administration and subsequent standard pharmacokinetic analysis by noncompartmental approaches. In addition, a detailed compartmental analysis based on concentration-time profiles will be useful in evaluating the systemic distribution processes in sufficient detail. This will be especially important if deconvolution procedures (see later) are included for the assessment of the pulmonary absorption profiles.

In addition to intravenous studies, estimates of the oral bioavailability of the drug need to be provided. For glucocorticoid studies, often very large doses of steroid have to be given to be able to obtain measurable drug levels. The percent oral bioavailability can then easily be obtained by comparing the dose-adjusted area under the concentration-time profiles after oral and IV administration:

$$\text{Oral bioavailability } (\%) = \frac{\text{AUC}_{\text{oral}} \times D_{\text{IV}}}{\text{AUC}_{\text{IV}} \times D_{\text{oral}}} \times 100$$

An elegant way of obtaining information on IV and oral dosing at the same time (with the advantage of reducing the variability of such estimation by deleting the interassay variability) is to use unlabeled drug for one form of administration and to dose at the same time a deuterated form of the drug for the other form of administration [85].

Degree of Systemic Availability.   The overall degree of drug absorbed into the systemic circulation is a parameter quantifying the systemic exposure after inhalation. Systemic drug exposure (systemic availability) can easily be determined using noncompartmental approaches by comparing the area under the plasma concentration–time profile, extrapolated to infinity (AUC_∞), observed after intravenous administration of the drug (AUC_{IV}) with that after inhalation (AUC_{inh}). To calculate these parameters, standard techniques for the determination of the AUC_∞ (trapezoidal rule and extrapolation to infinity) can be used. Correlation of the AUC_∞ obtained after inhalation with that after IV administration allows calculation of the systemic availability after inhalation.

The following equation provides such a correlation if doses after IV administration (D_{IV}) and inhalation (D_{inh}) differ:

$$\text{Systemic availability } (\%) = \frac{\text{AUC}_{inh} \times D_{IV}}{\text{AUC}_{IV} \times D_{inh}} \times 100$$

For drugs with zero oral bioavailability this method also provides a direct estimate of the pulmonary deposition efficiency of the device. For drugs with distinct oral bioavailability, this method, combined with charcoal-block, enables calculation of both pulmonary and oral availabilities [86].

This method can also provide important information on the degree of systemic exposure for the assessment of bioequivalence, by comparing the AUC_{∞} for innovator and generic products, using the following equation for the relative systemic availability:

$$\text{Relative systemic availability } (\%) = \frac{\text{AUC}_{generic}}{\text{AUC}_{innovator}} \times 100$$

Area-under-the-curve determinations allow one to estimate the degree of accumulation of drug during therapy by comparing the AUC during one dosing interval obtained after the first dose and at steady state.

Urine data, as previously described, might also be used for the assessment of the degree of systemic absorption through the lung (early urine data) and the total systemic exposure (total urine excretion). Resolution of such data will, however, depend on the correct cutoff time points defining pulmonary and oral absorption. For total systemic exposure, the amount of drug found in the urine after a single inhalation (Amount_{inh}) and the amount found after a single IV injection (Amount_{IV}) found in the urine (during a time period encompassing the total elimination of drug) allows the determination of the percentage of systemic exposure after inhalation. This percentage for an inhalation dose of D_{inh} and an injection dose D_{IV} can be calculated by the following equation:

$$\text{Relative systemic exposure } (\%) = \frac{\text{Amount}_{inh} \times D_{IV}}{\text{Amount}_{IV} \times D_{inh}} \times 100$$

C_{max}. C_{max} (maximum observed concentration) is also a parameter being affected by dose reaching the systemic circulation, absorption, and distribution kinetics. Since it is affected by a number of parameters, the interpretation of results depends on the nature of the study performed. For example, the differences in C_{max} between two devices delivering a solution-based drug with negligible oral bioavailability might indicate differences in the respirable fraction between the two devices. In other studies (that evaluate immediate-release and sustained-release preparations but similar deposition efficiencies), differences in C_{max} might indicate differences in the absorption profile. Thus, additional information (deposition efficiency, delivered dose) might be necessary to evaluate the results correctly.

Pharmacokinetic Tools to Characterize Absorption Kinetics. The sustained character of lung absorption is important for the degree of pulmonary selectivity. It is therefore important to evaluate lung absorption with pharmacokinetic tools. Several tools have been used to provide this information, including the time to reach the maximum plasma concentration (t_{max}), the mean absorption time (MAT), flip–flop, and deconvolution. These approaches are described next.

T_{MAX}. The time to reach maximum concentrations (t_{max}) has been used to evaluate how fast the drug is absorbed. This is done under the assumption that the slower the absorption from the lung, the longer will be t_{max}. The following equation, derived for a drug whose systemic distribution can be described by a one-compartment body model, shows that t_{max} depends not only on the absorption rate (k_a) but also on the elimination rate (k_e):

$$t_{max} = \frac{\ln\dfrac{k_e}{k_a}}{k_e - k_a}$$

Thus, for a given drug, a formulation with a slower absorption rate should show an increased t_{max} value. Because of the relatively fast absorption often seen after inhalation, sampling at early time points has to be frequent, in order to obtain reliable estimates of t_{max}. However, one cannot necessarily use t_{max} to determine whether two different drug entities are being absorbed with different rates because t_{max} is determined not only by k_a but also by k_e (which is likely to be different for two different drugs). In this case, knowledge of k_e (obtained after IV administration) and t_{max} can be used to calculate k_a. It is even more complicated for drugs with multicompartmental distribution properties. In these cases, t_{max} is determined by the absorption process and k_{10} (elimination rate of systemically available drug) and by rate constants governing the distribution among all systemic compartments. Also in these cases, an early t_{max} might not always indicate a fast absorption and a later t_{max} might not indicate a slow absorption process if two drugs differ in their systemic compartmental distribution pattern (differences in the rate constants among systemic compartments) [87]. Thus, the use of t_{max} to characterize the absorption pattern must be carefully considered.

MEAN ABSORPTION TIME (MAT). A much more robust parameter than t_{max} seems to be the estimation of the mean absorption time (MAT). This parameter can easily be obtained by noncompartmental analysis by estimating the mean residence time after inhalation (MRT_{inh}) and comparing it with the mean residence time after IV administration (MRT_{IV}):

$$MAT = MRT_{inh} - MRT_{IV}$$

The MRT is calculated from $AUC_{0-\infty}$ and the area under the first momentum curve ($AUMC_{0-\infty}$):

$$MRT = \frac{AUMC_{0-\infty}}{AUC_{0-\infty}}$$

This approach is robust because it does not rely on any pharmacokinetic assumptions and allows the characterization of absorption processes among different drugs if IV data are available. For example, differences in the absorption profiles between fluticasone propionate and budesonide can easily be identified with this method, while differences in t_{max} were not able to readily provide this information. The mean residence time without availability of intravenous data should not be used to compare absorption profiles of different drug entities, because it is also determined by the systemic elimination of the drug. This approach is, however, suitable for evaluating the differences of different formulations of the same drug.

THE "FLIP–FLOP" APPROACH. Assuming that the absorption rate is much slower than the elimination rate, concentration-time profiles of an inhaled drug will show a terminal slope (slope of the semilogarithmic plot at late time points) that reflects k_a rather than k_e. This phenomenon is called "flip-flop" (Fig. 11). For drugs that are absorbed slowly from the lung, the terminal elimination phase after inhalation should be slower than after IV administration. Monitoring the occurrence of flip-flop has been used to prove or disapprove the distinct slow absorption of pulmonary drugs [88]. While the concept is correct for drugs that are absorbed much more slowly than they are eliminated, drugs with a small k_e can

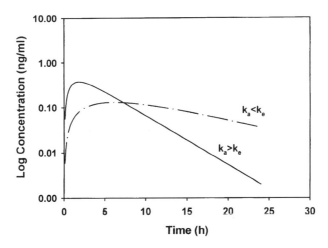

FIGURE 11 Effect of varying absorption rate constant (k_a) on the concentration time plots for two hypothetical drugs with similar dose, bioavailability, clearance, and volume of distribution. Case 1 (smooth line): $k_a > k_e$; and Case 2 (broken line): $k_a < k_e$ (flip-flop situation).

show similar terminal slopes after IV administration and inhalation, despite the fact that the drug is absorbed slowly from the lung. In this case, other PK parameters are more suitable for assessing the absorption properties.

DECONVOLUTION APPROACHES. Concentration-time profiles have also been analyzed by deconvolution methods [89]. Application of deconvolution methods to inhalation drugs must consider the multicompartmental distribution processes observed for most inhalation drugs. This makes it necessary to use PK estimates after intravenous administration within the deconvolution process. Thus, deconvolution of concentration-time profiles are based on the comparison of data obtained after IV administration and inhalation. This allows the generation of an input function, which describes the systemic absorption process and will generate full absorption profiles similar to those obtained from the isolated perfused lung preparations. Because of the compartmental approach used in these deconvolution processes, this method gives information not readily available from the noncompartmental analysis. Using deconvolution, Brindley and coworkers [89] were able to identify that 50% of the pulmonary-deposited dose of fluticasone propionate (FP) is absorbed within 2 hours, while the rest is absorbed more slowly, with 90% being absorbed by 12 hours. It is likely that differences in the absorption processes might reflect drug deposited in different regions of the lung (central or peripheral). Brindley and coworkers were able to show that, independent of the inhalation device, FP is multiexponential and that slow absorption into the systemic circulation provides a long pulmonary residence time [89]. Deconvolution of such data can be performed relatively easy with software such as PCDCON [90]. Similar approaches were able to show that after inhalation of fenoterol, parts of the delivered dose were absorbed relatively fast while the other fraction was absorbed more slowly [91]. This observation might be linked to differences in the absorption rate of a drug deposited into the lung vs. in the GI tract. In summary, deconvolution of inhalation data has the potential for analyzing the absorption processes in detail and with high resolution. It depends, however, on a somewhat complex data analysis.

Potential Role of Pharmacokinetics in Bioequivalence Studies. With more and more generic drugs entering the inhalation market, the industry [International Pharmaceutical Aerosol Consortium on Regulation and Science (IPAC-RS)], professional organizations (e.g., Inhalation Technology Focus Group of the AAPS), and the FDA are currently trying to streamline bioequivalence testing. Potential methods to be considered include pure in vitro studies, imaging techniques, and pharmacokinetic and pharmacodynamic studies. Pharmacokinetics is the standard for establishing bioequivalence of orally administered products; however, pharmacokinetic studies did not play a major role in early discussions of bioequivalence studies for inhalation drugs because analytical tools were judged not sensitive enough to provide reliable information and so clinical studies were proposed. Today, with the availability of sensitive analytical techniques, pharmacokinetics studies are able to provide information relevant for bioequivalence testing. Table 3 indicates potential applications of pharmacokinetic approaches within bioequivalence evaluations.

For drugs with zero oral bioavailability, a number of parameters important for bioequivalence testing can be extracted from pharmacokinetic studies. Comparison between $AUC_{0-\infty}$ estimates for innovator and generic products will provide direct information on the degree of pulmonary deposition because drug can enter the systemic circulation only through the lung. The resulting concentration-time profiles can be used to calculate the mean residence time, a parameter allowing conclusions on the absorption characteristics of the formulations.

TABLE 3 Questions Relevant for Bioequivalence Studies and Potential for Pharmacokinetic Approaches

Questions	Can PK be useful?
Factors determining the pulmonary effect	
• How much drug is deposited in the lung?	• Yes[a] (blocking of oral absorption[b] might be necessary for drugs that are absorbed orally)
• Where is the drug deposited in the lung?	• No (only if absorption rates differ in central and peripheral areas of the lung)
• How long does the drug stay in the lung?	• Yes[a] (blocking of oral absorption might be necessary for drugs that are absorbed orally)
Factors determining the systemic exposure	
• How much drug is absorbed systemically	• Yes
• How much drug is absorbed through the GI tract?	• Yes[b] (study with and without blocking of oral absorption are necessary for drugs that are absorbed orally)
• How much drug is absorbed from the lung?	• Yes[b] (blocking of oral absorption might be necessary for drugs that are absorbed orally)
• Is the time profile of systemic exposure similar?	• Yes

[a] Only true for drugs lacking significant oral absorption.
[b] Or other methods to differentiate between pulmonary and oral components might have to be used (e.g., time delay between oral and pulmonary absorption).

The role of the pharmacokinetic assessment of generic drugs showing a distinct oral absorption component is limited, because plasma levels cannot clearly be related to the oral and pulmonary pathways. Information on the systemic exposure, however, can be obtained without any problems if pharmacokinetic methods exist that allow differentiation between pulmonary-absorbed and orally absorbed drug (see earlier section on the charcoal method and the link of early drug levels to pulmonary absorption). Under these conditions, estimates can be derived for how much drug enters the systemic circulation through pulmonary and GI absorption, and information on the pulmonary absorption kinetics can be obtained. It is, however, vital for such approaches that, for example, the charcoal-blocking procedure is fully validated and effective.

It seems that PK studies for bioequivalence testing represent a middle ground between in vitro studies and clinical studies assessing pharmacodynamic equivalency, because they provide relevant information without the need to perform clinical studies. However, clinical studies showing the equivalence between PK and PD studies should also be performed.

Methods for Assessing Pulmonary Targeting

Inhalation therapy has been introduced into the clinics to ensure pulmonary effects with reduced systemic side effects. Animal and human studies for assessing pulmonary targeting are summarized next. Table 4 summarizes approaches for assessing pulmonary targeting.

Assessment of Pulmonary Targeting in Animal Models. Animal models are important tools in assessing the pharmacodynamic performance of antiasthma drugs. Pulmonary models have been developed for rat and mice, which allow the assessment of anti-inflammatory properties of a drug after antigen challenge. Alternatively, pulmonary eosinophilia can be induced by nonallergic modes,

---

TABLE 4 Methods to Quantify Pulmonary Targeting

Assessment of pulmonary targeting in animal models
- Sephadex-based models (eventually in conjunction with thymus weight)
- Receptor occupancy (or other pharmacodynamic markers) in lung and systemic circulation

Assessment of pulmonary targeting in humans
- Comparison of pulmonary effects after inhalation and systemic administration of doses inducing similar systemic effects
- Comparison of pulmonary effects after inhalation of different drugs at doses achieving identical systemic effects
- PK/PD-based approaches in humans

---

e.g., by administering sephadex [92–94]. This results in an increase in lung weight. The topical activity of inhaled glucocorticoids has been tested in such models by administering the glucocorticoid into the left lung lobe of rats, followed by administration of sephadex to the whole lung. Observing the differential effects of the glucocorticoid on left and right lobe weight can assess targeting. Targeting is observed when the effects on the left lobe are more pronounced than the effects on the right lobe, which will be exposed only to systemic glucocorticoid concentrations [95]. Alternatively, systemic effects of glucocorticoids have been assessed by monitoring the effects on thymus weight and comparing those with the local effects in the sephadex assay with the drug administered to the whole lung [95].

Other targeting models in rats or mice are based on the ex vivo monitoring of receptor occupancy after intratracheal administration of the drug, described here for glucocorticoids. Such models are based on the finding that the glucocorticoid receptors are similar in different tissues, resulting in identical receptor occupancy-time profiles when free levels in different tissues are identical, e.g., after systemic administration of a drug. Pulmonary targeting after intratracheal administration can then be assessed by comparing the receptor occupancy in the lung to a systemic organ such as the liver or kidney. A more pronounced receptor occupancy in the lung after intratracheal administration would then indicate pulmonary targeting. Similar approaches could be designed for cell membrane receptors, for example, for the beta-adrenergic receptors, using ex vivo receptor-binding approaches developed for other membrane receptors [96].

Assessment of Pulmonary Targeting in Humans. The direct assessment of pulmonary targeting in humans is not trivial. Quite often it is reduced to separately monitoring pharmacodynamic effects in the lung and systemic circulation. Comparing these properties with other drugs or dosing regimens often allows some conclusion on pulmonary selectivity. Because of the importance of assessing systemic and pulmonary effects, the following sections will first review approaches to assessing pulmonary and systemic effects and then discuss clinical approaches to quantifying targeting.

NONCOMPARTMENTAL ANALYSIS TO ASSESS SYSTEMIC EFFECTS IN HUMANS. The degree of systemic side effects can easily be measured for most inhalation drugs. This includes, for example, the change in plasma potassium levels [97,98] and increase in heart rate for beta-2-adrenergic drugs. Other parameters, such as lymphocyte numbers, the suppression of 24-hour urine cortisol [70,99] and 24-hour serum cortisol levels [100] (a more sensitive parameter) have been used for inhaled glucocorticoids.

In addition, linear growth measurements by stadiometry or knemometry, long-term bone density measurements, and the monitoring of bone markers have been used (for review see Refs. 101 and 102). As shown in Fig. 12 for the cortisol suppression by inhaled steroids, comparison between baseline and treatment-time profiles permits the calculation of the degree of suppression:

$$\% \text{ Suppression} = \frac{100(\text{AUC}_{\text{Baseline}} - \text{AUC}_{\text{Treatment}})}{\text{AUC}_{\text{Baseline}}}$$

PK/PD-BASED MODELS TO ASSESS SYSTEMIC EFFECTS IN HUMANS. While "noncompartmental" approaches are purely descriptive, PK/PD models for the evaluation of systemic side effects have been developed for a number of drug classes, including beta-2-adrenergic drugs (effects on potassium [97]), increase in heart rate [91], and glucocorticoids (cortisol suppression [103]), as well as effects on lymphocytes and granulocytes [104]. These approaches have the advantage of being useful in clinical trial simulations, thereby helping to streamline drug development. In general, plasma levels after inhalation are linked through

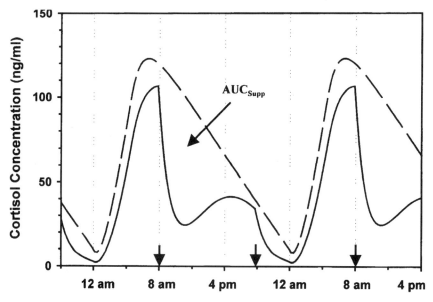

FIGURE 12   Illustration of the quantification of 24-hour cortisol suppression during multiple dosing of an inhaled steroid given b.i.d. The difference between placebo, or baseline (dashed line), and active treatment (solid line) can be used to calculate the degree of cortisol suppression. (Generated using an Excel spreadsheet developed by S. Krishnaswami et al., Ref. 114.)

a PK/PD approach with the pharmacodynamic effects either directly (through an E_{max} model) or, in the case of hysteresis between plasma concentrations and effect, through a so-called effect-compartment model (e.g., drug concentration in a hypothetical effect compartment is linked to the effect) or through an indirect-response model (e.g., drug modulates the synthesis rate of a hormone).

For other models, such as indirect-response [105] and effect-compartment models [106], it is necessary to model more complex effect–time relationships.

For example, such simple PK/PD models as described in Fig. 13 have been used to describe the effects of beta-2-adrenergic drugs on the heart rate, but models incorporating an effect-compartment [106] or indirect-response model [105] are necessary for other drug actions, such as the effects of glucocorticoids on lymphocytes and endogenous cortisol suppression (for review see Ref. 107).

Major advantages of such models are that they enable the identification of dosing regimens with given characteristics. They also enable the identification of equivalent doses of two different drugs or the prediction of how changes in doses and delivery devices will affect the systemic side effects.

ASSESSMENT OF PULMONARY EFFECTS IN HUMANS. In order to fully characterize an inhalation drug, knowledge of the topical-to-systemic-effect ratio is desirable. Thus, in addition to systemic side effects, pharmacodynamic assessments of the pulmonary effects need to be generated. Various lung function tests, including forced expiratory volume in one sec (FEV_1), peak expiratory flow rate (PEFR), forced vital capacity (FVC), mid-expiratory flow rate (MEFR), and use of airway hyperresponsiveness, have been used to measure the degree of pulmonary effects in asthmatics using the spirometer or body phlethysmography. Besides these, biomarkers of local effects, such as the reduction in certain cytokines, and modulation of nitric oxide [108,109] can be useful. In addition, the use of more traditional clinical parameters, such as diary scores, the need of rescue medication, treatment failures, progression of disease, and other routinely measure clinical parameters, are useful.

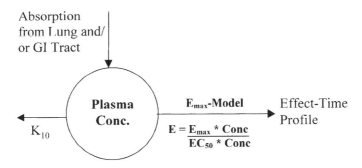

FIGURE 13 Simple PK/PD model linking plasma concentration directly to the effect.

For beta-2-adrenergic drugs, pulmonary effects, such as the reduction in FEV_1, are "hard parameters" that have been used for the assessment of pulmonary bioequivalence. As an example, detailed information has been given by the Endocrinology, Metabolism and Allergy Unit Bureau of Pharmaceutical Assessment Therapeutic Products Programme Health Canada (http://www.hcsc. gc.ca/hpb-dgps/therapeut/zfiles/english/guides/mdi/mdiatt_e.html) to use lung function parameters (FEV_1) for establishing equivalence or relative potency and safety of a second-entry short-acting beta-2-agonist metered-dose inhaler in asthmatic patients with defined severity.

For glucocorticoids, monitoring the pulmonary effects is made difficult because the time profile of glucocorticoid effects takes days or weeks to detect, and consequently time resolution of the pulmonary effects is low. Suitable surrogate markers of the pulmonary effects have not yet been fully described. This makes studies to quantify the pulmonary effects challenging, because dose–effect relationships obtained by using clinical outcome parameters are often very flat, and differences among different inhaled steroids are not easy to establish. Some data seem to suggest that pulmonary effects after exercise-induced asthma or stimulation with adenosine phosphate [110,111] is more sensitive, and dose–response curves are easier to obtain [112]. Typical results of such studies include the assessment of the comparative efficacy of different doses of the same drug or clinically relevant doses of different inhalation drugs.

Pk/pd-based models to assess pulmonary effects in humans. Currently, direct PK/PD methods for pulmonary effects have not been established, because the assessment of free drug concentration in the lung is very difficult, especially in humans.

Using systemic and pulmonary effects to assess pulmonary targeting in humans. Using markers for both systemic and pulmonary effects, attempts have been made to quantify or demonstrate pulmonary targeting. In one possible clinical design, pulmonary effects observed after systemic administration of the drug and after inhalation are compared. In this case (and without the availability of a robust PK/PD model), doses after systemic administration and inhalation have to be selected in such a way that systemic drug levels and systemic side effects are equivalent after both forms of administration. Pulmonary effects are then quantified after oral administration and inhalation. If pulmonary targeting is observed after inhalation, one would expect similar systemic effects after oral absorption but more pronounced systemic effects after inhalation (Fig. 14).

Toogood and coworkers used such an approach for the assessment of budesonide [113]. Patients were pretreated with beclomethasone dipropionate and then randomized to oral or inhaled budesonide, at doses expected to yield similar systemic budesonide levels. At these doses, the time to relapse

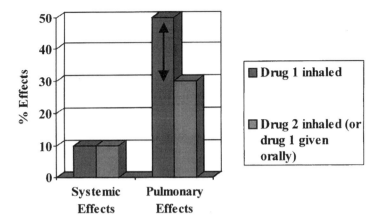

FIGURE 14 Clinical differences in pulmonary targeting. Doses of inhaled drugs are identified that will produce equipotent systemic effects. The drug with the higher degree of pulmonary effects will show more pronounced targeting. In a similar design, the same drug could be given orally and through inhalation. More pronounced pulmonary effects after inhalation snow targeting.

(the primary pulmonary outcome parameter) was longer for inhaled budesonide than after oral budesonide or placebo. This clinical approach showed, for the first time, targeting of an inhaled steroid. Such noncompartmental approaches for pulmonary targeting can be easily demonstrated for beta-2-adrenergic drugs, which show much steeper dose–response curves.

Pharmacokinetic/Pharmacodynamic modeling approaches might also be useful in demonstrating pulmonary targeting after inhalation. Such approaches have the advantage that one does not depend on the realization of similar systemic drug levels after systemic and pulmonary drug administration or on the difficulties to find such equivalent doses. A PK/PD-based approach to quantify the degree of pulmonary targeting was described for the beta-2-adrenergic drug fenoterol. Fenoterol was given systemically and after inhalation. The pharmacokinetic and pharmacodynamic (heart rate, change in FEV_1) data obtained after intravenous drug administration allowed the establishment of a robust PK/PD model with high predictive power for both systemic side effects and pulmonary effects. Figure 15 shows a discrepancy between PK/PD-derived predicted and clinically measured pulmonary effects. The differences between the PK/PD-based predicted pulmonary effects and the actual clinical responses (composite of systemic and local effects) allow the quantification of the degree of pulmonary targeting, because these effects must be induced by the higher pulmonary drug concentrations.

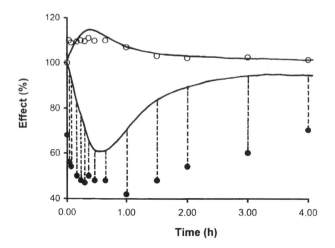

FIGURE 15 Effects of inhaled fenoterol (400 μg) on the heart rate (HR, open circles) and on reduction in pulmonary resistance (closed circles). Although the plasma levels of fenoterol are a good descriptor for systemic effects (HR), plasma levels cannot be used to predict effects on the pulmonary resistance. The area between the closed circles and the lower smooth line represents pulmonary selectivity.

SUMMARY

Inhaled-drug therapy will keep a central role in asthma therapy despite the development of new drug entities with oral administration routes. New developments in the inhalation area will further improve the local-to-systemic-effect ratios of inhalation drugs. This will involve the use of slow-release formulations, optimizing the deposition efficiency, and regional deposition of inhalation drugs (peripheral or central deposition) and further developments to improvement patient compliance (e.g., once-daily dosing). With the availability of more and more generic inhalation devices, questions on how to test bioequivalence will remain. Pharmacokinetic and pharmacokinetic/dynamic approaches will play an important role in streamlining such developments.

REFERENCES

1. Gonda I. J Pharm Sci 1988; 77:340–346.
2. Byron P, Phillips EM. In: Dalby R, Byron P, Farr SJ, eds. Respiratory Drug Delivery, Boca Raton, FL, 1990.
3. Byron PR. J Pharm Sci 1986; 75:433–438.

4. Hochhaus G, Mollmann H, Derendorf H, Gonzalez-Rothi RJ. J Clin Pharmacol 1997; 37:881–892.

5. Hochhaus G, Derendorf H, Moellmann H, Talton J, In: Schleimer RP, O'Byrne PM, Szefler SJ, Brattsand R, eds. Inhaled Steroids in Asthma: Optimizing Effects in the Airways. New York: Marcel Dekker, 2002:283–307.

6. Hochhaus G, Suarez S, Gonzales-Rothi RJ, Schreier H, In: Dalby R, Byron P, Farr SJ, eds. Respiratory Drug Delivery VI. Buffalo Grove, IL: Interpharm Press, 1998:45–52.

7. Mobley C, Hochhaus G. Drug Discov Today 2001; 6:367–375.

8. Dahlberg E, Thalen A, Brattsand R, Gustafsson JA, Johansson U, Roempke K, Saatok T. Mol Pharmacol 1984; 25:70–78.

9. Druzgala P, Hochhaus G, Bodor N. J Steriod Biochem Mol Biol 1991; 38:149–154.

10. Beato M, Rousseau GG, Feigelson P. Biochem Biophys Res Commun 1972; 47:1464–1472.

11. Hochhaus G, Moellmann H. Beta-Agonists: Terbutaline, Albuterol, and Fenoterol. New York: CRC, 1995:299–322.

12. Hochhaus G, Mollmann H. Int J Clin Pharmacol Ther Toxicol 1992; 30:342–362.

13. Falcoz C, Mackie A, Mcdowall J, McRae J, Yogendran L, Ventresca G, Bye A. Br J Clin Pharmacol 1996; 41:459P.

14. Ventressca G, Mackie A, Moss J, Mcdowall J, Bye A. Am J Respir Crit Care Med 1994; 149:A214.

15. Hochhaus G, Chen LS, Ratka A, Druzgala P, Howes J, Bodor N, Derendorf H. J Pharm Sci 1992; 81:1210–1215.

16. Ryrfeldt A, Andersson P, Edsbacker S, Tonnesson M, Davies D, Pauwels R. Eur J Respir Dis Suppl 1982; 122:86–95.

17. Dickens G, Wermeling D, Matheney C, John W, Abramowitz W, Sista S, Foster T. J Allergy Clin Immunol 1999; 103:S132.

18. Derendorf H, Hochhaus G, Rohatagi S, Mollmann J, Barth M, Erdmann M. J Clin Pharmacol 1995; 35:302.

19. Daley-Yates PT, Price AC, Sisson JR, Pereira A, Dallow N. Br J Clin Pharmacol 2001; 51:400–409.

20. Rohatagi S, Rhodes GR, Chaikin P. J Clin Pharmacol 1999; 39:661–663.

21. Mackie AE, Ventresca GP, Fuller RW, Bye A. Br J Clin Pharmacol 1996; 41:539–542.

22. Chaplin MD, Rooks W 2nd., Swenson EW, Cooper WC, Nerenberg C, Chu NI. Clin Pharmacol Ther 1980; 27:402–413.

23. Derendorf H, Hochhaus G, Rohatagi S, Mollmann H, Barth J, Sourgens H, Erdmann M. J Clin Pharmacol 1995; 35:302–305.

24. Biggadike K, Angell RM, Burgess CM, Farrell RM, Hancock AP, Harker AJ, Irving WR, Ioannou C, Procopiou PA, Shaw RE, Solanke YE, Singh OMP, Snowden MA, Stubbs RJ. J Med Chem (ASAP Article) 1999; 42.

25. Hill MR, Vaughan LM, In: Dalby RN, Byron PR, Farr SJ, eds. Respiratory Drug Delivery, 1998:53–60.

26. Newman SP, Brown J, Steed KP, Reader SJ, Kladders H. Chest 1998; 113:957–963.

27. Toogood JH. Ann Allergy 1985; 55:2–4.
28. Burton JA, Schanker LS. Steroids 1974; 23:617–624.
29. Burton JA, Schanker LS. Proc Soc Exp Biol Med 1974; 145:752–756.
30. Lanman RC, Gillilan RM, Schanker LS. J Pharmacol Exp Ther 1973; 187:105–111.
31. Gardiner T, Schamker L. Xenobiotica 1974; 725:731.
32. Burton JA, Schanker LS. Xenobiotica 1974; 4:291–296.
33. Schanker LS, Burton JA. Proc Soc Exp Biol Med 1976; 152:377–380.
34. Enna SJ, Schanker LS. Am J Physiol 1972; 223:1227–1231.
35. Burton JA, Gardiner TH, Schanker LS. Arch Environ Health 1974; 29:31–33.
36. Enna S, Schanker L. Life Sci 1973; 12:231–239.
37. Byron PR, Sun Z, Katayama H, Rypacek F. Pharm Res 1994; 11:221–225.
38. Hardy JG, Chadwick TS. Clin Pharmacokinet 2000; 39:1–4.
39. Suarez S, Gonzalez-Rothi RJ, Schreier H, Hochhaus G. Pharm Res 1998; 15:461–465.
40. Shek PN, Suntres ZE, Brooks JI. J Drug Target 1994; 2:431–442.
41. Fielding RM, Abra RM. Pharm Res 1992; 9:220–223.
42. Bot AI, Tarara TE, Smith DJ, Bot SR, Woods CM, Weers JG. Pharm Res 2000; 17:275–283.
43. Dellamary LA, Tarara TE, Smith DJ, Woelk CH, Adractas A, Costello ML, Gill H, Weers JG. Pharm Res 2000; 17:168–174.
44. Edwards DA, Hanes J, Caponetti G, Hrkach J, Ben-Jebria A, Eskew ML, Mintzes J, Deaver D, Lotan N, Langer R. Science 1997; 276:1868–1871.
45. Edwards DA, Ben-Jebria A, Langer R. J Appl Physiol 1998; 85:379–385.
46. Talton J, Fitz-Gerald J, Singh R, Hochhaus G. In: Dalby R, Byron P, Farr SJ, eds. Respiratory Drug Delivery VII. Buffalo Grove, IL: Interpharm Press, 2000:67–74.
47. Stefely JS, Hameister WM, Myrdal PB, Leach CL. AAPS Pharm Sci 1999; 1.
48. Green SA, Spasoff AP, Coleman RA, Johnson M, Liggett SB. J Biol Chem 1996; 271:24029–24035.
49. Thorsson L, Thunnisen F, Korn F. Am J Respir Crit Care Med 1998; 157:A404.
50. Miller-Larsson A, Mattsson H, Hjertberg E, Dahlback M, Tunek A, Brattsand R. Drug Metab Dispos 1998; 26:623–630.
51. Nilsson F, Strandberg P, Brattsand R, Miller-Larsson A. High airway selectivity of budesonide due to endogenous reversible esterification. ATS 2001, San Francisco, 2001.
52. Wieslander E, Delander EL, Jarkelid L, Hjertberg E, Tunek A, Brattsand R. Am J Respir Cell Mol Biol 1998; 19:477–484.
53. Mathias NR, Yamashita F, Lee VHL. Adv Drug Delivery Rev 1996; 22:215–249.
54. Forbes B. Pharm Sci Technol Today 2000; 3:18–27.
55. Kobayashi S, Kondo S, Juni K. Pharm Res 1995; 12:1115–1119.
56. Elbert KJ, Schafer UF, Schafers HJ, Kim KJ, Lee VHL, Lehr CM. Pharm Res 1999; 16:601–608.
57. Byron PR, Roberts NS, Clark AR. J Pharm Sci 1986; 75:168–171.
58. Byron PR, Niven RW. J Pharm Sci 1988; 77:693–695.
59. Ryrfeldt A, Nilsson E. Biochem Pharmacol 1978; 27:301–305.

60. Brazzell RK, Kostenbauder HB. J Pharm Sci 1982; 71:1274–1281.

61. Pavia D, Bateman JR, Sheahan NF, Clarke SW. Eur J Respir Dis 1980; 61:245–253.

62. Winters SL, Yeates DB. J Appl Physiol 1997; 83:1348–1359.

63. Sakagami M, Byron PR, Venitz J, Rypacek F. J Pharm Sci 2002; 91:594–604.

64. Esmailpour N, Hogger P, Rabe KF, Heitmann U, Nakashima M, Rohdewald P. Eur Respir J 1997; 10:1496–1499.

65. Van den Bosch JM, Westermann CJ, Aumann J, Edsbacker S, Tonnesson M, Selroos O. Biopharm Drug Dispos 1993; 14:455–459.

66. Digenis GA, Sandefer GP, Page RC, Doll WJ. Pharm Sci Technol Today 1998; 1:100–107.

67. Newman SP, Wilding IR. 1999; 2:181–189.

68. Berridge MS, Heald DL, Muswick GJ, Leisure GP, Voelker KW, Miraldi F. J Nucl Med 1998; 39:1972–1977.

69. Falcoz C, Mackie AE, Moss J, Horton J, Venetresca GP, Brown A, Field E, Harding SM, Wire P, Bye A. J Allergy Clin Immunol 1997; 99:S505.

70. Daley-Yates PT, Tournant J, Kunka RL. Clin Pharmacokinet 2000; 39:39–45.

71. Thorsson L, Edsbacker S, Kallen A, Lofdahl CG. Br J Clin Pharmacol 2001; 52:529–538.

72. Agertoft L, Andersen A, Weibull E, Pedersen S. Arch Dis Child 1999; 80:241–247.

73. Agertoft L, Pedersen S. Arch Dis Child 1993; 69:130–133.

74. Wildhaber JH, Devadason SG, Wilson JM, Roller C, Lagana T, Borgstrom L, LeSouef PN. Eur J Pediatr 1998; 157:1017–1022.

75. Chege JK, Chrystyn H. Respir Med 2000; 94:51–56.

76. Borgstrom L, Nilsson M. Pharm Res 1990; 7:1068–1070.

77. Thorsson L, Edsbacker S, Conradson TB. Eur Respir J 1994; 7:1839–1844.

78. Argenti D, Shah B, Heald D. J Clin Pharmacol 1999; 39:695–702.

79. Mollmann H, Derendorf H, Barth J, Meibohm B, Wagner M, Krieg M, Weisser H, Knoller J, Mollmann A, Hochhaus G. J Clin Pharmacol 1997; 37:893–903.

80. Hindle M, Chrystyn H. Br J Clin Pharmacol 1992; 34:311–315.

81. Hindle M, Newton DA, Chrystyn H. Thorax 1993; 48:607–610.

82. Aswania OA, Corlett SA, Chrystyn H. Eur J Clin Pharmacol 1998; 54:475–478.

83. Aswania OA, Corlett SA, Chrystyn H. J Chromatogr B Biomed Sci Appl 1997; 690:373–378.

84. Nasr H, Chrystyn H. Eur Respir J 1997; 10:129S.

85. Lundin P, Naber T, Nilsson M, Edsbacker S. Aliment Pharmacol Ther 2001; 15:45–51.

86. Borgstrom L. J Aerosol Med 1998; 11:55–63.

87. Krishnaswami S, Hochhaus G, Derendorf H. Br J Clin Pharmacol.

88. Kaellen A, Thorsson L. ALA/ATS International Conference, San Diego, CA, April 23–28, 1999.

89. Brindley C, Falcoz C, Mackie AE, Bye A. Clin Pharmacokinet 2000; 39:1–8.

90. Gillespie W. University of Texas, Austin, 1992.

91. Hochhaus G, Schmidt EW, Rominger KL, Mollmann H. Pharm Res 1992; 9:291–297.

92. Haddad el B, Underwood SL, Dabrowski D, Birrell MA, McCluskie K, Battram CH, Pecoraro M, Foster ML, Belvisi MG. J Immunol 2002; 168:3004–3016.
93. Bjermer L, Cai YG, Sarnstrand B, Brattsand R. Sarcoidosis 1994; 11:52–57.
94. Bjermer L, Sandstrom T, Sarnstrand B, Brattsand R. Am J Ind Med 1994; 25:73–78.
95. Brattsand R, Axelsson BI In: Schleimer RP, Busse WW, O'Byme PM, eds. Inhaled Glucocorticoids in Asthma. New York: Marcel Dekker, 1997:351–379.
96. Sadee W, Richards J, Grevel J, Rosenbaum JS. In vivo characterization of four types of opoid binding sites in rat brain. Life Sci 1983; 33:187–189.
97. Jonkers R, van Boxtel CJ, Koopmans RP, Oosterhuis B. J Pharmacol Exp Ther 1989; 249:297–302.
98. Braat MCP, Jonkers RE, van Boxtel CJ. Eur J Clin Pharmacol 1989; 36:A183.
99. Argenti D, Shah B, Heald D. J Clin Pharmacol 2000; 40:516–526.
100. Rohatagi S, Bye A, Mackie AE, Derendorf H. Eur J Pharm Sci 1996; 4:341–350.
101. Szefler SJ, Martin RJ. In: Schleimer RP, O'Byrne PM, Szefler SJ, Brattsand R, eds. Inhaled Steroids in Asthma: Optimizing Effects in the Airways. New York: Marcel Dekker, 2002:389–418.
102. Boulet L-P. In: Schleimer RP, O'Byrne PM, Szefler SJ, Brattsand R, eds. Inhaled Steroids in Asthma: Optimizing Effects in the Airways. New York: Marcel Dekker, 2002:465–490.
103. Rohatagi S, Bye A, Falcoz C, Mackie AE, Meibohm B, Mollmann H, Derendorf H. J Clin Pharmacol 1996; 36:938–941.
104. Rohatagi S, Hochhaus G, Mollmann H, Barth J, Galia E, Erdmann M, Sourgens H, Derendorf H. J Clin Pharmacol 1995; 35:1187–1193.
105. Rohatagi S, Hochhaus G, Moellmann H, Barth J, Derendorf H. Pharmazie 1995; 50:610–613.
106. Holford NHG, Sheiner LB. Clin Pharmacokinet 1981; 6:429–453.
107. Derendorf H, Meibohm B. Pharm Res 1999; 16:176–185.
108. Geller DA, Nussler AK, Disilvio M, Lowenstein CJ, Shapiro RA, Wang SC, Simmons RL, Billiar TR. Proc Natl Acad Sci USA January 15, 1993; 90:522–526.
109. Byrnes CA, Dinarevic S, Shinebourne EA, Barnes PJ, Bush A. Pediatr Pulmonol 1997; 24:312–318.
110. Van Den Berge M, Kerstjens HA, Meijer RJ, de Reus DM, Koeter GH, Kauffman HF, Postma DS. Am J Respir Crit Care Med 2001; 164:1127–1132.
111. De Meer G, Heederick D, Postma DS. Am J Respir Crit Care Med 2002; 165:327–331.
112. Pedersen S, Hansen OR. J Allergy Clin Immunol 1995; 95:29–33.
113. Toogood JH, Frankish CW, Jennings BH, Baskerville JC, Borga O, Lefcoe NM, Johansson SA. J Allergy Clin Immunol 1990; 85:872–880.
114. Krishnaswami S, Hochhaus G, Moellmann H, Derendorf H. AAPS PharmSci 2000; 2:Article 22 (http://www.pharmsci.org/).

8

Theoretical Principles and Devices Used to Generate Aerosols for Research

Keng H. Leong
Diodetec, Allison Park, Pennsylvania, U.S.A.

INTRODUCTION

Experimental aerosol research frequently requires the controlled generation of an aerosol. A particular property of the aerosol, such as a certain size distribution, may be required to ascertain its transport properties. The control of aerosol generation may extend beyond size distribution and concentration to the physical and chemical properties of the particles. In particular, the effective dose in aerosol therapy is a function of the physical and chemical properties of the aerosol particles in addition to the mass concentration delivered. The size, shape, and structure of the aerosol particles determine their aerodynamic or transport properties and, hence, affect the site and efficiency of deposition. After deposition, these same physical properties of the particles, in addition to the chemical properties, control the surface area of the particles and, hence, the rate of dissolution and absorption of the drug. Consequently, the control of the physical and chemical properties of the aerosol particles and of the number or mass concentration is a prerequisite for the accurate determination of the effective dose in aerosol therapy.

Numerous techniques have been developed to aerosolize liquids, resuspend particles, or generate aerosol particles. Descriptions of these aerosol generation techniques can be found in the literature of diverse fields such as powder technology, chemical engineering, defense technology, and atmospheric science, in addition to the journals of aerosol science, industrial hygiene, and medicine. Several reviews of aerosol generation methods have been published [1–7].

Consequently, some duplication of material in this current review is unavoidable. This chapter discusses aerosol generation methods based on the capability or the need to produce an aerosol with a desired property. Descriptions of generation methods use commercially available models as examples, although endorsement of the instruments is not necessarily to be inferred. This review is not intended to be comprehensive on the variety of aerosol generation methods but focuses on methods that have been proven to produce stable aerosols over a long duration and the parameters that control their stability. Generation methods that produce aerosols intermittently, such as the exploding-wire technique, or methods that are less well controlled or developed, such as generation from chemical reaction of gases, are not covered in this chapter. The reader is referred to the references for details on generation methods that are not discussed.

METHODS OF AEROSOL GENERATION

Given a continuous method of aerosol generation, the size distribution and mass concentration of the aerosol produced will remain constant if the parameters that affect the generation and dilution of the aerosol are held constant. In practice, some variation of these controlling parameters will occur, and the desired properties of the generated aerosol will degrade with time. The variation of the controlling parameters is affected by the choice of the particular method of generation and also by the duration of generation.

The size distribution of the aerosol is usually of primary importance, and the concentration is often controlled by dilution. However, some generation methods may produce aerosols with the desired distribution but with concentration that may be too dilute. The discussion of aerosol generation methods given in the following sections focuses on the control of size distribution and concentration. Control of particle shape and structure is discussed in the context of generation methods.

Evaporation–Condensation Methods

Methods of stable aerosol generation by evaporation of the bulk material and subsequent condensation to the aerosol form have generally evolved from the method developed by Sinclair and La Mer [8]. The aerosol was formed from the mixing of a flow of condensation nuclei with condensable vapor produced from heating a liquid with a relatively high boiling point and subsequent cooling. The output from this original method of aerosol generation was typically 10^5–10^6 particles cm^{-3} with particle sizes from 0.1 to several micrometers, but this was not very stable or reproducible. Enhancements and improvements to the stability and reproducibility have since been developed (see Ref. [3]). The evaporation–condensation method of aerosol generation that has evolved is depicted in Fig. 1.

The primary requirement is a source of vapor and a less volatile material that serves for condensation nuclei. Sodium chloride is commonly used to produce nuclei in the 10-nm-size range. This can be accomplished by heating the bulk material or by atomizing a dilute solution and drying the aerosol. The nuclei source can be a component (impurity) of the bulk material used, such as in the Rapaport–Weinstock generator, in which the impurity in the nebulized liquid serves as the condensation nuclei [9]. The use of heterogeneous nucleation for the formation of particles leads to a substantially more controllable and monodisperse aerosol than without the use of nuclei, that is, homogeneous nucleation.

The size of the particles is determined by the particular material selected and the vapor concentration used. In practice, limited variation in particle size can be achieved for a particular aerosol material because conditions for stable aerosol formation require a particular set of thermal and vapor concentration conditions. The monodispersity of the aerosol can be improved by revaporization and recondensation. In systems in which the condensation occurs in a container with a high ratio of volume to surface areas, relatively monodisperse particles can be obtained ($\sigma_g \sim 1.1$). Otherwise, the particle size varies with the proximity to the wall. In cylindrical or tubular systems, such as in the condensation aerosol generator developed by Liu et al. [10] or the falling-film generator, the particle size that is produced varies radially (see Ref. [3]). A more monodisperse aerosol can be produced by extracting the central portion of the flow, which is less subject to wall effects. Liu et al. [10] found that the monodispersity improved from a σ_g value of 1.35 to 1.15 by using only the central 5% of the aerosol flow. A commercial version of a modified Sinclair–LaMer generator is available with particle size control suited for inhalation studies [11].

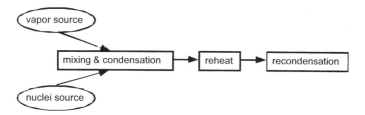

FIGURE 1 Schematic of evaporation–condensation method of aerosol generation.

The bulk material used for the vapor source is not restricted to liquids, because solids and even refractory materials have been used [12]. The difficulty is the requirement of higher temperatures (high-temperature furnaces) and a suitable material for the nuclei. Solid particles produced by the evaporation–condensation method tend to be spherical.

Temperature control is essential for maintaining a constant vapor or nuclei concentration. The vapor flux is controlled by the exposed surface area of the bulk material in addition to the temperature. If the vapor source is derived from heating the bulk material, the exposed surface area of the bulk material used in the furnace will change as the material is consumed. After the furnace is turned off, condensation of the vapor will occur on the walls. Consequently, stability and reproducibility problems usually occur in generator systems using furnaces. These problems can be overcome by using a constant-output atomizer or nebulizer system, but a liquid is required. The vapor is obtained by heating the aerosol. Prolonged heating of the bulk liquid, which may lead to decomposition, is avoided. A low concentration of a less volatile substance is usually added to liquid to serve as a stable nuclei source. Impurities in the liquid may also act as nuclei [11]. Otherwise, an external source of nuclei is used. Condensation to form the aerosol takes place in a long tube, where laminar flow is established. Use of the central core of the aerosol flow may be required for a mere monodisperse aerosol. Long-term operation of several hours can easily be achieved by using a large liquid reservoir for the atomizer. Additional control of the vapor source can be obtained by using a solution instead of a pure liquid. Hence, solids can vaporized by this method if a suitable solvent is available. A diffusion dryer may be required to lower the vapor concentration of the solvent. Buildup of the aerosol material on the tube wall of the condensation section will occur from condensation, and particle deposition from long duration operation. Degradation in the output may occur, and the section will have to be cleaned.

The evaporation–condensation method of aerosol generation can be used to produce particles with coatings. Espenscheid et al. [13] generated coated particles by condensing linolenic acid on silver chloride particles. Several other researchers have used similar techniques for the generation of coated particles. More recently, Lee et al. [14] generated diesel particles coated with polycyclic aromatic compounds. In principle, any aerosol particle can be coated by condensing a more volatile substance on it. The thickness of the coating will depend on the vapor concentrations and the coating time. In addition to the increase in particle size after coating, a less monodisperse aerosol can be expected. However, a recent technique developed by Couper et al. [15] produced a monodisperse aerosol ($\sigma_g = 1.1$) of hydrophobic particles with a hydrophilic core. The standard coating technique of using two separate components was combined into a single step by using a modified Rapaport–Weinstock generator with a collision atomizer to disperse a solution of the two components in ethanol.

A different technique was used by Durand Keklikian and Partch [16] to generate particles with a surface coating. Previously, a more volatile substance was coated on a less volatile particle. For their case, oil droplets coated with metal oxide were generated. This was accomplished by nebulizing solutions of titanium or aluminum alkoxides in oil. Hydrolysis of the alkoxide to the oxide occurred in the presence of water vapor, forming a solid shell encapsulating the oil droplet.

Nebulizers and Atomizers

Nebulizers and atomizers used in aerosol research produce a polydisperse aerosol consisting of particles under $10 \mu m$ in diameter. Most nebulizers use compressed air for atomization, whereas some use ultrasonics. Many models of compressed-air nebulizers have been developed, but they basically use the principle of air blast atomization of liquids issuing through a small orifice. Impaction plates or baffles are used to remove the larger droplets. Mass median diameters normally range from 2 to $5 \mu m$, with a compressed-air pressure of $20-30$ psig. A detailed discussion of nebulizers can be found in Raabe [5]. Most nebulizers or atomizers tend to have a small liquid reservoir and cannot be used for long duration unless the reservoir is refilled continuously.

A model that is of high stability and capable of long duration operation is that developed by Liu and Lee [17]. The principle of operation is illustrated in Fig. 2 for a commercially available version of the atomizer. Air is forced through an orifice to a small passage where the liquid is fed in. The liquid is atomized by the high-velocity airstream. The larger droplets impact on the wall of the passage and flow down to the excess liquid reservoir. The smaller droplets are carried up by the airflow. The droplet size in the aerosol stream that is produced can be controlled by varying the compressed-air pressure. Submicrometer particles or droplets can be produced by using solutions. The solution droplets are then dried by heating the aerosol and passing them through a diffusion dryer. In the case of water as the solvent, a simple but effective dryer can be made by using a bed of silica gel. Submicrometer-particle concentrations generated by this method range from 10^6 to $10^7 \, cm^{-3}$. The size distributions have a nominal σ_g value near 2. Larger aerosol output volume can be obtained with multiple-nozzle generators.

The compressed-air pressure is controlled by a pressure regulator. A syringe pump can be used to regulate the liquid feed. The excess liquid is not recycled back to the liquid reservoir as in many other designs. Evaporation of the solvent occurs rapidly after atomization because dry air is normally used. This will concentrate the solution droplets produced, and recycling of the larger droplets back to the liquid reservoir will change the concentration of the solution and cause the particle size produced to increase with time. Improvements to the design of Liu and Lee have been made by Leong et al. [18]. The constriction at

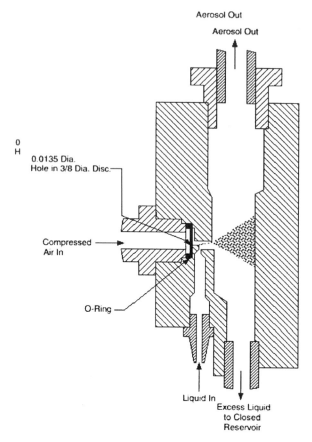

FIGURE 2   Schematic of an atomizer (TSI Model 3076).

the outlet of the atomizer was eliminated to prevent collection of droplets that may drip down. A low-pressure constant-liquid feed was used with a large reservoir for long-duration operation. Liquid feed control was achieved with a set pressure on the liquid reservoir and a flowmeter with a micrometer valve. Stable operation was obtained at a minimum liquid feed rate of 0.4 mL/min with very low liquid flow to the excess liquid reservoir.

The technique of nebulization of solutions to produce aerosols can also be used for suspensions. Insoluble or inert particles can be resuspended by nebulizing a suspension and by heating the aerosol to drive off the volatile liquid. A monodisperse aerosol of polystyrene particles can be generated with this method. To avoid having doublets or triplets of the primary particles, the suspension concentration should be less than that necessary to have less than one particle for the largest droplet produced. Otherwise, an impactor may be used to remove the larger particles. The nebulizers thus considered produce droplets of a few micrometers or less in diameter. Consequently, micrometer-size particles, such as bacteria and pollen, cannot be resuspended by this technique because they will be retained by the impaction plate in the nebulizer system. An atomizer capable of generating larger droplets is required. This is easily accomplished for the case of the atomizer shown in Fig. 2 by redesigning the atomizer so that the impaction wall is eliminated. If this is the case, the modal diameter of the droplets produced is approximately 10 μm at a pressure of 30 psig. The largest droplets are about 60 μm in diameter. The particle concentrations produced by atomizing suspensions can approach that of nebulizers for the case of submicrometer sizes, and the concentrations decrease substantially for larger particles because of the size distribution of the droplets produced. Higher concentrations of monodisperse particles in the micrometer-size range are more easily produced by other methods of generation, such as a fluidized-bed generator or a vibrating-orifice aerosol generator.

Ultrasonic nebulizers produce droplets in the micrometer-size range and are frequently used in aerosol drug therapy. Concentrations at $10^7 \, cm^{-3}$ are easily obtained for micrometer-size particles [19,20]. A simple ultrasonic nebulizer is shown in Fig. 3. Acoustic waves are generated in the liquid with a transducer. A coupling fluid is frequently used to prevent overheating of the transducer, which may occur when the liquid reservoir is empty. The frequency used is normally 100 kHz or higher. Disturbances on the surface of the liquid result, and droplets are formed. The airflow that is used can affect the size of the aerosol transported out of the nebulizer [5,20]. This occurs either through the decrease in coagulation of the droplets or the more efficient transport of larger droplets out of the nebulizer at higher flowrates [19,21].

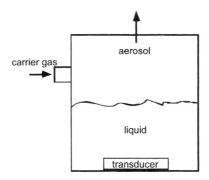

FIGURE 3 A simple ultrasonic nebulizer.

The mechanism of droplet formation from ultrasonic excitation of the liquid depends on the frequency and intensity applied [21]. At an intensity of $10\,\text{W/cm}^2$, capillary surface waves are formed from cavitation at frequencies less than $100\,\text{kHz}$. Cavitation can occur at lower-power intensities when dissolved gases are present. Droplets are thrown outward by the rupture of the cavitation bubbles or the wave crests. For such conditions, the droplet diameter can be related to the capillary wavelength [21,22].

$$d = 0.34\left(\frac{8\pi\sigma}{\rho_l f^2}\right)^{1/3}$$

where σ is the surface tension, ρ_l is the density of the liquid, and f is the ultrasonic frequency. For a given intensity level, the amplitude of wave motion decreases at higher frequencies, and cavitation becomes more difficult. However, the acceleration on the liquid surface increases with the applied frequency. This force causes miniature fountains or geysers to be formed. At power intensities less than $30\,\text{W/cm}^2$, droplets are thrown off intermittently by the geysers, at higher intensities, the droplets are produced continuously [23]. For this geyser mode of droplet formation, a reliable correlation of droplet size with applied power or frequency is not available, although many researchers have found that the droplet size tends to decrease with the frequency (see Ref. [21] and Ref. [22]). The previous equation for the cavitation mode probably can be used to estimate the droplet size, even though most commercially available ultrasonic nebulizers operate in the megahertz frequency range and droplets are produced by the geyser mode.

Although ultrasonic nebulizers produce substantially higher concentration of droplets than pneumatic-type nebulizers in the micrometer range, they have not found wide use in fundamental aerosol research. This is due largely to several inherent characteristics of the ultrasonic nebulizers. Given the modes of droplet formation and the physical phenomena, the parameters controlling droplet production have been shown to be the viscosity (static and dynamic), surface tension, and vapor pressure of the liquid [23,24]. Increased droplet production can be expected for liquids with high vapor pressure or low viscosity. The presence of dissolved gases will also contribute positively to droplet formation. Viscous liquids with low vapor pressure, such as oils, are difficult to nebulize. On the other hand, liquids with low surface tension, such as surfactants, are also difficult to nebulize, because of foaming. Most of the energy introduced into the liquid by the ultrasonic transducer goes into heating the liquid. Temperature increases of 10K have been observed for small commercial nebulizers [19]. For this temperature change, small changes in droplet size can be expected unless drastic change in the viscosity or surface tension occurs. In addition, increased vaporization of the liquid will occur. At high power levels, breakdown of organic molecules has been observed in addition to expected increases in temperature and vaporization rates (see Ref. [21]). For most aerosol studies, a low-volatility substance is preferred. Ultrasonic nebulization of a low-volatility liquid is difficult. The use of solutions avoids this difficulty, but, with time the increased vaporization of the solvent changes the concentration and, hence, the particle size generated.

Electrical Mobility Classification

The stable polydisperse output of an atomizer can be used with an electrical mobility classifier to generate monodisperse streams of submicrometer aerosols with diameters ranging from 0.001 to 1 µm [25,26]. A schematic of a commercially available electrical mobility classifier is shown in Fig. 4. It consists of a controller platform for charge neutralization and flow control of the aerosol source to a differential mobility analyzer (DMA) unit. Three DMA units are available that provide classification over a range of two orders of magnitude in particle size for each unit. The polydispersed aerosol is passed through a bipolar charger to bring the charge state of the aerosol to a Boltzmann equilibrium. The neutralized aerosol is made to flow on the outer annular region between two coaxial cylinders. The outer cylinder is grounded, and the inner cylinder is charged to a selected potential. Clean-sheath airflows surround the inner electrode. Stable flowrates are maintained by mass flow controllers. The electrical field set up in the coaxial region cause charged aerosol particles to migrate toward the inner electrode. Only charged particles within a narrow mobility range determined by the potential on the inner electrode and the flow

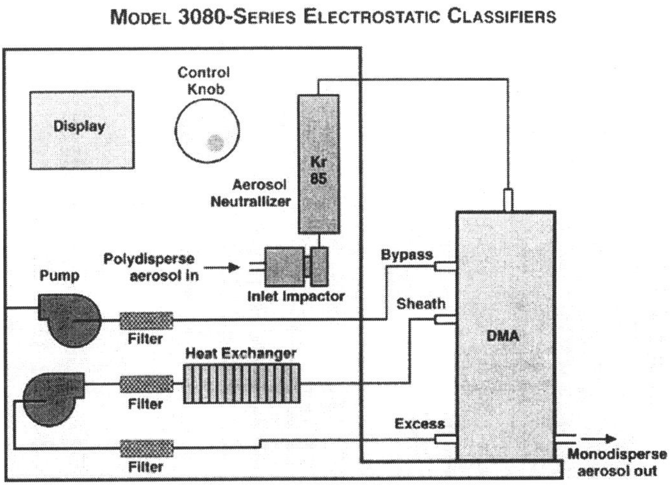

MODEL 3080-SERIES ELECTROSTATIC CLASSIFIERS

FIGURE 4 Schematic of an electrostatic classifier (TSI Model 3080).

rates can exit the slit near the end of the inner electrode. Hence, a particular size of particle corresponding to an electrical mobility value can be selected by the appropriate choice of an inner electrode voltage. The monodisperse particle concentration output for a particular size from a constant-output atomizer-mobility classifier system can be optimized by the selection of an appropriate solution concentration or operating conditions to match the modal size of the atomizer output to the selected monodisperse size. Monodisperse particle output up to $10^6 \, cm^{-3}$ can be obtained in the size range from 0.05 to 0.08 μm. Diffusion losses for smaller particle sizes restrict the concentrations to less than $10^4 \, cm^{-3}$ for particle sizes of about 0.01 μm. The output for particle sizes larger than 0.1 μm is limited by the output of the atomizer. Frequently, an atomizer evaporation–condensation technique is used to generate a polydisperse aerosol with particle sizes larger than 0.1 μm. Extension of particle size to 1 nm can be achieved using a DMA modified for ultrafine aerosols.

The output of the mobility classifier is monodisperse by mobility classification. The aerosol will then be monodisperse if all the particles are singly charged. A doubly charged particle will have the same mobility as a singly charged particle half its diameter. Occurrence of multiply charged particles is negligible for particle sizes less than 0.02 μm but becomes significant for larger particles. At a mobility size of 0.2 μm, more than 20% of the particles may possess a charge of two or more electrons. This is particularly troublesome because more than two-thirds of the mass of the aerosol particles reside on the particles that are 0.4 μm or larger. This problem in monodispersity can be alleviated by using two or more mobility classifiers in series, but the output will be reduced by losses in the additional classifier. Gupta and McMurry [26,27] have developed a method to minimize this problem of multiply charged particles. A charged condenser was used to remove the charged particles from the aerosol before subjecting the aerosol to a low-activity radioactive source. The particles exiting this arrangement were mostly uncharged or singly charged. At a particle size of 1.0 μm, only 25% of the particles were multiply charged, in contrast to 72% of the particles when the aerosol was at a Boltzmann equilibrium. Although monodispersity is improved, more than one order-of-magnitude reduction in particle concentrations can be expected with this method.

Electrospray Aerosol Generator

Generation of liquid aerosols by electrospraying has been a well-studied technique [28,29]. Electrostatic charges are used to decrease the surface tension of a liquid to facilitate or cause breakup of the surface. The placement of charge on the surface in practice necessitates a sufficiently conductive liquid for electric current flow to replenish charge carried away by the aerosol released. In an assist mode, a potential difference is placed on the liquid to decrease the droplet size for pneumatic atomization or vibrating-orifice droplet generation. For an electrostatic spray where a high potential at a liquid surface causes droplets to be ejected, different modes of droplet formation occur where polydisperse or mono-disperse droplets are produced. Recent work has shown that with a combination of a constant-pressure feed through a capillary tube and electrospraying, a stable, high-concentration ($\sim 10^7 \, \text{cm}^{-3}$), ultrafine ($\sim 10 \, \text{nm}$) aerosol can be produced [30]. A commercial version of an electrospray aerosol generator is shown in Fig. 5. A small volume of the liquid (conductivity $\sim 0.2 \, \text{S/m}$) to be sprayed is placed in the sample vial. Nonvolatile liquids, solutions, or suspensions of ultrafine particles can be used. Pressurizing the chamber forces a slow flow of the liquid up the capillary tube. A high voltage of several kilo volts applied to the platinum wire causes electrospraying of the liquid surface exiting the capillary tube, producing droplets approximately 200–2000 nm in diameter. The aerosol flow of a few liters per minute consist of highly charged droplets that are neutralized in the ionizer chamber. Careful control of the process parameters result in a monodisperse aerosol.

Vibrating-Orifice Monodisperse Aerosol Generator

The vibrating-orifice monodisperse method of aerosol generation is based on the principle of the disintegration of a jet of liquid issuing from an orifice that is

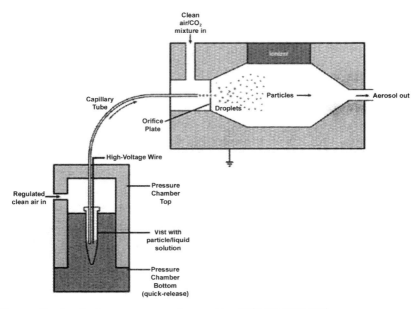

FIGURE 5   An electrospray aerosol generator (TSI Model 3480).

driven by a periodic vibration of the appropriate frequency and amplitude. The phenomenon of the breakup of a liquid jet into uniform droplets was studied by Plateau [31] and Rayleigh [32,33]. Castleman [34] observed that a jet can be made to disintegrate into uniform droplets on the application of a vibration of a suitable frequency and amplitude. This principle of uniform droplet production has been used by several groups of researchers to produce droplet generators [35–40]. Uniform droplets can be produced by vibrating the liquid, the container holding the liquid, or the orifice. The droplet size is primarily controlled by the size of the orifice. Droplet diameters produced are nominally twice the orifice diameter. The name *vibrating orifice* is commonly used because of the success of the commercial version of the generator developed by Berglund and Liu [40].

An illustration of the design of the vibrating-orifice generator head is shown Fig. 6. Liquid is fed into the generator head and forced out of the orifice.

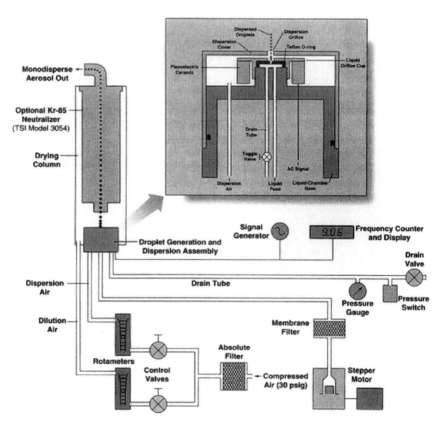

FIGURE 6   A vibrating-orifice aerosol generator (TSI Model 3450).

A syringe pump is usually used, and the liquid is filtered through a 0.5-μm, 13-mm-diameter filter in the commercial version of the generator manufactured by TSI, Inc. A drain tube is available for flushing the cavity upstream of the orifice. The piezoelectric ceramic is excited by a sinusoidal signal from a function generator. The vibration produced is transmitted to the orifice and breaks up the liquid jet into uniform droplets. The monodispersity of the jet can be verified by deflecting the jet of droplets with a jet of air that is a simple version of an inertial spectrometer [39]. Multiple deflected streams indicate that the droplets are not monodisperse. The jet of droplets passes through an aperture where dispersion air flows to disperse the jet to prevent coagulation of the droplets. Dilution air is supplied through a perforated plate around the base of a generator head. A radioactive bipolar ion source is frequently used to neutralize the charged particles produced, to decrease particle loss to the wall of the transport tubing. If a solution is used for the liquid, the dilution air aids in evaporating the solvent. The aerosol is usually heated, to ensure dry particles are produced. The aerosol produced by this method is very monodisperse, with $\sigma_g < 1.05$. The deviation from monodispersity is caused by the presence of a few percent of doublets formed from the coagulation of two droplets. The vibrating-orifice aerosol generator possesses an inherent advantage over other aerosol generators, in that the particle diameter, d, can be computed directly from the ratio of the liquid feedrate, Q, to the frequency of vibration, f, applied if the particle density, ρ_P, is the same as that of the bulk material used:

$$d = \left(\frac{cQ}{\pi f \rho_P} \right)^{1/3}$$

where c is the mass concentration of the solute per unit volume of the solution. For the case of a pure liquid, c has the value of 1. Particle diameters that can be produced range from 0.5 to 50 μm for solutions. The production of larger particles is not practical because of the difficulties in evaporation and transport, high particle losses, and low concentrations at large orifice sizes. Smaller particles can be produced if a very pure solvent is used. The particle concentrations obtainable using a 10-μm orifice are about $10^3 \, \text{cm}^{-3}$. The particle concentration decreases monotonically with the orifice size because the optimum exciting frequency also decreases. For a given orifice, a stable monodisperse stream of droplets may be obtained at more than one frequency of vibration. Schneider and Hendricks [36] determined experimentally that uniform droplets can be produced if the wavelength of the disturbance (applied signal) is between 3.5 and 7 times the diameter of the liquid jet, which is approximately the diameter of the orifice. The optimal wavelength for the disturbance to be most unstable is given by Rayleigh as 4.508d [32,33]. Hence, several monodisperse particle sizes can be obtained with a given orifice, particularly for larger orifices. It becomes more difficult to obtain a stable stream at frequencies other than the fundamental for orifice sizes less than 50 μm.

In practice, most researchers use a 20-μm orifice and obtain stable operation of the generator for longer than 5 hr. Difficulties are encountered for orifices 10 μm or less, which are preferred for the generation of higher concentrations. For these orifice sizes, pressures over 20 psig are required to maintain a stable jet. Conventional syringe pumps are inadequate, and special pumps are required when syringe feed is used. Many users have resorted to the economical method of pressure feed of the liquid using a liquid reservoir and a compressed gas tank (e.g., see Ref. [41]). Large liquid reservoirs can easily be used, in contrast to the limited capacity of syringes, but the feedrate has to be determined by weighing the output of the generator over a time interval. This is not a serious disadvantage if the orifice does not plug and the feedrate remains stable for a fixed pressure. Another alternative liquid feed method superior to the syringe pump is a high-pressure metering pump, which is commonly used in liquid chromatography [42]. The length of operation is not limited by the large refill reservoir that can be used.

Plugging of small orifices has been encountered by many users, even though the liquid was filtered. Special techniques have been developed by several users to overcome plugging of orifices to obtain stable operation of the generator for orifice sizes of 10 μm or lower. A point-of-use filtration technique was developed by Kreyling and Erbe [43] in which a filter was inserted immediately upstream of the orifice. Stable operation for several hours was achieved for a 5-μm orifice. Leong [41,44] developed a pressure-feed method using a 0.2-μm capsule filter with a 500-cm^2 filtration area and a flushing procedure to prevent plugging. Stable operation for up to 6 hr was achieved for 10-μm orifices and a few hours for an 8.7-μm orifice. Examination of the orifices, after the jet became unstable, by microscopy showed no plugging, and the reason for the instability was unclear. Orifices became unusable after an extended period, even though they appeared round and were not plugged.

The vibrating-orifice aerosol generator is commonly used to produce micrometer-size monodisperse aerosols. When solid particles are required, a solution of the substance is used, and the solvent has to be evaporated. Particles formed from the evaporation of solution droplets are not necessarily spherical and solid, as has been observed for submicrometer-size particles generated by nebulizers. Charlesworth and Marshall [45] examined the morphology of particles derived from solution droplets and found that different particle shapes and densities can arise, depending on the mode of evaporation. Leong [46,47] studied in detail the morphology of particles produced by a vibrating-orifice aerosol generator. The particle morphology is determined by the chemical properties (particularly the solubility) of the compound used and the conditions controlling the evaporation of the solvent. The variation in morphology was more diverse for compounds of lower solubility. An aerosol was generated that was monodisperse in mass but nonuniform in shape. A bimodal aerosol was also generated where the primary particles were hollow, with a small hole, and the secondary (in mass) component was derived from the fragment that left the hole. For most compounds, monodispersity in both mass and shape was obtained.

Particles derived from the evaporation of solution droplets are spheroidal. Shape (primarily in surface features), density, and size control of particles can be achieved by the appropriate selection of the compound, the concentration of the solution, the size of the droplet generated, and the conditions for the evaporation of the droplets. Fast evaporation rates tend to produce less solid and rough-surface particles, but this is tempered by the chemical properties of the compound. Smooth, spherical particles call for compounds with high solubility and slow evaporation rates. These requirements were used by Vanderpool and Rubow [48] to produce solid, smooth spheres of up to 70 μm in diameter. The different types of particles that can be produced from the evaporation of solution droplets include solid spheres with surfaces that are smooth, cracked, or wrinkled; hollow spheres, shells, and spheroidal particles that have a wrinkled surface like raisins; porous-type particles that are perforated with holes, and single crystals and particles composed of several crystals, which may be angular or spheroidal in shape.

Spinning-Disk Aerosol Generator

The spinning-disk method of droplet generation is based on the breakup of ligaments of liquid created at the periphery of a rapidly rotating disk when liquid is fed slowly to the center and top of the disk. Under appropriate conditions of stable liquid feed and rotation, the ligament thrown out by the rotating disk breaks up into a primary (large) and a satellite (small) droplet. This is illustrated in Fig. 7. The satellite droplet is deflected away by an airflow and is usually rejected.

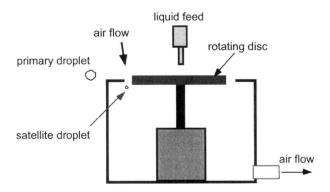

FIGURE 7 Illustration of a spinning-disk aerosol generator.

The primary stream of droplets is monodisperse. Walton and Prewett [49] demonstrated this principle of uniform droplet generation. An improved version with a spinning top was developed by May [50,51]. Further improved versions have been developed since then, and droplet sizes that are produced range from 15 to 150 μm (e.g., see Ref. [52]). A recent version produced monodisperse droplets between 10 and 60 μm in diameter [53]. Similar particles can be obtained using solutions. Toivonen and Bailey produced solid particles up to 40 μm in diameter [54]. Rotation speeds used are up to 70,000 rpm. Improvements in particle concentrations have been obtained by Cheah and Davies [55] but are still nominally less than $100\,cm^{-3}$. A detailed study of the mechanism of droplet formation was provided recently by Davies and Cheah [56]. Eisner and Martonen [57] demonstrated that if the primary and satellite droplets can be effectively separated, then two monodisperse aerosol streams can be generated simultaneously.

The particle diameter derived from the primary droplets can be predicted with the following expression [49]:

$$d = \frac{K}{\omega}\left(\frac{T}{D\rho_l}\right)^{1/2}\left(\frac{C}{\rho_P}\right)^{1/3}$$

where K is an empirical constant dependent on several factors, including the roughness of the spinning disk or top, ω is the radial frequency of the spinning top, T is the surface tension of the liquid, D is the diameter of the spinning top, ρ_l is the density of the liquid or solution, c is the concentration of the solution, and ρ_P the density of the particle. The value of K has been determined to vary from 2.3 to 7.0 with several different solutions for a spinning-top generator used by Mitchell [52].

The spinning-disk aerosol generator suffers from the low concentrations of particles achievable and the need for checking the particle size for a given set of operating conditions, in comparison to the vibrating-orifice aerosol generator. However, this method of generation is superior to that of the vibrating-orifice method in that it is not subject to the problems of orifice plugging. In addition, suspensions can easily be used, in contrast to the vibrating-orifice method, where stable operation cannot be expected, particularly for small orifices. The problem of particle morphology from the evaporation of solution droplets also applies here as in the previous method of aerosol generation.

Dust Generators

Dry powders are commonly resuspended to form an aerosol by pneumatic means. High concentrations are readily attainable, but stability of output and the presence of agglomerated particles are common problems. The basic requirements of a dust generator are a constant powder feed rate and a method of deagglomerating the powder. Many techniques have been used to develop a stable dust generator, and a recent review of different dry dispersion methods can found in Hinds [58]. Powder feed methods include scraping off the surface layer of a plug of powder such as in the Timbrell dust generator or the Wright dust feeder, vibrating sieve, screw feed, chain feed, and gravity feed mechanisms (59,60). The two methods of deagglomerating powders that have proven successful are the fluidized-bed and air-impaction methods.

The most stable method developed is the fluidized-bed aerosol generator. Initial work by Guichard [61] and Willeke et al. [62] has led to the development of a commercial model based on the prototype by Marple et al. [63]. The commercial version is shown in Fig. 8. Powder is fed to a fluidized bed of bronze beads by

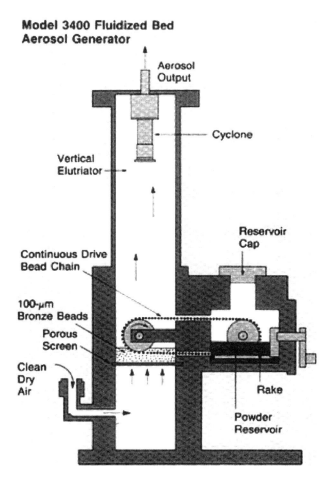

FIGURE 8　Schematic of a fluidized-bed aerosol generator (TSI Model 3400).

a continuous-bead-chain drive. Other types of metallic or ceramic beads can be used. The powder is deagglomerated by the fluidizing action and carried out of the bed by the airflow. A cyclone is used to remove agglomerated particles, especially when a fine aerosol is preferred. A period of 2–4 hr is required for the generator to reach a stable output. The recommended size ranges from 0.5 to 40 μm, and a mass concentration of up to 100 mg cm^{-3} is possible. Up to 15 L/min of airflow can be used with the fluidized bed of 100-μm beads. A higher-output fluidized-bed generator was developed by Boucher and Lua [64]. The stability of this improved generator was demonstrated for submicrometer-size basic oxygen furnace dust. The generator used a bed of nickel beads of 125–212 μm. The dust-feeding mechanism was a vibrating mesh system that used steel balls above the mesh to provide some milling and deagglomeration of the dust. The time required to reach a stable output was reduced to 30 min, and an aerosol loading of 4 g/m^3 was achieved at a flow rate of 70 L/min. Aerosols generated by fluidized beds tend to be highly charged, and an aerosol neutralizer is usually used [65].

Generation of asbestos or other fiber aerosols has been developed using fluidized beds. Early methods, though successful in aerosolizing the fibers, were not capable of a stable output for long durations (e.g. see Ref. 66 and Ref. 67). A stable fibrous aerosol generator was developed by Tanaka and Akiyama [68] using a continuos screw feeder. Glass fibers obtained by milling a binderless filter were mixed well with glass beads with diameters of 210–297 μm in distilled water. The mixture was dried in an oven. This two-component powder was fed into a hopper and transported to the fluidized bed by a screw feed. An overflow channel similar to that used by Guichard [61] maintained a constant bed height. This method of powder preparation avoided any clumping that might arise were the fibers fed directly into the bed. Stability and reproducibility of the generator were demonstrated on an hourly and a weekly basis.

The fluidized-bed method worked well, and it thoroughly deagglomerates dry and relatively noncohesive powders, such as coal, Arizona road dust, silica, copper ore, and potash [63]. The fluidizing action of the bed alone was inadequate for deagglomerating flocks of fibers and cohesive powders, such as dyes, that consist of relatively flat particles [69]. Air-impaction methods worked better.

The Timbrell dust generator was initially developed to generate asbestos fibers and was later modified for other powders [59]. The aerosols were generated by using two revolving rotor blades to cut or scrape an advancing plug of powder. Air jets dispersed the powder, which was scraped off. The stability of the output was controlled primarily by the packing of the powder plug. The particles might not have been thoroughly deagglomerated at higher feed rates because the air-impaction action was not strong. A commercial model was available but is no longer manufactured.

A more widely used dust generator has been the Wright dust feeder [60]. A diagram of the commercially available model is shown in Fig. 9. The powder

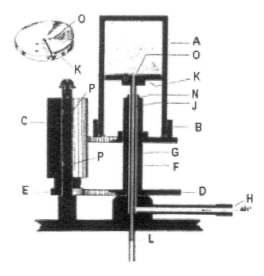

FIGURE 9 Commercial version of the Wright dust feeder. (A) dust chamber, (B) cap, (C) long pinion, (D) gear, (E) small pinion, (F) treaded spindle, (J) inner tube, (G) main spindle, (K) scraper head, (M) impaction plate, (N) spring ring, (O) scraper blade.

plug in chamber A is fed into inner tube 3 by scraper K when the chamber is rotated. Air fed in through opening H carries the dust down inner tube 3. The aerosol is accelerated through the orifice at L, and agglomerates are broken up by impaction plate M. Particle sizes greater than 10 μm are not recommended because of variability in the packing of the dust plug. Airflow rates can vary from 10 to 40 L/min, and output mass concentrations are about 10 g/m^3. The time to reach stable output is approximately 5 min, which is much shorter than for a fluidized bed.

Higher output both in mass loading and flowrates can be achieved with an NBS-II dust generator. The model name is somewhat generic, and the original design was by Dill at the Bureau of Standards [70]. A commercial version was previously available but has been discontinued. Dust in the hopper flows down by the action of gravity, aided by an agitator. The dust is fed into the spaces between the teeth of a rotating cog. Excess dust is removed by the contoured spreader plate. The dust is carried to a slit that covers three consecutive teeth. The dust is sucked up by the compressed-air ejector. Strong turbulent motions within the ejector nozzle serve to deagglomerate the dust. Fewer agglomerates are present in the aerosol at higher operating pressures of the ejector. Particle sizes ranging from 1 to 100 μm can be aerosolized. Airflow rates are 50–90 L/min, and aerosol mass concentrations are about 100 g/m^3.

Another method of dust generation uses the rotating-brush method. The design follows that of the German standard VDI-3491 (e.g., see Ref. [71]). A rotating brush with a high-velocity airflow of 150 m/see is used to disperse the dust from an advancing plug. Particle sizes up to 100 μm can be dispersed. Airflow rates are specified from 10 to 50 L/min. Aerosol loadings of up to 100 g/m^3 can be obtained. The duration of operation is limited by the volume of the powder plug and the rate of feed. Cohesive particles, such as carbon black, can be dispersed. Intermittent generation of large agglomerated particles from buildup on the brush has been found [72]. As in all plug feed methods, the stability of the output is determined by the uniformity of the packing of the powder. An additional consideration is the required cleaning of the brush after operation [71]. Fibrous particles can also be dispersed by this method [71].

Conditioning and Transformation of Aerosol Particles

Conditioning of the aerosol produced by a particular generator is frequently required for a specific application to prevent coagulation or loss of the particles. Particle concentration and size distribution are commonly modified. Aerosol particles generated are frequently charged and are usually neutralized with a bipolar ion source. Aerosol particle concentrations can easily be diluted after generation with the addition of clean dilution gas. The size distribution of the original aerosol can be modified with the use of cyclones, impactors, or electrical mobility classifiers. The intent is the elimination of undesired agglomerates or large particles. The morphology of particles generated from the evaporation of solution droplets can be controlled, as described previously, by controlling the conditions of evaporation.

An aerosol may be conditioned by heating to modify the physical, chemical, and morphological properties of the particles. Such a technique is often used to produce insoluble particles from generation techniques that require solutions or liquids. Kanapilly et al. [73] generated metal oxide particles by nebulizing solutions of metal chelates and thermally decomposing the particles to solid oxide particles. Hollow particles and shells were obtained under some conditions of drying of the solution droplets and heating of the particles. Jenkins et al. [74] generated monodisperse cerium oxide particles from colloidal suspensions using a spinning-top generator.

Ramamurthi and Leong [75] applied a similar technique to generate monodisperse aerosols of metallic, metal oxide, and carbon particles. The primary particles were generated using the vibrating-orifice aerosol generator. Metal oxide particles were obtained by thermal decomposition of the primary particles. The conversion of the metal oxide to metal was achieved by the use of a reducing gas (hydrogen). Particles obtained were generally spheroidal, with wrinkled or dimpled surfaces. Hollow copper oxide particles were produced when copper sulfate particles were thermally decomposed. The monodisperse hollow spheres fragmented to polydisperse copper particles when reduced, indicating the need for relatively solid particles for monodispersity to be maintained. Monodisperse carbon particles were generated by pyrolysis of polystyrene spheres.

The technique of using a gaseous reactant to modify an aerosol was studied by Robbins and Cadle [76] for a sulfuric acid aerosol and ammonia gas system. A sulfuric acid aerosol was produced by an evaporation–condensation technique and was reacted with ammonia gas. The uptake of ammonia by the acid particles was examined. Movilliat [77] generated silica aerosols by reacting a water aerosol with silicon chloride gas. Further treatment of the aerosol with heat yielded silica gel particles. At higher temperatures, silica particles were obtained. This technique of modifying particle properties was used by Durand-Keklikian and Parteli [16] to generate oil droplets coated with a ceramic. Water vapor reacted with the alkoxides (titanium or aluminum) in solution to form a coating of oxide. Hence, the use of a vapor-phase reactant can be exploited for the generation and transformation of the physical and chemical properties of an aerosol.

SUMMARY

Several stable methods of aerosol generation have been discussed. Their characteristics are summarized in Table 1. Commercial sources of these generators are listed in Table 2. These methods are suitable for aerosolizing bulk materials that are either liquids or powders. Solids can be converted to a liquid by the use of solvents or to a powder by grinding. The generators listed in Table 1 offer methods of producing polydisperse and monodisperse aerosols. Each method has certain characteristics that may be suited for a particular application. The electrostatic classifier and the vibrating-orifice and spinning-disk generators produce monodisperse aerosols. The evaporation–condensation generator can also produce monodisperse aerosols under controlled conditions. The vibrating-orifice and spinning-disk generators are usually used for producing micrometer-size particles, whereas the other monodisperse generators are used for submicrometer-size particles. Polydispersed particles are generated by nebulizers and evaporation–condensation generators. The dust-resuspension generators listed in Table 1 produce aerosols at different rates. Low stable output is best achieved by a small fluidized-bed generator, although equilibration time may be long. Improved equilibration time and higher output are characteristic of the air-impaction type of dust generators. However, the stability is controlled by the packing of the power column.

The usual constraints for using these generators are that the liquids be sufficiently inviscid and that the powders be noncohesive. In the case of liquids

TABLE 1 Comparison of Aerosol Generation Methods

Parameter	E–C	N	EC	VO	SD	FD	RB	WDF	NBS
Aerosol output (1/min)	1–10	1–10	1–5	>20	>10	5–15	10–50	10–40	50–85
Particle concentration/ loading	10^4–10^8 cm^{-3}	10^7–10^8	10^2–10^6	<10^3	$10 \sim 10^2$	0.01–0.1 g/m	0.07–100	0.01–25	10–200
Particle size (μm)	0.005–5	0.01–5	0.002–0.3	0.5–100	0.3–100	0.5–40	1–100	0.5–10	1–100
Size distribution (σ_g)	1.1–1.5	~2	<1.1	1.05	>1.05	Determined by powder used			
Output stability (%)	5	<5	5	<5	<5	5	10–30	7	10
Equilibration time after startup (min)	30–100	~1	~1	~1	<5	100–200	100	~5	~1

E–C, evaporation–condensation; N, nebulizer; EC, electrostatic classifier; VO, vibrating orifice; SD, spinning disc; FD, fluidized bed; RB, rotating brush; WDF, Wright dust feeder; NBS, NBS dust generator. Values of parameters given are from specifications listed by TSI, Inc., and BGI, Inc. Stability data are from the references. A density of I g/m^3 is assumed for the mass concentration values.

TABLE 2   Commercial Sources of Aerosol Generation Instruments

Source	Instruments
BGI Incorporated 58 Guinan Street Waltham, MA 02154 www.bgiusa.com	Collision nebulizer, spinning-top aerosol generator, NBS dust generator, Timbrell dust generator, Wright dust feeder
Dante Measurement Technology www.dantecmt.com	SAFEX fog generators
TSI Incorporated 500 Cardigan Road P.O. Box 64394 St. Paul, MN 55164 www.tsi.com	Constant-ouput atomizer, tri-jet aerosol generator, electrostatic classifier, vibrating-orifice aerosol generator, fluidized-bed aerosol generator, small-scale powder disperser

that are too viscous for practical aerosolization, heat may be applied to decrease the viscosity (e.g. wax). An alternative is the use of an appropriate solvent. Similarly, methods may be devised to decrease the cohesiveness of a powder. For most powders, the use of a low-humidity environment (carrier gas) generally helps. Alternatively, the powder may be heated to ensure its dryness. However, triboelectric effects may increase, and the use of aerosol neutralizers is required to neutralize the highly charged particles produced. Even under dry conditions, powders that are composed of flakes are difficult to deagglomerate because of the relatively large surface area of contact between particles. Combined fluidization and air impaction may be required to ensure deagglomeration.

The modification of the physical properties of the bulk material can be used to allow aerosol generation that is otherwise impractical. However, in many cases a property of the original powder or resulting aerosol particles is compromised. The use of a solution in the generation of an aerosol results in spheroidal particles that may not represent the shape or the density of the original powder. In addition, the generation of dry particles frequently requires the application of heat and absorption of the solvent. The solvent may also interfere with the experiment. Deagglomeration techniques to resuspend particles may break up fragile particles, changing the original size distribution.

For many application, high output of aerosol in both concentration and flowrate is preferred so that ease of detection can be achieved and lengthy experiments need not be conducted. Increasing the number of generators or, in the case of nebulizers, the number of nozzles, is a direct and relatively easy solution. However, the cost of several generators may be prohibitive. For example, the monodisperse aerosol generators listed in Table 1 are relatively costly. Increase in flowrate can easily be achieved by the addition of carrier gas, but at the expense of aerosol particle concentration. An alternative is the use of a high-output polydisperse generator and a virtual impactor to select and concentrate the larger particles for the experiment.

In general, the selection of a particular aerosol generation method requires careful consideration of the physical properties of both the bulk material and the aerosol required and of the number concentration and flowrate of the aerosol. In many cases, commercial aerosol generators may not be able to meet all the requirements and, thus, need to be modified. Customized generators are frequently the norm, and some experiments may even require the development of new methods.

ACKNOWLEDGMENTS

The assistance of Bob Gussman of BGI, Inc., and the staff of TSI, Inc., in supplying schematic drawings, photographs, and descriptions of instruments is very much appreciated.

REFERENCES

1. Whitby KT, Lundgren DA, Peterson CA. Int J Wat Poll 1965; 9:263.
2. Bailey AGJ. Mater Sci 1974; 9:1344–1362.
3. Kerker M. Adv Colloid Interf Sci 1975; 5:105.
4. Dennis R, ed. Handbook on Aerosols, TID-26608. National Technical Information Service, U.S. Dept of Commerce, 1976.
5. Raabe OG. In: Liu BYH, ed. Fine Particles: Aerosol Generation, Measurements, Sampling and Analysis. New York: Academic Press, 1976:57–110.
6. Tillery MI, Wood GO, Ettinger HJ. Environ Health Perspect 1976; 16:25.
7. Pui DYH, Liu BYH. TSI Q 1979; 5:5.
8. Sinclair D, La Mer VK. Chem Rev 1949; 44:245.
9. Rapaport E, Weinstock SE. Experentia 1955; 11:363.
10. Liu BYH, Whitby KT, Yu HHS. J Rech Atmos 1966; 3:97.
11. Peters C, Altmann J. J Aerosol Med 1993; 6:307.
12. Jacobsen RT, Kerker M, Matijevic E. J Phys Chem 1967; 71:514.
13. Espenscheid WF, Willis E, Matijevic E, Kerker M. J Colloid Sci 1965; 20:501.
14. Lee PS, Gorski RA, Johnson JT, Soderholm SC. J Aerosol Sci 1989; 20:627.
15. Couper A, Ryan K, Richardson RB. J Colloid Interf Sci 1989; 128:96.
16. Durand-Keklikian L, Partch RE. J Aerosol Sci 1988; 19:511.
17. Liu BlYH, Lee KW. J Am Ind Hyg Assoc 1975; 36:861.
18. Leong KH, Wang HC, Stukel JJ, Hopke PK. J Am Ind Hyg Assoc 1980; 43:135.
19. Mercer TT, Goddard RF, Flores RL. Ann Allergy 1968; 26:18.

20. Denton MB, Swartz DB. Rev Sci Instrum 1974; 45:81.
21. Boucher RMG, Kreuter J. Ann Allergy 1968; 26:591.
22. Lang RI. J Acoust Soc Am 1962; 34:6.
23. Illin BI, Eknadiosyants OK. Sov Phys Acoust 1966; 12:310.
24. Gershenzon EL, Eknadiosyants OK. Sov Phys Acoust 1964; 10:156.
25. Liu BYH, Pui DYH. J Colloid Interf Sci 1974; 47:155.
26. Gupta A, McMurry PH. Aerosol Sci Technol 1989; 10:451.
27. Chen D, Pui DYH, Humes D, Fissan H, Quant FR, Sem GJ. J Aerosol Sci 1998; 29:497.
28. Grace JM, Marijnissen JCM. J Aerosol Sci 1994; 25:1005.
29. Marijnissen J, ed. J Aerosol Sci 1999; 30(Special issue: electro-hydrodynamic atomization).
30. Chen D, Pui DYH, Kaufman SC. J Aerosol Sci 1995; 26:963.
31. Plateau. In: Rayleigh JWS, ed. Theory of Sound, Vol. 2. NY: Dover, 1945.
32. Lord Rayleigh. Proc Lond Math Soc 1878; 10:4.
33. Lord Rayleigh. Proc R Soc 1879; 29:71.
34. Castleman RA. Bur Std J Res 1931; 6:369.
35. Fulwyler MJ. Science 1965; 150:910.
36. Schneider JM, Hendricks CD. Rev Sci Instrum 1964; 35:1349.
37. Linblad NR, Schneider IM. J Sci Instrum 1965; 42:635.
38. Dabora EK. Rev Sci Instrum 1969; 38:502.
39. Strom L. Rev Sci Instrum 1969; 40:778.
40. Berglund RN, Liu BYH. Environ Sci Technol 1973; 7:147.
41. Leong KH. J Aerosol Sci 1986; 17:855.
42. Wang HC, private communication, 1989.
43. Kreyling WG, Erbe F. J Aerosol Sci 1985; 16:261.
44. Leong KH. J Aerosol Sci 1981; 12:417.
45. Charlesworth DH, Marshall WR. A I Che E 1960; 6:9.
46. Leong KH. J Aerosol Sci 1987; 18:511.
47. Leong KH. J Aerosol Sci 1987; 18:525.
48. Vanderpool RW, Rubow KL. Aerosol Sci Technol 1988; 9:65.
49. Walton WH, Prewett WC. Proc Phys Soc (Lond) 1949; 62:341.
50. May KR. J Appl Phys 1949; 20:932.
51. May KR. J Sci Instrum 1966; 43:841.
52. Mitchell JP. J Aerosol Sci 1984; 15:35.
53. Melton PM, Burnell PKP, Harrison RM. J Aerosol Sci 1989; 20:1605.
54. Toivonen H, Bailey MR. Aerosol Sci Technol 1989; 11:196.
55. Cheah PKP, Davies CN. J Aerosol Sci 1984; 15:741.
56. Davies CN, Cheah PKP. J Aerosol Sci 1984; 15:719.
57. Eisner D, Martonen TB. Aerosol Sci Technol 1988; 9:105.
58. Hinds WC. In: Willike K, ed. Generation of Aerosols and Facilities for Exposure Experiments. Ann Arbor, MI: Ann Arbor Science, 1980:171–187.
59. Timbrell V, Hyett AW, Skidmore JW. Ann Occup Hyg 1960; 11:273.
60. Wright BM. J Sci Instrum 1950; 27:12.

61. Guichard JC. In: Liu BYH, ed. Fine Particles: Aerosol Generation, Measurement, Sampling and Analysis, New York. Academic Press, 1976:173–193.
62. Willeke K, Lo CSK, Whitby KJ. J Aerosol Sci 1974; 5:449.
63. Marple VA, Liu BYH, Rubow KL. Am Ind Hyg Assoc J 1978; 39:26.
64. Boucher RF, Lua AC. J Aerosol Sci 1982; 13:499.
65. Yeh HC, Carpenter RL, Cheng YS. J Aerosol Sci 1988; 19:147.
66. Griffis LC, Pickrell JA, Carpenter RL, et al. Am Ind Hyg Assoc J 1983; 44:216.
67. Myojo T. Ind Health 1983; 21:79.
68. Tanaka I, Akiyama T. Ann Occup Hyg 1987; 31:401.
69. Henderson RF, Cheng YS, Dutcher JS, Marshall TC, White JE. Final Report for Phase I Studies: Generation and Characterization of Dye Aerosol, Fort Derrick, Frederick, MD: U.S. Army Medical Research and Development Command, 1984. Project Order 3807, AD A1422491. .
70. Dill RS. Trans Am Soc Heating Ventilation Eng 1938; 44:379.
71. Hollander W, Hollander M, Beyer A, Koch W. J Aerosol Sci 1987; 18:903.
72. Barr EB, Cheng YS. Evaluation of TSI model 34-10 dry powder disperser. Inhalation Toxicology Research Institute Annual Report. 1987:61–64.
73. Kanapilly GM, Raabe OG, Newton GJ. J Aerosol Sci 1970; 1:313.
74. Jenkins RA, Mitchell JP, Nichols AL. Fifth Particle Size Analysis Conference, University of Bradford, September 16–19, 1985.
75. Ramamurthi M, Leong KH. J Aerosol Sci 1987; 18:175.
76. Robbins RC, Cadle RD. J Phys Chem 1958; 62:469.
77. Movilliat P. Ann Occup Hyg 1962; 4:275.

9

The Design and Development of Inhalation Drug Delivery Systems

Paul J. Atkins and Timothy M. Crowder
Oriel Therapeutics Inc., Research Triangle Park, North Carolina, U.S.A.

INTRODUCTION

The inhalation delivery of therapeutic agents has been known, though poorly understood, for many years. A wide variety of agents has been administered to the lung via oral inhalation, for the treatment of diverse disease states. The most frequent use of inhalation therapy is for the treatment of obstructive airway diseases, such as asthma and chronic obstructive pulmonary disease (COPD), using drugs such as short- and long-acting β sympathomimetics, corticosteroids, and anticholinergic agents. However, the respiratory route has been receiving increased attention since the early 1990s as a portal route for systemic drug delivery, most notably for the delivery of inhaled insulin [1,2].

Common to all inhalation dosage forms and delivery systems is the need to generate the optimum "respirable dose" (particles $< 5.0\,\mu\text{m}$) of a therapeutic agent, and this is a central performance feature in the rational design and selection of a delivery system. Moreover, this performance, in terms of aerosol quality, should be demonstrated throughout the product's shelf life, in addition to the more usual chemical and physical stability criteria. Thus, particularly in the development of metered-dose inhalers (MDIs) and dry powder inhalers (DPIs), device design is integrated with formulation work in the overall product development strategy. Frequently, therefore, such inhalation delivery systems tend to be compound specific. Thus, the physicochemical properties and the pharmacological profile (dose) of a given compound will occasionally predispose the choice of inhalation system. Hence, a good basis of preformulation information is essential for the rational design, selection, formulation, and development of inhalation drug delivery systems.

Within the pharmaceutical industry, inhalation drug delivery system selection is a pivotal commercial decision. This should be based on factors such as:

Overall clinical objective (acute or chronic treatment)
Target patient population (e.g., ambulatory, infants, elderly)
Regulatory requirements
Competitor activity

Three basic types of commercially available inhalation drug delivery systems exist, and each is specifically addressed in this chapter.

Nebulizers: Traditionally used for the acute care of nonambulatory, hospitalized patients, particularly with coordination or dexterity difficulties. Solutions or suspensions can be nebulized by ultrasonics or an air jet and administered via a mouthpiece, ventilation mask, or tracheostomy.

Metered-dose inhalers: A versatile, multidose inhaler where the drug is formulated in a propellant mix, under pressure, with the drug being expelled (by a valve) in a metered volume from the volatile mixture as the propellant evaporates. These products have been the subject of much research interest since the early 1990s as pharmaceutical companies have sought to replace their CFC formulations with newer formulations containing the non-ozone-depleting gases (hydrofluroalkanes—HFAs).

Dry powder inhalers: These are inhalers that typically fall into two general types of commercially available systems: single-dose and multidose systems. The multidose systems have been finding increased use in recent years and are generally either "passive" devices, where the patient provides the energy to disperse the drug powder in a stream of inspired air, or "active" devices, in which the energy comes from the device.

This chapter presents an overview of formulation design, describes device function, and addresses product operation in relation to inhalation delivery system performance for nebulizers, MDIs, and DPIs. Methods of manufacture of dosage form are also briefly discussed to highlight critical features of each inhalation delivery system.

PREFORMULATION ASPECTS ON INHALATION DRUG DELIVERY SYSTEM DESIGN

Due to the diverse nature of inhalation dosage forms, preformulation as applied to the development of inhalation formulations can be extremely broad in scope. Although a good deal of relevant information of a generic nature (i.e., pK_a, log P) would typically be generated during preliminary physicochemical profiling of a drug substance [3], specialized information specific to the intended dosage form is also required.

The importance of identifying the mode of delivery to the lung (i.e., nebulizer, MDI, DPI) as early as possible cannot be overemphasized. A drug salt form selected assuming development of a propellant-based MDI suspension formulation may be wholly unsuited for application in an aqueous-based nebulizer suspension on the basis of solubility and crystal growth potential. Physicochemical properties and stability issues considered to be of importance in the development of inhalation formulations are discussed later, as they relate to the individual dosage forms.

Particle Engineering

Since the early 1990s, the notion of producing particles of a specific size, density, and morphology has evolved, and it has the potential to lead to significant advances in pulmonary drug delivery [4]. Typically, particles for use by inhalation would be produced by a milling (micronization) process that would result in a batch of material with a size range between 1.0 and 3.0 microns (necessary for inhalation). Scientists have realized that there may be more elegant techniques available for the production of small particles, including supercritical fluid recrystallization, spray-drying, or controlled precipitation, in which size control could be achieved and other desirable properties (e.g., extended release of the drug) may be realized [5]. There are a number of companies that have developed specialist processes to manufacture these types of particles (e.g., Alkermes; Eiffel; Nektar Therapeutics). These methods now provide formulators with the capability to have small quantities of material in a defined particle size readily available.

Formulations for Nebulization

The development of a nebulizer solution or suspension formulation is contingent on the same core preformulation data as would be required to support the development of any formulation. Physicochemical parameters such as pK_a, log P, isoelectric pH (proteins and peptides), and solubility (vs. pH, ionic strength, buffer, and cosolvent level) are all important. Tonicity and solution pH, though typically regarded as formulation issues, must be investigated during preformulation to ensure selection of an appropriate salt form for development. For example, acidic (pH < 2) hypertonic and hypotonic aerosols have been demonstrated to induce bronchoconstriction in asthmatic subjects [6]. A hydrochloride or sulfate salt of a weakly basic drug that forms a strongly acidic solution, therefore, may not represent the optimum choice if the tonicity of the formulation is compromised as a result of pH adjustment using buffers.

It is important to profile the solution stability of the drug candidate as early as possible to identify the pH of optimum stability. The influence of light, oxygen, and trace metals on compound degradation also needs to be considered to assess the requirement for antioxidants (sodium metabisulfite, ascorbic acid, etc.) or chelating agents (EDTA, citric acid, etc.). Inclusion of such agents, though required to improve the chemical stability, must be weighed against the potential for adverse effects on the lung. Drug stability in solution should be monitored using a stability-indicating assay, following stress storage as a function of elevated temperature. In addition, conditions that promote hydrolysis (pH extremes), photolysis (ultraviolet and visible light), oxidation (O_2, O_2/light), and trace metal ion catalysis (Fe^{+2}, Fe^{+3}, Cu^{+2}, Co^{+2}, etc.) all merit consideration [3]. Temperature cycling is also useful as a means of assessing potential problems relating to complexation or hydrate formation as manifested by precipitation or crystal growth.

As a guide to formulation development, studies should be undertaken to evaluate the contribution of candidate excipients, including preservatives, antioxidants, chelating agents, cosolvents, and buffers on compound stability and solubility. This is particularly important in the development of suspensions for nebulization. Compatibility with packaging components also needs to be considered as a matter of priority. Peptides and proteins in particular are notorious in their ability to adsorb onto a variety of surfaces, particularly plastic.

Dry Powder Inhalation Formulations

Of critical importance in the development of DPI products is the evaluation, optimization, and control of flow and dispersion (deaggregation) characteristics of the formulation. These typically consist of drug blended with a carrier (e.g., lactose). The properties of these blends are a function of the principal adhesive forces that exist between particles, including van der Waals forces, electrostatic forces, and the surface tension of adsorbed liquid layers [7]. These forces are influenced by several fundamental physicochemical properties, including particle density and size distribution, particle morphology (shape, habit, surface texture), and surface composition (including adsorbed moisture) [8]. In addition, the combination of dry powder formulations and plastics poses the additional problem of offering electrostatically charged surfaces for collection of drug particles. Interparticle forces, which influence flow and dispersion properties, are particularly dominant in the micronized or microcrystalline powders required for inhalation therapy ($< 5 \, \mu m$). It is obvious that the particle size distribution of the drug and the diluent (excipient) need to be optimized during early preformulation and formulation development studies to ensure consistent aerosol cloud formation.

It is imperative, during early development, to characterize the moisture sorption and desorption attributes of the drug in relation to available salt forms. Assuming solubility is sufficient to ensure adequate absorption, a nonhygroscopic form should be explored. This would confer a number of advantages, including improved flow properties and dispersion as well as enhanced physical stability in the bulk and final dosage forms due to minimal moisture transfer between the drug, immediate container (e.g., gelatin capsule shell), and the environment. Furthermore, improved chemical stability may result in the case of hydrolytically labile drugs. Hygroscopic growth during administration would also be minimized. Although inherently attractive, the approach of using nonhygroscopic drug forms must be applied with caution, because, in the case of insulating particles, the level of adsorbed moisture may not be sufficient to dissipate attractive electrostatic forces, resulting in particle adhesion. Particle morphology, including attributes such as crystal habit, surface texture, and porosity, also influences particle adhesion [9]. Anisometric particles, that is, those with extreme "elongation" or "flatness" ratios, tend to build up packing of high porosity, but they are also more readily deformed by compression than packing of isometric particles. Anisometric particles tend to align along their long axis during flow and, thus, to exhibit less internal friction than isometric particles [8]. Powder flow tends to be adversely affected by surface roughness and porosity.

A particle engineering approach that has been the subject of much recent attention is one in which sub-unit-density particles are produced. These particles are attractive because it is the aerodynamic diameter, rather than any other measure, that determines the site of deposition for inhaled particles. The aerodynamic diameter is the characteristic dimension of a hypothetical sphere, of unit density, with an identical setting velocity (the velocity at which a particle moves downward when acted upon only by the force of gravity) to that of the particle in question [10]. Many pharmaceutical aerosol particles are spherical with density of $1 \, g/cm^3$, most certainly in the case of liquid aerosols. For these particles, the aerodynamic and geometric diameters are equivalent. However, particles with other than unit density can be "respirable" particles even if their geometrical diameter is not $1-3 \, \mu m$ in size [11]. Thus, the aerodynamic diameter, rather than the geometric diameter, must be given careful consideration when predicting deposition efficiency of a given inhaled aerosol. The distribution of sizes around the aerodynamic median size is also an important parameter in the efficiency of deposition [12].

The efficiency of dispersion, in the case of dry powder aerosols, relative to varying geometric diameters of the particles may also be an important factor. Specifically, dispersion requires the powder to overcome interparticulate forces binding particles in bulk powder and to become entrained as single particles in the inhalatory airstream. Interparticulate forces are dominated by the van der Waals force for particles in a respiratory size range. All other factors being equal, the van der Waals force will decrease as the geometric particle size increases (Fig. 1). Thus, in general terms, probability of deposition in the deep lung is at odds with efficiency of dispersion for dry powder inhalers. Sub-unit-density particles provide a means to decrease interparticulate forces due to their larger geometric diameters, while their aerodynamic diameter is still in the respirable size range.

It should be apparent, based on the brief overview just presented, that prediction of powder rheology based on the potential interplay of a number of physicochemical properties is extremely complicated. Instead, flow and dispersion properties are generally characterized using appropriate derived properties, including, but not limited to, angle of repose, bulk density, compressibility, and dustability. It is important to identify and control critical

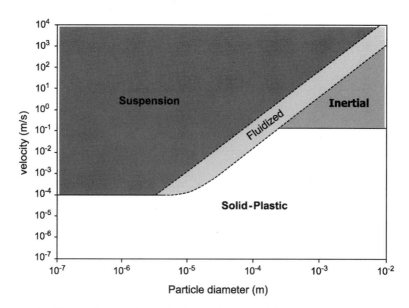

FIGURE 1 Phase diagram for typical granular material interactions.

parameters, both fundamental and derived, to ensure optimum and consistent product performance, although this may not always be possible [13].

Environmental factors, including temperature, humidity, and light, are essential considerations during formulation development. Therefore, it is imperative to evaluate the influence of these factors on the physical and chemical stability of the formulation during early preformulation studies. Light exposure can usually be controlled by judicious choice of product packaging; however, temperature and humidity are not so easily controlled, and they often act in concert to promote product degradation. The effects of elevated temperature and humidity on product stability can be assessed after stress storage. Some years ago Yoshioka and Carstensen [14] proposed several useful kinetic models for the accelerated testing of solid pharmaceuticals based on isothermal storage at controlled elevated temperature and controlled elevated humidity. Temperature- or humidity-cycling experiments can also be useful, particularly for assessing potential physical changes.

Chemical degradation after stress storage is assessed using an appropriate stability-indicating assay. In addition, physical changes are evaluated using an array of techniques available to the preformulation scientist, including polarized light microscopy (aggregation, crystal growth), differential scanning calorimetry, infrared spectroscopy, x-ray diffractometry, solution calorimetry, thermogravimetric analysis, and hot-stage microscopy (moisture uptake, polymorph interconversion, pseudopolymorph formation). Stressed stored samples should also be evaluated for evidence of caking and discoloration.

Metered-Dose Inhaler Formulations

The development of MDI formulations requires the same core preformulation data as described previously. However, additional parameters must also be evaluated, including solubility in propellant vs. concentration and nature of dispersing agent, crystal growth potential (related to solubility), and, most importantly, suspension properties (sedimentation, redispersibility). These issues have been studied very carefully since the early 1990s as pharmaceutical scientists have gained further experience with the "new" pressurized gases HFA134a and HFA 227, which have very different physicochemical properties from the more widely used CFCs that they replaced. Issues relating to physical stability must be addressed early during the development of an MDI suspension formulation. In addition to dispersibility, of particular importance is the potential for the drug to undergo crystal growth. Because this process is solution mediated, the solubility of the active in prospective formulations must be assessed. The influence of crystal and salt form, propellant composition, and surfactant should be evaluated with the objective of minimizing solubility. Although no general rules apply, it is prudent to limit drug solubility to the range of low parts per million to avoid significant problems with crystal growth for suspension formulations.

The solubility of a solute is a function of the particle size of the solute. Small particles, possessing high surface free energy, are more soluble than larger particles. The increase in solubility is dramatic for particles of less than one micrometer [15]. This phenomenon is particularly relevant to the development of MDI suspension formulations because the drug is present as a microfine, polydisperse powder. Preferential dissolution of smaller particles results in localized supersaturation and crystal growth after deposition on larger particles (Ostwald ripening). The propensity of the drug to undergo growth is typically assessed by cycling prototype formulations over a range of temperatures that the product is likely to be subjected to (e.g., 2°C ↔ room temperature ↔ 40°C). Samples are evaluated microscopically for evidence of crystal growth after a predetermined number of cycles. Other techniques, including differential scanning calorimetry, solution calorimetry, infrared spectroscopy, and x-ray powder diffraction, can be used to characterize changes in crystal form.

Water should always be regarded as a hostile impurity in propellant-based MDI formulations. Although only sparingly soluble in CFC propellants, it is much more soluble in the HFA propellants (typically 600–2200 ppm, depending on the propellant [16]), and water can act as a powerful cosolvent. As such, it can induce aggregation and catalyze processes described previously. In addition, it can promote degradation of hydrolytically unstable drugs. Because water cannot usually be rigorously excluded from MDI formulations, it is important to evaluate its influence on product integrity and performance [17]. Temperature-cycling experiments should be conducted on formulation prototypes as a function of added water.

From the standpoint of the number and diversity of excipients generally used, propellant MDI formulations are relatively simple formulations. The current technology comprises either propellant-drug-based formulations, suspension formulations that contain one or more solvents (typically ethanol) to aid the solubility of the surface active agents, or solution formulations using known excipients, including glycerol [18]. Excipient compatibility studies can, therefore, be extended at an early stage to include actual formulation prototypes. Factors to be considered as part of the excipient selection process include solubility, chemical and physical compatibility with the drug, and potential interactions with container and valve components. This issue is reported to have affected formulation development activities to the extent that internally coated canisters are now being used for some MDI products.

Chemical compatibility is appropriately assessed by evaluating drug and surfactant blends, using a stability-indicating assay, following storage at elevated temperature of prototype formulations. Potential interactions of the drug with prospective containers and valve components can be evaluated by comparing assay results for samples stored at elevated temperature in plastic-coated glass aerosol bottles with corresponding results for samples stored in contact with prospective packaging components, including aluminum as well as intact or dismantled valves. The oxygen and water content of the test samples should be controlled to establish their role in drug degradation and to avoid misleading results.

Criteria considered so far in the selection of a suitable drug form for MDI development include drug solubility and excipient and component compatibility. In addition to these parameters, suspension properties need to be carefully considered in the selection process. These are discussed in more detail later in this chapter in the section on the development of MDIs.

INHALATION DRUG DELIVERY SYSTEM DESIGN—NEBULIZED DRUG DELIVERY

Nebulizers are widely used today for drug delivery to the respiratory tract and are particularly useful for the treatment of hospitalized or nonambulatory patients. Fundamentally, there are two general types of nebulizer systems, the ultrasonic and the air jet.

In ultrasonic nebulizers, ultrasound waves (Fig. 2) are formed in an ultrasonic nebulizer chamber by a ceramic piezoelectric crystal that vibrates when electrically excited. These set up high-energy waves in the solution, within

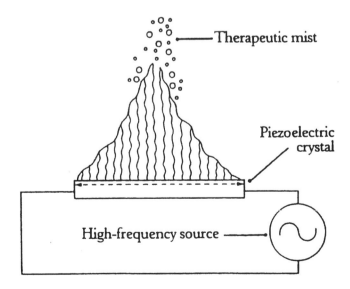

FIGURE 2 Schematic of an ultrasonic nebulizer.

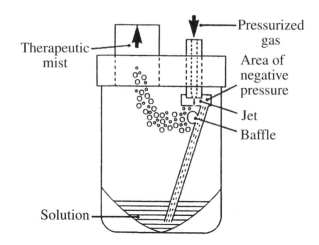

FIGURE 3   Schematic of an air-jet nebulizer.

the device chamber, of a precise frequency that generates an aerosol cloud at the solution surface.

The aerosol produced by an air-jet nebulizer (Fig. 3) is generated by a completely different principle. When compressed air is forced through an orifice, an area of low pressure is formed where the air jet exists. A liquid may be withdrawn from a perpendicular nozzle (the Bernoulli effect) to mix with the air jet to form droplets. A baffle (or baffles) within the nebulizer is often used to facilitate the formation of the aerosol cloud. Carrier air (oxygen) can be used to generate the "air jet." Alternatively, compressors may be used to generate the airstream.

The nebulized aerosol may be administered during a normal breathing pattern via a mouthpiece, inserted into a ventilation circuit or via a tracheostomy. Alternatively, a ventilation mask can be used. Air-jet nebulizers are far less convenient than ultrasonic nebulizers, which is the principle advantage of the latter. Although major improvements have been made using microelectronics to minimize and produce handheld nebulizers, and a number of specialized companies are known to be working on developing portable liquid-based delivery devices (e.g., Aerogen, Aradigm, BattlePharma) [19–22], these systems are still not widely commercially available. Furthermore it is believed that such systems will still be less portable than the MDI or contemporary DPI devices.

Nebulizer Performance

When a therapeutic agent is formulated into a nebulizer solution or suspension, the quality of the aerosol generated, in terms of aerodynamic particle size, can be markedly dependent on the type of nebulizer used and its operation. This issue has been studied for over 30 years but is still a major challenge for the pharmaceutical industry today. Although having absolute control of the nebulizer formulation per se, the formulator (or the pharmaceutical company supplying the solution for nebulization) has very little control over the nebulizer system prescribed to the patient and of the operational parameters used by the health care professional during dosing. However, there is a strong desire on the part of drug regulators to control the patient's exposure by having drug products (nebulizer formulations) that have operational data collected during the development phase with one or more suitable nebulizers (e.g., DNAase™ [23]).

The literature abounds with examples of nebulizer performance variability, in terms of both output and aerodynamic particle size generated. Furthermore, frequently the manufacturer's information provides inadequate detail. Newman and colleagues [24,25] investigated 11 air-jet nebulizers in terms of mass median aerodynamic diameter (determined by Malvern laser light scattering), geometric standard deviation, and the respirable aerosol mass (i.e., particles $< 5\,\mu m$). Considerable performance variation was noted between the nebulizer brands and, indeed, within different units of the same brand. Aerodynamic particle size also decreased with increasing compressed gas flowrate. As a consequence, they concluded that the quantity of drug available to the subject was dependent on the choice of air-jet nebulizer and its operation in terms of compressed gas flow. Other investigators have evaluated different drug/nebulizer combinations and reached similar conclusions [26].

Drug delivery from an air-jet nebulizer is a complex process. Here are some of the various issues that merit careful consideration when evaluating nebulizer delivery.

The variability between different nebulizer brands and of individual units within a given brand

The calculation of a true dose delivered (in relation to evaporative losses, residual volume, etc.)

The aerodynamic particle size of the nebulized dose (i.e., respirable dose delivered)

The airflow (and the variability thereof) and its effect on nebulizer output (mass) and the respirable dose

Changes in ambient and nebulizer solution temperatures during the time course of nebulization and their effect on evaporative losses

Changes in drug concentration during nebulization (i.e., potential changes in drug delivered versus time)

These parameters may compound those inherent intersubject and intrasubject variables, such as breathing pattern, respiratory performance (e.g., tidal volume), and airway function, and thus further complicate pulmonary drug delivery. As a consequence, given such variables (to provide standardization), various studies have concluded that a designated nebulizer should be calibrated before use. Guidelines are now available for the effective and consistent clinical use of these devices [27].

The performance of ultrasonic nebulizers has received less attention than that of air-jet nebulizers, perhaps because they are perceived as being intrinsically less variable [28]. However, it is important to note that brands of the ultrasonic nebulizer have significantly different features. Transducer frequency (based on manufacturer's information) varies over a range of several megahertz. This operating frequency may also shift slightly in aged units. Many ultrasonic nebulizers have electrical "power" settings and variable-airflow features. As a consequence, the nebulizer solution output per liter of air under extreme operating conditions can vary considerably between different device brands [29].

In general, ultrasonic nebulizers are capable of greater output (when parameters are optimized) than air-jet units, although they often retain a higher dead volume. Intrinsically, the aerodynamic particle size generated by ultrasonic nebulizers is dependent on the brand used and its operational parameters. Similarly, ultrasonic nebulizers produce a coarser aerosol (higher median aerodynamic diameter) than air-jet nebulizers. It is critical that careful evaluation of the performance of the pharmaceutical product with the nebulizer that is ultimately designed for use with be conducted prior to clinical use. Differences in dosing of potent drugs may result if the inappropriate operating conditions are used [30].

Nebulizer Solution Formulations

Nebulizers are designed primarily for use with aqueous solutions or suspensions. Typically the drug suspensions use primary particles in the range of 2–5 microns. As a consequence, pharmaceutical solution technology, consistent with that used for parenteral products, may be applied to nebulizer solution or suspension formulation and processing.

Nebulizer solutions are usually formulated in water, although other cosolvents, for example, glycerin, propylene glycol, and ethanol, may be used. However, it is important to note that any excipients with possible airway toxicological implications might compromise a drug product; thus, such additional excipients should not be introduced unless essential and, if so, formulated at the lowest feasible concentration. The range of suspending agents in approved products is limited.

Nebulizer solution pH may be an important factor in determining compound physical or chemical stability. It has been recommended [31] that solution pH be greater than 5.0, because there is considerable evidence to show that bronchoconstriction is a function of hydrogen ion concentration.

Nevertheless, the formulation "buffer capacity" and "titratable acid content," in addition to the nature of the acid present, are perhaps the most important factors for nebulizer solutions of greater than pH 2.0.

With the advent of the potential of using the inhaled route to deliver macromolecules there has been considerable interest in the development of nebulized formulations of macromolecules [32]. Compound stability is a significant issue for these biotechnology products; as such, aqueous nebulizer solutions do not provide an inert vehicle. Moreover, the high shear experienced with an air-jet nebulizer may induce secondary or tertiary structural changes in peptide or proteins. In addition, reservoir temperature changes during nebulization may compound problems in physical or chemical stability with biotechnology products. Furthermore, macromolecules often produce viscous solutions, with modified interfacial and surface tension. A complete investigation of these factors is critical during early product development.

Nebulizer solutions are typically filled as unit dosages in plastic containers. The latter uses blow-fill-seal technology [33]. Thus drug formulation compatibility with plastics is an important factor. Characterization of any sorption processes of plasticizer, monomer, and "extractables" or "leachables" is critical during long-term product-evaluation studies. Such sterile unit-dose formulations, in essence, do not require chemical preservation.

In summary, although widely used, nebulizers are a highly variable, in general poorly understood means of achieving respiratory drug delivery despite their successful therapeutic use for many years.

INHALATION DRUG DELIVERY SYSTEM DESIGN—METERED-DOSE INHALERS
Introduction

A metered-dose inhaler (MDI) is a complex system designed to provide a fine mist of medicament, generally with an aerodynamic particle size of less than 5 microns, for inhalation directly to the airways for the treatment of respiratory diseases such as asthma and COPD.

The main components of all MDIs (Fig. 4) are:

- The active ingredient
- The propellant (a liquefied gas)
- A metering valve
- A canister
- An actuator/mouthpiece

The active ingredient (the drug) may be either dissolved in the propellant or a cosolvent (e.g., ethanol) or suspended in the propellant. A surface-active agent

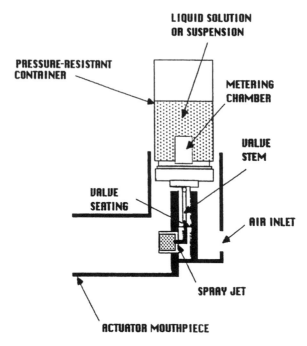

FIGURE 4   Essential components of a metered-dose inhaler.

may be included to ensure that the drug is well suspended and to help lubricate the metering valve.

The metering valve is the key to measuring and presenting a consistent and accurate dose to the patient; it is made up of a number of precision-made plastic or metal components. The valve is crimped onto a canister, which is ordinarily made of aluminum. Finally, there is the actuator, which holds the canister and through which the patient inhales the dose.

Marketed MDIs usually contain either CFCs or, more recently, HFCs as propellants. CFC-containing MDIs contain CFC-12 and CFC-11 and sometimes CFC-114. HFCs 134a and 227 have been developed as replacements for CFCs and are used in newer MDIs. In addition, some preliminary work has been conducted with MDIs using hydrocarbons as propellants.

Formulation Components

There are two types of MDI formulations: suspension formulations, in which microparticulate drug (typically micronized material) is dispersed in a combination of propellants, and solution formulations, in which the drug freely dissolves in either the propellant or a combination of propellant and an acceptable cosolvent, typically ethanol [34]. Both types of formulations have inherent advantages and disadvantages. Traditionally, suspension formulations have been the more common dosage form, but with the advent of the hydrofluroalkane propellants (HFA 134a, HFA227), which have poor solvency characteristics, the use of cosolvents has become more common, and solution formulations are increasing in use.

Suspension formulations typically have few problems with chemical stability because the drug is dispersed rather than being a homogeneous solution. Furthermore, they are also capable of delivering relatively high drug loads [e.g., Tilade™ (Aventis) is an MDI that delivers 2 mg of nedocromil sodium per actuation]. However, suspension formulations suffer from one major drawback: They need to be physically stable to ensure formulation homogeneity and, thus, uniform medication delivery. Particularly for HFA formulations in the absence of suspending agents, there may be rapid separation of the heterogeneous mixture, resulting in either creaming or flocculation, which can lead to poor reproducibility of medication dosing, particularly if the interval between dosing and shaking is inconsistent [35].

In addition, because the respirable fraction of the aerosol cloud that is emitted from a suspension MDI is highly dependent on the geometric size of the bulk drug particles (i.e., the aerodynamic size cannot be smaller than the initial geometric size of the primary particles), there are limitations to the respirable fraction that can be achieved. As such, solution formulations offer opportunities to circumvent some of these problems, particularly with drugs that have a significant solubility in the volatile propellants, where greater respirable fractions can be obtained [36].

Since the late 1980s it has become increasingly apparent that CFCs have a detrimental effect on the Earth's ozone layer [37]. This has lead to an extensive search for propellants that could be used as alternatives that have much less of an effect on the environment. The hydroflurocarbons (HFA 134a and 227) are both now being widely used in the pharmaceutical industry [16] as propellants for MDIs. These materials are pharmacologically inert and have similar properties to the CFC propellants they replaced. However, they are sufficiently different from the CFCs that there has been a significant investment in formulation strategies for the range of drugs traditionally delivered by MDIs.

HFC-134a and -227 are novel pharmaceutical excipients (inactive ingredients) developed for widespread and long-term use as replacements for CFCs in MDIs. Because the propellants in MDIs comprise the large majority of the formulation, often in excess of 98%, and the patients using these drugs are particularly vulnerable to airway irritation or toxicities, extensive testing had to be conducted on these propellants. Thus, both of these HFCs have undergone the same toxicological testing as any new chemical drug substance. Both are now widely approved as propellants suitable for MDI use [38] (Table 1).

All HFC MDIs contain the same physical components as the CFC MDI products (e.g., drug, propellant, canister, metering valve, and actuator); however, the very different physical properties of the HFC propellants has meant that significant changes have had to be made to the technology for these components. Although the active ingredient remains the same in most cases, whereas almost all CFC MDIs were presented as suspensions, there is now a growing number of HFC-propelled MDIs that have the drug in solution. Some formulations contain a cosolvent such as ethanol to help dissolve the surfactant or drug. There are also products on the market that do not contain a surfactant, simply being a suspension of micronized drug in propellant. Changes in hardware for the formulation has also necessitated changes to the equipment and processes used to manufacture HFA MDIs.

There are a number of companies involved globally in developing HFA MDIs, these include: 3M Pharmaceuticals (USA); GlaxoSmithKline (UK); Boehringer Ingelheim (Germany); Aventis (France/Germany); Cipla (India); Asta-Medica (Germany); Ivax-Norton Healthcare (USA/UK); and Chiesi (Italy). Table 2 outlines a list of some of the currently available formulations (by company) for the most widely prescribed inhaled drugs: salbutamol, beclomethasone, and budesonide.

The first introduction of an HFA MDI for the widely prescribed short-acting β-agonist salbutamol, occurred in the United Kingdom in 1994. Today there are over 60 countries where there is at least one salbutamol (short-acting β-agonist) containing MDI approved and marketed. Another β-agonist (fenoterol—Boehringer Ingleheim) is now also available in a number of European countries.

TABLE 1 Hydrofluroalkane (HFC) Propellants Used in MDIs

Propellant structure	$CL-\overset{\overset{\displaystyle CL}{\vert}}{\underset{\underset{\displaystyle CL}{\vert}}{C}}-F$	$Cl-\overset{\overset{\displaystyle F}{\vert}}{\underset{\underset{\displaystyle F}{\vert}}{C}}-Cl$	$F-\overset{\overset{\displaystyle F}{\vert}}{\underset{\underset{\displaystyle F}{\vert}}{C}}---\overset{\overset{\displaystyle H}{\vert}}{\underset{\underset{\displaystyle F}{\vert}}{C}}-H$	$F-\overset{\overset{\displaystyle F}{\vert}}{\underset{\underset{\displaystyle F}{\vert}}{C}}---\overset{\overset{\displaystyle F}{\vert}}{\underset{\underset{\displaystyle H}{\vert}}{C}}---\overset{\overset{\displaystyle F}{\vert}}{\underset{\underset{\displaystyle F}{\vert}}{C}}-F$
Name	CFC-11	CFC-12	HFA-134a	HFA 227
Density	1.49	1.33	1.21	1.41
Vapor pressure (psig at 20°C)	− 1.8	67.6	68.4	56.0
Boiling point (°C)	23.7	− 29.8	− 26.5	− 17.3

TABLE 2   Typical HFA MDI Formulations

Drug compound	Formulation	Company producing
Salbutamol	Ethanol/surfactant/134a	3M Pharmaceuticals
		Ivax-Norton Healthcare
	134a alone	GlaxoSmithKline
		Cipla
Beclomethasone	Ethanol/134a	3M Pharmaceuticals
		Ivax-Norton Healthcare
	Ethanol/134a/glycerol	Chiesi
Budesonide	Ethanol/134a/glycerol	Chiesi
	134a alone	Cipla

In addition to the introduction of beta-agonist HFC MDIs, there is a growing number of controller medications available as HFC MDIs. These include beclomethasone, fluticasone, disodium cromoglycate, and nedocromil sodium. Further product introductions are anticipated in the coming years; however, it should be noted that some products cannot or will not be reformulated with HFCs as MDIs and so alternatives (such as DPIs) are being developed. It was estimated that in 2002 there were over 100 million HFA MDIs produced globally, representing approximately 25% of worldwide MDI production.

The degree to which a high-respirable dose can be achieved with an MDI is dependent on obtaining a low, uniform primary particle size of the active agent. Often, material is milled (ball milled) or micronized (jet milled) using any one of the suitable systems that are commercially available. Clearly, this becomes difficult if small amounts of bulk material are available, as is often the case in early formulation development studies. Several smaller jet mills are available and can be used for this purpose [39]. However, it needs to be recognized that the use of high-energy forces on the bulk material may impart undesirable physical change, so this should be monitored carefully. Other methods of producing small particles can be explored, including controlled crystallization, because this can sometimes be the only way to produce sufficiently small material, particularly if the active material is thermally unstable or has a low melting point.

MDIs, be they solution or suspension formulations, typically contain a surfactant or dispersing agent. These materials generally need to have some solubility in the propellant blend. Commonly used surfactants include sorbitan trioleate (SPAN 85), oleic acid, and lecithins, at levels between 0.1% and 2.0% wt/wt [40]. These agents are required both to maintain the disperse nature of the drug (in suspension formulations) and to provide lubrication for operation of the metering valves. However, these surfactants have poor solubility in the HFA propellants, so alternate formulation strategies, using cosolvents, have been developed, with some success [18,36].

The fundamental requirement of an MDI formulation is that the drug dose be delivered accurately and reproducibly as an aerosol containing a significant fraction of drug particles in the respirable range (aerodynamic diameter $< 5\,\mu m$) [41]. This requirement can be met only by a suspension formulation, if the drug can be homogeneously distributed, in a deaggregated state, with minimal segregation during the period before administration. The extent and rate of drug separation (sedimentation or creaming) can in theory be reduced to some extent by manipulating the physicochemical properties of the formulation. According to Stokes' law, the rate of settling of a spherical particle, in a fluid medium, is directly proportional to the difference in density of the particle and the medium and the square of the particle's radius. Balancing the density of the drug and continuous phase of an MDI formulation as a means of eliminating settling would appear to be one option for achieving effective formulations, although the ranges are limited given the nature of the new HFA propellants.

As anticipated by Stokes' law, the rate of drug separation in an MDI suspension is also related to the particle size and particle size distribution. Within this context, it is important to define *particle* in its broadest sense to include primary drug particles and multiparticulate aggregates that may coexist or even predominate in suspension. The extent of aggregation is moderated by the use of appropriate nonionic surfactants, which adsorb on particle surfaces, reducing solid–liquid interfacial tension. Repulsion, due to steric interaction of hydrophobic surfactant chains projecting from particle surfaces, is viewed as the dominant mechanism in inhibiting particle aggregation in low-dielectric propellants [42]. Aggregation to form stable, loosely adherent masses (flocs) occurs when van der Waals forces of attraction slightly override electronic and steric forces of repulsion. Stability is conferred because the interacting particles reside in a secondary potential energy minimum. The forces of cohesion are generally small enough that the particles can be readily redispersed on mixing. The technique of controlled flocculation is often used as a means of optimizing oral suspensions. The principal involves increasing the size of the flocs by manipulation of zeta potential and surfactant concentration, to a point where the sedimentation ratio (sediment volume/total volume) is maximized (ideally $F = 1$). This approach has been widely used in developing HFA formulations. What is clear is that in developing an MDI suspension, the suspension properties must be viewed in terms of their relevance to aerosol output (maximized respirable fraction) as well as content homogeneity and redispersibility (optimized dose-to-dose reproducibility). These parameters can be reliably assessed only by the appropriate testing of trial formulations.

Typical Containers

There are essentially two types of containers that are currently used for MDI products. These are either glass, which are typically laminated or plastic coated so that they can withstand high pressures, or aluminum products. The latter are generally preferred and much more widely used because they are lighter, robust, and impervious to light. However, in some cases the inert nature of glass containers makes them a more suitable choice for use in solution formulations. These containers are sufficiently robust to withstand internal pressures of up to 150 psig without deformation.

Aluminum containers for use in MDI products are typically in the range of 15 to 30 mL in capacity, with a neck diameter of 20 mm. They are prepared in one of two ways: either from a monobloc of aluminum, by rapid impact slugging, or from a more precise deep-drawing process [39]. This gives the canisters more wall uniformity and, thus, greater weight uniformity, which is important in the multistage filling process. Both of these processes result in seamless canisters, which makes them more robust. The cans should be thoroughly cleaned before use because they may often contain residual particulates or a small oily residue as a result of the manufacturing process. A variety of can finishes (internal and external) are available. These are typically either epoxy or epoxy-type resins [40] or, more recently, fluoropolymer coated and, as such, either assist in conferring a more aesthetic appeal to the product or minimize drug adhesion to the canister walls.

Metering Valves

The metering valve in an MDI is the critical component in the design of an effective delivery system. The main function of the metering valve is to reproducibly deliver a portion of the liquid phase of the formulation in which the medication is either dissolved or dispersed. The valve also forms the seal atop the canister to prevent loss of the pressurized contents. The valves generally comprise at least seven components that are constructed from a variety of inert materials. Typical materials of construction are acetal or polyester for the valve body, stainless steel or acetal for the valve stem, generally anodized aluminum for the ferrule, and butyl, nitrile, or neoprene for the elastomers used in the seals and gaskets [43].

These valves are essentially designed to work in the inverted (stem down) position. Depression of the valve stem allows the contents of the metering chamber to be dispensed through the orifice in the valve stem. After actuation, the metering chamber refills from the bulk liquid formulation, once the metering chamber is sealed from the atmosphere and is ready to dispense the next dose. This is essential; otherwise, continuous spray would be achieved. Typical volumes that are dispensed range from 25 to 100 µL. The accuracy of the dosing is dependent on the selection of suitable components within the valve that show compatibility with the formulation and the design of a stable (physically) formulation. Incorrect assembly of the valve would result in poor metering performance. Thus, exhaustive tests are carried out on stratified samples of each batch of valves manufactured by the suppliers.

It should be pointed out, however, that because these valves are designed to dispense volumetrically, changes in the formulation density (by varying the propellant ratios) can affect the amount (by weight) that is dispensed. Hence, during the formulation design process, say, for a nominal target dose of 100 μg, these need to be taken into account. Key components of the metering valve are the elastomer seals and gaskets. As discussed previously, these form the barrier to the external environment, preventing ingress of materials (e.g., water) into the formulation, but they also minimize product leakage. They are selected for their durability during repeated use and for their compatibility with the formulation (propellants). A typical valve could be actuated up to 200 times during the lifetime of the product, and the seals and gaskets need to perform equally well throughout this cycle, with minimal deformation.

Where the pressurized propellant is charged through the valve (pressure-filled products), there needs to be a high degree of deformation of the filling gasket to occur for the filling to be easily accomplished. Thus, these valves are complex in their requirements and in design. Furthermore, the elastomer components also need to have suitable swelling characteristics when in contact with the propellants. This issue has been highlighted during the development of the HFA propellants, where new elastomeric materials were required to maintain value functionality [42]. Elastomers also need to have low levels of extractable materials. When there is a tendency for materials to be leached out of the valve by components within the formulation, this tendency can be minimized by prewashing or extracting of the valves (or their components).

Actuators and Inhalation Aids

The actuator (or mouthpiece) of an MDI is generally constructed from a range of polyethylene or polypropylene materials by injection-molding techniques. The actuator is the means by which the valve stem in the metering chamber is depressed and patients, by cupping their lips around the squat end (Fig. 4), inhale the dose. The aerosol cloud generated after the depression of the valve stem is dependent on the vapor pressure (propellant ratio) of the formulation, the geometric size of the active drug if the product is a suspension formulation, the volume of the metering chamber, and, critically, the diameter of the jet orifice in the mouthpiece. The diameter of this orifice also controls the rate of spray formation [44]. The free flow of the expanding aerosol cloud through this orifice is essential. To ensure that this critical orifice does not become partially blocked during repeated use of the actuator, regular washing of the actuator is recommended [45]. Studies conducted during formulation development can mimic patient use and, thus, establish the frequency with which buildup of drug on the orifice is likely to occur.

The common design of actuators is the classic "L" shape [39]. However, despite very clear instructions, many patients (in particular, children) find it difficult to coordinate the actuation and inspiration essential for the effective use of MDIs. This has led to the development of a variety of spacer and extension types of mouthpieces. The original concept of the plume- (or cone-) shaped device came from the work of Moren [46]. These devices aid patient coordination by allowing them to actuate into the reservoir and then, subsequently, to inhale from the resulting cloud. The inclusion of a small vent in the spacer prevents exhaling into the reservoir. Today the most widely used spacer is the AeroChamber™ (Monohagan Medical), which has been widely studied for its effectiveness in aiding drug delivery (see Fig. 5). In addition it comes with a wide range of face masks for use with infants.

Extended mouthpiece devices are also available (e.g., Azmacort™, Aventis). With this device, the point of inspiration is removed further from the point of actuation, allowing greater evaporation time for the less volatile propellants, plus large particle sedimentation in the airstream, with a concomitant

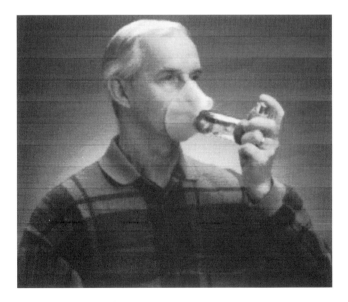

FIGURE 5 Photo of an AeroChamber™.

decrease in aerodynamic particle size of the cloud and a reduction in oropharyngeal impaction.

Another very elegant and highly portable device that aids patient coordination is the breath-actuated inhaler, originally developed by Riker Laboratories (3M) [47] and further enhanced by Ivax-Norton (EasiBreathe). In this type of device, a mechanical release mechanism is used, firing the MDI when a certain threshold inspiratory flowrate is reached. Once the dose has been dispensed, the device is then reprimed, ready for use. This type of device has gained wide acceptance in Europe and has been introduced for several MDI products.

Manufacture and Evaluation of Metered-Dose Inhalers

There are essentially two processes for the filling of MDIs, pressure-filling and cold-filling. In the pressure-filling process, typically a concentrate of drug (after comminution), excipients, and propellant is prepared in a suitable batching vessel. These are almost always in suspension, so the contents of the vessel need to be thoroughly mixed using a high-shear mixer. Often, this will then be recirculated from the batching vessel through the filler and back to the vessel to maintain the homogeneity of the suspension. This concentrate is then filled into purged canisters using a volumetric filler, and the valve is crimped into place. Additional propellant is then added through the metering valve, under pressure, using high-speed fillers. This process is known as *gassing*. A modification to this approach is to prepare the whole formulation in a pressure vessel and then to volumetrically fill this into a prepurged canister through the metering valve, which has already been crimped in place. Filling at subambient temperatures may aid precision of the process.

The alternative approach is to use cold-filling. As the term suggests, cold temperatures are applied in order to liquefy all the propellants. These are then filled volumetrically into canisters, and the valve is crimped into place. Cold-filling has some advantages in small batch manufacture. However, as in any process of scale-up, it is important to recognize that there may be subtle differences in performance between one product manufactured by a process on a laboratory scale and another on a full production scale.

One feature critical to both filling processes is that manufacturing conditions must be at low humidity so that the level of condensed water within the product is kept to a minimum. The significance of water, and the destructive role that it can play in MDI formulations, has been described in some detail by Miller [17] and is critically important, particularly for HFA formulations, where the solubility of water is far greater than with CFCs.

After filling, the canisters are leak tested. This can be accomplished by passing the filled canisters through a heated waterbath (typically at 50°C) to raise the vapor pressure. The canisters will be cleaned during this process, and any "gross leakers" are identified. Furthermore, container integrity can be assessed, and canisters showing structural weakness can be rejected. The canisters are then dried and stored under ambient conditions to allow equilibration of the components within the metering valve. After, equilibration, canisters are check weighed, and latent leakers (those that fall below the specified minimum fill weight based on the storage condition) are detected and discarded. This is an important check on processing conditions, in particular, valve damage during the filling process or the use of inappropriate valve crimp dimensions. The canisters are then spray tested and inserted into their actuators and final package.

As in any pharmaceutical manufacturing process, careful control and inspection of the various product components are essential. Dimensional checks on the can, valve, and actuator need to be carried out. In addition, standard identity and purity tests for active and excipients, including propellants, must be performed. In-process checks also need to be made regarding the active concentration in the concentrate and also the level of dispersion. A careful check on valve crimp dimensions will minimize latent leakers. In a two-stage filling process, precision of fill at each stage is critical to the concentration of active in the finished product. Thus, gravimetric determination of the fill weights of both stages is also required.

There is a range of tests that need to be carried out on MDIs during formulation development and stability evaluation. The scope and nature of these tests have been widely debated for several years, and they are still being discussed. A detailed discussion on the merits of these tests is beyond the scope of this text; the FDA has issued a guidance document on these tests [41] and how they should be applied; this should be carefully reviewed before embarking on any inhaled-product development activity. It is, however, important to highlight some of the more crucial tests for MDIs. Clearly, many of the standard tests for other pharmaceutical dosage forms also apply to MDIs. These include stability, purity, and dose uniformity; however, MDIs require special consideration because of their uniqueness. The two most important tests, in addition to those described previously, are the metering performance of the valve and the aerodynamic particle size of the dispersed aerosol cloud.

There is much debate about these particular tests and their appropriateness. However, the concept of the use of aerodynamic particle size testing as a compendial test is now well established. Both impactor testing and impingers testing have a role in the development of MDIs, because they are useful tools in studying aerosol clouds and can provide information that leads to formulation optimization (at least in terms of respirable dose). It should be emphasized that these data should not be taken in isolation, and other appropriate particle-sizing techniques should also be used. A more complete discussion of this topic can be found in Chapter 11.

In summary, the MDI is a safe and well-established inhalation delivery system. The transition from CFC propellants has begun but has been plagued with technical challenges and has taken far longer than many expected. This has encouraged scientists to look for alternate means of delivering drugs to the lungs. MDIs containing HFA propellants where the drugs are dissolved in a mixture of propellant and cosolvent are being proposed as a means to achieve efficient delivery of drugs, including macromolecules, to the lung [38].

INHALATION DRUG DELIVERY SYSTEM DESIGN—DRY POWDER INHALERS
Introduction

Today there are essentially two types of DPIs, those that use drug filled into discrete individual doses, e.g., either a gelatin capsule or a foil–foil blister, and those that use a reservoir of drug that meters out doses when required. Both are now widely available around the globe and are gaining broad acceptance. There is clearly considerable interest in these devices because they do not require CFC propellants to disperse the drug and, as such, can be regarded as ozone-friendly delivery systems. Furthermore, although these devices do overcome the need for coordination of actuation and inspiration because they are essentially breath actuated, this is also one of their disadvantages. It is known that some DPIs require inspiratory flowrates of 60 L/min [48,49] to effectively deaggregate the powder. This certainly cannot always be achieved by all asthmatic patients, particularly infants. This section discusses each of these types of device in turn and some of the common themes in relation to developing formulations for use in such devices (see Fig. 6).

Unit-Dose Devices

Single-dose powder inhalers are devices in which a powder-containing capsule is placed in a holder. The capsule is opened within the device and the powder is inhaled. The capsule residue must be discarded after use and a new capsule inserted for the next dose. The concept of the Spinhaler™ was first described in the early 1970s by Bell and colleagues [50], who had developed this device for the administration of powdered sodium cromoglycate. Briefly, the drug mixture, which often includes a bulk carrier to aid powder flow, is prefilled in a hard gelatin capsule and loaded into the device. After activation of the device, which pierces the capsule, the patient inhales the dose, which is dispensed from the vibrating capsule by means of inspired air.

A similar device (Rotahaler™, GlaxoSmithKline) has also been available for many years, delivering salbutamol and beclomethasone dipropionate powders. Here, the drug mixture is again filled in a hard capsule, and

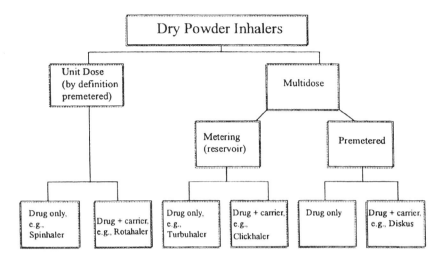

FIGURE 6   Types of DPIs.

the capsule is inserted into the device; however, the capsule is broken open in the device, and the powder is inhaled through a screened tube [51]. Another device that dispenses drug loaded into hard gelatin capsules (fenoterol) is the Berotec Inhalator™ (Boehringer Ingelheim) [52]. Several introductions of single-dose DPIs have occurred over the past few years using similar designs (e.g., Aerolizer™—Novartis; Handihaler™—Boehringer Ingelheim).

Single-dose devices have performed well in clinical use for over 30 years. However, one criticism of these devices is the cumbersome nature of loading, which may not be easily accomplished if a patient is undergoing an asthma attack and requires immediate delivery of drug. This is clearly pertinent to devices that deliver short-acting bronchodilators. In addition, elderly patients may not have the manual dexterity to accomplish all the necessary maneuvers. Hence there has been considerable focus on developing multidose devices.

Multidose Devices

The development of multidose DPIs was pioneered by A. B. Draco (now a division of AstraZeneca) with their Turbuhaler [53]. This device is truly a metered-dose powder delivery system. The drug is contained within a storage reservoir and can be dispensed into the dosing chamber by a simple back-and-forth twisting action on the base of the unit (Fig. 7). The device is capable of working at moderate flowrates and also delivers carrier-free particles [54]. However, one of the drawbacks of the Turbuhaler has been the fact that it has

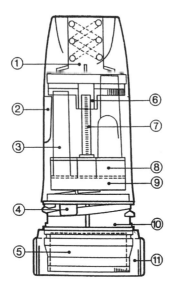

(1) mouthpiece with insert

(2) bypass air inlet

(3) inhalation channel

(4) air inlet

(5) desiccant store

(6) window for dose indicator

(7) dose indicator

(8) storage unit for drug compound

(9) dosing unit

(10) operating unit

(11) turning grip

FIGURE 7 Components of the Turbuhaler, a multidose dry powder inhaler. (1) mouthpiece with insert, (2) bypass air inlet, (3) inhalation channel, (4) air inlet, (5) desiccant store, (6) window for dose indicator, (7) dose indicator, (8) storage unit for drug compound, (9) dosing unit, (10) operating unit, (11) turning grip.

a highly variable delivery at different flowrates. This has also been the major criticism of several recently developed reservoir-type powder devices (e.g., Clickhaler™—ML Laboratories).

To address issues associated with a need for multiple dosing and consistent performance, Glaxo developed the Diskhaler™ [55], which was used to deliver a range of drugs, including salbutamol and beclomethasone. This device uses a circular disk that contains either four or eight powder doses on a single disk. This typically would be treatment for one to two days. The doses are maintained in separate aluminum blister reservoirs until just before inspiration. On priming the device, the aluminum blister is pierced, and the contents of the pouch are dropped

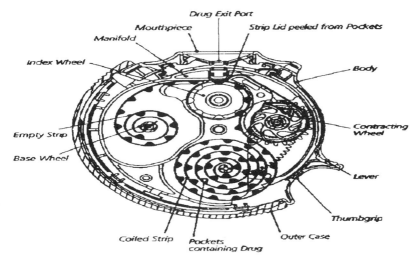

FIGURE 8 Schematic of the Diskus™ powder inhaler.

into the dosing chamber. This product had limited commercial success and was superceded in the late 90's by the Diskus™. This device (see Fig. 8) is a true multidose device, having 60 doses in a foil–foil aluminum strip that is opened only at the point just prior to patient inspiration [56]. Consistent performance [57] and broad patient acceptance has allowed the Diskus™ to become the gold standard of multidose powder delivery devices.

Formulation Aspects

Dry powder formulations either contain the active drug alone or have a carrier powder (e.g., lactose) mixed with the drug. The drug particles must be of sufficiently small aerodynamic diameter to make it to and deposit on the airways. Micronized dry powder can be inhaled and deposited in the airways effectively from DPIs by patients with adequate breathing capacity because they can pull sufficient air through the device. However, young children, some patients with severe asthma, and elderly COPD patients may not always be able to achieve adequate inspiratory flow to ensure optimal medication delivery from DPIs.

Brown [58] alluded to the complexities involved in the design and development of a DPI. In much the same way as for an MDI, the combination of formulation (drug and carrier), the way that it is presented to the device, and the design of the dosing device itself all contribute to the overall performance of the dosage form. The requirement to use micronized drug with small (ideally less than 5.0-μm) particles, to achieve good aerodynamic properties of the dispersed powder, is confounded by the need to develop formulations that fill easily and accurately [59]. It is also important that changes in the physical nature of the formulation on transportation and storage not adversely affect the product performance. This needs to be investigated during formulation development. The inclusion of a carrier (often lactose) can aid in the handling of the formulation and may impart some aerodynamic benefits also. A further factor that aids in the design of optimal formulations is a close interaction of preformulation scientists and process chemists to provide materials (active drug) that have the desirable physical properties. This then allows delivery systems to be designed in which the drug forms stable aggregates that can be readily handled and are easily dispersed in the dosing device. However, there is still likely to be a need to achieve sufficient inspiratory flowrates in order to attain good respirable doses [60].

Peart and Clarke [4] in 2002 reviewed extensively the range of DPI developments, in terms of both device and formulation work that has been undertaken in the preceding decade. This is clearly an active area of interest for scientists as they strive to develop efficient delivery systems that do not contain environmentally harmful propellants. The goal of delivering micronized powders is a challenging one. Because of their very nature, these types of powders are highly cohesive. Their high interparticulate forces make them difficult to deaggregate, hence the need for high inspiratory flowrates and turbulent airflow within DPIs. Inclusion of a carrier may aid the deaggregation process, but it can also lead to problems with absorption of atmospheric moisture. Controlled temperature and humidity studies of salt forms and lactose (or other suitable carrier) combinations are essential during formulation development. In the Turbuhaler™, the effects of moisture uptake are moderated by the inclusion of a desiccant (see Fig. 7).

In 1988 Vidgren and colleagues [61] showed that spray-dried particles of disodium cromoglycate had better (at least in vitro) aerodynamic properties (i.e., a higher fraction of the dose in a smaller-size range) than micronized material, and others have continued these investigations using other methods of particle generation [61]. Staniforth et al. [62] have looked at various techniques to improve formulation performance by the development of tertiary mixtures. All the formulation development work is typically focused on achieving better aerosol performance.

Much interest has been focused recently on developing delivery systems that deaggregate the powder [63], for this effectively minimizes formulation development work. Some of these systems are extremely complex in operation and may prove difficult to achieve in everyday operations. In addition, some designs that have already been achieved (e.g., Nektar Therapeutics' Enhance™

device for the delivery of inhaled insulin) are likely to be bulky and too large to be portable.

In summary, DPIs are a widely accepted inhaled delivery dosage form, particularly in Europe, where they currently are used by approximately 40% of asthma patients, for the delivery of medications used to treat asthma and COPD. They may find use in a much broader spectrum of diseases as targeted delivery to the lung begins to be more widely accepted. Their lack of propellants makes them a desirable, environmentally friendly alternative.

SUMMARY

The design and development of inhalation drug delivery systems is a highly complex task. Optimization of the choice of compound polymorph and salt form is highly desirable, and an effective method of making small particles with consistent properties is essential. Adequate preformulation characterization of the chosen powder is essential. Formulation development should ideally be directed toward a specific objective predefined in terms of the system deployed for its clinical usefulness. Nebulizer solutions are perhaps the simplest formulations because the drug is water soluble. MDIs and DPIs require an understanding of both the chemical and physical attributes of the drug in relation to excipients, vehicles, and diluents and polymer components. However, common to the development of all systems is an appreciation that one of the most important factors in pulmonary delivery from an inhalation dosage form is the requirement for a good-quality aerosol (in terms of the aerodynamic particle size of cloud generated) and its potential to achieve the desired regional deposition in vivo.

REFERENCES

1. Ganderton D, Jones TM, eds. Drug Delivery to the Respiratory Tract. UK: Ellis Horwood, 1987.
2. Phillips EM, Hill M. Proceedings Respiratory Drug Delivery VIII, 2002; 61–69.
3. Wells JI. Pharmaceutical Preformulation: The Physicochemical Properties of Drug Substances. UK: Ellis Horwood, 1988:152–181.
4. Peart J, Clarke MJ. Am Pharm Rev 2001; 4:37–45.
5. Vanbever R, et al. Pharm Res 1999; 16:1735–1742.
6. Snell NJC. Respir Med 1990; 84:345–348.
7. Hickey AJ, Concessio NM, van Oort MM, Platz RM. Pharm Tech 1994; 18:58–64.
8. Hinds WC. Aerosol Technology: Properties, Behavior and Measurement of Airborn Particles. New York: Wiley, 1982:127–132.
9. Hickey AJ, Concessio NM. Adv Drug Delivery Rev 1997; 26:29–40.
10. Reist PC. Aerosol Science and Technology. New York: McGraw-Hill, 1993.

11. Edwards DA, Hanes J, Caponetti G, Hrkach J, Ben-Jebria A, Eskew ML, Mintzes J, Deaver D, Lotan N, Langer R. Science 1997; 276:1868–1871.
12. Musante CJ, Schroeter JD, Rosati JA, Crowder TM, Hickey AJ, Martonen TB. J Pharm Sci 2002; 91:1590–1600.
13. Crowder TM, Hickey AJ. Pharm Tech 2000; 24:50–58.
14. Yoshioka S, Carstensen JT. J Pharm Sci 1990; 79:943–944.
15. Higuchi WI, Ho NFH, Goldberg AH. In: Lachman L, Lieberman H, Kanig JL, eds. The Theory and Practice of Industrial Pharmacy. Philadelphia: Lea & Febiger, 1971:134.
16. Pischtiak AH, Pittroff M, Schwarze T. Aerosol Eur 2001; 9(10):44–47.
17. Miller NC. In: Byron PR, ed. Respiratory Drug Delivery. Boca Raton: CRC Press, 1990:249.
18. Acerbi D, et al. Proceedings Respiratory Drug Delivery VIII, 2002; 391–395.
19. www.aerogen.com
20. www.aradigm.com
21. www.battellepharma.com
22. Goldberg J, et al. Eur Respir J 2001; 17:225–232.
23. Physicians Desk Reference. 53rd ed. 1999; 1070.
24. Newman SP, Pellow PG, Clarke SW. Clin Phys Physiol Meas 1986; 7:139–146.
25. Newman SP, Pellow PG, Clay MM, Clarke SW. Thorax 1985; 40:671–676.
26. Alvine GF, Rodgers P, Fitzsimmons KM, Ahrens RC. Chest 1992; 101(2):316–319.
27. European Respiratory Society guidelines on the use of nebulizers. Eur Respir J 2001; 18:228–242.
28. Reisner C, et al. Ann Allergy, Asthma, Immunol 2001; 86(5):566–574.
29. Flament MP, Leterme P, Gayot A. Drug Dev Ind Pharm 2001; 27(7):643–649.
30. Hess D. Respir Care 2000; 45(6):609–623.
31. Beasley R, Rafferty P, Holgate ST. Br J Clin Pharmacol 1988; 25:283–287.
32. Niven RW. Pharm Tech 1993; 16:72–82.
33. Sharp J. J Parent Sci Tech 1990; 44:289–292.
34. June, DS, Schultz, RK, Miller, NC. Pharm Tech 17:40–52.
35. Cyr TD, Graham SJ, Li KY, Lovering EG. Pharm Res 1991; 8(5):658–660.
36. Leach CL, Davidson PJ, Boudreau RJ. Eur Respir J 1998; 12(6):1346–1353.
37. Molina MJ, Rowlands FS. Nature 1974; 249:810–812.
38. Szkudlarek Brown BA. Drug Delivery Technol 2002; 2(7):52–59.
39. Hallworth GW. In: Ganderton D, Jones TM, eds. Drug Delivery to the Respiratory Tract. UK: Ellis Horwood, 1987:87–118.
40. Sciarra JJ, Cutie AJ. In: Banker GS, Rhodes CT, eds. Modern Pharmaceutics. 2nd ed. New York: Marcel Dekker, 605–634.
41. Guidance for industry metered-dose inhaler (MDI) and dry powder inhaler (DPI) drug products. www.fda.gov/CDER/guidance/index
42. Byron PR, Dalby RN, Hickey AJ. Pharm Res 1989; 6:225–229.
43. Metering valve information. Bespak plc and Valois
44. Byron P. In: Byron P, ed. Respiratory Drug Delivery. Boca Raton, FL: CRC Press, 1990:167–205.
45. Physicians Desk Reference. 53rd ed. 1999; 2879.

46. Moren F. Int J Pharm 1978; 1:205–212.
47. Kirk WF. Pharm Int 1986; June:150–155.
48. Hindle M, Byron PR. Int J Pharm 1995; 116:169–177.
49. de Boer AH, Gjaltema D, Hagedoorn P. Int J Pharm 1996; 138:45–56.
50. Bell JH, Hartley PS, Cox JSG. J Pharm Sci 1971; 60:1559–1564.
51. Newman SP. In: Clarke SW, Pavia D, eds. Aerosols and the Lung: Clinical and Experimental Aspects. Stoneham, MA: Butterworths, 1984:87.
52. Ribeiro LB, Wiren JE. Allergy 1990; 45:382–385.
53. Wetterlin K. Pharm Res 1988; 5:506–508.
54. Newman SP, Moren F, Crompton GK, eds. A New Concept in Inhalation Therapy. UK: Medicom, 1987.
55. Plover GM, Langdon CG, Jones SR, Fidler C. J Int Med Res 1988; 16:201–203.
56. Boulet LP, et al. J Asthma 1995; 32(6):429–436.
57. Prime D, et al. Adv Drug Delivery Rev 1997; 26:51–58.
58. Brown K. In: Ganderton D, Jones TMT, eds. Drug Delivery to the Respiratory Tract. UK: Ellis Horwood, 1987:119–123.
59. Tan SB, Newton JM. Int J Pharm 1990; 61:145–155.
60. Auty RM, Brown K, Neale MG, Snashall PD. Br J Dis Chest 1987; 81:371–380.
61. Vidgren M, Vidgren P, Uotila J, Paronen P. Acta Pharm Fenn 1988; 97:187–195.
62. Lucas P, Clarke MJ, Anderson K, Tobyn MJ, Staniforth JN. In: Dalby RN, Byron PR, Farr SJ, eds. Respiratory Drug Delivery VI. Interpharm Press, 1998:243–250.
63. Crowder TM, Louey MD, Sethuraman VV, Smyth HDC, Hickey AJ. Pharm Tech 2001; 25:99–113.

10

Aerosol-Filling Equipment for the Preparation of Pressurized-Pack Pharmaceutical Formulations

Christophe Sirand

BLM Associates, Inc., Greenwich, Connecticut, U.S.A.

Jean-Pierre Varlet

Valois S.A., Le Neubourg, France

Anthony J. Hickey

University of North Carolina, Chapel Hill, North Carolina, U.S.A.

INTRODUCTION

Changes to manufacturing processes of propellant-based metered-dose inhalers (pMDIs) due to the transition to hydrofluoroalkane- (HFA-) based formulations from chlorofluorocarbon- (CFC-) based systems are under way. These changes are proceeding concurrently with reformulation efforts of the pMDI systems themselves. In some cases, this may result in changes to the formulation [1].

Although the general principles of pMDI manufacture have remained the same during the transition to HFA systems, several processes and technology-related modifications have been required. In general, the manufacturing process is modified according to the final formulation used and the properties of this propellant system.

CFC 11 previously played an important role in the manufacturing process by facilitating the preparation of a concentrate at room temperatures and ambient pressures [2]. There were several technical advantages of manufacturing with nonpressurized systems [3].

The frequent use of ethanol in HFA systems is an example of a required process modification. These systems have required alterations to the elastomers used in the valves and seals of filling equipment due to different extraction and solvent profiles. Also, ethanol is corrosive to unprotected aluminum, and this must be taken into consideration [1]. In terms of manufacturing environment, large quantities of potentially flammable solvents must also be a factor in process design. For pressure filling of HFA propellants, the piston ram system may be replaced by the diaphragm displacement system [1].

Broad reviews of aerosol packaging and production may be found in the literature [4–9]. The following sections focus specifically on the process of placing the components of the aerosol formulation into a sealed container. Thus, it is beyond the scope of this chapter to consider the physicochemical aspects to the development of the formulation itself, the selection of actuators for the value or any other packaging materials (labels, boxes, and package inserts), or subsequent quality control issues.

DEFINITION OF TERMS

The terms used to describe the equipment in the manufacture of pressurized-pack pharmaceutical aerosols may not be within everyone's experience. Therefore, it is appropriate to define some of these terms before discussing packaging in detail.

The term *concentrate* or *concentrate product* has been defined as all of the components that are included in the aerosol formulation with the exception of the propellant [6–8]. The concentrate would, therefore, include the active ingredient, surfactant, solvent, and any additional materials, such as antioxidants or antimicrobials. It may also include low-vapor-pressure propellants such as propellant 11 or cosolvents such as ethanol.

Propellants are generally high-vapor-pressure CFCs and HFAs. Until recently the most common examples were the CFC propellants 11, 12, and 114. These propellants have been superceded in new formulations by HFA 134a and 227. The HFA propellants are intended to replace CFC 12. Some of the physicochemical characteristics of these propellants are shown in Table 1. The use of atmospheric-ozone-depleting CFCs in inhalers was a hotly debated issue in the late 1980s and early 1990s [11,12]. This may be followed in the professional literature [13–23]. It is now clear that CFCs will

TABLE 1 Vapor Pressure and Molecular Weights of Common CFC Propellants

Propellant	Number	Vapor pressure (psia) at 25°C	Molecular Weight
Trichloromonofluoromethane	11	13.4	137.4
Dichlorodifluoromethane	12	94.5	120.9
Dichlorotetrafluoroethane	114	27.6	170.9
Tetrafluoroethane	134a	96.0	102.0
Heptafluoropropane	227	72.6	170.0

Source: Ref. 10.

be phased out in favor of HFAs, and the FDA has stated its position on the subject [24].

An aerosol container consists of a number of components. The *container* may be constructed of aluminum or coated aluminum (to prevent interactions with the product). Other materials have been employed, including tinplate, glass, plastic-coated glass, and polycarbonate. The *valve* that is attached to the opening of the container may be constructed of aluminum or tinplate, in the main, with additional components, such as valve stem and gaskets, being made of a variety of polymers or rubbers [1,3–5].

A *collet* is used to crimp the valve to the top of the container. The collet consists of a number of "teeth" arranged in an open circle (with gaps between them) of larger diameter than the valve ferrule. The gaps between these teeth enable them to be drawn together to form a closed circle of smaller diameter than the valve ferrule. If the valve is seated on the container and the collet is placed over the valve and the "teeth" are drawn together, the pressure applied to the valve ferrule results in a crimp that attaches the valve to the container. This is described in detail in the following.

A *filling nozzle* or *head* is used to deliver either the concentrate or the propellant to the container in a controlled and quantitative fashion.

LABORATORY OR PILOT PLANT EQUIPMENT
Concentrate Product–Filling Equipment
General Description of Product Filler

Existing machines for filling concentrate products are analogous to the piston motion of a plunger within a syringe. These machines are operated pneumatically. Throttle valves on each of two inlets to the pneumatic cylinder allow the adjustment of the filling and refilling speeds. Figures 1 and 2 show the positions of these inlet valves. Where a high level of dosage accuracy is

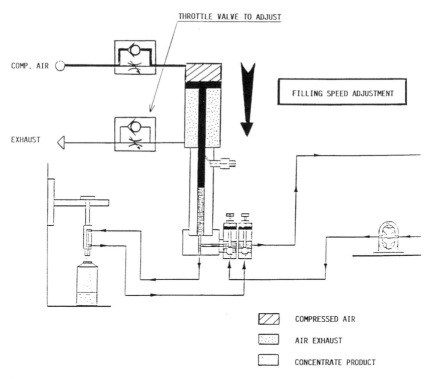

COMP. AIR ◯

THROTTLE VALVE TO ADJUST

EXHAUST ◁

FILLING SPEED ADJUSTMENT

▨ COMPRESSED AIR

▨ AIR EXHAUST

▨ CONCENTRATE PRODUCT

FIGURE 1 Concentrate product–filling equipment in filling position.

required of the fillers, a purging device is added to eliminate all vapor trapped in the metering cylinder of the filler.

A filling nozzle connected to the outlet of the metering cylinder releases the concentrate product into the container to be filled. The appropriate filling nozzle is selected according to several criteria. These fall under these general headings:

Type of activity: pharmaceutical, chemical, other
Dosage accuracy required
Speed of filling

For pharmaceutical products, the major criterion is that of accuracy. Mass market aerosols, such as paints, insecticides, and cosmetics, prioritize speed.

Two different types of filling nozzles are usually available. Figures 3, 4, and 5 show a filling nozzle type in which the canister must be present for the filling to occur. The container mechanically operates this nozzle when the filling unit is lowered. Figures 6 and 7 show a filling nozzle that is

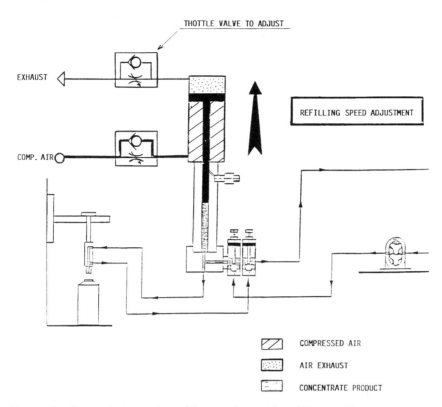

THOTTLE VALVE TO ADJUST

EXHAUST

REFILLING SPEED ADJUSTMENT

COMP. AIR

COMPRESSED AIR

AIR EXHAUST

CONCENTRATE PRODUCT

FIGURE 2 Concentrate product–filling equipment in refilling position.

operated by a servomotor. Servomotor nozzle filling occurs automatically as the concentrate product–filling pressure is increased. At the end of the filling, instantaneous closing occurs that results in no loss of product due to dripping, as shown in Fig. 8. This has been adopted for pharmaceutical purposes.

Suspension Filling. The major difficulty in filling with a suspension, which may consist of a number of components, is maintaining the homogeneity of the mixture. A recirculation loop is fitted on the installation to avoid any drug sedimentation in the tank, tubings, or filling device. During each filling cycle, this recirculation is interrupted to completely isolate the filling unit, as shown in Fig. 9. Between filling cycles, the recirculation is fully operational, which allows the concentrate product to flow freely through the filler and return to the tank, as shown in Fig. 10.

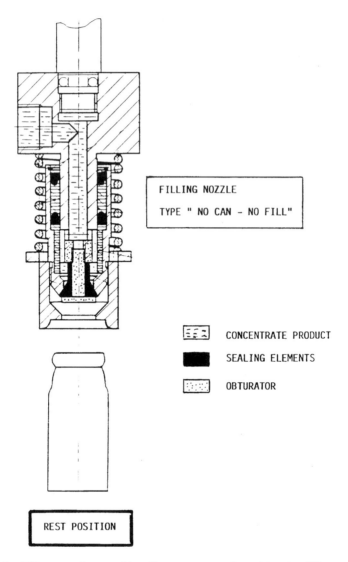

FILLING NOZZLE

TYPE " NO CAN - NO FILL"

	CONCENTRATE PRODUCT
	SEALING ELEMENTS
	OBTURATOR

REST POSITION

FIGURE 3 Filling nozzle, requiring the presence of canister for filling to occur, before filling.

The suspension concentrated product must be chilled to obtain accuracy during filling with propellant 11. Slow evaporation of propellant results in a vapor lock in the tubing and metering cylinder of the filler. This ultimately results in inaccurate filling. The simplest solution to this problem is to chill

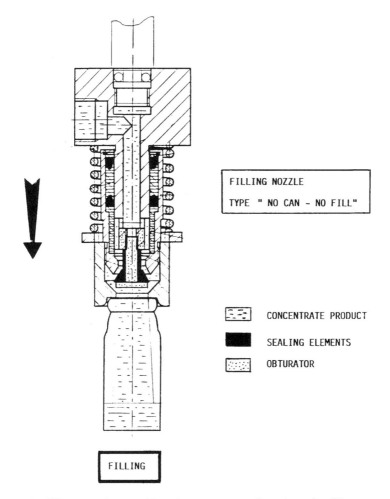

FILLING NOZZLE

TYPE " NO CAN - NO FILL"

CONCENTRATE PRODUCT

SEALING ELEMENTS

OBTURATOR

FILLING

FIGURE 4 Filling nozzle, requiring the presence of canister for filling to occur, during filling.

the product in a double-jacketed tank around which cold water is circulated at 2–4°C (35–40°F), as shown in Figs. 9 and 10. Figure 11 shows the approach when propellant 114 is also used in the concentrate; then not only does it have to be refrigerated, but the tank must be maintained under compressed nitrogen at 40–50 psig.

As indicated previously, a pump is necessary to render the recirculating system operational. The capacity may be small. One pint per minute

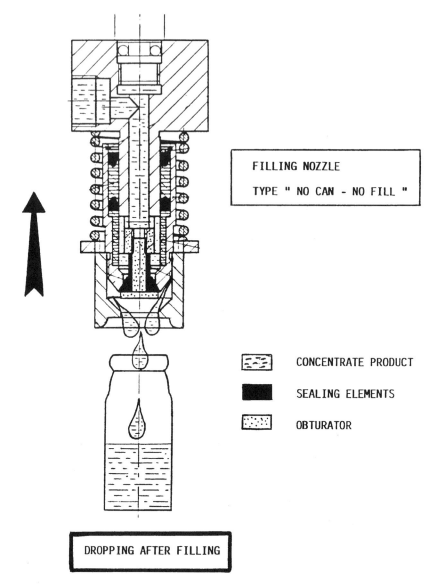

FIGURE 5 Filling nozzle, requiring the presence of canister for filling to occur, after filling.

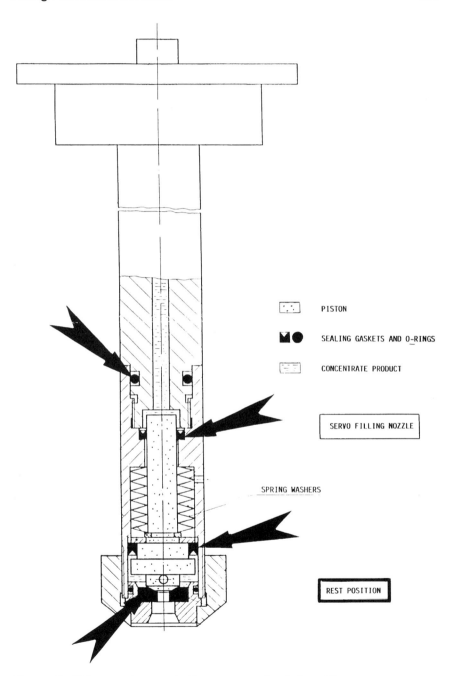

PISTON

SEALING GASKETS AND O-RINGS

CONCENTRATE PRODUCT

SERVO FILLING NOZZLE

SPRING WASHERS

REST POSITION

FIGURE 6   Filling nozzle operated by a servomotor, before filling.

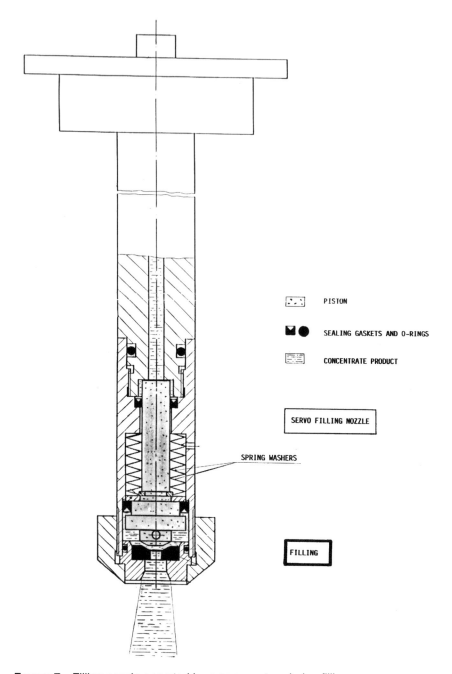

FIGURE 7   Filling nozzle operated by a servomotor, during filling.

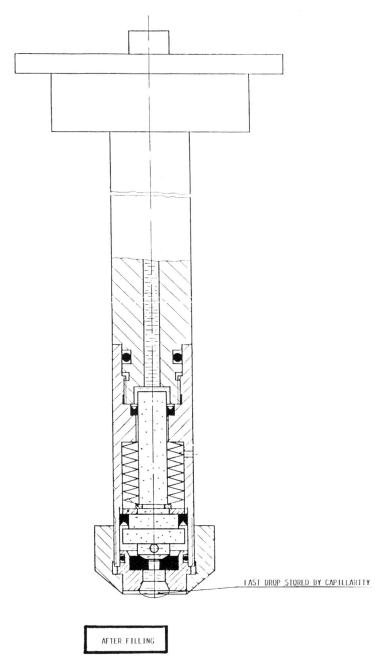

LAST DROP STORED BY CAPILLARITY

AFTER FILLING

FIGURE 8 Filling nozzle operated by a servomotor, after filling.

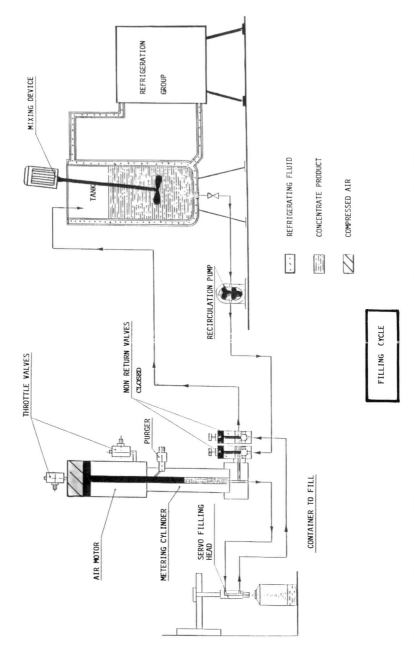

FIGURE 9 Suspension-filling equipment showing interrupted recirculation system during filling.

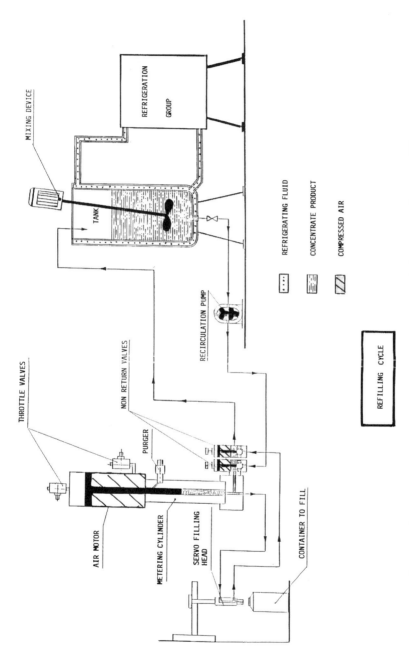

FIGURE 10 Suspension-filling equipment showing operational recirculation system between fillings.

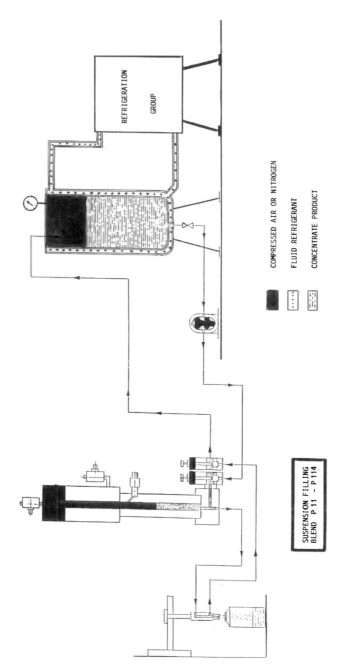

COMPRESSED AIR OR NITROGEN

FLUID REFRIGERANT

CONCENTRATE PRODUCT

SUSPENSION FILLING
BLEND P 11 - P 114

REFRIGERATION GROUP

FIGURE 11   Suspension-filling equipment for high-vapor-pressure propellant.

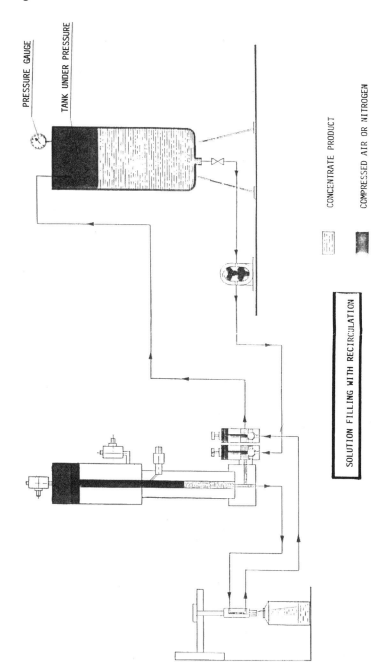

PRESSURE GAUGE

TANK UNDER PRESSURE

CONCENTRATE PRODUCT

COMPRESSED AIR OR NITROGEN

SOLUTION FILLING WITH RECIRCULATION

FIGURE 12   Solution-filling equipment.

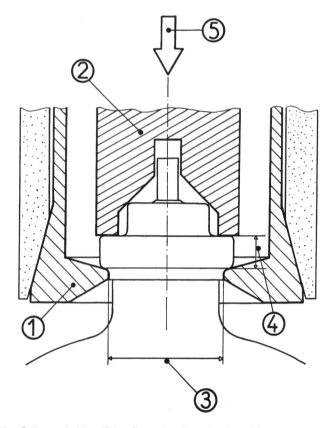

FIGURE 13 Schematic identifying five rules for crimping. (1) Well-adapted shape of crimp collet, (2) well-adapted depth stop, (3) crimping diameter, (4) crimp height, (5) sufficient vertical force.

(0.47 L/min) is sufficient. The maximum pressure provided by the pump must remain far under the servomotor filling nozzle operating pressure. When the quantity of concentrate product in the tank exceeds 1 gallon, a pump delivering a larger flow should be selected to guarantee product homogeneity. Gear pumps, diaphragm pumps, and piston pumps are recommended. Centrifugal pumps are not suitable for this purpose. Pump selection also requires consideration of possible component swelling after contact with propellant. The pump should be arranged in the system to allow gravity feed. Thus, risks of vapor-phase formation in the inlet tubing will be eliminated, as shown in Figs. 9 and 10.

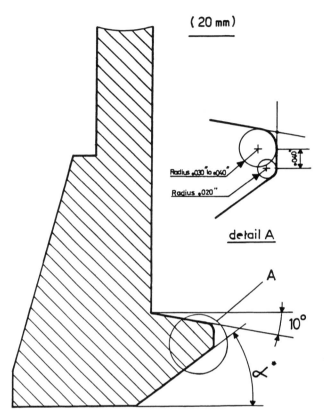

(20 mm)

Radius .030" to .040"

Radius .020"

detail A

A

10°

α°

FIGURE 14   Recommended shape for crimp collet. The angle, α, varies according to the type of bottle or can being crimped.

Solution Filling.   Solutions generally do not involve products subject to fast evaporation, such as chlorofluorocarbons, and therefore they do not require chilling and recirculation. Figure 12 shows a solution-filling system.

With product fillers that are not equipped with a purging device, it may be difficult to purge all air remaining in the metering cylinder and tubings. As a result, the first hundred fillings may be inaccurate. The addition of a recirculation system prevents this inconvenience, and, in practice, fillings become more accurate after the first five actuations.

Crimping Equipment

Five rules must be observed to perform correct crimping. These rules are illustrated schematically in Fig. 13 and are described as follows.

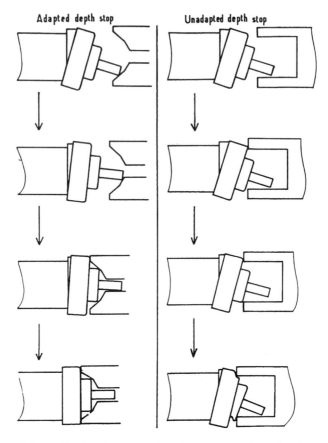

FIGURE 15 Schematic showing correct and incorrect action of a depth stop.

TABLE 2 Vertical Force Applied to Valve Ferrule During Crimping and the Extent of Compression of the Sealing Gasket Required for Different Containers

Container gasket (%)	Force provided, N (lb)	Compression of the scaling
Glass bottle	578–667 (130–150)	20
Coated bottle	578–667 (130–150)	20
Aluminum cannister	400–578 (90–130)	40

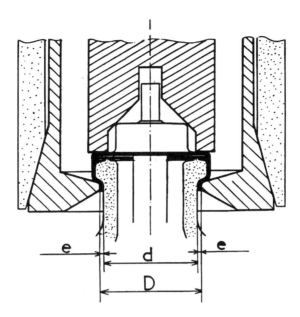

FIGURE 16 Adjustment of the crimping diameter.

Rules Governing Correct Crimping

Crimp Collet. Use an appropriate crimp collet. This must have a shape perfectly adapted to the various kinds of bottles or cans to be crimped. Figure 14 shows a recommended shape for a crimp collet.

Depth Stop. Use a depth stop adapted to various kinds of valves and pumps. The shape of the depth stop must be designed according to the external shape of the valve ferrule. The depth stop has three functions. It transmits the necessary force to compress the sealing gasket; it enables adjustment of the crimping height; and it positions the valve ferrule correctly inside the crimp collet. The result is a good concentric crimp.

On the inside of the depth stop profile, it is often better to provide an inlet cone on which the stem and the dome of the valve will slide. A precise and gentle placement of the valve ferrule into the depth stop will, thus, be obtained, as shown in Fig. 15.

Crimping Diameter. The theoretical crimping diameter must be determined to adjust the crimp collect closing. Figure 16 shows a schematic of the adjustment of crimping diameter. The theoretical crimping diameter can be determined according to a simple equation. Assuming a glass bottle

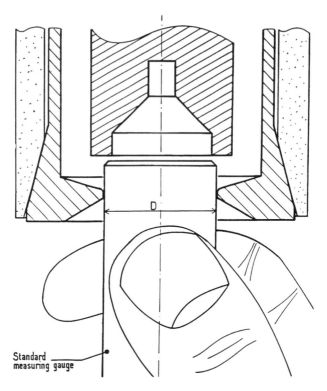

FIGURE 17   Adjustment of the crimp collet closing using a standard-diameter (*D*) measuring gauge. (*D* is the theoretical diameter.)

configuration, the diameter of crimp collet, with tongs in their closed position, is:

$$D = d + 2e + 0.008 \text{ in.}$$

where *d* is the bottle diameter beneath the neck, *e* is the thickness of the valve ferrule metal, and 0.008 in. is the clearance necessary to avoid breakage risk of the bottle and the crimp collet.

   The practical adjustment of the crimp collet closing is performed by putting the machine in its low position (tongs closed). The crimp collet closing is then adjusted using a standard-diameter measuring gauge, as in Fig. 17.

   Crimping Height.   Calculate the theoretical crimping height to determine the position of the depth stop in the crimp collet. Knowledge of the theoretical

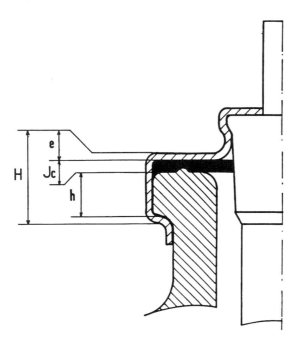

FIGURE 18 Adjustment of crimping height. *H* is the crimping height, *h* is the height of the glass neck, *e* is the thickness of the valve ferrule metal, and *Jc* is the thickness of the compressed gasket.

crimping height allows the adjustment of the depth stop to the correct position in the crimp collet. Figure 18 illustrates the crimp parameters. In a glass bottle configuration, the crimping height can be adjusted according to the following equation:

$$H = 2e + Jc + h$$

where H is the crimping height, h is the height of the glass neck, e is the thickness of the valve ferrule metal, and Jc is the thickness of the compressed gasket.

Compression.   To prevent leaks resulting from an imperfect crimp of the valve ferrule on the neck of the container, the thickness of the seal must be reduced. The seal will, thus, be compressed, providing sufficient vertical force that is applied to the ferrule just before crimping (Table 2). The object of the compression is to provide a sufficient vertical force on the valve ferrule during the crimping.

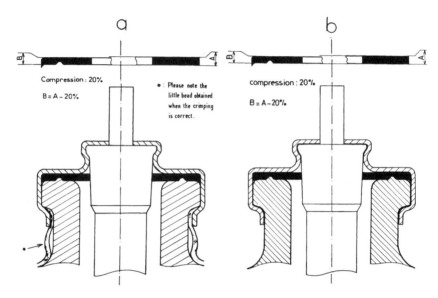

FIGURE 19   Valve seating on (a) a coated and (b) an uncoated glass bottle.

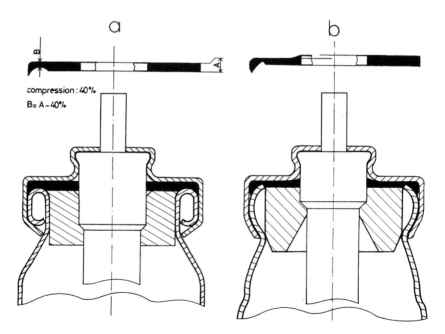

FIGURE 20   Valve seating on an aluminum (a) roll-neck and (b) cut-edge canister.

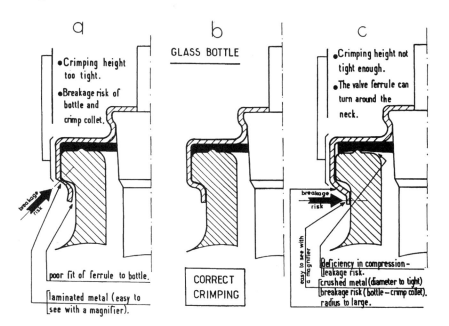

FIGURE 21 Valve seating on glass bottle indicating (a) loose, (b) correct, and (c) tight crimp.

To obtain sufficient compression of the sealing gasket, it is necessary to respect the values given in Table 1. Compression of the sealing gasket is shown in Figs. 19 and 20 for a glass bottle, a coated glass bottle, and roll-neck (Cebal Safet) and cut-edge (Presspart) aluminum cans.

Control of Quality of Crimping

Figure 21 shows a crimp on a glass bottle indicating a correct crimp, a crimp that is too tight, and a crimp that is not tight enough. Figure 22 shows the same range of crimping phenomena for an aluminum can. A crimper control Socoge may be used to monitor crimp height. This device aims to define and control a size of crimping height on valves and pumps that are currently used on bottles in the perfumery and pharmaceutical industries.

The recommended crimp dimensions vary according to the types of container and valve being considered. The following discussion of dimensions for crimping is appropriate for Valois metering valves, type DF10 or DF30. Taking these examples, the precision with which valves may be attached to the containers can be indicated. Figure 23 refers to the 20-mm FEA standard glass bottle. The crimp collet closing diameter (D) may be

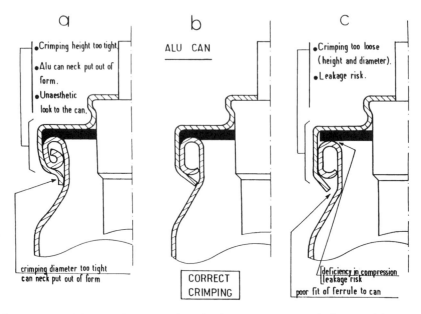

FIGURE 22   Valve seating on roll-neck aluminum canister indicating (a) loose, (b) correct, and (c) tight crimp.

easily determined according to d, the diameter beneath the neck, which can be measured with a caliper gauge. As measured with a Socoge crimper control gauge, the crimping height is $H = 0.209 \pm 0.002$ in. $(5.3 \pm 0.05$ mm). These dimensions are valid only with a 1-mm gasket. Figure 24 refers to an aluminum can type of Cebal Safet. The crimp collet closing diameter should be $D = 0.65$ in., and the crimping height is the same as that for the FEA standard glass bottle. Figure 25 refers to the aluminum can type of Presspart. The crimp collet closing diameter is 0.697 in., whereas the crimping height is 5.7 mm.

Propellant-Filling Equipment

Propellant-Filling Methods

Pressure Filling.   The propellant is introduced under high pressure into the container through the valve, as shown in Fig. 26. Most valve manufactures design their valves for this method.

Cold Filling.   The propellant is cooled to a very low temperature and poured into an open container. However, this procedure creates the inconvenience of requiring equipment able to produce an extremely low temperature ($-50°F$).

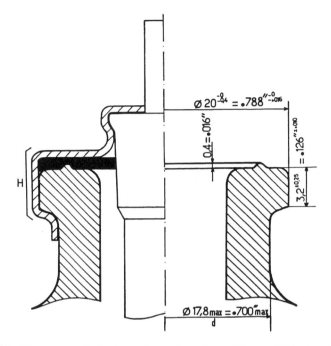

FIGURE 23 Recommended crimp dimensions for a 20-mm FEA standard glass bottle. *H* is crimp height, and *d* is the diameter beneath the neck as measured with a caliper gauge.

Undercap Filling. The propellant is filled under the valve immediately before crimping. This technique is used mainly for the 1-in-opening containers, because large quantities of propellant can be filled very quickly. Nevertheless, this method results in large losses of propellant.

General Description of a High-Pressure Propellant Filler

A high-pressure propellant-filling installation consists of two main units: a propellant compressor pump and a propellant-filling machine.

Propellant Compressor Pump. To feed the propellant-filling machine properly, a propellant compressor pump is necessary. The pump guarantees a regular amount of propellant pressure supply and helps prevent the formation of a vapor phase in the metering cylinder of the filler and in the tubings of the system. When filling with propellant 12, for instance, an average pressure of 170–200 psig should be delivered at the outlet of the propellant pump.

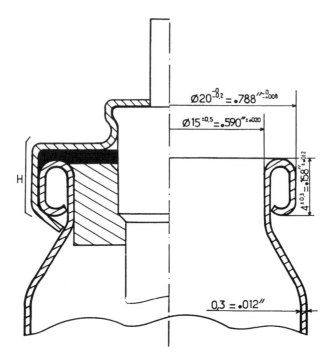

$\varnothing 20^{-0.2} = .788''^{-0}_{-.008}$

$\varnothing 15^{\pm 0.5} = .590''^{\pm .020}$

$4^{\pm 0.3} = .158''^{\pm .012}$

H

$0.3 = .012''$

FIGURE 24   Recommended crimping dimensions for a roll-neck aluminum canister (Cebal Safet).

When setting up or using a propellant-filling installation, the inlet of the pump must be connected to the liquid phase outlet of the propellant tank. On most of the propellant tanks that are commercially available, two valves allow the selection of either the vapor phase or the liquid phase of the propellant. It is important when using such a system to ensure that the vapor-phase valve of the propellant tank is correctly turned off. It is also important to avoid long pieces of tubing between the pump and the propellant tank. The maximum length of tubing should be 1 m (3 ft). This is shown in Figs. 26 and 27, which indicate a pressure-filling process.

Propellant Filler Unit.   The propellant filler may also be compared with a syringe piston system, as was the concentrate-product filler. When the pneumatic pump pushes on the piston, a very high pressure builds up in the metering cylinder of the filler. A filling head is connected to the outlet of the metering cylinder and allows the introduction of the propellant into the container through the valve. As seen previously, this technique is called pressure filling.

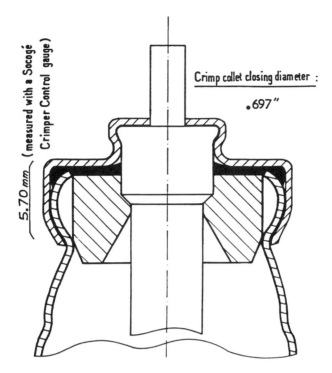

FIGURE 25 Recommended crimping dimensions for a cut-edge aluminum canister (Presspart).

To control the propellant pressure injection, that is, the pressure necessary to inject liquid propellant through the valve, an air regulator is fitted on the inlet of the pneumatic cylinder, as shown in Figs. 27 and 28. By adjusting the amount of air pressure allowed in the pneumatic cylinder, it is possible to decrease or increase the propellant pressure injection. This pressure injection varies, according to the type of valve, between 500 and 800 psi. Manufactures of valves usually recommend specific pressure injection for their products.

Filling Head. The filling head is the device that allows the propellant to be introduced into the container. Because valve manufacturers design their products differently, technical filling specifications cannot be the same for every valve on the market. Thus, it is not possible to use a standard filling head for all valves. Each valve requires an appropriate filling head to be pressure filled correctly. This filling head must also be designed according to the pressure-filling equipment used.

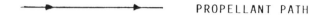

PROPELLANT PATH

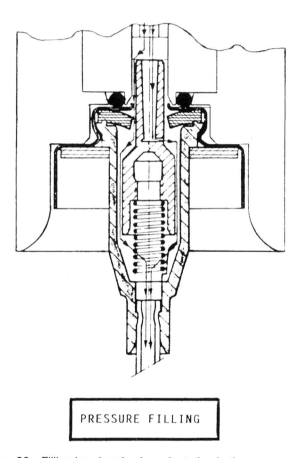

PRESSURE FILLING

FIGURE 26   Filling head and valve orientation in the pressure-filling process.

MANUFACTURING FACILITIES

Fundamentally, the manufacturing facilities do not differ from the laboratory or pilot plant. The same rules regarding installation and use principles must be respected to perform proper concentrate filling, crimping, and propellant charging. The only difference is the product output capacity of the equipment, which is, of course, greatly superior in the case of the manufacturing facilities.

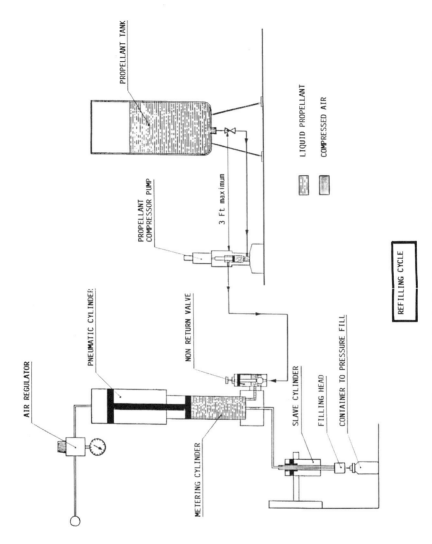

PROPELLANT TANK

PROPELLANT
COMPRESSOR PUMP

3 Ft maximum

LIQUID PROPELLANT

COMPRESSED AIR

AIR REGULATOR

PNEUMATIC CYLINDER

METERING CYLINDER

NON RETURN VALVE

SLAVE CYLINDER

FILLING HEAD

CONTAINER TO PRESSURE FILL

REFILLING CYCLE

FIGURE 27 Pressure-filling system illustrating the propellant-filler unit in refilling position.

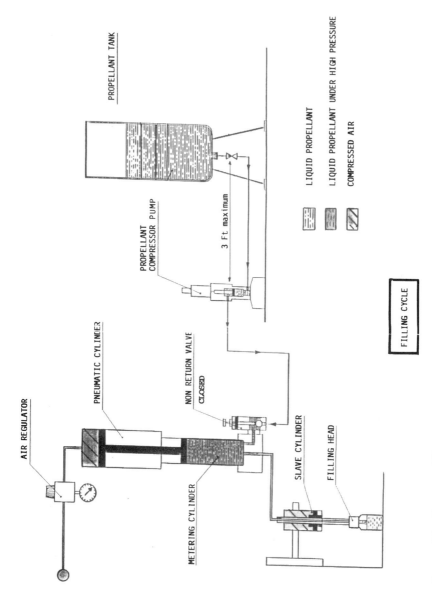

FIGURE 28 Pressure-filling system illustrating the propellant-filler unit in filling position.

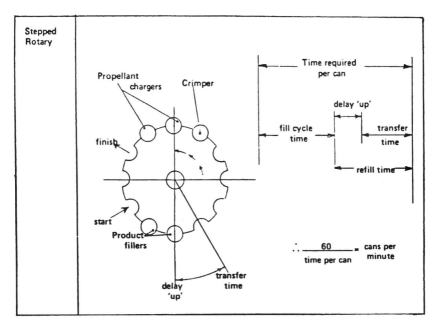

FIGURE 29 Stepped rotary machines for large-scale manufacturing.

According to the desired production output capacity, two main types of machines can be selected: stepped rotary and continuous rotary.

Stepped Rotary Machines

On the stepped rotary machines, the maximum output is related directly to the type of valve used. Effectively, when using a metered valve, such as those used for bronchodilator aerosols, you should not expect an output production of more than 35–40 cans/min. A stepped rotary machine is shown schematically in Fig. 29. With other valves, designed for fast filling, output capacity can reach 60–70 cans/min. Figure 29 shows how to calculate the time required per container.

Continuous Rotary Machines

Continuous rotary machines, unlike the stepped rotary machines, do not perform concentrate filling, crimping, and propellent charging on the same indexing unit. Each operation in the aerosol packaging process is carried out on a different continuous rotary station. As a result, high production output capacity is obtained (100–200 containers/min). Figure 30 shows a continuous rotary machine.

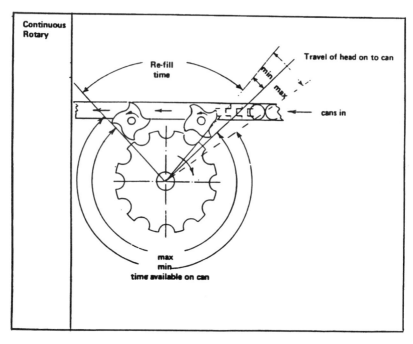

FIGURE 30   Continuous rotary machines for large-scale manufacturing.

It is of prime importance to pinpoint the total production expected before investing in manufacturing facilities. When significant production is required, it would be appropriate to select a continuous rotary system rather than multiple stepped rotary machines.

REFERENCES

1. Smith IJ. J Aerosol Med 1995; 8:S19–S27.
2. Wilkinson A. Metered-Dose Inhaler Technology. Buffalo Grove, IL: Interpharm Press, 1998:69–116.
3. IPAC. Ensuring patient care: the role of the HFC MDI. International Pharmaceutical Aerosol Consortium, 2nd ed. 1999.
4. Sanders PA. Principles of Aerosol Technology. New York: Van Nostrand Reinhold, 1970.
5. Gorman WG, Popp K. In: Tyle P, ed. Specialized Drug Delivery Systems. New York: Marcel Dekker, 1990:451–471.

6. Sciarra JJ, Cutie AJ, In: Lieberman HA, Rieger MM, Banker G, eds. Pharmaceutical Dosage Forms: Disperse Systems. Vol. 2. New York: Marcel Dekker, 1990:417–460.
7. Sciarra JJ, Cutie AJ. In: Banker G, Rhodes C, eds. Modern Pharmaceutics. 2nd ed. New York: Marcel Dekker, 1990:1–30.
8. Sciarra JJ. In: Lachmann L, Lieberman HA, Kanig JL, eds. Theory and Practice of Industrial Pharmacy. Philadelphia: Lea & Febiger, 1970:605–638.
9. Sciarra JJ, Stoller L. The Science and Technology of Aerosol Packaging. New York: Wiley Interscience, 1974.
10. Hickey AJ, Evans RM. In: Hickey AJ, ed. Inhalation Aerosols. New York: Marcel Dekker, 1996:426.
11. Dalby RN, Byron PR, Shepherd HR, Papadopoulos E. Pharm Technol 1990; 14:26–33.
12. Fischer FX, Hess H, Sucker H, Byron PR. Pharm Technol 1989; 13:44–52.
13. Chem Eng News 1990; 68(29):5.
14. Ainsworth SJ. Chem Eng News 1990; 68(17):23–52.
15. Zurer PS. Chem Eng News 1990; 68(14):21–22.
16. Chem Eng News 1990; 68(11):27.
17. Chem Eng News 1990; 68(10):21.
18. Chem Eng News 1989; 67(50):16.
19. Chem Eng News 1989; 67(33):5.
20. Chem Eng News 1989; 67(30):7–13.
21. Chem Eng News 1989; 67(28):17.
22. Chem Eng News 1989; 67(27):8.
23. Chem Eng News 1989; 67(17):5–6.
24. Fed Regist 2002; 67:48370–48385.

11

Methods of Aerosol Particle Size Characterization

Anthony J. Hickey
University of North Carolina, Chapel Hill, North Carolina, U.S.A.

INTRODUCTION

The most important physicochemical parameter influencing the deposition of aerosols in the lungs is particle or droplet size. Consequently, it is necessary to understand the principles and the methods of estimating particle size, allowing meaningful interpretation of the data. In addition, therapeutic effect is related to the mass of particles having a specific size, which relates to the distribution of particles in a range of sizes fully describing the aerosol.

A reappraisal of the particle size characterization of pharmaceutically relevant materials, including therapeutic aerosols, was advocated in the late 1980s [1]. This led to a reevaluation of compendial standards for particle size measurement [2]. By the late 1990s most pharmacopoeia had adopted new standards for the testing of inhalation aerosols.

Particle size analysis of pharmaceutical aerosols has a strong foundation based on other disciplines. Most of the analytical techniques used were in existence before the development of the modern pharmaceutical aerosol dosage form. However, some significant challenges have to be overcome in the use of these techniques for assessing pharmaceutical systems.

The following sections focus on the principles of collection and characterization of pharmaceutical aerosols. Instruments have been selected to illustrate the methods that they typify.

PARTICLE SIZE

A wide variety of methods have been used to measure the particle size of aerosols, and most of these have found an application in the specialized field of pharmaceutical product characterization. In general, these approaches result in the measurement of a particular diameter that may be defined according to the principle underlying the measurement [3].

Definitions of particle diameters derived by different methods have been described in detail [4]. The *aerodynamic* diameter is defined as the diameter of a unit-density sphere having the same settling velocity, generally in air, as the particle. This encompasses particle shape, density, and physical size, all of which influence the aerodynamic behavior of the particle. As a dynamic parameter, it can generally be linked with aerosol deposition and specifically with that in the lung [5].

An aerosol rarely consists of particles that are the same size, and usually a distribution of sizes around a mean is observed. The observed data may be fitted by statistical approximation to a distribution. The number of particles in a size range when plotted against the logarithm of the particle diameters frequently exhibit a normal (Gaussian) distribution. This is known as a *log-normal distribution* and is described by a parameter known as the *geometric standard deviation*. Theoretically, a monodisperse aerosol will exhibit a geometric standard deviation of 1; in practice, however, an accepted limit is 1.2 [6].

INERTIAL IMPACTION

Inertial impaction has been used to sample and size fractionate aerosol particles and droplets for many years [7,8]. The original devices were designed to sample atmospheric air for pollutants, and many are still used for this purpose [9–18]. The nature of the development of these devices has had some implications for their use by the pharmaceutical scientist. The interest in their theoretical performance and practical application resulted in many of their limitations being understood before their use for characterizing pharmaceutical products. However, they were designed and calibrated to sample aerosol particles over a larger size range than is necessary for therapeutic purposes and, in some cases, under airflow conditions far in excess of physiological conditions (Sierra 23-L, Sierra Instruments, Inc., Carmel Valley, CA) [19]. Complications in data interpretation may arise from the sampling techniques used specifically to assess pharmaceutical aerosols. These are discussed in later sections.

Calibration

Inertial impactors are calibrated using monodisperse aerosols. Generation of monodisperse aerosols is discussed in detail elsewhere in this book (Chap. 8) [20]. The most commonly used methods are the vibrating orifice [21,22] and the spinning disk (or top) [23–25]. The spinning-disk method has the advantage of generating large concentrations of aerosol. The production and removal of secondary droplets [25], necessarily of a different size than the primaries, by the latter method requires close monitoring to ensure that a truly monodisperse aerosol is being generated. The vibrating-orifice generator produces a low-concentration aerosol output. Consequently, calibration can take considerable time. The most significant source of polydispersity in this device is a tendency of the orifice to clog. The experienced investigator can avert this error by monitoring at intervals for deposits. The droplet size may deviate from theoretical expectations when there are any imperfections in the orifice. Microscopic examination before initiation and upon completion of the study should show a perfectly circular orifice. This procedure allows the condition of the orifice to be established over the time frame of the study.

The method of calibration involves investigating each stage independently [26,27]. Monodisperse aerosols of a known particle size may be generated and collected on a single stage. The fraction of the aerosol that is not collected on the stage is collected on a filter to allow estimates of the total mass of aerosol being generated. The filter used for this purpose collects particles 0.2 μm in diameter and larger. The amount deposited on each stage can then be expressed as a percentage of the total collected (stage plus filter). By plotting the percentage collected against the particle size, a sigmoid curve is obtained, as shown in Fig. 1. The middle portion of this curve indicates the 50% cutoff diameter. This is the diameter at which it was determined experimentally that 50% of the particles were collected and that the remaining 50% were passed to the absolute filter. The curve differs from that derived theoretically, which is a step function, with a cutoff diameter indicated by the vertical portion of the curve, also shown in Fig. 1.

Filtration
Filter Holders

Filter holders are required to facilitate sampling and are made by a variety of companies (Millipore, Cambridge, MA; BGI, Waltham, MA). These are usually made of stainless steel, with machined inner surfaces to allow the unperturbed

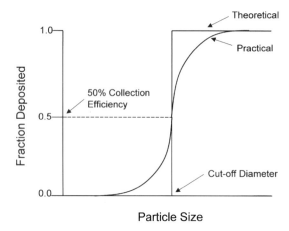

FIGURE 1   Hypothetical collection efficiency of a stage of an impactor. Fraction deposited plotted against particle size. The step function indicates the theoretical deposition, and the curve indicates the practical characteristics.

passage of air through the device. Fig. 2 shows a general design of a filter housing. The aerosol inlet (A) is conical to direct the aerosol to the filter. A central mesh (B) supports the filter selected for sampling the aerosol. The outlet is not subject to the same design constraints as the inlet because it does not carry aerosol. Thus, the body of the housing may be reduced to the dimension of the outlet orifice over a short distance (C). Air is drawn through the filter by means of a vacuum pump connected at the outlet. The filter housings may be grounded to prevent electrostatic deposition of charged particles.

Filters

Fiber Filters.   Fibers have proven efficient surfaces on which to deposit particles. Glass fiber filters are frequently used as "absolute" filters to collect particles 0.22 µm in diameter and greater. The advantage of fiber filters is their ability to allow the passage of the large volumes of air usually accompanying an aerosol while retaining the particles. As the particle size of the aerosol to be collected increases, the filter required to collect it uses larger-diameter fibers and will allow the passage of larger volumes of air. The operational pressure drop across a fiber filter is relatively small [28].

The principle of filtration combines many of the individual mechanisms of collection on which other methods are based. Thus, diffusion (Brownian motion), inertia, interception, charge, and sedimentation may all contribute to deposition of particles on filters. The inertial and interception effects are illustrated in Fig. 3.

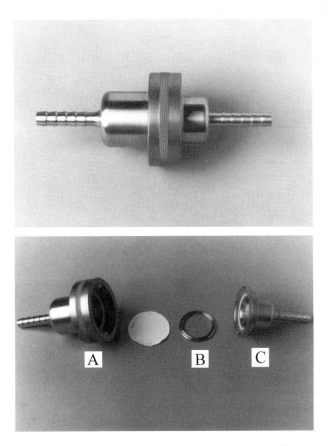

FIGURE 2 Photograph of a filter holder for aerosol sampling. Disassembled view shows (A) conical inlet, (B) mesh support for filter, and (C) outlet.

A large particle will follow a path deviating from the streamline as it approaches the fiber and will impinge on the fiber surface. If the particle follows a path approximately perpendicular to the fiber surface, it is deposited as a result of its inertia. Those particles that do not follow a path directly to the surface of the fiber but that enter the airstream passing within the distance equivalent to the radius of the particle from the fiber will be intercepted. It is only necessary for the surface of the particle to touch the fiber for capture to take place [29].

The theory of deposition on fibers, or cylinders, lying transverse to the direction of airflow has been studied thoroughly [9,28–32]. Fiber filters have been placed in specialized pharmaceutical aerosol sampling tubes that can

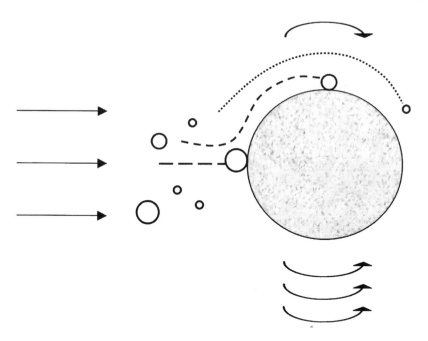

FIGURE 3 Principle of interception of particles by fibers showing large particles impacting, small particles being intercepted as they pass close to the surface, and the smallest particles passing beyond the fiber.

be used to collect particles emitted from inhalers. Such a device, shown in Fig. 4, is identified in the *United States Pharmacopoeia* [33,34]. The recommended operating conditions are unique to this device and require a fixed pressure drop (4 kPa) to be generated across the device from which the aerosol is sampled in a fixed volume of 4 L.

Membrane Filters. The cellulose-derivative membrane filters, as we know them, have been available since 1927 and are now commonplace [29,32,35–38]. The classic membrane filters are prepared by means of a colloid chemical process: gelation of concentrated colloidal solutions of polymers and removal of solvent to leave pores. Although porous, in practice they differ from the capillary model of a pore in that their structure is not regular. A classic membrane filter has three different structures: the upper surface structure, the inner structure, and the lower surface structure [29,35–38]. These filters contain tortuous channels, and the pore sizes inside the filter are larger than those on the surface of a membrane filter. The diameters of these channels can be closely controlled during manufacture. The mechanisms involved in the capture of

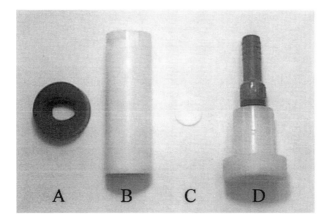

FIGURE 4   Emitted dose sampling tube (Nephele). Disassembled view shows (A) rubber mouthpiece for connection to (B) inhaler cylindrical inlet, (C) filter, and (D) outlet through which vacuum is employed to draw air.

particles are diffusion, sieving, and impaction with little influence of charge [28,29]. The pressure drop across these filters is high, and they are usually used at relatively low airflow velocities.

Membrane filters are particularly appropriate for use in conjunction with microscopy because most particles are deposited on the upper surface. This is shown in Fig. 5, which is a scanning of aerosol particles on a membrane filter. High-power light microscopy is also possible, because the filter becomes transparent on the application of immersion oil.

The nucleopore membrane filters are more recent developments, being available since 1965 [35–37]. Nucleopore membrane filters are prepared by means of a nuclear physical process: neutron irradiation in a nuclear reactor followed by chemical etching. The structure of the resulting filters is geometrically regular. The capillary filter model fits a nuclear membrane filter well [38].

Both classic membrane filters and nucleopore membrane filters are made of organic materials soluble in many nonaqueous solvents. Types of metallic membrane filters are also available, for example, silver metal membrane filters. These filters are made by means of a powder metallurgy process. They are useful for organic microanalysis of aerosol samples [39].

The optimal mean filtration radius is an arithmetic average of pore radii measured on the surface of a membrane filter by means of electron microscopy and is used to characterize cellulose, nucleopore, and silver membrane filters.

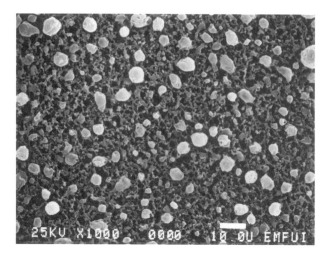

FIGURE 5 Scanning electron micrograph of particles deposited on membrane filter.

Collecting aerosol particles on different filters allows particles to be segregated by size. A graded sequence of filters may be used, providing the pressure drop at each stage is monitored.

Cascade Impactors

Cascade impaction is one of the oldest methods for the dynamic characterization of aerosol particles. The method is used daily for the characterization of pharmaceutical aerosols, despite not currently being a pharmacopoeial requirement. The Food and Drug Administration first recognized the popularity of this type of sizing device by setting a standard for its use in the assessment of generic pharmaceutical aerosols for bioequivalence [40]. This has been superceded by pharmacopoeial and regulatory standards, as described in the last paragraph of this chapter. Other methods have been described in the literature [41–43].

Dynamic Particle Behavior

The principle on which inertial impactors operate is based on the aerodynamic behavior of aerosol particles. Fig. 6 shows a schematic diagram of particle collection by an inertial collection device. When the direction of a gas flow changes, the suspended particles continue to move in the original direction of flow until they lose inertia as a result of friction with the molecules in the surrounding medium. They are then said to "relax" into the new direction of flow, and the time taken for this to occur is known as the "relaxation time." A collections surface is placed in the path of the original direction of gas flow. Large particles will impact the surface. Small particles relax more quickly into a new direction of flow than the larger ones and, therefore, do not encounter the collection surface. The diameter at which a transition occurs from complete deposition to little or no collection of particles can be established by sampling particles of known size. This calibration will apply to known gas flows and linear velocities and assumes a fixed distance to the collection surface at each stage. Cascade impactors and impingers use these principles. Placing a series of jets and corresponding obstacles in the path of a single gas flow allows the removal of aerosol particles according to their size. Subsequently, the distribution may be reconstructed, based on the calibration for each stage. More Specifically, this is achieved by passing the gas flow through a series of orifices of decreasing diameter, thus producing an increased linear velocity, resulting in increased particle inertia. The collection surfaces may also be placed closer to the jets, or the point at which the direction of gas flow changes, at each consecutive stage.

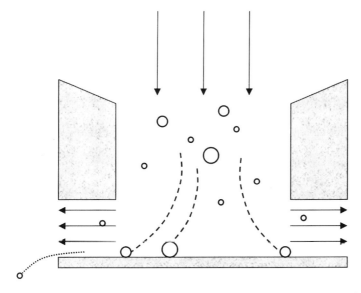

FIGURE 6 Schematic diagram of the method of collection of aerosol particles by an impactor. Solid arrows show direction of movement of airflow. Large particles impact on the collection surface, while small particles pass around it.

This does not allow particles of certain size to travel far enough or does not give them enough time to follow the new direction of flow before encountering a collection surface.

The relaxation time corresponding to the distance traveled by a particle until it follows the new direction of flow, the "stopping distance," can be derived from the equation for the terminal settling velocity [19]:

$$V_T = \frac{d^2 \rho g C_c}{18\eta}$$

and the relaxation time is

$$t = \frac{d^2 C_c \rho}{18\eta}$$

where d is the aerodynamic diameter, ρ is unit density ($I = g/cm^3$), η is the viscosity of air, g is the acceleration due to gravity, and C_c is the slip correction factor.

The chief design parameter for impactors is the plate collection efficiency, ideally a function of a single dimensionless parameter, the ratio of the stopping distance of the particle to the width of the impactor jet. This parameter is called the Stokes number and is defined as

$$\text{Stk} = \frac{S}{d_c} = t\frac{U_o}{d_c}$$

where S is the "stopping distance," U_o is the initial velocity, and d_c is a critical dimension, in this case orifice diameter. The Stokes number may be thought of as the ratio of the particles "persistence" to the size of the obstacle. A well-designed impactor has a sharp cutoff at a Stokes number of 0.2, for a circular jet. Ideally, the cutoff is a step change from an efficiency of 0 to 1, as shown in Fig. 1. Ideal behavior can be achieved [44] if (1) in the region between the jet exit plane and the impaction plate the component of the air velocity parallel to the centerline of the nozzle (y) is a function of y only and (2) the y-component of the velocity of the particles at the jet exit plane is uniform across the jet. In real impactors, these conditions are only approximated. The chief departures from the ideal lie in the fluid boundary layers near the impactor walls. Particle behavior in these zones causes nonideal cutoff characteristics at large efficiencies in real devices.

The methods of handling data are based mainly on a log-normal fit to the particle size distribution data [45,46]. To eliminate some of the vagaries surrounding the derivation of the median diameter and geometric standard deviation from log-probability plots, computer methods have been developed to derive these parameters from the data [47,48]. These methods use nonlinear curve-fitting programs that result in error maps of the least mean square analysis from which the best fit can be derived. Some methods have been suggested that involve the use of a programmable pocket calculator [49].

Types of Cascade Impactors

A cascade impactor that seems to be among the most commonly used in the pharmaceutical industry is the Delron [10]. This is a Batelle-type instrument, named after the place of development. There are two models, the Delron Cascade Impactor (DCI) DCI-6 and the DCI-5. As the model numbers suggest, the DCI-6 is a six-stage and the DCI-5 a five-stage device. Each has an additional "absolute" (0.22-μm) filter to collect particles that are not deposited on each of the stages. The DCI-5 has a low airflow rate of 1.25 L/min. Conversely, the DCI-6 has a high airflow rate of 12.5 L/min. The DCI-6 seems to be the more popular model for pharmaceutical aerosol sampling. Fig. 7 shows a schematic diagram of the DCI-6. The stages are arranged vertically; thus, this type of impactor is sometimes referred to as "stacked" or "in-stack." Each stage has a single circular orifice beneath which resides a glass slide 38 mm in diameter. The nominal cutoff points for each stage of the impactor, based on a 50% collection efficiency, are 16, 8, 4, 2, 1, 0.5, and 0.2 μm [10]. It has been pointed out, however, that if the collection surfaces are coated to enhance the collection efficiency, the cutoff diameters change. Thus, the device has been reported to have cutoff diameters of 11.2, 5.5, 3.3, 2.0, 0.9, 0.5, and 0.2 μm when silicone fluid–coated glass slides were used [48]. Although this instrument is no longer mass-produced, the number in existence have given it prominence for assessing pharmaceutical aerosols.

Another cascade impactor commonly used in pharmaceutical aerosol characterization is the Andersen 1 CFM Ambient Sampler, of which a number of models exist [50–53] (Andersen Samplers, Inc., Atlanta, GA). This is also a stacked impactor, operating at an airflow rate of 1 ft^3/min, or 28.3 L/min. It differs from the Delron instrument in the number of stages, the number of circular orifices at each stage, and the size of the collection surfaces. Fig. 8 illustrates the arrangement of the eight stages in the Anderson impactor. These stages are preceded by a preseparator that removes large particles (>9.9 μm). The device uses a perforated plate rather than a single jet. This plate contains as many as 400 orifices per stage. Beneath the plate is situated a stainless steel collection plate 80 mm in diameter. The nominal cutoff diameters for each stage are 9.0, 5.8, 4.7, 3.3, 2.1, 1.1, 0.7, and 0.4 and the filter 0.2 μm [52,53]. The foregoing conditions are chosen for metered-dose inhaler and nebulizer sampling. This impactor has also been utilized at a flow rate of 60 L/min for the evaluation of dry powder inhaler performance. Since the cutoff diameters shift as a function of increased

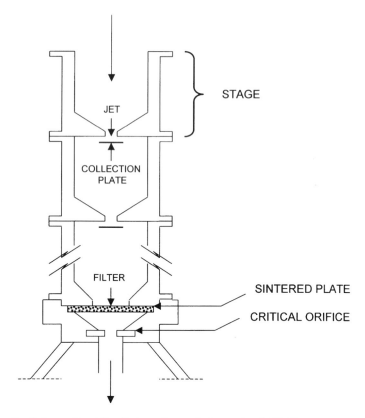

FIGURE 7   Schematic of the Delron Cascade Impactor (DCI-6).

flowrate, the instrument was recalibrated by the manufacturer, stage 7 was removed, and stage − 1 inserted above stage 0, to give values as follows, 6.2, 4.0, 3.2, 2.3, 1.4, 0.8, and 0.5 and the filter 0.2 μm [54]. The Marple Miller Impactor (MSP Corp.) was developed for ease of use and suitability for inhalation aerosol samples over a range of operating flowrates (30, 60, and 90 L/min) [55].

The Sierra 210 Series of impactors (Andersen Samplers, Inc.) consist of 10-, 8-, and 6-stage devices. These use radial slots rather than circular jets as described in the previous examples. The device is designed to offer the advantage of a greater number of stages in the submicrometer range at a selected flowrate that effectively renders it of little relevance to pharmaceutical aerosols.

A significant effort occurred at the end of the 1990s to develop a new method of inertial sampling that had a greater application in pharmaceutical product development. This resulted in the manufacture of a the Next Generation Cascade Impactor. This device has the advantage of chambers that collect aerosol

AMBIENT AIR FLOW

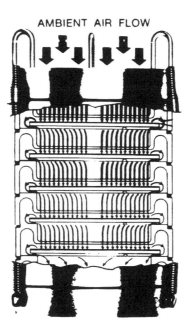

FIGURE 8 Schematic of the Andersen Sampler. (With permission of Andersen Samplers, Inc.)

particles and that can act as vessels into which a fluid can be placed to dissolve these particles for subsequent chemical analysis. Fig. 9 shows a photograph of the new impactor [56]. Although significant for the environmental sciences, this is somewhat unnecessary for the study of pharmaceutical products. At a flow rate of 0.3 L/min, the cutoff values for stages 4–10 are 13, 8.5, 4.8, 2.9, 1.9, 1.3, and 0.58 μm, respectively. Thus, six stages are in the size range of interest. At flow rates of 10 and 21 L/min, approaching those of the Delron and Andersen devices, eight stages may be used, three of which are submicrometer and four of which are in the size range of interest. There are other cascade impactors and inertial devices, most of which find application in the fields of environmental and occupational health [57–61].

Most cascade impactors do not give data in real time. The collection surfaces must be removed from the device and subjected to chemical or gravimetric analysis. However, one impactor does give data in real time. The Model PC-2 Air Particle Analyzer (California Measurements, Inc., Sierra Madre, CA) achieves a real-time measurement by using piezoelectric quartz crystal microbalance (QCM) mass sensors to electronically weigh particles at each impactor stage [62,63]. The device has 10 stages and separates the aerosol into

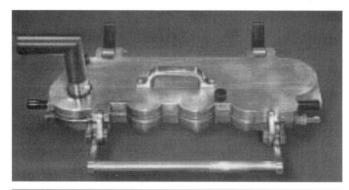

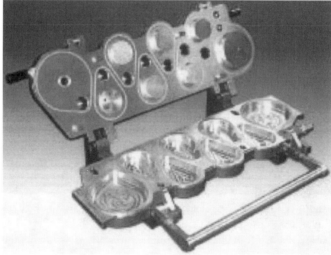

FIGURE 9 Next Generation Cascade Impactor, showing some of the unique design features intended to render the system automatable.

fractions between 25 and 0.5 μm. Its lower stages operate at reduced pressures to accurately separate smaller particles. Fig. 10 shows the arrangement operating portions of the device at a single stage. Only one of two unsealed crystals collects particles. The other acts as a reference to null out temperature and humidity effects. The frequency difference between the crystals is the QCM signal, and it changes in proportion to particle collection on the sensing crystal. A microcomputer process the QCM signals and provides the data output in a printout. An additional advantage of this device is that the crystals at each stage may be removed and subjected to scanning electron microscopy and energy-dispersive x-ray spectroscopy without disturbing the sample.

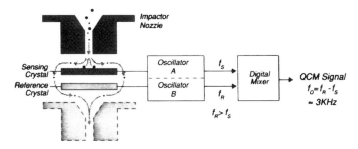

FIGURE 10 Schematic of the Quartz Crystal Microbalance Sensor System. (With permission of California Measurements, Inc.)

Limitations of Cascade Impactors

Humidity. Winkler [64] showed that in atmospheric relative humidities greater than 75% adhesion of particles to the plates is good, but in drier air, less than 75% relative humidity, there is often a loss of particles. He also studied [65] the growth of various particles with rising humidity, demonstrating the very important point that particles of mixed constitution, as found in the atmosphere, gradually increase in weight. Another complication is the effect on cascade impactor performance of the growth of particles. Hanel and Gravenhorst [66] showed theoretically that the cutoff radius can nearly double over the whole range of humidity. The number of particles per stage is not affected to the same extent, and the problem is eliminated at relative humidities less than 70% [67,68]. This effect has been used to investigate hygroscopic growth of aerosol particles [69].

Overload. The tendency to overload the collection surface in the small-particle stages in an attempt to collect measurable sample masses has been observed [67]. Attempts to avoid this problem by the use of adhesive layers or fibrous filters on the impaction plates create other, unanticipated complications [51,57,70–73].

Sampling. Sampling practices play an important role in particle size characterization using cascade impactors. Short-duration sampling may result in unrepresentative size estimates [74]. This is also the case for anisokinetic sampling [19].

Impingers

Impingers were the first devices operating on a dynamic principle to be adopted for aerosol sampling and particle characterization by the *British Pharmacopoeia* (BP) [75]. The data derived from these devices are intended to reflect the fraction of a pressurized inhalation aerosol emitted dose with a particle size likely to result in its deposition in the lower airways. The particles passing to the lower portion of the device are considered to be respirable. As such, this is the therapeutically desirable fraction of the aerosol. The two devices described in the BP operate on slightly different principles [75]. Apparatus A is a liquid impinger and requires solvent in both chambers to collect the aerosol. Apparatus B is a virtual impactor that uses a sintered glass disk and glass fiber filter to collect the two aerosol fractions. The liquid impinger has frequently appeared in the literature [76–80]. These devices are illustrated schematically in Fig. 11.

These types of devices are not a recent development, and the debate over their value in comparison with a cascade impactor was evident 25 years ago [5]. Knowing the respirable mass fraction of an aerosol, derived from an impinger, does not inform the investigator of the total size distribution as derived from cascade impaction. Of note, the respirable fraction as estimated by the inertial impingers, BP Apparatus A, has been correlated with the clinical performance of bronchodilator aerosols [81]. In the debate concerning the merits of the two impingers, their recommended use may need to be drug specific. Table 1 [82] shows data for the deposition of sodium cromoglycate (Intal) in vivo [83,84] and in vitro. This illustrates the capacity of the BP Apparatus B to reproduce the estimated dose of this drug to the lung, unlike Apparatus A. Two-stage impinger methods have given way to cascade impaction as a routine method of evaluating pharmaceutical aerosols. A more sophisticated impinger, the four-stage system (with cutoff diameters of 13.3, 6.7, 3.2, and 1.7 μm at a flowrate of 60 L/min) has been adopted for evaluation of dry powder aerosols [85]. Its value lies in the fact

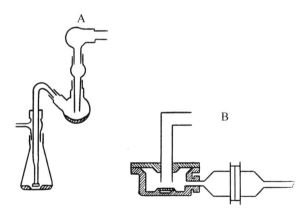

FIGURE 11   Diagrams of apparatus (A) twin impinger and (B) metal impinger as described Condenser Lens in the *British Pharmacopoeia*. (From Ref. 98, with permission of Fisons Corp.)

TABLE 1 Comparison of the Metal Impinger and Twin Impinger for the Dispersion Analysis Secondary Electron Detector of Intal (Sodium Cromoglycate) Metered-Dose Inhalers

Formulation	In vivo % in lung	In vitro % "fine" particles	
		Metal impinger	Liquid impinger
Intal (1 mg)	11.0	25	33
Intal (5 mg)	8.8	20	9
Dose[a]	4.0	4.0	1.36

[a] Dose $= (\% \times 5\,mg)/(\% \times 1\,mg)$.
Source: Ref. 100.

that the additional stages give more information regarding the particle size distribution, and the liquid sampling avoids re-entrainment of particles [54].

MICROSCOPY TECHNIQUES

The microscope uses lenses to magnify and focus the image of objects that are beyond the resolution of the human eye. These lenses may be optical, as in the case of the light microscope, or electromagnetic, as in the case of the electron microscope. The practical limit to the resolution of the image of a particular object is dependent on the wavelength of light or the energy of emitted electrons. Fig. 12 shows schematic diagrams of the complex optical microscope and the scanning electron microscope [86].

Particle Collection

Filtration is a suitable method for the collection of aerosols for microscopy, as mentioned previously. Particles may also be collected using inertial devices and may be examined by microscopy [73]. A third method that has not been mentioned is electrostatic precipitation, or sampling.

Electrostatic Precipitation

Electrostatic precipitators collect particles that may subsequently be examined by microscopy. The method precipitates particles according to the charge they carry. The aerosol is passed between two plates or surfaces across which is a large potential difference. Deposition occurs as a function of the ratio of the charge to the inertia (mass and velocity) of the particles [87]. The principle on which this method is based considers the motion of particles in planes directly perpendicular to and parallel to the plane of the condenser [88].

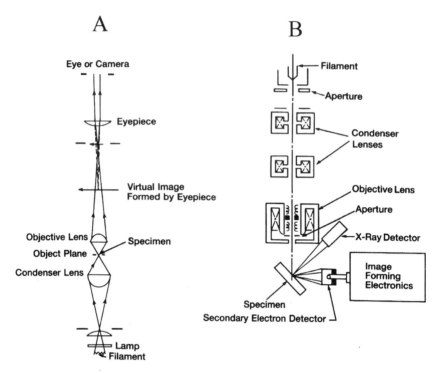

FIGURE 12 Schematic of (A) compound optical and (B) combined scanning electron microscope–microprobe analyzer. (From Ref. 82, with permission of VCH Publishers, Inc.)

The charge on a particle may originate in various ways. In crushing powders, the particles receive electric charges, as might occur in jet milling; the atomization of liquids produces droplets that are charged owing to fluctuations in the concentration of ions in the liquid, such as occurs in nebulization; aerosols formed at high temperature are charged by thermoionic emission; and precipitation of gaseous ions and electrons or aerosol particles produces charges. At the moment when aerosols are formed, particles may be highly charged, but, whatever the initial distribution of charges, a stationary state is gradually approached due to precipitation of the particles or ions that are constantly being formed.

The TSI Model 3100 Electrostatic Aerosol Sampler collects and deposits particles ranging from 0.02 to 10 μm onto a collection substrate. It does not collect large samples quickly. The samples may be collected directly onto glass slides, metal foil, plastic sheets, or coated electron microscope grids.

This has the advantage of eliminating the hazard of contaminating the samples during transport. Fig. 13 shows a diagram of the arrangement of the instrument. The aerosol is drawn into the chamber of the instrument at a rate of 5 L/min, which must be precalibrated by the operator. Positive ions are generated by corona discharge from a fine, positively charged tungsten wire. As aerosol passes through the charging section, intermittent pulses of these ions impart a positive charge to the particles. The intermittent pulses are produced by an alternating voltage. During the negative phase, positive ions mingle with aerosol particles that, in turn, become positively charged. As the aerosol leaves the charging section, it enters the collecting section. If no voltage difference exists between the top and bottom of the collecting section, the aerosol passes through and does not deposit. In the instrument's intermittent, precipitation mode, particles are located on the substrate in an unbiased (by morphological characteristics, including particle size) manner during collection. The sampler applies a positive square-wave voltage to the upper polished charging plate. The positive square wave is "on" for 1.5 sec and "off" for 3 sec per cycle. The lower plate remains at ground potential. When the square wave is "off," the particles pass through the collection section in the airflow. When the square wave is "on," the particles migrate from the upper to the lower plate. While the positive precipitating voltage is "on" (not in the intermittent mode), particles that are entering the collection section deposit, predominantly according to size and shape. There is an area on the

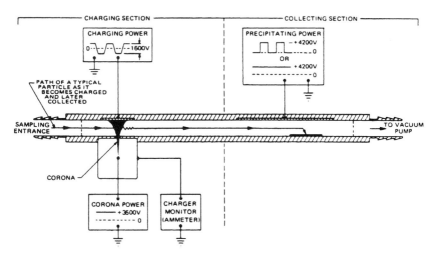

FIGURE 13 Schematic of an electrostatic precipitator. (With permission of TSI, Inc.)

lower plate that is unbiased by these particle characteristics, and it is marked for the convenience of the investigator. The preferential deposition at the entrance does not exhibit the sensitivity required for this to be useful as a particle-sizing technique per se. Particle deposition in the entrance region is concentrated enough to allow collection for chemical or radioactivity analysis. Particle sizing must be performed using an independent technique, such as optical or electron microscopy [89].

Light Microscopy

Traditionally, particles were sized by "looking at them." Initially, as indicated by early pharmaceutical requirements [90,91], the compound, transmission light, microscope, and its various corollaries were used. These include bright- and dark-field, polarized, reflectance (incident), differential-interference, and phase-contrast illuminations. These techniques pose some immediate questions of data interpretation. Heywood [92,93] was one of the first investigators to suggest that to avoid the complexities of shape, a standard should be adopted that normalized the image of the particle to circular disks of equivalent area. Specialized graticules were developed in which circular disks were placed in the field of view of the microscope for direct comparison with the particle being examined [9,19,94]. Fig. 14 shows one example of the numerous similar graticules that were developed.

There are many limitations to this technique. It is a subjective measure that is open to observer errors. The time taken to measure individual particles in this way restricts the total number of size estimates that can be collected, allowing statistical errors to occur [95]. Indeed, the American Society for Testing and Materials (ASTM) recommends that the modal class of the size distribution should contain at least 100 particles and that at least 10 particles should be present in each size class [96]. Another approach, that of "stratified sampling," recommends at least 10 particles in every size class that has a significant influence on the size curve [97]. Microscopy, as a static method, can identify irregular shapes but cannot fully predict their effects on particle behavior. Similarly, it does not take into account density, which plays a role in the dynamic behavior of particles. Both of these factors influence aerosols entering the lung [98]. There are practical limits to the accuracy of measurements. The resolution of the optical microscopes make them suitable for measurement of particles 1 μm or larger in size. Finally, microscopy examines particles in their plane of maximum stability, and this two-dimensional view may not accurately reflect the three dimensions of the particle.

Image-splitting optical microscopy was developed to reduce observer error [Watson image-shearing eyepiece [4], Fleming particle size analyzer [99]]. These

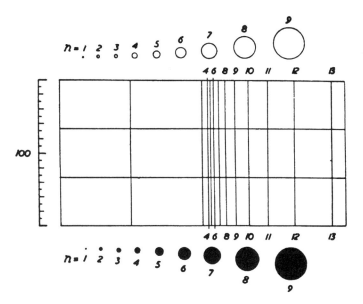

FIGURE 14 Diagram of the modified Patterson–Cawood globe and circle graticule used for counting and sizing particles. (From Ref. 7, with permission of the *Journal of Scientific Instrumentation.*)

methods use mirrors or prisms that may be combined with a video camera to create two images of the particles being viewed. One image may be displaced with respect to the other, which remains stationary. By displacing the particle image so that its opposite sides touch (i.e., moving the right edge to touch the left edge of the stationary particle, or vice versa), the distance the image is moved represents a measure of the particle size. This method is still limited by the resolution of the microscope, although the subjectivity of the estimate of the particle size is much reduced.

The wavelength of the visible spectrum used in optical microscopy, 400–700 nm [100], is much larger than that of an electron of Compton wavelength, 0.386 pm [101]. Materials approaching in size the wavelength of the energy form used will have a reduced tendency to absorb or interfere with its path. Ultimately, a limit to detection, where no absorbance or interference occurs, will be reached in which the material will become essentially "invisible." It is apparent that this will happen at much larger sizes for visible light, photons, than for electrons. Indeed, there is an approximately 1000-fold difference between the two techniques. Thus, electron microscopy allows greater resolution and, in turn, magnification than optical microscopy.

Electron Microscopy

Scanning electron microscopy is open to some error due to the gold-, palladium-, or platinum-coating methods used [86]. The coating not only adds slightly to size of the particles but may mask morphological features that could influence particle behavior. Transmission electron microscopy does not exhibit this drawback. Figure 15 shows scanning and transmission electron micrographs of samples from the same population of particles. The particles appear relatively smooth by scanning electron microscopy and rough by transmission electron microscopy. The smoothness in this instance may be an artifact of gold coating, which in this case may have allowed greater definition of surface morphology. However, this example is given to indicate the care in preparation and the caution that should be exercised in interpreting electron micrographs.

The major advantage of microscopic methods is their direct measurement of particle size. In many of the alternative methods, at least one automated data-interpretation or calculation step is inserted between the instrumental analysis and establishing the estimate of particle size. This reduces the subjectivity of the measurement while increasing the likelihood of interpretive errors.

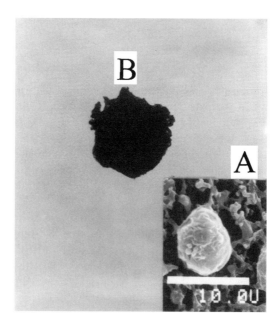

FIGURE 15   (A) Scanning and (B) transmission electron micrographs of particles from the same population, indicating the smoothing effect of gold coating in the scanning electron micrograph.

Image Analysis

One of the earliest imaging systems to be used in conjunction with microscopy was the Quantimet Model 720 system, an automated image analyzer [102,103]. The pattern recognition modules of the image-analyzing computer allowed features to be classified by orientation-independent size criteria, such as area and perimeter. By application of a wide range of complex shape, size, and density criteria, it was also possible to separate features by shape.

More recently, the Brinkmann Model 2010, shown schematically in Fig. 16, has been used for "on-line" determinations of particle size. It combines a scanning laser and particle size analyzer, based on time of transition, with a shape analyzer. A video camera takes still images every 3 sec. Samples in any state can be measured by interchanging sample modules. The He–Ne laser beam passes through a rotating wedge prism that rotates the beam. The rotating beam goes through the sample and falls on a photodiode that measures beam intensity. When a particle interrupts the beam, the time of interaction, along with the rotational speed of the beam, can be translated into the particle diameter.

Shape Factors and Particle Morphology

Image analysis techniques have also been used to derive information concerning particle shape. The topic of shape factors and particle morphology has been of considerable interest to aerosol scientists. Some particle measurement techniques require a correction factor that accounts for the particle shape, to allow interpretation of the data. A range of approaches have resulted in a number of shape-factor definitions, many of which have been named after their proponents. The most recent approaches to assessing shape factors appear to derive from Fourier or fractal analysis of particle boundaries. It is impossible to do justice to the wealth of literature on this subject in this brief discussion. However, some references are given that may be reviewed at leisure [104–119]. Many physicochemical factors, such as surface area, density, charge, and wettability, are related to the particle surface, and these have implications for particle flow, aggregation, aerodynamic, and dissolution behavior. The shape of particles is known to play an important role in the generation, deposition, and therapeutic activity of aerosol particles [118–121]. The impact of shape on the investigation of materials that pose a respirable hazard suggests that this may be a useful approach pharmaceutically [112]. It is, therefore, worth considering the information on particle shape that is available from image analysis [122].

Other instruments using principles similar to those described previously are the Optomax V image analysis system (Optomax, Burlington, MA) and Imageplus (Dapple Systems, Sunnyvale, CA). This is by no means a comprehensive list of companies supplying equipment of this nature.

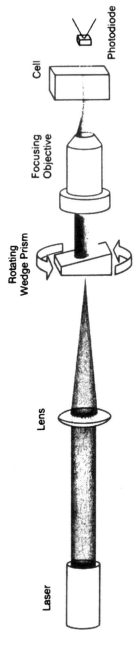

FIGURE 16 Schematic of the laser optic measuring system used in an imaging analyzer. (With permission of Brinkmann Instruments.)

LIGHT-SCATTERING METHODS

Young's observation that the maxima and minima in a shadow behind an obstacle were caused by interference waves began the interest in the phenomenon of light scattering early in the nineteenth century. In the latter part of the nineteenth century, Maxwell developed the electromagnetic theory of light that linked electrical and optical phenomena. Lord Rayleigh used the new theory of electromagnetic radiation to investigate the scattering of white light by small particles. He formulated an approximation applying to very small particles whose refractive index was small. In order for Rayleigh scattering to apply, the particles also must be small in comparison to the wavelength of the radiation. Rayleigh's approximation is valid for particles of diameter less than one-tenth the wavelength of the incident light. This restriction assumes that the particle has a uniform internal field when the wave passes through, resulting in only one scattering center.

Light scattering was further investigated by Mie, who published his complete theory in 1908. Unlike Rayleigh scattering, Mie accounted for the complete light-scattering pattern by taking into account the electric field inside and outside the particle. As particles increase from 0.10 to 10 times the wavelength of the incident radiation, scattering occurs from more than one point in a single particle and is out of phase. This results in interference and reduced light intensity. The scattering of light was calculated as a power series that takes into consideration the different angles of scattering, wavelength of incident light, differences in refractive indices, and the diameter of a sphere. The Mie theory, unlike the Rayleigh approximation and Debye approximations, may be applied to absorbing and nonabsorbing particles. Although the Mie theory could be used to determine particle size distributions, the calculations are so complex that it was not feasible until the advent of the computer.

Debye's approximation was published in 1909, and it applies to slightly larger particles than the Rayleigh approximation but to a narrower range of refractive indices. As the particle size approaches the wavelength of the incident radiation, different regions of the same particle will behave as scattering centers. There will be interference between the waves of light scattered from the same particle. Therefore, the Rayleigh approximation must be multiplied by a correction factor to account for the interference. This approach accounts for particles with more than two scattering centers and recognizes the tendency for the number of centers to increase with particle size. It also considers that coordinates must be described by a radial distance and two angles.

Another approximation that can be applied to particles larger than the Rayleigh region is the Rayleigh–Gans approximation. For Rayleigh scattering, the vertical components of scattered light remain constant. However, as the particle size increases, the light intensity is inversely proportional to the angle to observation and passes through a minimum. This requires radiation to undergo a small phase shift when passing through the particle. The addition of the phase shift term results in an asymmetric scattering pattern about 90°.

For particles approaching the wavelength of light, the complex Mie theory is required. However, for much larger particles, the contribution of the radiation refracted within the particle diminishes in relation to the radiation diffracted external to the particle. Furthermore, the amount diffracted is independent of the particle's refractive index because it involves rays external to the particle. When particles are four or five times greater than the wavelength of the incident radiation, Mie theory can be reduced to the simpler Fraunhofer diffraction theory. This theory explains that the intensity of light scattered by a particle is proportional to the particle size, whereas the size of the diffraction pattern is inversely proportional to the particle size. Fraunhofer determined that a central stop blocked light proportional to the fourth power of the particle diameter. The transmission filter permitted scattering light proportional to the volume, or third power, of the particle diameter to be measured.

Rayleigh scattering, the Rayleigh–Gans and Debye theories, and diffraction are all well-known limiting cases to the complex Mie theory of light scattering. Two inventions contributed significantly to the use of light scattering for particle analysis. These were the laser, in 1961, and the computer, in the late 1960s. The computer was necessary to perform the manipulations required by Mie theory. The laser was important because it provided coherent monochromatic light of high intensity that allowed the development of dynamic-scattering techniques. Pusey was responsible for the development of the scattering theory concerning lasers. *Coherent* light means that the phase relationships in a beam are maintained, and random diffraction patterns are formed after striking the particles. The particles in the array are undergoing Brownian motion, and the fluctuations in the scattered light give information about the particle size. The particles are diffusing around their equilibrium positions, resulting in a fluctuation in the number of scattering centers seen by the photodetector. The spectrometer analyzes these fluctuations and obtains the diffusion coefficient, which is related to the particle diameter by the Stokes–Einstein equation.

Calibration

Calibration of optical devices is most frequently performed using polystyrene latex spheres that can be generated from dilute aqueous suspensions and dried before measurement. The ASTM developed a standard for the use of reticles, or disks, that can be placed in the path of the beam of a laser diffraction device for the purpose of calibration. Some manufacturers maintain that their instruments do not require calibration. The "calibration" step may then be regarded as a verification of the alignment of the optics of the instrument.

Forward Light-Scattering Particle Counters

Hodgkinson's [123] exposition on the optical measurement of aerosols, though dated with respect to instrumentation, contains an excellent review of the theoretical aspects of this subject. Fig. 17 illustrates a classic forward light-scattering arrangement.

Optical particle counters have been used for a number of years. The forward scattering of light minimizes the effects of shape and refractive index. The Royco 4100 series (4101 and 4102, Royco Instruments, Inc., Menlo Park, CA) use the near forward light-scatter region (7–17°) and, thus, have the previously mentioned advantage [124,125]. The Royco 4130 and Climet 7000 series (Climet instrument Co., Redlands, CA) minimize the effects of shape and refractive index by using an ellipsoid mirror to collect light scattered from the forward direction [126]. Older models of the Royco and Climet devices, the Royco 220 and Climet 208, are described in detail by Allen [4]. The PMS ASASP-X laser aerosol spectrometer system (Particle Measuring Systems, Inc., Boulder, CO) uses a parabolic mirror to collect all light scattered by a particle over an angular region (35–120°) [127,128]. The particle diameter obtained by these techniques is a projected area diameter. Each of these devices has a small sensing volume, for example, 2.63 mm^3 for the Royco 220 [4] and 0.004 mm^3 for the PMS ASASP-X [127,128]. Each of these manufacturers markets a number of devices, each targeted at the measurement of airborne particles in a specific size range. Table 2 lists some of the instruments that may be of interest for pharmaceutical purposes. Additional instruments measure particles up to 5.0 μm, for example, Models Turbo-110 and Micro LPCA (PMS), 5120 (Hiac/Royco), CI-7400 (Climet), and 3755 laser particle counter (TSI, St. Paul, MN). However, this does not cover the entire size range of interest for therapeutic purposes. Of note, many of these instruments are designed for use in cleanrooms where monitoring and environmental control of submicrometer particles are the greatest concerns.

Laser Diffraction

As indicated, Fraunhofer diffraction is a special case of Mie theory that can be used to obtain the volume of particles. The Malvern Instruments Model 2600c series of sizers (Malvern Instruments, Southborough, MA) use a laser diffraction method. The instruments are equipped with an IBM-compatible computer that controls the collection, manipulation, and presentation of data. The principle of operation is illustrated in Fig. 18. The instruments consist of a low-power laser transmitter and receiver detector units mounted 50 cm apart. Particles or spray

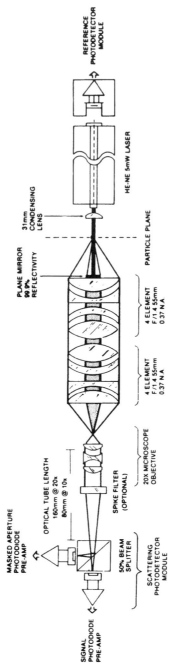

FIGURE 17   Classic forward light-scattering instruments. (With permission of Particle Measuring Systems, Inc.)

TABLE 2 Manufacturers and Specifications of Some Light-Scattering Instruments

| | Manufacturer and model | | | | | |
| | Particle-measuring systems | | | HIAC/Royco | | Climet |
	LAS-250X	CSASP-100	5130	5250	4130	CI-7300
Size range (μm)	0.2–12	0.3–20	0.3–10	0.5–25	0.3–15	0.3–10
Channels (n)	15 (+1)	15	6	8	6	6
Resolution (μm)	0.1	0.03	0.1	0.5	0.3	0.3
Sampling flow rate (L/min)	2.83	0.08	28.3	28.3	28.3	28.3
Light source	He–Ne laser	He–Ne laser	He–Ne laser	Laser diode	He–Ne laser	Quartz halogen polychromatic
Optics	Parabolic mirror collects 35–120°	Near forward-angle scatter	Wide-angle 90° scattering	Near forward-angle scatter	Elipsoid mirror collects 30–170°	Elipsoid mirror collects 15–150°

droplets passing through the laser beam scatter light that is focused on a ring diode array detector. Each detector is radially optimized for a particular band size. The output signal is digitized and converted into a particle size distribution by means of the integral computer. Depending on the configuration of the instrument, the size range that can be measured is $0.5-300\ \mu m$ for dry powders and $0.5-1800\ \mu m$ for sprays. Results are presented in 32 size classes. The instrument can be arranged to synchronize the spray and data collection. This has been specifically developed to analyze metered-dose inhalers. The data are expressed in terms of volume percentiles. However, other statistical diameters are calculated. The data are manipulated so that many of the parameters that are of interest are automatically available to the investigator.

Laser Doppler Velocimetry
Jet Acceleration

Laser Doppler velocimetry may be used in a decelerating flow where the aerosol particles are traveling at low speed [129]. However, accelerating the particles through a jet or nozzle seems the most popular method among instrument manufacturers. The principle of using a nozzle to accelerate particles and laser Doppler velocimetry to measure the particle velocity near the nozzle exit is seen as a rapid method for determining the aerodynamic diameter [130,131]. This technique eliminates the time-consuming analysis required to obtain the same parameter by cascade impactor or impinger.

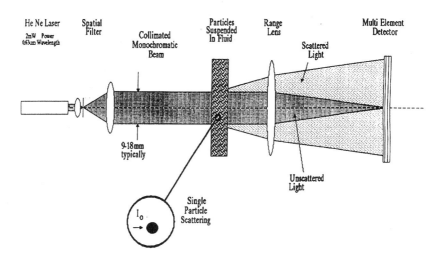

FIGURE 18   Principle of operation of a Fraunhofer diffraction laser particle sizer. (With permission of Malvern Instruments, Inc.)

The TSI Model APS34 powder-sizing system, shown in Fig. 19, measures powders dispersed in air and measures aerodynamic diameter. It is combination of the TSI Model 3433 disperser and Model APS33B aerodynamic particle sizer. The Model APS33B aerodynamic particle sizer, as its name suggests, can be used independently to size aerosol powders and sprays. A time-of-flight measurement technique is used where larger particles have a greater inertia and, thus, longer transit times than smaller particles. Particles accelerate and cross a two-spot laser velocimeter. A photomultiplier collects the scattered-light pulses generated by particles crossing the laser beams and activates a high-speed digital clock. There are 58 channels that collect transit times and calculate the size distribution. It can accurately measure particles from 0.5 to 30 μm. The operating flowrate is 5 L/min.

The Malvern API Aerosizer (Malvem Instruments Ltd., Southborough, MA) operates on the principle of supersonic flow in a jet, followed by laser Doppler velocimetry to measure the aerodynamic diameter of particles in the size range from 0.5 to 200 μm using 50 channels. The operating flowrate is 6 L/min. The Atcor Net-2000 is a similar device for determining aerodynamic diameter, except that it is capable of sizing particles up to only 5.0 μm in diameter at a flowrate of 0.1 ft^3/min (2.83 L/min).

The Insitee particle velocimeters include PCSV-E and PCSV-P, which provide two independent measurement volumes. The PCSV-E has three configurations, is nonintrusive, and can span a flow of stream up to 1.5 in diameter. The PCSV-P extends measurement to a larger scale. Both operate using a low-power He−Ne laser that illuminates particles, and a photomultiplier then measures the scattered light from each particle. The amplitude of the scattered-light signal is dependent on the particle size as well as the trajectory. A deconvolution algorithm solves the sizing ambiguity and is capable of sizing particles from 0.2 to 200 μm.

Acoustic Vibration

Laser Doppler velocimetry has been combined with acoustic excitation to allow the derivation of the relaxation time for particles, from which the aerodynamic diameter can be calculated [132–136]. The particle relaxation time is derived from the velocity amplitude of the aerosol particle and that of the medium while the aerosol is subjected to acoustic excitation of a known frequency. A differential laser Doppler velocimeter is used to measure the velocity amplitude of the particle, and a microphone is used to measure the velocity amplitude of the medium. The aerodynamic diameter of the particle can be derived from the relaxation time and the known particle density. The method can be applied to real-time in situ measurement of the size distribution of an aerosol containing both solid and liquid droplets in the diameter range of 0.1–10 μm.

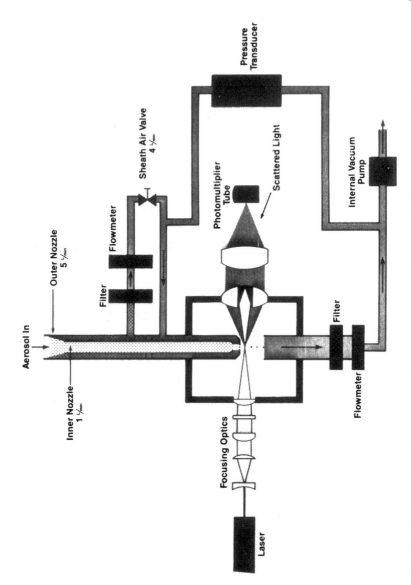

FIGURE 19 Principle of operation of laser Doppler velocimetry (LDV) instrument. (With permission TSI, Inc.)

Limitations to Laser Techniques

Most laser techniques are not capable of examining the entire aerosol. This means that the sampling technique must be included in the interpretation of the data obtained. Isokinetic sampling is imperative, and sampling conditions must, therefore, be considered of the utmost importance [19]. During the measurement of the particle size by this method, the aerosol does not encounter an impaction surface as is the case during inhalation. Thus, the assignment of a particle size representing the nominal cutoff for the respirable fraction does not have the same meaning as the same size in inertial sizing systems. It is likely that some of the small particles are removed from the airstream in the upper airways by aggregation, droplet coalescence, and impaction. This is not mimicked by the laser technique. The laser technique will, however, give some insight into droplet dynamics during passage from the actuator. Therefore, it is possible to investigate the size as a function of the time after leaving the actuator, which will result in information concerning the dynamics of evaporation and aggregation effects.

PHARMACEUTICAL PRODUCT ASSESSMENT

The consideration of major importance in the use of various particle measurement techniques for the assessment of pharmaceutical aerosols is the method of sampling. Unlike most aerosols for which the sizing techniques were originally developed, pharmaceutical aerosols occur in very high concentrations in the carrier airstream. Additionally, the particle size may vary as a function of the position of sampling of the aerosol with respect to the generating orifice or mechanism. Because this is also the case when aerosols are presented to the patient for inhalation, the importance of the design of the sampling port may not be in obtaining the "absolute" or equilibrium particle or droplet size. It is, perhaps, of more significance to estimate the particle size of the aerosol as it would be presented to the patient or the lung. There are a variety of physiological parameters to consider in a true model of this situation. Thus, a pragmatic approach is to adopt a geometry for the sampling port that results in realistic estimates of the respirable fraction as defined by a correspondence with pulmonary deposition or bioequivalence studies. The sampling port does not necessarily require dimensions bearing any relationship to the upper respiratory tract [137]. This is still a topic of much debate that is unlikely to find its solution in a single method. As with most approaches to scientific discovery, the use of a number of methods will yield a broad database, enabling the investigator to make informed judgments with respect to optimizing the dosage form.

SUMMARY

A number of methods are available for estimating the particle or droplet size of pharmaceutical aerosols.

1. The aerosol output may be sized using inertial techniques. These methods may involve impaction, centrifugation, or sedimentation. The most popular techniques for the assessment of the particle size of pharmaceutical aerosols are techniques that use a filter, impactor, or impinger.
2. The particles can be visualized using optical or electron microscopy, and specific dimensions can be measured with less subjectivity. The advent of computers also allows particles to be sized by image analysis techniques based on optical or electron photomicrographs.
3. Laser-scattering techniques have been used in a variety of operational modes to size pharmaceutical aerosols. These may be listed as forward scattering, Fraunhofer diffraction, and laser Doppler velocimetry, in conjunction with either accelerating nozzles or acoustic excitation.

These techniques use different operating principles and often express the size of the particles according to different definitions. It is important that the investigator understand the size parameter being measured. It is valuable to estimate particle size using different techniques to obtain a broad view of the behavioral characteristics of an aerosol. For this reason, the pharmaceutical aerosol scientist should combine techniques from the previously mentioned groups.

PERSPECTIVE ON RESEARCH SINCE THE EARLY 1990s

There has been significant research in the area of particle size characterization of pharmaceutical aerosols since the early 1990s. The focus has been not only on methods but on data presentation, analysis, and requirements for regulatory submissions.

A series of review articles were published by the Inhalation Technology Focus Group of the American Association of Pharmaceutical Scientists describing the range of methods that have been employed to measure the particle size of pharmaceutical inhalation aerosols. These methods include: microscopy [138], impingers [139], impactors [140], holography [141], laser light techniques, including right-angle light scattering [142], time-of-flight [143], diffraction [144], and phase Doppler anemometry [145]. New instruments have been developed, including the Next Generation Inertial Impactor, which has been designed for ease of use [56]. With regard to laser optical techniques, one of the most significant advances is the use of Mie theory in the algorithm for laser diffraction rather than Fraunhofer, which had been employed for almost two decades. Nevertheless, the debate surrounding the appropriateness of the methods, diffraction, time-of-flight, phase Doppler analysis, etc. continues. It is as relevant now as in early '90s to remind the reader of the complementary nature of all sizing methods. There is a need for regulatory and pharmacopoeial standards on which to base the quality of the product, but for development purposes the more approaches that are used to evaluate the product the better is the understanding of its true nature.

Data presentation had rarely been the subject of scrutiny in the years prior to the previous edition of this book. However, in the intervening years it has become clear that no single mathematical fit approximates all particle size distributions [146]. Consequently, the suitability of a log-normal distribution must be assessed prior to deriving the standard parameters of median diameter and geometric standard deviation to describe the data. Moreover, if there is no good mathematical fit to the data, alternative analyses that do not invoke a model may be more appropriate. Under these circumstances, simply stating a fine particle mass (fraction) in addition to the median diameter or presenting the data in blocks of size ranges may be more meaningful. Indeed, the latter approach may be less misleading to any reviewer than using descriptors of a distribution that may be a poor approximation to the raw data.

Following the debate surrounding sampling by inertial impaction in the early 1990s, the apparatus required for propellant-driven metered-dose inhalers and dry powder inhalers has been specified by the USP [33] and EP [147]. In addition, the FDA has issued guidelines on the methods to be employed for both pulmonary and nasal delivery products [148].

REFERENCES

1. Group IP. Pharm J 1990; 244:22.
2. Hickey AJ, Jones LD. Pharm Technol 2000; 24:48–58.
3. Davies CN. J Aerosol Sci 1979; 10:477.
4. Allen T. Particle Size Measurement. London: Chapman and Hall, 1981:103.
5. Hatch TF, Gross P. Pulmonary Deposition and Retention of Inhaled Aerosols. New York: Academic Press, 1964:27–43.
6. Fuchs NA, Sutugin AG. In: Davies CN, ed. Aerosol Science. New York: Academic Press, 1966:1–30.
7. May KR. J Aerosol Sci 1982; 13:37–47.
8. May KR. J Sci Instrum 1945; 22:187.
9. Green HL, Lane WR. Particulate Clouds, Dusts, Smokes and Mists. London: E. and F.N. Spon, 1964:258.
10. Mitchell RI, Pilcher JM. Ind Eng Chem 1959; 51:1039.

11. Martonen T, Clark M, Nelson D, Willard D, Rossignol E. Fundam Appl Toxicol 1982; 2:149–152.

12. Lundgren DA, Balfour WD. J Aerosol Sci 1982; 13:181–184.

13. Rao AK,. In: Lundgren DA, Lippmann M, Harris FS, Clark WE, Marlow WH, Durham MD, eds. Aerosol Measurement. Gainesville, FL: University Presses of Florida, 1979:117.

14. Reist PC. Introduction to Aerosol Science. New York: Macmillan, 1984:80.

15. Marple VA, Willeke K. In: Lundgren DA, Lippmann M, Harris FS, Clark WE, Marlow WH, Durham MD, eds. Aerosol Measurement, Gainesville. FL: University Presses of Florida, 1979:90.

16. Zaiacomo TD, Tarroni G, Prodi V, Melandri C, Formignani M, et al. J Aerosol Sci 1983; 14:314.

17. Odgen TL, Birkett JL. In: Walton WH, ed. Inhaled Particles. Oxford: Pergamon Press, 1977:93.

18. Marple VA. J Aerosol Sci 1978; 9:125–134.

19. Hinds WC. Aerosol Technology: Properties, Behavior, and Measurement of Airborne Particles, Second Edition. New York: Wiley, 1999.

20. Leong KH. In: Hickey AJ, ed. Pharmaceutical Inhalation Aerosol Technology. New York: Marcel Dekker, 1992:129–154.

21. Berglund RN, Liu BYH. Environ Sci Technol 1973; 7:147–152.

22. Liu BYH. In: Lundgren DA, Lippmann M, Harris FS, Clark WE, Marlow WH, Durham MD, eds. Aerosol Measurement. Gainesville, FL: University Presses of Florida, 1979:40.

23. Byron PR, Hickey AJ. J Pharm Sci 1987; 76:60–64.

24. Mercer TT. Arch Intern Med 1973; 131:39–50.

25. Walton WH, Prewett WC. Proc Phys Soc 1949; 62:341.

26. Ranz WE, Wong JB. Ind Eng Chem 1952; 44:1371–1381.

27. Groom CV, Gonda I. J Pharm Pharmacol 1980; 32(suppl.):93.

28. Dorman RG. In: Davies CN, ed. Aerosol Science. New York: Academic Press, 1966:195.

29. Pich J. In: Davies CN, ed. Aerosol Science. New York: Academic Press, 1966:223.

30. Rance RW. J Soc Cosmet Chem 1974; 25:545–561.

31. Weber ME, Paddock D. J Colloid Interface Sci 1983; 94:328.

32. Pich J. In: Matteson MJ, Orr C, eds. Filtration Principles and Practices. New York: Marcel Dekker, 1987.

33. USP24. The United States Pharmacopoeia and National Formulary. 2000:1895–1912.

34. Hickey AJ, Swift D. In: Baron PA, Willeke K, eds. Aerosol Measurement: Principles, Techniques, and Applications. New York: Wiley, 2001:1031–1052.

35. Spurny K. Z Biol Aerosol-Forsch 1965; 12:369.

36. Spurny K. Z Biol Aerosol-Forsch 1966; 12:3.

37. Spurny K. Z Biol Aerosol-Forsch 1967; 13:398.

38. Spurny KR. In: Mercer TT, Morrow PE, Stober W, eds. Assessment of Airborne Particles: Fundamentals Applications and Implications to Inhalation Toxicity. Springfield, IL: Charles C Thomas, 1972:54.

39. Richards RT, Donovan DT, Hall JR. Am Ind Hyg Assoc J 1967; 28:590.
40. Division of Bioequivalence of the Food and Drug Administration. Informal communication under 21 CFR 10.90 (b)(9), 1989.
41. Hunke WA, Yu ABC. Am J Hosp Pharm 1987; 44:1392.
42. Hallworth GW, Andrews UG. J Pharm Pharmacol 1976; 28:898.
43. Kim CS, Trujillo D, Sackner MA. Am Rev Respir Dis 1985; 132:137–142.
44. Marple V, Willeke K. In: Liu BYH, ed. Fine Particles. New York: Academic Press, 1976.
45. Raabe OG. Environ Sci Technol 1978; 12:1162–1167.
46. Cooper DW. J Aerosol Sci 1982; 13:111–120.
47. Cooper DW, Spielman LA. Atmos Environ 1976; 10:723.
48. Gonda I, Kayes JB, Groom CV, Fildes FJT. In: Stanley-Wood N, Allen T, eds. Particle Size Analysis. New York: Wiley, 1982:31.
49. Carpenter RL, Barr EB. Am Ind Hyg Assoc J 1983; 44:268.
50. Vaughan NP. J Aerosol Sci 1989; 20:67–90.
51. Rao AK, Whitby KT. J Aerosol Sci 1978; 9:87–100.
52. Andersen AA. Am Ind Hyg Assoc J 1966;27.
53. Andersen AA. J Bacteriol 1958; 76:471.
54. Dunbar CA, Hickey AJ, Holzner P. KONA 1998; 16:7–44.
55. Miller NC. In Byron PR, Dalby RN, Farr SJ eds. Kespiratory Drug Delivery IV. Buffalo Grove, IL: Iterpharm Press, 1994:37.
56. Roberts DL, Romay FJ, Marple VA. Expected aerodynamic performance of commercial next generation pharmaceutical impactors. Presented at Respiratory Drug Delivery VIII, Tuscon, AZ, 2002.
57. Rao AK, Whitby KT. J Aerosol Sci 1978; 9:77–86.
58. Martonen TB. Am Ind Hyg Assoc J 1982; 43:154–159.
59. Hering SV, Flagan RC, Friedlander SK. Environ Sci Technol 1978; 12:667.
60. Lippmann M. In: Lundgren DA, Lippmann M, Harris FS, Clark WE, Marlow WH, Durham MD, eds. Aerosol Measurement. Gainesville, FL: University Presses of Florida, 1979:66.
61. Hsu SI. Atmos Environ 1983; 17:1029.
62. Chuan RL, Woods DC. Geophys Res Lett 1984; 11:553.
63. Chuan RL. In: Liu BYH, ed. Fine Particles. New York: Academic Press, 1976:763.
64. Winkler P. J Aerosol Sci 1974; 5:235.
65. Winkler P. J Aerosol Sci 1973; 4:373.
66. Hanel G, Gravenhorst G. J Aerosol Sci 1974; 5:47.
67. Esmen NA, Lee TC. Am Ind Hyg Assoc J 1980; 41:410.
68. Willeke K, McFeters JJ. J Colloid Interface Sci 1975; 53:121.
69. Hickey AJ, Gonda I, Irwin WJ, Fildes FJT. J Pharm Sci 1990; 79:1009 1014.
70. Jupe H, Richter F-W, Watjen U. J Aerosol Sci 1981; 12:218.
71. Boulaud D, Diouri M, Madelaine G. J Aerosol Sci 1982; 13:187.
72. Hickey AJ. Pharm Res 1988; 5:S247.
73. Hickey AJ. Drug Dev Ind Pharm 1990; 16:1911–1929.
74. Blyth DA, Picknett RG. Particle Size Analysis. London: Society for Analytical Chemistry, 1967:188.

75. Pharmacopoeia B. London: Her Majesty's Stationary Office, 1988:A204–A207.

76. Meakin BJ, Stroud N. J Pharm Pharmacol 1983; 35:7P.

77. Hallworth GW, Clough D, Newnham T, Andres UG. J Pharm Pharmacol 1978; 30(suppl.):39P.

78. Hickey AJ, Fults K, Cyr TD. Pharm Res 1989; 6:S-48.

79. Fults K, Cyr TD, Hickey AJ. Characterization of pharmaceutical aerosols using inertial collection devices. Presented at Proceedings of the Second World Congress on Particle Technology, Kyoto, Japan, 1990.

80. Phillips EM, Byron PR, Fults K, Hickey AJ. Pharm Res 1990; 7:1228–1233.

81. Padfield JM, Winterborn JK, Pover GM, Tattersfield A. J Pharm Pharmacol 1983; 35:10P.

82. Clarke AR. Particle size of metered dose inhalers—current methodologies. Presented at Aerosol Technology Committee of the American Association of Pharmaceutical Sciences Forum, Keystone, CO, March 30, 1990.

83. Newman SP, Clarke AR, Talaee N, Clarke SW. Thorax 1989; 44:706.

84. Newman SP, Clarke AR, Talaee N, Clarke SW. Thorax. In press.

85. Asking L, Olsson B. Aerosol Sci Technol 1997; 27:39–49.

86. Reimschuessel AC, Macur JE, Marti J. In: Sibilia JP, ed. A Guide to Materials Characterization and Chemical Analysis. New York: VCH, 1988.

87. Oglesby S, Nichols GB. Electrostatic Precipitation. New York: Marcel Dekker, 1978.

88. Fuchs NA. Mechanics of Aerosols. New York: Pergamon Press, 1964.

89. Liu BYH, Whitby KT, Yu HHS. Rev Sci Instrum 1967; 38:100.

90. British Pharmaceutical Codex. London: Pharmaceutical Press, 1968:80.

91. US Pharmacopoeia. Presented at U.S. Pharmacopoeia Convention, Rockville, MD, 1985.

92. Heywood H. Inst Chem Engl Suppl 1947; 25:14.

93. Heywood H. Trans Inst Min Metall 1945/1976; 55:391.

94. Guruswamy S. Particle Size Analysis. London: Society for Analytical Chemistry, 1967:29.

95. Stockham JD. In: Stockham JD, Fochtman EG, eds. Particle Size Analysis. Ann Arbor, MI: Ann Arbor Publishers, 1977.

96. American Society for Testing and Materials, Philadelphia: The Society, 1973:28.

97. Yamate G, Stockham J. In: Stockham JD, Fochtman EG, eds. Particle Size Analysis. Ann Arbor, MI: Ann Arbor Publishers, 1977:28.

98. Raabe OG. J Air Pollut Control Assoc 1976; 26:856–860.

99. Rance RW. J Soc Cosmet Chem 1972; 23:197–208.

100. Weast RC, ed. Handbook of Physics and Chemistry. Boca Raton, FL: CRC Press, 1985:E-194.

101. Weast RC, ed. Handbook of Physics and Chemistry. Boca Raton, FL: CRC Press, 1985:F-195.

102. Gibbard DW, Smith DJ, Wells A. Microscope 1972; 20:37–50.

103. Hallworth GW, Hamilton RR. J Pharm Pharmacol 1976; 28:890.

104. Beddow JK, Vetter AF, Sisson K. Powder Mettal Intern 1976; 8:69.

105. Beddow JK, Vetter AF, Sisson K. Powder Mettal Intern 1976; 8:107.

106. Beddow JK, Philip GC, Vetter AF, Nasta MD. Powder Technol 1977; 18:19–25.
107. Meloy TP. Powder Technol 1977; 17:27.
108. Flook AG. In: Stanley-Wood N, Allen T, eds. Particle Size Analysis. New York: Wiley, 1982:255.
109. Anvir D, Farin D, Pfeiffer P. Nature 1984; 308:261.
110. Pfeiffer P, Anvir D. J Chem Phys 1983; 79:3558.
111. Anvir D, Farin D, Pfeiffer P. J Chem Phys 1983; 79:3566.
112. Kaye BH. A Random Walk Through Fractal Dimensions. New York: VCH, 1989:95.
113. Kaye BH, Clark G. Particle Particle Syst Characterization 1989; 6:1.
114. Kaye BH. In: Stanley-Wood N, Allen T, eds. Particle Size Analysis. New York: Wiley, 1982:3.
115. Meakin P. Adv Colloid Interface Sci 1987; 28:263.
116. Mandelbrot BB. Fractal Geometry of Nature. San Francisco: Freeman, 1983.
117. Anvir D, ed. Fractal Structures in Heterogeneous Chemistry. New York: Wiley, 1989.
118. Chan HK, Gonda I. Int J Pharm 1985; 37:99.
119. Chan HK, Gonda I. Int J Pharm 1988; 41:147–157.
120. Chan HK, Gonda I. J Aerosol Sci 1989; 20:157.
121. Gonda I, Khalik AFAE. Aerosol Sci Technol 1983; 4:233.
122. Tohno S, Takahashi K. KONA 1988; 6:2.
123. Hogkinson JR. In: Davies CN, ed. Aerosol Science. New York: Academic Press, 1966:287.
124. Davies PJ, Muxworthy EM, Pickett JM, Smith GA. J Pharm Pharmacol 1978; 30(suppl):40P.
125. Ettinger HJ, DeField JD, Bevis DA, Mitchell RN. Am Ind Hyg Assoc J 1969; 30:20.
126. Ho AT, Bell KA. J Aerosol Sci 1981; 12:239.
127. Hinds WC, Macher JM, First MW. Am Ind Hyg Assoc J 1983; 44:495.
128. Hinds WC, Macher JM, First MW. J Environ Sci 1982; 25:20.
129. Russo AJ, Hackett CE, Croll RH. Rev Sci Instrum 1979; 50:1391–1395.
130. Wilson JC, Liu BYH. J Aerosol Sci 1980; 11:139–150.
131. Agarwal JK, Remiarz RJ, Quant FR, Sem GJ. J Aerosol Sci 1982; 13:222.
132. Mazumder MK, Wilson JD, Wankum DL, Cole R, Northrop GM, et al. In: Crapo JD, Smolko ED, Miller FJ, Graham JA, Hayes AW, eds. Extrapolation of Dosimetric Relationships for Inhaled Particles and Gases. New York: Academic Press, 1989:211–234.
133. Kirsch KJ, Mazumder MK. Appl Phys Lett 1975; 26:193.
134. Hiller FC, Mazumder MK, Wilson JD, Bone RC. J Pharm Pharmacol 1980; 32:605–609.
135. Hiller FC, Mazumder MK, Wilson JD, Bone RC. J Pharm Sci 1980; 69:334–337.
136. Halbert MK, Mazumder MK, Bond RL. Food Cosmet Toxicol 1981; 19:85–88.
137. Fults K, Cyr TD, Hickey AJ. J Pharm Pharmacol 1991; 43:726–728.
138. Evans R. Pharm Technol 1993; 17:146–152.
139. Atkins PJ. Pharm Technol 1992; 16:26–32.
140. Milosovich SM. Pharm Technol 1992; 16:82–86.

141. Gorman WG, Carrol FA. Pharm Technol 1993; 17:34–37.

142. Jager PD, DeStefano GA, McNamara DP. Pharm Technol 1993; 17:102–120.

143. Niven RW. Pharm Technol 1993; 17:72–78.

144. Ranucci J. Pharm Technol 1992; 16:109–114.

145. Ranucci JA, Chen F-C. Pharm Technol 1993; 17:62–74.

146. Dunbar CA, Hickey AJ. J Aerosol Sci 2000; 31:813–831.

147. Medicines EDftQo. European Pharmacopoeia, The Stationery Office, 2001.

148. http://www.fda.gov/cder/guidance/index.html. FDA guidance for MDIs and DPIs.

12

Summary of Common Approaches to Pharmaceutical Aerosol Administration

Anthony J. Hickey
University of North Carolina, Chapel Hill, North Carolina, U.S.A.

INTRODUCTION

The use of aerosol delivery systems continues to be a desirable means of administering locally acting agents to the lungs. Since the early 1990s there has been a surge of interest in the pulmonary delivery of proteins and peptides for systemic activity but to date none of these products have made it to market [1]. During this period the major commercial successes have been in the form of dry powder systems [2] and alternative propellant systems [1], as will be discussed later in the chapter. The incidence of asthma and chronic obstructive disease continues to rise and the need for improvement and diversity of therapies remains a priority in their treatment [3].

Aerosol foams, sprays, and powders have been used in personal [4,5], household [6], engineering, food, cosmetic [7], and pharmaceutical products [8–10]. This technology has had a significant influence on society in the last 50 years. Many people have direct experience of the pharmaceutical aerosol systems used to treat asthma. The ability of the patient to use these aerosols properly is a serious concern in the treatment of this disease. This may in part be attributed to poor instruction in the use of the devices. However, underlying the problem is a general lack of understanding of the principles of operation and limitations of inhalation products.

Material discussed in previous chapters (notably in Chaps. 1, 3, and 6) has focused in a concise review of the methods of aerosol generation and administration, concluding with some comments on aerosol therapy. My intention is to place material that has appeared in previous chapters in context and to facilitate the discussions of clinical applications that appear in subsequent chapters.

PARTICLE SIZE AND OTHER PARTICLE CHARACTERISTICS

The factors influencing particle and droplet deposition in the lung are summarized as a preliminary to considering aerosol generation and administration.

The deposition characteristics and efficacy of an aerosol depend largely on the particle or droplet size [11–13]. The purpose for which the product will be used will dictate the most suitable particle size. Large droplets of significant mass may achieve high velocities as a result of spraying. Their momentum will carry them directly to the selected surface, for example, to the skin, where they will deposit, coalesce, and coat or coat on wiping. Smaller droplets would not have great enough momentum to pass directly to the surface and would hang in the atmosphere until, under the influence of gravity, they would deposit on any available surface. Very small particles might remain in the atmosphere for an extended period of time and present an inhalation hazard. In 1966, the Task Group on Lung Dynamics, concerned mainly with the hazards of inhalation of environmental pollutants, collated experimental and theoretical models from the literature and proposed a model for deposition and clearance of particles from the lung [14].

The aim was to identify the influence of particle size on deposition in different regions of the lung. In contrast to the approach of investigators in the fields of environmental health and industrial hygiene, the inhalation aerosol formulator wants the particles or droplets to be small enough to deposit in the lung [8,9]. The particles or droplets should be in a size range that allows them, suspended in air, to pass beyond the first surfaces they encounter on inspiration, those of the mouth, throat, and upper airways, and to pass to the lower airways.

The Task Group model suggested that particles larger than 10 μm in diameter are most likely to deposit in the mouth and throat. Between the sizes of 5 and 10 μm, a transition from mouth to airway deposition occurs. Particles smaller than 5-μm diameter deposit more frequently in the lower airways and, thus, would be appropriate for pharmaceutical inhalation aerosols. The Task Group model, based on nose breathing, illustrates the general principles of the relationship between particle size and lung deposition. However, it may overestimate the total deposition and the fraction of particles depositing in the alveoli by ignoring mouth breathing [15]. Deposition in the lung is the subject of continued speculation, but it is generally accepted that the formulator should target the 1- to 5-μm range as desirable for airway deposition.

Figure 1 shows graphically the Task Group on Lung Dynamics model for lung deposition. This figure is shown to illustrate a commonly held misconception about aerosol deposition. Three regions of deposition are shown: the nasopharyngeal, tracheobronchial, and pulmonary regions. Particles or droplets smaller than 1 μm deposit predominantly in the tracheobronchial and pulmonary regions. Little or none of the aerosol in this size range deposits in the nasopharynx.

This often leads to the potentially erroneous conclusion that submicrometer aerosols would generally be most appropriate for lower airway deposition of pharmacologically active agents to achieve the desired therapeutic effect.

The mass of material reaching the site of action is related directly to the therapeutic effect. Small individual particles carry very little mass. These are difficult to generate in high concentrations and are subject to a varying degree, depending on particle size, to exhalation. The fraction deposited at the site of action is only of value when the total mass is equal to or exceeds the therapeutic

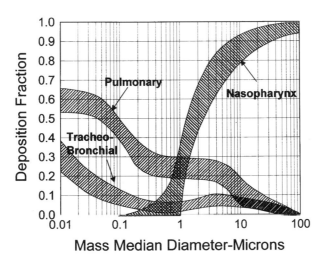

FIGURE 1 Task Group on Lung Dynamics model for lung deposition. The shaded area represents the range of effects when the σg varies between 1.2 and 4.5 at a tidal volume of 1450 mL. (With permission of *Health Physics*.)

dose. Thus, the largest particles capable of penetrating into the deep lung offer the greatest therapeutic advantage, and the target size range of 1–5 μm is generally accepted as the formulator's guide to optimized lung deposition [16,17]. To some extent, this range has been dictated by the technology available for aerosol generation [10,18]. However, if it were possible to generate submicrometer pharmaceutical aerosols easily, the time period required for delivery of a therapeutic dose would generally be prohibitively long.

It is rarely the case that the sizes of all particles in an aerosol are the same, or monodisperse [19]. An aerosol consists of particles of numerous sizes, and each one of these will deposit in different regions in the lung. The range of particle sizes is known as the *distribution*. Figure 2 shows a typical distribution. The skew to the left of this distribution is indicative of log normality [20,21]. This expression refers to the fraction of particles of a particular size that, when plotted against logarithms of the particle sizes, exhibit a normal, bell-shaped, or Gaussian, distribution. A narrow distribution indicates an aerosol whose particles have similar sizes. The most common expression of particle sizes divides the distribution in half (50% above and 50% below that size and is known as the *median* size) according to statistical convention. A broad distribution may have the same median particle size as the narrow one, but there will be a considerable range of particle sizes.

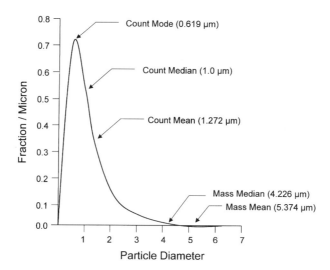

FIGURE 2 Representative log-normal particle size distribution. The values in parentheses are based on a count median diameter of 1.0 μm and a σg of 2.0. (With permission of *Health Physics*.)

Assuming a median diameter in the respirable range, then a larger proportion of a narrowly distributed aerosol will be respirable than for a broad distribution. It would seem that a broad distribution is not desirable to achieve the goal of targeting the lower airways. The conventional measure of the log-normal distribution of particle size is the geometric standard deviation [22,23]. Given the median diameter and geometric standard deviation of aerosol particles, the size distribution can be constructed.

As with all dosage forms, it is the amount of drug reaching the site of action that dictates the therapeutic effect. The importance of this observation to a formulator can be emphasized by two examples: [1] When expressing the particle size of an aerosol, it might seem appropriate to count the number of particles of each size and to plot the distribution as shown in Fig. 2. In a hypothetical aerosol sample consisting of one 10-μm particle and 1000 1-μm particles, the number of particles of a particular size leads to the belief that the vast majority ($>99.9\%$) of the aerosol is respirable. Unfortunately, from a therapeutic standpoint, one 10-μm particle carries the same mass as 1000 1-μm particles. Thus, only 50% of the mass of the aerosol (mass of 1-μm particles divided by the mass of 1- and 10-μm particles combined) would reach the lung. [2] A solution aerosol droplet of an appropriate size will not carry the same amount of drug as a solid particle because part of its composition is solvent. Both of these examples are important formulation considerations when considering the dose.

Gonda [24] described the influence of polydispersity on deposition of aerosol particles in the lung assuming a variety of distributions ($\sigma g = 1, 2,$ and 3.5). Figure 3 shows that a small median diameter results in the highest deposition in the pulmonary region. The narrow distribution ($\sigma g = 1$) results in maximum deposition in the pulmonary region when the median diameter is 2 μm. As the distribution is increased and as the aerosol becomes more polydisperse, the maximum at 2 μm disappears into a general trend toward increased deposition in the pulmonary region as the median diameter is reduced. One interpretation of this observation is that, as referred to earlier, aerosols formulated to achieve a small median diameter and a narrow distribution will be most effective in penetrating the lower airways. It is also true that the narrow distribution is more sensitive to a change in the median diameter, with a 10-fold variation in the range 1–10 μm. A highly polydisperse aerosol is less sensitive to changes in median diameter but does not achieve maximum pulmonary deposition. These are important considerations because an aerosol may be subject to changes in median diameter resulting from manufacture storage or generation.

Other characteristics of particles that influence their deposition are density, charge, shape, solubility, and hygroscopicity. These play a secondary role to particle size. The density of the particle contributes to its mass and, thus, inertia [20,23]. Increasing density will result in increased, or more rapid, deposition of particles. Charge has a number of effects. First, particles may aggregate as

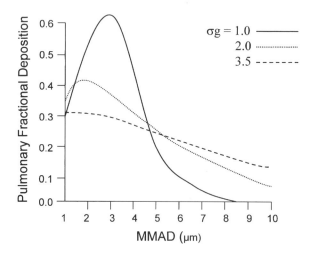

FIGURE 3 Theoretical pulmonary deposition as a function of particle size for a range of distributions. (With permission of *Journal of Pharmacy and Pharmacology.*)

a result of their charge characteristics and become larger "particles," reduced in number, with the concomitant effect on deposition [25–27]. Second, the airways sometimes have charged areas at their surface that may influence charged particles to deposit [28]. Shape seriously influences deposition only when particles deviate significantly from sphericity. This is rarely the case with pharmaceutical inhalation aerosol particles or droplets. Hygroscopicity is the tendency of particles to associate with water in the atmosphere. Considerable effort has been expended in elucidating the behavior of hygroscopic environmental aerosols [29–37]. The airways of the lung have a relative humidity of 99.5% at a body temperature of 37°C [38–41].

Hygroscopic particles will grow in diameter as they associate with water [42,43]. Drugs that exhibit aqueous solubility will dissolve in the water, and this brings about further rapid association [6,17,42,44–46]. It has been suggested, for example, that cromolyn sodium and isoproterenol sulfate dihydrate grow to more than 2.5 times their original diameter in the lung [47]. Because this growth occurs rapidly, it influences deposition of particles in the respiratory tract [48–55].

This chapter is not concerned with specific formulation issues; however, referring to the prospect of controlled release of drugs from aerosols in the lung is worthwhile. The immediate benefit of this approach stems from the occurrence of nocturnal asthma and the need to treat this condition [56]. Several approaches have been taken to achieve this aim, ranging from reformulation [57] to the use of drug-carrier systems [58–64]. Although oral controlled-release theophylline exists, circadian pharmacokinetics may result in toxic systemic levels of the drug [65]. There would be great merit in developing a controlled-release inhaled product because this would target the site of action and present drug in small quantities, thus reducing the incidence of unwanted side effects. It has been suggested, however, that the maximum residence time of pharmaceutical aerosol particles in the lung is 12 hr [66]. This observation is based on lung deposition of particles and their removal by mucociliary clearance. Materials that prolong the residence time of drug in the lung should be viewed with some caution because they may pose a toxicity problem [67]. Therefore, some limitations to the effectiveness of a controlled-release delivery system may exist.

COMPOUNDS COMMONLY ADMINISTERED TO THE LUNG

Chapters 2 and 4 thoroughly reviewed the compounds administered to the lung and their chemical origins and activity.

Most compounds administered to the lung are bronchodilators [68–76]. These fall in the general categories of catecholamines [74,77], resorcinols [74,78–80], saligenins [74,81], and prodrugs [74,82,83], all of which exhibit or result in P-adrenergic receptor agonist activity. Other common agents are anticholinergic and corticosteroid agents [44,84–88] and cromolyn sodium [89–91], which is known to stabilize mast cells to inhibit the production of histamine, leukotrenes, and other substances known to cause hypersensitivity. Combination therapy with P-adrenergic receptor agonists and anti-inflammatory agents has been used [91,92]. These agents are administered to the lung for their local activity. Ergotamine tartrate, an α-adrenergic receptor antagonist, is administered to the upper airways for the treatment of vascular headaches, or migraines, indicating the potential of this route for the administration of systemically acting agents [9,64]. Antibiotic agents have also been administered to the lung, notably for the treatment of cystic fibrosis [93–98]. In recent years the approval of tobramycin has added another antibiotic to the therapy for cystic fibrosis [99,100]. In addition, DNAase was approved for aerosol administration as a means of cleaving leukocyte DNA to reduce the viscosity of mucus and facilitate expectoration by cystic fibrosis patients [101,102]. Some more common materials have been administered to relieve respiratory distress, including water, saline, detergent, mucolytics, and proteolytics [103]. A variety of additives are used in the formulation of pharmaceutical aerosols [104]. Some of these are shown in Table 1. Oleic acid is included as a suspending agent and valve lubricant in pressurized-pack inhalers. Although there is no evidence that this material has toxic effects when delivered in small quantities from an aerosol to the airways, it is known to induce pulmonary edema at high systemic concentrations [105,106]. Sodium metabisulfite and benzalkonium chloride have been included in some nebulizer aerosol formulations as a preservative. Recent

TABLE 1   Additives in Currently Manufactured Oral and Nasal Inhalants

Inhalant	Manufacturer	Use	Additives
Oral			
Beclovent	Glaxo	Anti-inflammatory[a]	Complex: trichloromono fluoromethane clathrate
Norisodrine sulfate aerohaler	Abbott	Bronchial dilator[b]	Lactose
Proventil inhaler	Schering	Bronchial dilator[c]	Oleic acid
Acrobid	Key	Bronchial dilator[c]	Sorbitan trioleate
Ventolin	Glaxo	Bronchial dilator[c]	Oleic acid
Alupent inhalant solution	Boehringer Ingelheim	Bronchial dilator[c]	Saline
Duo-Medihaler	Riker	Bronchial dilator[c]	Sorbitan triolcate, cetylpyridinium chloride
Isuprel hydrochlo-ride solution	Breon	Bronchial dilator[c]	Sodium chloride, citric acid, glycerin chlorbutanol, sodium bisulfite
Isuprel Mistometer	Breon	Bronchial dilator[c]	Alcohol, ascorbic acid
Medihaler-ISO	Riker	Bronchial dilator[b]	Sorbitan trioleate
Norisodrine Aerotrol	Abbott	Bronchial dilator[b]	Alcohol, ascorbic acid
Primatene mist	Whitehall	Bronchial dilator[b]	Alchol, ascorbic acid
Nasal			
Beconase	Glaxo	Anti-inflammatory[a]	Complex: Trichloronionofluoroniethane clathrate
Dristan	Whitehall	Relieve nasal congestion	Thimersol preservative, benzalkonium chloride, alcohol
Nasalcronm	Fisons	Treat allergic rhinitis[d]	Benzalkonium chloride, EDTA

Nasalide	Syntex	Treat allergic rhinitis	Propylene glycol, PEG 3350, citric acid sodium citrate, butylated hydroxyanisole, EDTA, ben-zalkonium chloride, NaOH/HC
Vancenase	Schering	Anti-inflammatory[a]	Complex: trichlorotnonofluoromethane clathrate, oleic acid
Decadron turbinaire	Merck, Sharp & Dohme	Anti-inflammatory[a]	Alcohol
Syntocinon	Sandoz	Induce lactation	Dried sodium phosphate, citric acid, sodium chloride, glycerin, sorbitol solution, methylpa-raben, propylparaben chlorbutanol

[a]Corticosteroid.
[b]Sympathomimetic.
[c]β-Adrenergic stimulant.
[d]Cromolyn sodium.
Source: *Physicians' Desk Reference*, 1985.

studies focused on bronchoconstriction induced by the presence of these materials [107–109]. In light of these observations, the addition of preservatives has been frowned upon, and regulatory agencies prefer nebulizer solutions to be prepared as sterile products. Propylene glycol and ethanol are used in nasal aerosols and have been suggested as solvents in oral aerosol formulations [110,111]. Other carboxylic acid additives, selected to improve drug delivery, may also be included in powder aerosol formulations [112]. Propylene glycol and carboxylic acids are known to irritate mucous membranes when present at certain concentrations, and alcohols will cause bronchoconstriction. Manipulating the drug molecule may achieve the same ends as reformulating. Pentamidine is used to treat *Pneumocystis carinii* pneumonia infections in AIDS patients. This has been prepared in various salt forms to improve the bioavailability [113]. In circumstances such as this, it is essential to establish that the increased bioavailability does not increase the toxicity of the drug. These examples, of additives and formulations, are given to indicate that great caution must be exercised in the selection and use of materials in the lung because the potential for local toxicity exists.

METHODS OF GENERATION

Many drugs are formulated in a variety of ways to enable the use of all of the common methods of generation. The explanation for this approach is that each of the methods offers certain advantages, either as a fundamental characteristic of the devices used or in concert with the nature or gravity of the disease state being treated.

Nebulizers

A variety of nebulizers are used, usually in hospital settings. The two major types of nebulizers are the jet and ultrasonic devices shown in Figs. 4 and 5, respectively. Jet nebulizers operate on the principle that by passing air at high speed over the end of a capillary tube, liquid may be drawn up the tube from a reservoir in which it is immersed (Venturi or Bernoulli effect) [114]. When the liquid reaches the end of the capillary, it is drawn into the airstream and forms droplets that disperse to become an aerosol. An ultrasonic generator uses a piezoelectric transducer to induce waves in a reservoir of solution [115]. Interference of these waves at the reservoir surface leads to the production of droplets in the atmosphere above the reservoir. An airstream is passed through this atmosphere to transport the droplets as an aerosol. Both of these methods successfully produce droplets in the size range for inhalation [116–119]. The success of these devices can be measured by their use in the treatment and diagnosis of respiratory disease. Because of the size of the droplets,

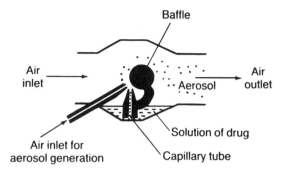

FIGURE 4 Schematic of jet nebulizer. (With permission of Drug Topics.)

approximately $1-2\,\mu$m, the mass carried is small, and, therefore, the dose is administered over an extended period, which on average is 10–15 min. The droplets produced are small enough to penetrate to the lung periphery. Early nebulizer therapy involved the generation of mists of water or saline for inhalation [120–124]. By radiolabeling the droplets with a gamma-emitting radioisotope and by having patients inhale the aerosol, the lungs can be imaged by gamma scintigraphy [125,126]. This method enables areas of poor ventilation, symptomatic of a disease state, to be identified. Standardized provocation tests for allergy studies also use this method of delivery [127,128]. Nebulizers are commonly used with solutions of bronchodilators, such as albuterol and terbutaline, for patients who cannot use metered-dose inhalers (MDIs) or who are suffering from severe asthma that requires hospitalization [129–132].

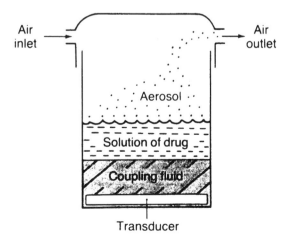

FIGURE 5 Schematic of ultrasonic nebulizer. (With permission of Drug Topics.)

Additionally, sodium cromoglycate [90,133], corticosteroids [91], and pentamidine [134] have been administered by nebulizer. These devices are more effective generators of small particles than both MDIs and dry powder generators [8]. This results in a greater proportion of the dose reaching the lower airways, although each solution droplet contains less drug than each particle generated from an MDI or dry powder generator. As an example of the adult dose administered by nebulizer therapy, 1.25–5 mg albuterol sulfate is administered in 2–5 mL or more of 0.9% sodium chloride every 46 hr. Often, nebulizers are operated continuously, and the patient is asked to take intermittent breaths from each dose. Between breaths, the aerosol may be vented into the room. This approach leads to inconsistent and unpredictable dose administration to the patient. Some variation in total output, particle size, and overall efficiency exists among different generators [116,119,135–139].

Figure 6 shows a photograph of three jet nebulizers. Numerous jet nebulizers are being marketed, and, indeed, some concern has been expressed about the "nebulizer epidemic" [140,141]. The first two nebulizers shown were selected because they are both used to deliver pentamidine to patients suffering from *Pneumocystis carinii* pneumonia, a secondary infection in AIDS. Of note, ultrasonic nebulizers have also been used for this purpose. Treatment of this particular disease is the most notable example of nebulizer therapy in recent years. Significantly, no other method of pentamidine aerosol generation is currently available.

Modifying two hospital jet nebulizers, a Bird Micronebulizer and an Acorn II, to allow a solution feed, at 0.1–0.6 mL/min, showed that the respirable (% <5 μm) output characteristics of these devices varied between 70–87% and

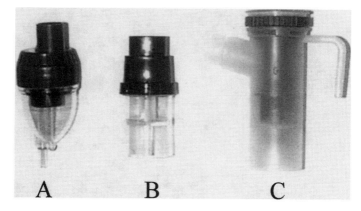

FIGURE 6 Photograph of (A) Aeromist, (B) Respigard II, and (C) Pari LC Star nebulizers, the first two of which are used to deliver pentamidine.

97–99%, respectively [139]. The airflow rate was fixed at 8.3 and 9.1 L/min for the Bird and Acorn nebulizers, respectively. The nebulizers shown in Fig. 6 were assessed in their conventional orientation at different airflow rates [142]. The Respigard II that was operated in the range of airflow rates between 4.9 and 8.5 L/min produced an aerosol with a respirable fraction of 76–87%. The Aeromist that was operated at 7.6–11.8 L/min produced an aerosol with a respirable fraction of 91–93%. Therefore, the operating conditions have only a slight effect on the respirable fraction of the aerosol. However, solution flowrate and airflow rate both significantly influence total output of these devices [139,142]. Low flowrates result in low total output. The implication of these observations is that high flowrates are more likely to result in a therapeutic effect.

A device using an alternative principle to that of the jet and ultrasonic nebulizers has been described but has not been adopted to any extent. The Babington nebulizer, shown in Fig. 7, uses a principle that was first devised for fuel atomization [143]. Liquid (for the purposes of this discussion, a drug solution) is supplied to the outer surface of a hollow sphere. A thin film forms over the entire surface of the sphere. Compressed air supplied to the interior of the sphere expands through a small rectangular orifice at the top of the dome. Fine liquid particles form as escaping air ruptures a portion of the liquid film

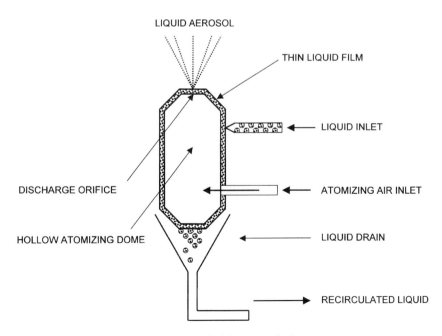

FIGURE 7 Schematic diagram of the Babington nebulizer.

flowing over the spherical surface. Excess liquid is collected and recirculated. Smaller quantities of liquid are required for use in the Babington than ultrasonic devices due to the need for more material to saturate the atmosphere at the elevated ambient temperatures in the latter nebulizer. Jet nebulizers, in general, require a higher operating pressure than the Babington system to produce therapeutic aerosols. Of note, however, is that in recent years, improvements in jet and ultrasonic nebulizer design have rendered these advantages of less significance than originally.

Different auxiliary methods of administration can be used in conjunction with nebulizers to deliver aerosol to the patient [144]. A mouthpiece may be inserted in the mouth or a face mask may be attached tightly to the face. A large-bore inlet adapter attaches tubing from the nebulizer outlet to the mouthpiece or mask. It is possible to compensate for exhaled aerosol without increasing resistance to prevent condensation. A face tent fits more loosely around the patient's mouth, allowing speech. The latter arrangement is frequently used with ultrasonic nebulizers. A tracheostomy mask may be fitted to the patient's tracheostomy tube directly and requires a T-shaped adapter. Environmental chambers are used to enhance therapy and include incubators, pediatric croup tents, and hoods.

There appear to be many contradictions in the literature concerning the efficacy of nebulizer therapy. It has been suggested that although an MDI delivers a much smaller dose than a nebulizer, the same effect is observed clinically. This may be explained in terms of the time taken to administer a dose using a nebulizer. The generally smaller-particle-size output from nebulizers in comparison with that of MDIs and the delivery as solution rather than as suspension explains the time required to deliver the dose by this method. The particle size advantage of nebulizers leads to their use when patients are admitted to hospitals with severe airways obstructions. Once their condition has stabilized, the patients are placed on MDI aerosol therapy, which is more convenient.

Clinical complications related to the use of nebulizers have been observed. Facial dermatitis with superimposed bacterial infections have been described and are caused by the prolonged use of a face mask [145]. Contamination of the small-volume nebulizers has been linked with oropharyngeal colonization [146,147]. In one report, infections were seen four times more frequently in patients receiving inhalation therapy for respiratory diseases than in those who are not. At least one example of death resulting from contamination has been reported.

It has been suggested that the increased popularity of nebulizer treatment for asthma has been the cause of an elevation of the number of deaths due to asthma. An effect that has been observed is the paradoxical bronchoconstriction, in which compounds that are administered to the airways to cause bronchodilatation cause constriction [148–150]. It has been proposed that this effect is caused by a component of the nebulizer formulation. More specifically, the presence of preservatives, the possibility of contamination, and the effects of ionic strength have all been implicated. It seems appropriate, therefore, to suggest the development of a unit-dose form with increased likelihood of sterility, without preservatives and formulated as isotonic solutions.

Hypoxia resulting from the home use of nebulizers has been reported. This would appear to result from misuse of the devices. Indeed, patient misuse may not be the only problem. A poll of 67 physicians with a stated interest in chest disease showed that there was a significant difference in their prescribing of β-adrenergic receptor agonists for delivery by nebulizer [129]. There was a fivefold difference in the dose of albuterol, a 20-fold difference in the volume of the diluent solution, and a 10-fold variation in the flow of gas driving the nebulizer that the physicians used. Undoubtedly, some of this variation may be attributed to the use of different devices. However, implicit in these observations is a significant potential dose-delivery problem.

A completely new nebulizer principle was introduced in the late 1990s [151]. A vibrating multicrifice plate system was employed. This electronic system does not require the cumbersome air pump of the jet nebulizers and employs a principle that can be scaled up to handheld systems [152].

Despite some drawbacks, the successful use of these nebulizers in the treatment of serious incidents of asthma, which do not respond to MDI or dry powder treatment, renders them a useful method in respiratory therapy.

Metered-Dose Inhalers

Figure 8 shows a schematic diagram of an MDI. These devices are most frequently used to deliver suspension aerosols, consisting of solid particles of drug suspended in a liquid propellant. The original particle size of the suspended powder is very important because this dictates the smallest particle size generated from the device. The powder is prepared by milling to the appropriate size. Micronized powders prepared in this fashion are approximately 3–5 μm in size. The powder is suspended in the propellant by means of a surfactant, for example, oleic acid. Because of the size of the particles, the suspension is not colloidal and, therefore, is stable for only minutes. This means that it is important to shake the suspension to redisperse the particles before use. The propellant, in which the particles are suspended, in either a CFC blend or HFA/ethanol mixture. These have high vapor pressure and must be packed under pressure, at room temperature, or cold-filled as a liquid at a temperature well below their boiling point [153]. The most common propellants used are propellants 11, 12, and 114 [154]. The containers that are available for packaging are numerous, but aluminum cans or plastic-coated glass bottles are most common for pharmaceutical products. The cans are crimp-sealed with a valve through

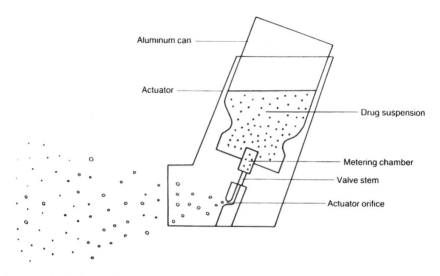

FIGURE 8 Schematic of diagram of a metered-dose inhaler. (With permission of Drug Topics.)

which the contents can be dispensed. The principle of operation of these devices is that (1) a metering chamber fills with suspension as the can is inverted; (2) by depressing the valve stem, the metering chamber is simultaneously closed to the reservoir within the container and opened to the atmosphere by the actuator jet; and (3) because atmospheric pressure is much lower than the equilibrium vapor pressure in the can, the propellent vaporizes rapidly, which propels the suspended particles, surfactant, and some unevaporated propellant through the jet into the atmosphere and eventually to the patient. A variety of physical and analytical tests have been described for characterizing these systems [155–158]. Metered-dose valves have been shown to deliver 10–15% of the mean valve delivery for each actuation [159]. Increasing the metering volume of an MDI has been shown to have no effect on the total lung deposition [160]. The same study showed that increasing the vapor pressure of the propellant mixture resulted in both increased total lung deposition and lower airways deposition. Doses administered in each bolus vary according to the active ingredient. Albuterol sulfate, for example, has a single dose of 200 μg (Ventolin), whereas beclomethasone dipropionate is 42 μg (Beclovent). Despite dose variation, most MDIs call for administration of one or two puffs three or four times daily for adults. Figure 9 shows a number of common MDIs. These deliver albuterol, beclomethasone, and sodium cromoglycate. The inverted canisters are seen protruding above the actuator

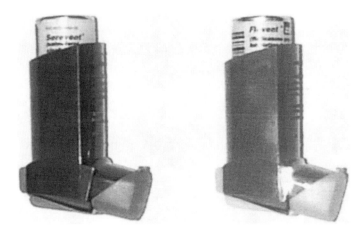

FIGURE 9 Photograph of common metered-dose pressurized-pack inhalers.

sheath. Although components may vary, the overall design is very similar from one product to another.

A number of studies comparing metered-dose pressure-packed inhalers with other methods of inhalation have been described [161–168]. In general, MDIs are considered appropriate for patients who are ambulatory and subject to mild or moderate bronchoconstriction. The rationale for this treatment is the ability of the aerosol produced by the MDI to penetrate the lungs of the patient. The dose delivered may result in immediate relief or serve as a prophylactic, depending on the drug used. In more severe cases, particularly those requiring hospitalization of the patients, the smaller droplets produced by the nebulizer systems may be required to deliver the drug to the lung. The dose will require some time to deliver; thus, relief may be delayed, but, notably, MDI treatment is unlikely to succeed under these circumstances.

MDIs, as with other devices, are subject to misuse by patients. The administration problems associated with the delivery of aerosols from MDIs generally appear to be related to inappropriate technique, particularly coordination of breathing and actuation [169–171]. There are particular problems in the use of this technique by children, who may not respond as readily to instruction [172]. Also of note, there is still some debate on the most appropriate methods of administration, particularly with respect to the use of different drugs.

To avoid the need for coordination in breathing and actuation of the inhaler, a breath-actuated system has been devised. Patients who inhaled at 50 L/min did not experience significantly greater bronchodilation using a breath-actuated device than those using a conventional MDI [173]. The Autohaler, shown in

Fig. 10, is a more recent version of the breath-actuated device. For those patients who find coordination of breathing and actuation difficult, this device is convenient, providing there is no therapeutic disadvantage.

The most significant developments in metered-dose inhaler technology to occur since the early 1990s have been the introduction of hydrofluoroalkane (HFA) systems as alternatives to chlorofluorocarbon (CFC) systems [174]. This has largely been caused by the link between the use of CFC systems and ozone depletion in the upper atmosphere [152,175]. Albuterol and beclomethasone have been reformulated in HFA products, but as yet the CFC products are still subject to an annually renewable medical exemption. The Food and Drug Administration has recently published its position on alternative propellant formulations, which should initiate the phase-out of CFCs [176]. In the meantime, a number of generic CFC products of albuterol have been manufactured. The opportunity for reformulation of products as they come of patent is likely to increase research and development in this area in the near future. New formulation opportunities will also arise from these developments, including solutions [177], micellar [178,179], and microemulsion [180].

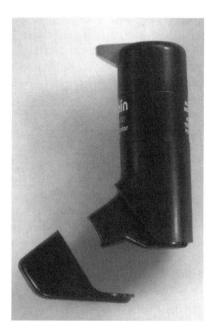

FIGURE 10 Photograph of a breath-actuated metered-dose pressurized-pack inhaler (Autohaler).

Dry Powder Generators

The delivery of aerosol powders by generation with minimal formulation has been an attractive prospect to many researchers. The early use of a dry powder artificial phospholipid in the treatment of neonatal respiratory distress syndrome proved very successful [181]. Because no delivery system was available to facilitate this treatment, a simple system was devised. A Laerdal neonatal resuscitation bag was modified to hold a capsule containing the artificial surfactant, as shown schematically in Fig. 11. However, where MDIs of the prescribed medication are available, both physicians and patients prefer their use. The powders themselves have to be prepared in the same way as those used in MDIs, by milling. Often, excipients are added to carry the fine powder. Lactose has been used in both cromolyn sodium and albuterol formulations. As a consequence of the interest in dry powders, a number of products have been

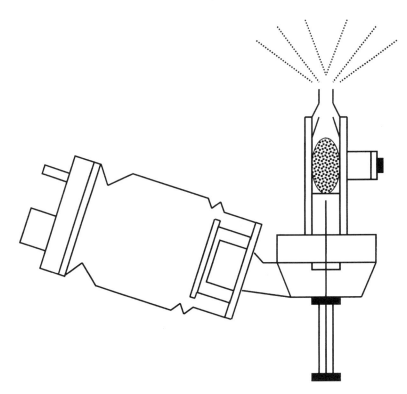

FIGURE 11 Modified Laerdal neonatal resuscitation bag. (With permission of *Lancet.*)

developed for this purpose. The principle of operation of this type of generator is to use the patient's breathing to govern the airflow in which the aerosol powder is dispersed. The Spinhaler (Fisons Pharmaceuticals) [19] for the delivery of cromolyn sodium, shown in Fig. 12, delivers the active ingredient from a capsule that is pierced before operation. The mechanism for piercing the capsule is incorporated in the device. The Spinhaler rotates the capsule under the influence of the patient's breath, ejecting aerosol particles into the airstream. These particles pass though rotor blades, driving the capsule rotation, and are collected or deaggregated to ensure that smaller particles are administered to the patient. The Turbuhaler (AB Draco) [182], for delivery of terbutaline sulfate and budesonide, uses a reservoir of drug that fills a series of conical-shaped holes with the powder. By twisting a grip at the base of the Turbuhaler, the holes are filled and scraped at the surface to eliminate excess material. Thus, the dose is governed by the volume of the holes. The preparation of drug in this device is important. Micronized powder is spheronized into soft aggregates that are easily handled, for loading, but readily deaggregate for inhalation. This drug is deaggregated and delivered to the patient in the turbulent flow of air passing the conical holes as inhalation occurs. Cromolyn sodium (Intal) is supplied in 20-mg capsules, which must be administered in one inhalation four times daily, for adults. The Turbuhaler delivers less than 1 mg per actuation. The Rotahaler (Glaxo) [163], for delivery of albuterol, and the Berotec (Boehringer Ingelheim) [183], for the delivery of fenoterol, operate on a similar principle. A twisting motion of the device cracks a gelatin capsule containing the drug, which is then available for inhalation. The Inhalator (Boehringer Ingelheim), of the Berotec system, involves blister piercing and inhalation. It has been shown that the pressure drop across these devices, the Rotahaler and Inhalator, represent the extremes of low and high values, respectively [184]. This observation is consistent with a shift in the focus of in vitro characterization based on pressure drop [185] as a relevant measure of performance. The importance of this feature can be considered in the following terms. A low-pressure-drop device offers little resistance to patient inspiratory flow; however, it does not induce significant shear in the powder bed. Consequently, inhalation is easy but the powder is not dispersed well. In contrast, a high-resistance device offers significant resistance to patient inspiratory flow; however, considerable shear is applied to the powder. Consequently, inhalation is more difficult but powder is dispersed well. Therefore, comparison of devices at the same pressure drop is a relevant measure of their performance, if not a truly controlled study. It is possible to go one step further to account for both pressure drop and airflow rate using a power performance criterion that then allows direct comparison of device performance, since all data are normalized for these variables [186].

Figure 13 shows the Spinhaler (Fisons), Rotahaler (GSK), and Diskhaler (GSK), and Fig. 14 shows a Turbuhaler (Astra-Zeneca) and Discus (GSK). While

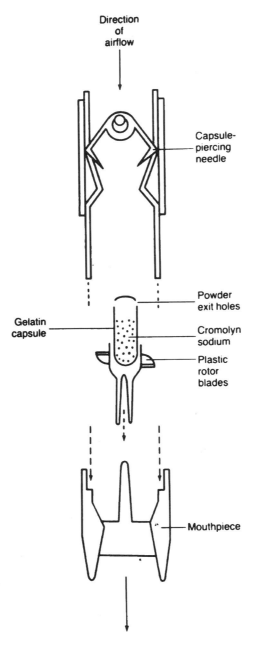

FIGURE 12 Schematic diagram of a Spinhaler (Fisons) dry powder generator. (With permission of Drug Topics.)

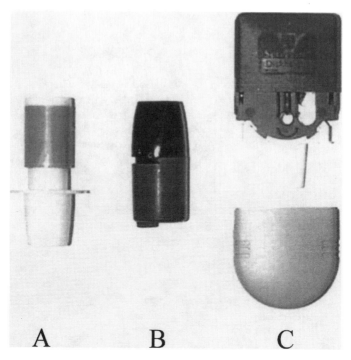

FIGURE 13 Photograph of the (A) Spinhaler, (B) Rotahaler, and (C) Diskhaler.

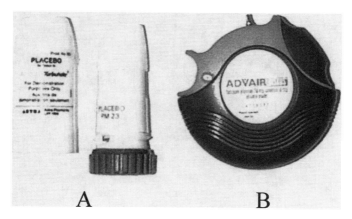

FIGURE 14 Photograph of the (A) Turbuhaler and (B) Diskus.

the original DPIs appear to be similar to the pressurized-pack inhalers, the newer products can now be distinguished as operating by different principles. Since this publication of the first edition of this volume, the Rotahaler product has been discontinued and the Diskhaler and Discus products have been more prominently employed to deliver different drugs. Figure 15 shows the original Inhalator Ingelheim, used in the Berotec system described in the previous paragraph, and the Handihaler (Boehringer Ingelheim), which operates on a similar principle but has a different configuration. In addition, the Foradil Aerolizer (Novartis), which is intended to deliver formoterol fumarate (12.5 mg) from a capsule, is shown, since its principle of operation is similar to that of the other two products, that is, piercing a gelatin blister containing the drug, which is then drawn, under the patient's effort, with high resistance from the device.

As with the metered-dose inhalers, some old drugs have been repackaged in new devices. For dry powder inhalers these are not true generics but have a similar impact on the marketplace. Most notable of these in the Clickhaler (Innovata Biomed), which is marketed in Europe, for the delivery of albuterol (salbutamol) and beclomethasone.

Dry powder generation is hindered by aggregation of the particles [20]. This property may be attributed to surface charge characteristics of the powder and van der Waals forces. A factor that exacerbates this problem is the hygroscopic nature of many pharmaceutical powders [43,45,47]. Hygroscopicity is known to change the powder flow properties [187]. Attempts have been made to modify the surface characteristics of dry powders to reduce both aggregation

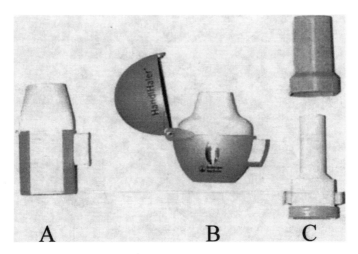

FIGURE 15 Photograph of the (A) Inhalator, (B) Handihaler, and (C) Foradil Aerolizer.

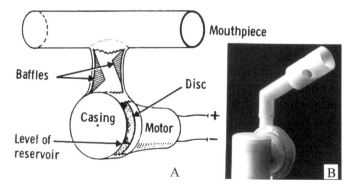

FIGURE 16 (A) Schematic (with permission of *Lancet*) and (B) photograph of prototype vertical spinning device (Nebulet).

[188] and hygroscopicity [48,189]. Such approaches may reduce the need for traditional excipients, such as lactose.

Dry powder aerosols must begin as a reservoir of free-flowing powder that can be dispersed in the airstream of the patient's inspiratory breath. To achieve a free-flowing powder, an excipient, lactose, is added as a carrier for the drug particles [190,191].

In dry powder delivery to the lung, recognizing the uniqueness of the complete system of formulation and generator is important. Certain design characteristics in the generators facilitate dispersion of the powder and capture of large particles that will not reach the lung. Thus, the success of the dry powder formulation depends to a large extent on the development of appropriate generators. Most methods have used a passive liberation of the powder into the patient's inhaled airflow. A prototype device has been described that employs a vertical spinning disk to project the aerosol in the airstream [192]. The device is shown in Fig. 16. This device has been used to produce dry powder aerosols but requires a large reservoir of drug to deliver a reproducible dose [48,193,194].

ADMINISTRATION ACCESSORIES
Baffles

Most aerosol delivery systems have surfaces that are designed to collect or disperse particles. Jet nebulizers have spheres, as shown in Fig. 4, or plates placed immediately in front of the jet to collector break up large droplets. Metered-dose inhalers do not traditionally have baffles; however, the surface of the actuator collects aerosol particles as they pass through the mouthpiece. Dry powder aerosol generators deliver aerosols by tortuous channels that collect or deaggregate large particles.

Spacer Devices

Metered-dose inhalers dispense a plume of aerosol that may extend as much as 40 cm beyond the outlet of the actuator [160,195]. It is known that propellants with lower vapor pressures require some time to evaporate. A spacer placed between the patient and the MDI gives large droplets time to evaporate to respirable sizes while allowing collection of large particles or aggregates, which slow down as they move further from the jet, thus losing inertia and sedimentation properties under the influence of gravity [196–198]. Thus, less material is deposited in the mouth and more in the lungs of individuals than is deposited by the conventional MDI alone. The therapeutic advantage of depositing more drug in the lungs is multifaceted. Oral candidiasis has been reported in patients using inhaled corticosteroids to treat their asthma. This results from deposition in the mouth and throat. Reducing drug deposition in areas outside the target organ is always desirable, especially when toxic side effects are known to occur. Thus, a spacer device may reduce toxicity [199,200]. In some devices, the flowrate for inhalation can be monitored and adjusted by the patient by means of an airflow-actuated whistle in the spacer device [201,202]. This produces a sound at airflow rates known to result in optimal deposition in the lung. The simplest spacer device can consist of a reservoir bag [203–205], which is a bag into which the aerosol is generated to allow sedimentation before administration to the patient. The InspirBase device, a collapsible reservoir bag, is shown in Fig. 17 [205–207]. Figure 18 shows an extended actuator tube spacer. Figure 19 shows a large-volume tube spacer and a holding chamber. There is some speculation concerning the effectiveness of tube spacers. Those with a volume of 80 mL may not be sufficiently large in design to give the patients enough air to inhale according to their own breathing pattern. Also, some of the respirable aerosol particles are thought to be removed by deposition in the actuator in such a device. Cone spacers, as shown in Fig. 20, with the correct aerosol formulation may be useful because there is no deleterious effect on the production of fine particles and because a sufficient volume of air, 700 mL, is present for the patient to breathe slowly. The cone shape is intended, to some extent, to enclose the plume of aerosol and, thus, offer reduced opportunity for impaction of particles, compared with MDIs alone or with tube spacers [198]. Because respirable particles will sediment unless they are removed by inhalation, the time from firing into the spacer to inhalation must be controlled. One such system sprayed into a large-volume spacer requires that inhalation be completed within 20 sec of firing. Manufacturer's specifications should be

A

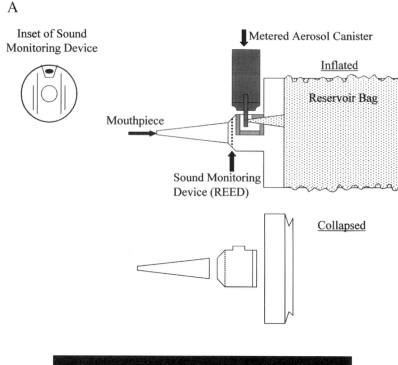

Inset of Sound
Monitoring Device

Metered Aerosol Canister

Inflated

Reservoir Bag

Mouthpiece

Sound Monitoring
Device (REED)

Collapsed

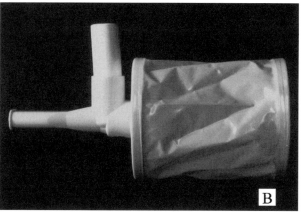

FIGURE 17 (A) Schematic (with permission of *American Review of Respiratory Disease*). (B) Photograph of reservoir bag spacer (InspirEase).

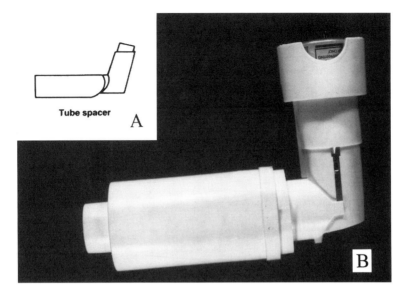

FIGURE 18 (A) Schematic (with permission of Drug Topics). (B) Photograph of an extended actuator tube spacer (Azmacort).

consulted for each device that is used, although this is probably a good estimate for cone devices. The most common cone spacer devices are the Nebuhaler [208–210] and the Aerochamber [211,212]. Studies using conical spacer devices occasionally result in contradictory results [213]. Thus, there have been reports of both reduced [208] and enhanced [209,210] efficacy of a

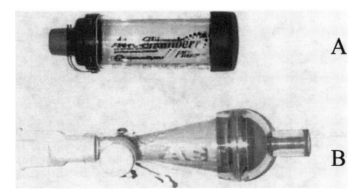

FIGURE 19 Photograph of the (A) AeroChamber Plus tube spacer. (B) ACE holding chamber.

A

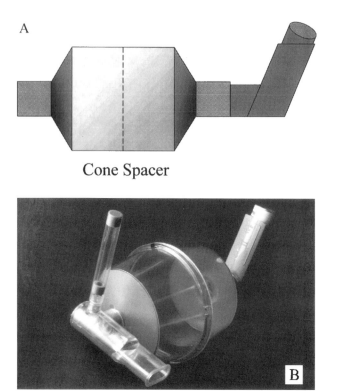

Cone Spacer

FIGURE 20   (A) Schematic and (B) photograph of cone spacer (Inhal-Aid).

device using a β-receptor agonist. Studies performed using spacers have focused initially on the advantage of their combination with an MDI rather than on the use of an MDI alone [214–217]. Beyond this, the comparison of jet nebulizers with the combination MDI and spacer system has been performed [206,211,212], with conflicting conclusions. Finally, the impact of the MDI and spacer system on therapy with different drugs has been considered [207].

AEROSOL ADMINISTRATION BIOLOGICAL FACTORS

Factors that also govern the therapeutic effect are the anatomy and physiology of the individual and diseases of the lung. These are uncontrollable variables that are important to be aware of. The lung divides dichotomously over 23 generations until it reaches the alveolar sacs. There are 300 million of these covering more than $140\,m^2$. The conducting airways are covered with smooth muscle and are innervated. Specialized cells produce mucus, and others carry cilia that transport the mucus to the trachea, where it exits and is swallowed. The purpose of these features of the lung is to prevent the entry of particulates and to maintain conditions suitable for gaseous exchange. This ensures that blood gases are maintained within prescribed limits. Thus, the pharmaceutical formulator is trying to overcome the natural housekeeping of the lung. It has been shown that the slow breathing in conjunction with a 10-sec breath hold gives improved deposition [218,219]. Why is this the case? Breathing slowly subjects particles to lower speeds, and, thus, they have less inertia. The likelihood that these particles will encounter a surface and impact in the mouth, throat, and upper airways is reduced, increasing their potential to deposit in the lower airways. At least one report suggests that the speed of inhalation may not be a significant factor [220]. Deep breathing in conjunction with breath holding has been correlated with increased aerosol persistence in the lung [219]. The breath hold allows a number of things to occur: Those particles that escape inertial impaction will be subject to sedimentation, failing under gravity, or to diffusion, random motion as a function of collisions with gas molecules. Each of these phenomena can transport the particles to a surface, where they will deposit. Thus, breath holding allows further deposition of aerosol particles that might otherwise be exhaled.

METHODS OF AEROSOL ADMINISTRATION

The most important factor in the effective use of inhalation aerosols is patient skill and correct instruction in the use of inhalers.

Nebulized aerosol is introduced to the patient by compressed air, either from a constant source or from a device known as intermittent positive-pressure ventilator. Nebulized aerosols rely less on the patient's own breathing pattern. Under some circumstances the dose administered to the patient by nebulizer is inconsistent or unpredictable. In a hospital setting, the aerosol administration can be supervised by qualified individuals. Home administration is not always supervised, and there is, therefore, a potential for misuse.

The method of administration of aerosols from MDIs is more important. The MDI should be inverted several times to ensure that the aerosol particles are suspended. The patient should exhale gently and then, tilting the head slightly, place the mouthpiece either, according to the conventional approach, in the mouth, closing the lips around it, or, according to a second approach, place the mouthpiece 6–12 in. directly in front of the open mouth. The latter suggestion is thought to aid evaporation and removal of large particles according to the principle of spacer devices. The patient should then begin to slowly inhale from resting lung volume. Just after beginning the inhalation, the inhaler must be depressed firmly. This releases the medicament, and continuing the inspiration carries the aerosol to the lung. At the end of the breath, the patient should hold for 10 sec or as long as is comfortable before breathing out slowly.

The administration of dry powder generators does not require the same degree of patient coordination as the MDI. Nevertheless, it is worthwhile considering the procedure that should be used. The device must be prepared to deliver the dose. This may mean, for example, in the case of a Spinhaler, piercing the capsule or, for the Turbuhaler, loading the base by twisting the grip at its base. The patient should exhale gently and then tilt the head and place the mouthpiece in the mouth, closing the lips around it. He should then inhale deeply and evenly. Because this device operates upon inhalation, slow breathing may not be adequate to generate the aerosol effectively. The aerosol will be transported to the lung on the breath of the patient.

Even if a patient conforms with the recommended techniques for administration of aerosols, as little as 10% of the dose reportedly reaches the site of action in the lung [221].

To summarize, aerosols have become a common sight in contemporary life. The efficiency of inhalation aerosols in the treatment of asthma relies, to a large extent, on characteristics of the particles or droplets generated. A number of devices are available for the administration of active compounds to the lung. These fall in the general categories of nebulizers, MDIs, and dry powder generators. The presence of baffles or other collection surfaces or the use of spacer devices may improve the size characteristics of aerosols generated to enhance the therapeutic effect and reduce the incidence of side effects. Finally, understanding the principles behind the methods of administration of drugs to the lung, combined with an awareness of anatomy and physiology and a knowledge of the advantages of certain breathing patterns, enables the patient to be instructed in the appropriate use of inhalation aerosols.

SUMMARY

After a brief explanation of the factors governing deposition of aerosol particles in the lung, the common methods of administration of inhalation aerosols have been described. The drugs most frequently delivered by this route are bronchodilators. Correct administration and the use of inhaler accessories, such as spacer devices, enhance the efficacy of inhaled drugs. It is essential that the patient be instructed in the correct use of the devices to optimize the therapeutic effect.

The discussion of products has deliberately been restricted to those that have been commercialized. There are several reasons for doing this. Firstly, this is consistent with the title of the chapter. Secondly, the author does not have to immerse himself in the plethora of information on technologies under development. Lastly, the reader has not been introduced to technologies that may be short-lived and ultimately irrelevant to progress in the field. Indeed, the benefit of having a decade between this edition and the last is that some technologies that were emerging in the early 1990s have since faded and the reader has no reason to be concerned about them.

The introduction of new drugs (salmeterol, fluticasone, budesonide, formoterol, for example) has caused a number of new aerosol systems to be introduced in each of the categories of propellant-driven metered-dose inhalers, dry powder inhalers, and nebulizers. Since existing nebulizers can be employed to deliver new drugs and metered-dose inhaler technology improvements are not apparent to the observer (changes in gasket materials, can coatings, etc.), the most prominent changes would seem to be evident in the emergence of new dry powder inhaler systems, mostly developed on a drug-specific basis. While a surprisingly small number of new products have been commercialized recently, the research since the early 1990s will give rise to a variety of new products hitherto not seen by patients and healthcare professionals.

REFERENCES

1. Crowder TM, Louey MD, Sethuraman VV, Smyth HDC, Hickey AJ. Pharm Technol 2001; 25:99–113.
2. Dunbar CA, Hickey AJ, Holzner P. KONA 1998; 16:7–44.
3. http://www.lungusa.org/.
4. Rance RW. J Soc Cosmet Chem 1972; 23:197–208.
5. Rance RW. J Soc Cosmet Chem 1974; 25:545–561.
6. Halbert MK, Mazumder MK, Bond RL. Environ Res 1982; 29:263–271.
7. Halbert MK, Mazumder MK, Bond RL. Food Cosmet Toxicol 1981; 19:85–88.
8. Byron PR. Drug Dev Ind Pharm 1986; 12:993–1015.
9. Gonda I. Crit Rev Ther Drug Carrier Syst 1990; 6:273–313.
10. Davies PJ. Soap Perfum Cosmet 1983; 56:78–81.
11. Newman SP, Clarke SW. Thorax 1983; 38:881–886.
12. Moren F. Eur J Respir Dis 1982; 63:51–55.
13. Clay MM, Pavia D, Clarke SW. Thorax 1986; 41:364–368.
14. Task Group on Lung Dynamics. Health Phys 1966; 12:173–207.
15. Camner P. Health Phys 1981; 40:99–100.
16. Byron PR. Pharm Technol 1987; 11:42–56.
17. Smith G, Hiller C, Mazumder M, Bone R. Am Rev Respir Dis 1980; 121:513–517.
18. Dalby RN, Byron PR. Pharm Res 1988; 5:36–39.
19. Fuchs NA, Sutugin AG. In: Davies CN, ed. Aerosol Science. New York: Academic Press, 1966:1–30.
20. Hinds WC. Aerosol Technology, Second Edition. New York: Wiley, 1983.
21. Reist PC. Introduction to Aerosol Science. New York: Macmillan, 1984:80.
22. Allen T. Particle Size Measurement. New York: Chapman and Hall, 1990.
23. Raabe OG. J Air Pollut Control Assoc 1976; 26:856–860.

24. Gonda I. J Pharm Pharmacol 1981; 33:52P.
25. Gonda I. Int J Pharm 1985; 27:99–116.
26. Gonda I, Chan H-K. J Pharm Pharmcol 1985; 37:56P.
27. Chan H-K, Gonda I. Int J Pharm 1988; 41:147–157.
28. Yu CP, Chandra K. J Aerosol Sci 1978; 9:175–180.
29. Cocks AT, Fernando RP. J Aerosol Sci 1982; 13:9–19.
30. Haenel G, Zankl B. Tellus 1979; 31:478–486.
31. Hanel G. Adv Geophys 1976; 19:73–187.
32. Martonen TB. Bull Math Biol 1982; 44:425–442.
33. Martonen TB, Bell KA, Phalen RF, Wilson AF, Ho A. Ann Occup Hyg 1982; 26:93–108.
34. Tang IN. In: Willeke K, ed. Generation of Aerosols and Facilities for Exposure Experiments. Ann Arbor, MI: Ann Arbor Science, 1980.
35. Tang IN, Munkelwitz HR, Davis JG. J Aerosol Sci 1977; 8:149–159.
36. Thudium J. Pure Appl Geophys 1978; 116:130–148.
37. Milburn RH, Crider WL, Morton SD. A M A Arch Ind Health 1957; 15:59–62.
38. Ferron GA, Haider B, Kreyling WG. J Aerosol Sci 1983; 14:196–199.
39. Scherer PW, Haselton FR, Hanna LM, Stone DR. J Appl Physiol 1979; 47:544–550.
40. Straubel H. In: Benarie MM, ed. Studies in Environmental Science. Amsterdam: Elsevier, 1980:239–244.
41. Muir DCF. Clinical Aspects of Inhaled Particles. William Heinemann, 1972:179.
42. Byron PR, Davis SS, Bubb MD, Cooper P. Pestic Sci 1977; 8:521–526.
43. Gonda I, Kayes JB, Groom CV, Fildes FJT. In: Stanley-Wood N, Allen T, eds. Particle Size Analysis. New York: Wiley, 1981:31–43.
44. Hiller FC, Mazumder MK, Wilson JD, Bone RC. J Pharm Pharmacol 1980; 32:605–609.
45. Hiller FC, Mazumder MK, Wilson JD, Bone RC. J Pharm Sci 1980; 69:334–337.
46. Hickey AJ, Martonen TB. Pharm Res 1993; 10:1–7.
47. Ferron GA. J Aerosol Sci 1977; 8:251–267.
48. Hickey AJ, Gonda I, Irwin WJ, Fildes FJT. J Pharm Sci 1990; 79:1009–1014.
49. Eisner AD, Graham RC, Martonen TB. J Aerosol Sci 1990; 21:833–848.
50. Persons DD, Hess GD, Muller WJ, Scherer PW. J Appl Physiol 1987; 63:1195–1204.
51. Persons DD, Hess GD, Scherer PW. J Appl Physiol 1987; 63:1205–1209.
52. Ferron GA, Oberdorster G, Henneberg R. J Aerosol Med 1989; 2:271–283.
53. Ferron GA, Kreyling WG, Haider B. J Aerosol Sci 1990; 21:611–631.
54. Ferron GA, Haider B, Kreyling WG. J Aerosol Sci 1988; 19:343–363.
55. Morrow PE. Physiol Rev 1986; 66:330–376.
56. Dethlefsen U, Repges R. Med Klin 1985; 80:44–47.
57. Feinstein W, Sciarra JJ. J Pharm Sci 1975; 64:408–441.
58. DeLuca PP, Gupta P, Hickey AJ, Mehta R. Pharm Res 1990; 7.
59. Gupta PK, Hickey AJ. J Control Release 1991; 17:129–148.
60. Farr SJ, Kellaway IW, Parry-Jones DR, Woolfrey SG. Int J Pharm 1985; 26:303–316.

61. Farr SJ, Kellaway IW, Carman-Meakin B. J Control Release 1987; 5:119–127.
62. Woolfrey SG, Taylor G, Kellaway IW, Smith A. J Control Release 1988; 5:203–209.
63. Taylor KMG, Taylor G, Kellaway IW, Stevens J. Int J Pharm 1990; 58:57–61.
64. Niven RW, Schreier H. Pharm Res 1990; 7:1127–1133.
65. Primrose WR. Lancet 1983; 8330–8927.
66. Byron PR. J Pharm Sci 1986; 75:433–438.
67. Gonda I. J Pharm Sci 1987; 77:340–348.
68. Hickey AJ. Drug Top 1989; 133:60–69.
69. Andersen SD. Med Sci Sports Exerc 1981; 13:259–265.
70. Miller WF. Arch Intern Med 1973; 131:148–155.
71. Wilson AF. Progress in Drug Research. Boston: Birkhauser-Verlag, 1984:111–125.
72. Woolcock AJ. Am Rev Respir Dis 1977; 115:191–194.
73. O'Donoghue DJ. Br Med J 1983; 286:1053.
74. McFadden ER. Inhaled Aerosol Bronchodilators. Baltimore: Williams and Wilkins, 1986.
75. Jenne JW, Murphy S, eds. Drug Therapy for Asthma. New York: Marcel Dekker, 1987.
76. Soler M, Imhof E, Perruchoud AP. Respiration 1990; 57:114–121.
77. Clarke SW, Newman SP. Thorax 1984; 39:1–7.
78. Nilson HT, Simonsson BG, Strom B. Eur J Clin Pharmacol 1976; 10:1–7.
79. Ruffin RE, Kenworthy MC, Newhouse MT. 1978; 23:338–343.
80. Salome CM, Schoeffel RE, Woolcock AJ. Thorax 1981; 36:580–584.
81. Maeson FPV, Smeets JJ, Gubbelmans HLL, Zweers PGMA. 1990; 97:590–594.
82. Pinnas JL, Bush RK, Dockhorn RJ, Repsher L, Neidl MJ. J Allergy Clin Immunol 1987; 79:768–775.
83. Walker SB, Kradjan WA, Bierman CW. Pharmacotherapy 1985; 5:127–137.
84. Meltzer EO, Kemp JP, Orgel HA, Izu AE. Pediatrics 1982; 69:340–345.
85. Slavin RG, Izu AE, Bernstein IL, Blumenthal MN, Bolin JF, et al. J Allergy Clin Immunol 1980; 66:379–385.
86. Carpentiere G, Marino S, Castello F, Baldanza C, Bonanno CT. Respiration 1990; 57:100–103.
87. Reed CE. Am Rev Respir Dis 1990; 141:S82–S88.
88. Brundage KL, Mohsini KG, Froese AB, Fisher JT. Am Rev Respir Dis 1990; 142:1137–1142.
89. Schoeffel RE, Andersen SD, Lindsay DA. Aust N Z J Med 1983; 13:157–161.
90. Weiner D, Saaid M, Rashef A. Am Rev Respir Dis 1988; 137:1309–1311.
91. Azeveoo M, Dacosta JT, Fontes P, Dasilva JPM, Arauso O. J Int Med Res 1990; 18:37–49.
92. Pavia D, Bateman JRM, Sheahan NF, Clarke SW. Eur J Respir Dis 1981; 61:245–253.
93. Morandini GC, Mauro M, Finiguerra M, Zanierato G. Drugs Exp Clin Res 1981; VII:513–520.
94. Hodson ME, Penketh ARL, Batten JC. Lancet 1981; 8256:1137–1139.

95. Møller NE, Eriksen KR, Feddersen C, Flensborg EW, Høiby N, et al. Eur J Respir Dis 1982; 63:130–139.
96. Itkin IN, ML M. J Allergy 1970; 45:146–162.
97. Brastburg J. Antimicrob Agents Chemother 1990; 34:381–384.
98. Hoiby N, Koch K. Thorax 1990; 45:881–884.
99. Standaert TA, Vandevanter D, Ramsey BW, Vasiljev M, Nardella P, et al. J Aerosol Med 2000; 13:147–153.
100. Geller DE, Pitlick WH, Nardella PA, Tracewell WG, Ramsey BW. Chest 2002; 122:219–226.
101. Shak S. Chest 1995; 107:65S–70S.
102. Fiel SB, Fuchs HJ, Johnson C, Gonda I, Clark AR. Chest 1995; 108:153–156.
103. Lourenço RV. Arch Intern Med 1982; 142:2299–2308.
104. Physicians' Desk Reference. Medical Economics. Oradell, NJ, 1985.
105. Julien M, Hoeffel JM, Flick MR. J Appl Physiol 1986; 60:433–440.
106. Halden E, Hedstrand U, Torsner K. Acta Anaesthiol Scand 1982; 26:121–125.
107. Lotvall JO, Skoogh B-E, Lemen RJ, Elwood W, Barnes PJ, Chung KF. Am Rev Respir Dis 1990; 142:1390–1394.
108. Boucher M, Roy MT, Henderson J. Ann Pharmacother 1992; 26:772–774.
109. Asmus MJ, Sherman J, Hendeles L. J Allergy Clin Immunol 1999; 104:S53–S60.
110. Davis SS. Int J Pharm 1978; 1:71–83.
111. Davis SS, Elson G, Whitmore J. Int J Pharm 1978; 1:85–93.
112. Chowhan ZT, Amaro AA. J Pharm Sci 1977; 66:1254–1258.
113. Debs R, Brunette E, Fuchs H, Lin E, Shah M, et al. Am Rev Respir Dis 1990; 142:1164–1167.
114. Perry RH, Chilton CH. New York: McGraw-Hill, 1975:5–11.
115. Boucher RM, Kreuter J. Ann Allergy 1968; 26:591–600.
116. Clay MM, Pavia D, Newman SP, Clarke SW. Thorax 1983; 38:755–759.
117. Clay MM, Newman SP, Pavia D, Jones TL, Clarke SW. Lancet 1983; 592–594.
118. Dennis JH, Stenton SC, Beach JR, Avery AJ, Walters EH, Hendrick DJ. Thorax 1990; 45:728–732.
119. Mercer TT, Tillery MI, Chow HY. Am Ind Hyg Assoc J 1968; 29:66–78.
120. Lewis RA, Ellis CJ, Fleming JS, Balachandran W. Thorax 1984; 39:712.
121. Asmundson T, Johnson RF, Kilburn KH, Goodrich JK. Am Rev Respir Dis 1973; 108:506–511.
122. Bau SK, Aspin N, Wood DE, Levison H. Pediatrics 1971; 48:605–612.
123. Wolfsdorf J, Swift DL, Avery ME. Pediatrics 1969; 43:799–808.
124. Laube BL, Swift DL, Addams GK. Aerosol Sci Technol 1984; 2:97–102.
125. Pillay M, Ackermans JA, Cox PH. Eur J Nucl Med 1987; 13:331–334.
126. Ishfaq MM, Ghosh SK, Mostafa AB, Hesselwood SR, Williams NR, Hickey AJ. Eur J Nucl Med 1984; 9:141–143.
127. Ryan G, Dolovich MB, Roberts RS, Frith PA, Juniper EF, et al. Am Rev Respir Dis 1981; 123:195–199.
128. Andersen SD, Schoeffel RE, Finney M. Thorax 1983; 38:284–291.
129. Staniforth JN, Lewis RA, Tattersfield AE. Thorax 1983; 38:751–754.
130. Crompton GK. Pharm J 1985; 237–238.

131. Cochrane GM, Prior JG, Rees PJ. Br Med J 1985; 290:1608–1609.
132. Shenfield GH, Evans ME, Walker SR, Peterson JW. Am Rev Respir Dis 1978; 108:501–505.
133. Newth CJL, Newth CV, Turner JAP. Pediatr Res 1981; 15:1216.
134. O'Dougherty MJ, Page C, Bradbeer C, Thomas S, Barlow D, et al. Lancet 1988; 2:1283–1286.
135. Matthys H, Köhler D. Respiration 1985; 48:269–276.
136. Douglas JG, Leslie MJ, Crompton GK, Grant IWB. Br Med J 1985; 290:29.
137. Kradjan WA, Lakshminarayan S. Chest 1985; 87:512–516.
138. Newman SP, Pellow PGD, Clarke SW. Chest 1987; 92:991–994.
139. Hickey AJ, Byron PR. J Pharm Sci 1987; 76:338–340.
140. Editorial. Lancet 1984; 8406:789–790.
141. Weinberg E, Klein M. S A M J 1988; 74:136–137.
142. Kuchel K, Hickey AJ. Unpublished data.
143. Litt M, Swift DE. Am Rev Respir Dis 1972; 105:308–310.
144. Steventon RD, Wilson RSE. Br J Dis Chest 1981; 75:88–90.
145. Redy DJ, Barton K, Stanford CF. Postgrad Med J 1988; 64:306–307.
146. Botman MJ, Kreiger RAD. J Hosp Infect 1987; 10:204–208.
147. Warachit B. J Med Assoc Thail 1988; 33–34.
148. Editorial. Lancet 1988; 2:202.
149. Rocchiccioli KM, Pickering CAC. Thorax 1984; 39:710.
150. Borland C, Chamberlain A, Barber B, Higenbottam TM. Thorax 1984; 39:240.
151. DeYoung L. *The AeroDose multidose inhaler device design and delivery characteristics.* Presented at Respiratory Drug Delivery VI, Hilton Head, FL, 1998.
152. Dunbar C, Hickey AJ. Pharm Technol 1997; 21:116–125.
153. Riker Laboratories R. UK Patent No. 837,465, 1960.
154. Weast RC, ed. Handbook of Physics and Chemistry. Boca Raton, FL: CRC Press, 1985/1986:E31-E42.
155. Porush I, Thiel CG, Young JG. J Am Pharm Assoc 1960; 49:70–72.
156. Young JG, Porush I, Thiel CG, Cohen S, Stimmel CH. J Am Pharm Assoc 1960; 49:72–74.
157. Fiese EF, Gorman WG, Dolinsky D, Harwood RJ, Hunke WA, et al. J Pharm Sci 1988; 77:90–93.
158. Rea AR, Drew RM, Wong SSL, Hailey DM. J Pharm Pharmacol 1982; 34:225–229.
159. Scharmach RE. Aerosol Age 1982; 8:36–40.
160. Newman SP, Morén F, Pavia D, Corrado O, Clarke SW. Int J Pharm 1982; 11:337–344.
161. Rivlin J, Mindorff C, Levison H. Am Rev Respir Dis 1983; 127(suppl):206.
162. Cushley MJ, Lewis RA, Tattersfield AE. Thorax 1983; 38:908–913.
163. Webber BA, Collins JV, Braithwaite MA. Br J Dis Chest 1982; 76:69–74.
164. Shim CS, Williams MH. J Allergy Clin Immunol 1984; 73:387–390.
165. Cissik JH, Bode FR, Smith JA. Chest 1986; 90:489–493.
166. Lourenco RV, Cotromanes E. Arch Intern Med 1982; 142:2163–2172.

167. Fuller HD, Dolovich MB, Postmituck G, Pack WW, Newhouse TM. Am Rev Respir Dis 1990; 141:440–444.
168. Patel UB, Bell AE, Martin GP, Marriott C. J Pharm Pharmacol 1985; 37(suppl):108P.
169. Orehek J, Gayrard P, Grimaud CH, Charpin J. Br Med J 1976; 1:76.
170. Paterson IC, Crompton GK. Br Med J 1976;76–77.
171. Saunders KB. Br Med J 1965; 5441:1037–1038.
172. Harper TB, Strunk RC. Am J Dis Child 1981; 135:218–221.
173. Morley CJ, Miller N, Bangham AD, Davis JA. Lancet 1981; 10:64–68.
174. Pischtiak AH. Chim Oggi 2002; 20:14–19.
175. Molina MJ, Rowland FS. Nature 1974; 249:1810.
176. Register F. 2002; 67:48370–48385.
177. Smyth HDC, Mejia-Millan EA, Hickey AJ. Respir Drug Delivery VIII 2002; 2:735–738.
178. Evans RM, Attwood D, Chatham S, Farr S. J Pharm Pharmacol 1990; 42:601–605.
179. Evans RM, Farr SJ, Armstrong NA, Chatham SM. Pharm Res 1991; 8:624–629.
180. Sommerville ML, Cain JB, Charles S, Johnson J, Hickey AJ. Pharm Dev Technol 2000; 5:219–230.
181. Coady TJ, Davies HJ, Barnes P. Clin Allergy 1976; 6:1–6.
182. Wetterlin KIL. Pharm Res 1988; 5:506–598.
183. Ribeiro LB, Wiren JE. Allergy 1990; 45:382–385.
184. Clark AR, Hollingworth AM. J Aerosol Med 1993; 6:99–110.
185. USP24. *The United States Pharmacopoeia and National Formulary*, 2000; 1895–1912.
186. Dunbar CA, Morgan B, VanOort M, Hickey AJ. PDA J Pharm Sci Technol 2000; 54:478–484.
187. Wolny A. Pr Inst Inzynierii Chemicznej Politechniki Warszawskiej 1979; 8:21–35.
188. Al-Chalabi SAM, Jones AR, Luckham PF. J Aerosol Sci 1990; 21:821–826.
189. Hickey AJ, Jackson GV, Fildes FJT. J Pharm Sci 1988; 77:804–809.
190. Bell JH, Hartley PS, Cox JSG. J Pharm Sci 1971; 60:1559–1564.
191. Byron PR, Jashnani R, Germin S. Pharm Res 1990; 7:81S.
192. Malem H, Ward M, Henry D, Smith WHR, Gonda I. Lancet 1981; 664–666.
193. Hickey AJ. Drug Dev Ind Pharm 1988; 14:337–352.
194. Hickey AJ. Ph.D. dissertation, University of Aston, Birmingham, England, 1984.
195. Hallworth GW. In: Ganderton D, Jones T, eds. Drug Delivery to the Respiratory Tract. New York: VCH, 1987:87–118.
196. Corr D, Dolovich M, McCormack D, Ruffin R, Obminski G, Newhouse M. J Aerosol Sci 1982; 13:1–7.
197. Newman SP. J Aerosol Sci 1983; 14:69.
198. Newman SP. In: Clarke SW, Pavia D, eds. Aerosols and the Lung: Clinical and Experimental Aspects. London: Butterworths, 1984:197–224.
199. Prahl PH, Jensen T. Clin Allergy 1987; 17:393–398.
200. Brown PH, Blundell G, Greening AP, Crompton GK. Thorax 1990; 45:736–739.
201. Anonymous. Aust J Pharm 1982; 63:636.
202. Shim C, Williams HM. Am J Med 1980; 69:891–894.

203. Kim CS, Berkeley BB, Sackner MA. Am Rev Respir Dis 1981; 123(suppl):71.

204. Sackner MA, Brown LK, Kim CS. Chest 1981; 80:915–918.

205. Tobin MJ, Jenoury G, Danta I, Kim C, Watson H, Sackner MA. Am Rev Respir Dis 1982; 126:670–675.

206. Morley TF, Marozsan E, Zappasodi SJ, Gordon R, Griesback R, Giudice JC. Chest 1988; 94:1205–1209.

207. Karpel JP, Pesin J, Greenberg D, Centry E. Chest 1990; 98:835–839.

208. Cox ID, Wallis PJW, Apps MCP. Br Med J 1984;288–1044.

209. Newman SP, Millar AB, Lennard-Jones TR, Moren F, Clarke SW. Thorax 1984; 39:935–941.

210. Hidinger KG, Dorow P. Curr Ther Res Clin Exp 1984; 337–341.

211. Salzman GA, Pyszczynski DR. Am J Respir Dis 1985; 133:A48.

212. Berenberg MJ, Baigelman W, Cupples LA, Pierce L. Am J Respir Dis 1985.

213. Corr D, Dolovich M, Obminski G, McCormack D, Newhouse MT. J Aerosol Sci 1983; 14:70.

214. Hodges IGC, Milner RP, Stokes GM. Arch Dis Child 1981; 56:787–788.

215. Ellul-Micallef R, Moren F, Wetterlin K, Hidinger KC. Thorax 1980; 35:620–623.

216. Gomm SA, Keaney NP, Winsey NJP. Thorax 1980; 35:552–556.

217. Bloomfield P, Crompton GK. Br Med J 1979; 2:1479.

218. Lawford P, McKenzie D. Br J Dis Chest 1982; 76:229.

219. Williams TJ. Br J Dis Chest 1982; 76:223–228.

220. Palmes ED, Wang CS, Goldring RM, Altshuler B. J Appl Physiol 1973; 34:356–360.

221. Newman SP, Pavia D, Moren F, Sheahan NF, Clarke SW. Thorax 1981; 36:52–55.

13

Therapeutic Aerosols: An Overview from a Clinical Perspective

F. Charles Hiller

University of Arkansas for Medical Sciences, Little Rock, Arkansas, U.S.A.

INTRODUCTION

The explosion of knowledge about aerosol medicine since the early 1990s is impressive. Who would have thought 10–15 years ago that we would be investigating aerosols for use in such things as lung transplantation, gene therapy, treatment of respiratory failure, nicotine for smoking cessation, and many others, as well as adding new and valuable information to currently utilized therapeutic modalities such aerosol bronchodilators, aerosolized steroids, and, for CF, antibiotic aerosols. The potential for aerosol science to contribute to medical care has never been greater. The focus of this review is on three broad topics: (1) certain basic aspects of aerosol deposition, (2) new information about "old" aerosols, i.e., bronchodilators and their delivery, and (3) new horizons for aerosols in the treatment of human diseases.

As we recognize the progress in management of diseases by inhalational delivery of drugs as aerosols, it is necessary to acknowledge that many of the human conditions we treat are caused directly by inhaled particles. In the United

States alone, about 450,000 deaths a year are directly attributable to toxins inhaled via tobacco smoke. The increasing use of tobacco in developing nations is now bringing the epidemic of diseases caused by tobacco to the rest of the world. Occupational exposure to minerals such as asbestos and silica is now very much reduced in the industrialized West, but exposure continues to be a problem in the Third World. Inhaled antigens cause allergic lung diseases such as asthma, and inhaled microbes cause infections ranging from viral to tuberculosis. The importance of inhaled particles in the pathogenesis of lung disease cannot be overemphasized.

Some of the diseases caused by inhaled toxins and antigens are treated with inhaled medications. Inhalation therapy has been a mainstay of the treatment of lung disease for centuries [1]. Although most such early therapies were worthless, a few were effective. The inhalation of smoke from plants containing stramonium has been used since antiquity to treat asthma [2].

In 1974, the Sugarloaf Conference [3] underscored the empiric nature of many applications of inhalation therapy, as it was called at that time. The scientific basis for many treatments was very weak. Although there has been considerable progress since the early 1980s, there are today still many uncertainties about inhaled drug delivery and many variations of delivery equipment and methods. A more recent consensus statement reviews some advances and describes continuing needs for investigation [4].

Given the current rising interest in aerosol treatment modalities, it is especially remarkable that nothing of consequence is taught in medical schools about particle generation or deposition in the lung. The vast majority of physicians who order aerosol treatments of any type for their patients know next to nothing about this process. This is not to say they are uninformed about the medications they prescribe, only the delivery method. Graduates of schools of pharmacy are probably similarly devoid of adequate teaching about inhaled medications. The changing knowledge about best delivery practices is not well disseminated.

PARTICLE DEPOSITION

The site and quantity of particle deposition in the respiratory tract depend mainly on particle size but are also affected by respiratory pattern and airway pathology. Understanding the terminology of particle deposition is essential. *Deposition* is the capture of particles on a surface. Some inhaled particles are deposited by the respiratory epithelium, and others are exhaled. *Clearance* is the removal of any deposited particles by any process and is not a major topic of this discussion, although it may be important for the efficacy of inhaled medications. *Total deposition* is the difference between the inhaled and exhaled mass of the substance of interest. *Regional deposition* defines mass in various anatomic levels in the respiratory tract [5]. Regions are defined as (1) the nasopharyngeal region, which is from the nose to the vocal cords, (2) the tracheobronchial region (tracheobronchial), from the vocal cords to and including terminal bronchioles (generations 0–17), and pulmonary region (pulmonary), from and including respiratory bronchioles to distal alveoli [5]. Throughout this chapter, these abbreviations are used to refer to these regions. Note that the Task Group model is a nasal inhalation model and is not representative of mouth inhalation. For some aspects of discussion, the tracheobronchial region may be considered in two parts, large airways (trachea through subsegmental airways) and small airways (generations 6–17). Deposition can also be considered on the basis of deposition per airway generation and deposition per unit surface area.

Surface Area Concentration
Respiratory Tract Dimensions

It is important that various anatomic dimensions be considered when the biological effects of deposition are assessed. This is especially important when deposition is reported only as total or regional respiratory tract deposition, which is usually the case, and not deposition by unit surface area. Anatomic dimensions of the respiratory tract are listed in Table 1. The total surface area per airway generation increases rapidly, so surface area concentrations (determined using lung models) of deposited aerosol decline several orders of magnitude from large airways to the pulmonary region [6,7]. The magnitude of this decline depends mainly upon the size of the inhaled particle. For example, the surface concentration decreases more than 10-fold from airway generation 3 to generation 15 for a 1.0-μm particle and more than 100-fold for a 5-μm particle over the same generations. For all respirable sizes, surface concentration is highest in airway generation 3 [9]. Expression of deposition as mass in a region can be misleading. This concept has received relatively little attention in the study of the efficacy of therapeutic aerosol.

Local Aberrations in Deposition

Calculation of surface area concentrations implies even distribution of particles on the airway wall, but this is probably not the case. Studies of deposition in lung models of large [12,13] and small airways [14] suggest that deposition on airway surfaces is uneven. At all airway generations, it is likely that flow kinetics cause heavy deposition at some points, especially at carinae but also along selected portions of the airways between branches. This creates "hot spots" and "cold spots" with respect to particle concentration on airway walls. The importance of uneven deposition with local "hot spots" with high drug concentration, and also "cold" spots with low concentration, is not known. That local deposition in the forms of "hot spots" could be detrimental is made plausible by the evidence that "hot spots" of tobacco smoke particulate deposition have been related to pre-dilection of lung cancer for those sites [12]. It is reasonable to speculate that such uneven deposition of a medication might be detrimental or might be a reason for less than maximal efficacy. This subject has not been sufficiently studied.

Central and Peripheral Deposition. Aerosol deposition in people with obstructive lung disease is shifted toward larger, more central airways. The extent to which airway obstruction reduces delivery to small airways and, thereby, limits drug efficacy is unclear.

Focal Irregularities in Deposition. Reference has already been made to the irregular deposition of aerosol in normal large vs. small airways. The effects of partial obstructions and irregularities in the airway surface configuration also disturb deposition, [15]. Airway obstruction, thus, impairs deposition in several ways. Total obstruction completely blocks deposition in some diseased airways. Local partial obstructions perturb deposition by causing irregularities in deposition at the level of single airways. In general, airway obstruction causes deposition to shift to more central areas. The effects of these various perturbations of deposition caused by airway pathology on efficacy of therapeutic aerosols are not sufficiently studied.

Postdeposition Drug Distribution. In considering the effects of irregular surface deposition, drug distribution after deposition must also be studied. Movement of drug on airway surfaces may occur. Such movement also might be a mechanism by which drug is distributed from hot spots to portions of airway surface that receive less aerosol. The effectiveness of surface activities such as surface diffusion and mucociliary movement in evening out deposition irregularities is not known. With the expectation that further study will confirm and clarify the current information regarding deposition irregularities, further study of surface events that might affect surface concentrations after deposition will become mandatory.

There are other reasons for understanding better what happens to drugs after deposition. There is little information describing movement of drugs from site of deposition to site of action. Movement to the site of action probably takes place, in part, by nonspecific mucociliary transport and by passive diffusion after deposition. Drugs must also move through the mucosa to the site of action, either on smooth muscle cells in the case of β_2-adrenergic receptor agonists or on various mediator cells in the mucosa and submucosa. The mechanisms and routes by which this movement takes place are insufficiently studied but may be very important for improving drug efficacy.

Targeting Deposition

Targeting of a certain region of the respiratory tract may be desirable from a therapeutic viewpoint. When bronchodilators are given to patients with asthma, small and medium airways are the target. When medication is given for systemic absorption, the target is the gas exchange region. Another reason for targeting has been the effort to minimize deposition in the upper airway and to maximize deposition below the larynx. There have been remarkable advances in targeting techniques in the last several years. Size has been the most important factor for targeting for many years, but new studies indicate that generation methods, other particle characteristics such as density, and delivery/inhalation modifications may greatly improve the deposition fraction.

Measurement of Deposition

If targeting is a goal, it must be based on a presumption that deposition can in some way be assessed to determine the outcome of targeting. Assessment of pharmacokinetic and pharmacodynamic effects is useful. Direct quantitative measurement of targeting, i.e., the measurement of deposition by airway generation, is generally not possible in human beings. A recent study of deposition of a stable isotope of triamcinolone is remarkable in the accomplishment because it accomplishes separation of deposition between conducting airways and acinar airways, i.e., generations 1–14 and 15–23, using PET scanning [16]. This technique is of great interest and has considerable research potential. Comparison of such measurements to changes in outcome measured by clinical parameters would add a new dimension in the assessment of therapeutic aerosol design.

Targeting by Size Control

The goal of most manufacturers has been to produce particles in the 2- to 3-μm size range, although this is not always achieved. This size seems most appropriate for delivering the greatest mass to small airways. Based on information about β_2-adrenergic receptor location, this is the proper area to target for treating asthma. Examination of plots of regional deposition indicates that 20–30% of particles of this size will deposit in the airways during normal breathing. Although ultrafine particles, those smaller than 0.1 μm, deposit in distal airways in progressively greater fractional quantities, the mass of 0.03- and 0.3-μm particles is, respectively, 10^{-6} and 10^{-3} that of a 3-μm particles. An aerosol of ultrafine particles needs to be much more concentrated or inhaled much longer to deliver an equivalent mass of drug. Such a particle concentration cannot be practically achieved. Consequently the 2- to 3-μm size is the most practical for best overall respiratory tract dosing. This size is also effective for delivering the greatest total mass to the pulmonary region. Traditional aerosols deliver heterodisperse aerosols, so if the size is stated as 3 μm, this in fact represents the mass median aerodynamic diameter (MMAD). Many particles are smaller and many larger. Knowledge of this distribution allows calculation of estimated deposition parameters based on lung models. If the size distribution can be narrowed, the aerosol can be targeted somewhat more tightly, and efficacy for a given dose may change. There is some evidence for this. Administration of ipratropium bromide, 8 μg, as a monodisperse 2.8-μm aerosol is as effective as administration of 40 μg as a heterodisperse aerosol from a metered-dose inhaler (MDI) and spacer [17]. In practice, standard medical devices cannot generate monodisperse aerosols.

Size can be controlled by many aspects of aerosol generation. These include control of hygroscopic growth, control of evaporation, and control of generation techniques. While manipulation of particle growth characteristics is not commonly studied, it has some potential as a means of aiding targeting. Control of generation and inhalation techniques are usually given more attention, and such will be our approach.

Targeting by Control of Hygroscopic Growth

Most inhaled medications are hygroscopic; that is, they accumulate water and grow in size. Some particles are deliquescent; that is, they become a droplet solution as water accumulates. Growth depends on relative humidity, and conversion to a droplet usually takes place rather abruptly at a specific humidity, termed the *deliquescent point*. Growth continues as humidity rises, with size increasing exponentially as humidity increases to greater than 95%. Respiratory tract temperature and humidity [18] and health implications of particle growth [19] have been reviewed. The size change caused by particle hygroscopic growth affects the total deposition and deposition site of inhaled hygroscopic particles.

Clinical studies indicate that smaller particles are more effective than larger particles when given for bronchodilation [20,21]. Optimal particle size has traditionally been chosen without regard for aerosol hygroscopic properties. Inhaled particles can grow considerably as they accumulate water in the humid respiratory tract. The size change would affect deposition pattern and quantity. Manipulation of hygroscopic growth to a slow growth rate that would allow better penetration to peripheral airways is the goal of most efforts to control growth.

Past efforts to target a specific deposition site were based on the control of particle size at inhalation. Also, efforts to control growth of particles by adding substances with surfactant properties have been reported. Addition of lauric and capric acids to disodium fluorescein markedly reduces particle growth [22], as does the addition of a cetyl alcohol monolayer to saline droplets [23]. Such a reduction of growth would be expected to facilitate particle penetration to more distal lung regions before deposition. The extent to which commonly used therapeutic aerosols grow at respiratory tract humidity needs further study.

Most MDIs contain surfactant materials that might be expected to affect growth. The shift in size distribution caused by exposure of MDI-produced aerosols to high (95–96%) humidity is modest. The MMAD of a metaproterenol sulfate aerosol from an MDI increased from 4.05 μm at 16% relative humidity to 5.22 μm at 98% relative humidity [23], and similar studies indicate growth also for sodium cromolyn [25]. The high humidity used in these studies was not as high as the 99.5% humidity present in distal lung [26].

Information from measurements at these high levels does indicate significant influence. Particles generated from a hypotonic solution penetrate further than do particles of similar initial size generated from a hypertonic solution [27]. Similar observations made using bronchodilators generated as supersaturated particles indicate a twofold to threefold growth from 0 to 99.5% RH, while disodium cromoglycate remains a crystalline structure up to 90% relative humidity and grows only 1.26-fold over this size range [28]. These data indicate, as one would predict, that hypotonic particles evaporate in vivo while the hypertonic particles presumably grow, so, in either case, particle concentration moves toward equilibrium at isotonicity. There are few studies documenting effects of hygroscopic size changes in vivo. There is probably potential for the application of growth control particle generation to medical aerosols, but we do not yet have sufficient understanding of the process to make clinical application practical.

Controlling Inhalation and Modifying Delivery Technology

Aerosolized medications are unique because of the complexity of their formulation requirements and the necessary engineering for their delivery devices. Medications loaded into MDIs or dry powder inhalers (DPIs) must be prepared so that they will disperse quickly and not reaggregate in the generation process, and the device must be easy to use and deliver accurate dose. There is no accurate control of the quantity reaching the target area. Intravenous medications are simpler—a known dose can be delivered and pharmacokinetic and pharmacodynamic properties examined. Ingested medications can be defined in terms of fraction absorbed from the gut and pharmacokinetic and pharmacodynamic performance. Inhaled particles must be created with less than full understanding of the factors that control dose: (1) physical properties of the particle, (2) the generation system, and (3) patient inhalation techniques. All of these lead to a much more "nebulous" design process than commonly encountered with intravenous or oral medications.

Because of the uncertainty in dose delivery and the relatively benign nature of many inhaled medications used in past years, large quantities were often delivered from nebulizers to assure results. The term *dose overkill* will occasionally be used, meaning the administration of such a large dose that, no matter how inefficient the delivery system, enough will get to the right place to cause maximum effect, as might be expected with receptor saturation when using beta adrenergic bronchodilators.

ADVANCES IN APPLICATIONS OF CONVENTIONAL AEROSOLS

This discussion includes two topics: (1) delivery of bronchodilators and glucocorticoids to patients with asthma and chronic obstructive pulmonary diseases (COPD) and (2) aerosols for the treatment of cystic fibrosis (CF).

Aerosols for Asthma and Chronic Obstructive Pulmonary Disease

There are a number of driving forces behind the considerable development in this subject since the early 1990s. Environmental concerns caused a move from chlorofluorocarbon (CFC) propellants to newer hydrofluoroalkane (HFA) propellants for metered-dose inhalers (MDIs). These concerns were also partially responsible for the creation of newer dry powder inhalers (DPI). Such DPI devices were also a response to a need for less demanding hand–chest coordination, which some patients found difficult with conventional MDIs. Coordination was also responsible in part for a move to the use of spacer devices, as was also the need to improve lung delivery of inhaled drug. The latter need also provided an impetus to improve nebulizer devices and inhalation techniques for their use. Perhaps the greatest incentive for product advancement is the marketplace; and for these common diseases for which patients take many medications, the marketplace is huge. Without this potential, there would not be nearly so much advancement in devices to deliver aerosols and new drugs to be delivered.

Advances in MDI and DPI Technology and Use

Enantiomer Preparations of Inhaled Drugs. There has been much interest in the differences in effects of enantiomers of many medications, and beta agonist adrenergic bronchodilators have received much attention. Evidence suggests that the (R)-enantiomer of albuterol is mainly responsible for bronchodilation while the (S)-enantiomer may stimulate airway reactivity. Data suggest, however, that after aerosol delivery, the systemic absorption for (R)-albuterol is faster than for (S)-albuterol and that, conversely, the lung retention of (S)-albuterol is longer, which may be detrimental [29]. The extent to which enantiomers will displace racemic preparations is not yet determined.

Generic Proliferation of Devices and Medications. The proliferation of new aerosol generators moves at a rapid pace. New MDI and nebulizer brands are introduced regularly. Even for those who watch this field, it is not unusual to hear a new, unfamiliar brand name regularly. One trend has been the move to generic MDIs and to over-the-counter availability. These are introduced in the literature by comparing them with well-known older devices. Often, documentation that generic brands or new devices are comparable to older ones is difficult to come by, so comparisons showing pharmacokinetic equivalency are useful [30]. One such, the Respimat, which is a multidose handheld nebulizer, appears to deliver more flunisolide to the lungs (9.9%) than does either an MDI (5.1%) or an MDI with spacer (7%) [31].

New CFC Substitutes for MDIs. The HFAs are rapidly replacing CFCs in MDIs. Numerous clinical studies have focused on documenting efficacy and safety. Some data suggest that the lung deposition fraction of beclomethasone dipropionate using HFA-134a MDI is much higher than that for CFC MDI [32]. The major reason for this difference is the particle size of the HFA aerosol, 1.1 μm, compared to the CFC aerosol, with a size of 3.5 μm. Evidence indicates that pulmonary deposition can be significantly influenced by HFA chosen and by actuator design. Lung deposition for fenoterol was significantly influenced by the actuator nozzle designed for HFA-134a [33]. The convenience of MDIs, in use since the 1950s, will ensure a major continuing role despite anticipated inroads by dry powder inhalers.

Inhalation Technique. Inhalation technique receives much attention even today. Proper use is important for MDIs and DPIs. Modifications of delivery techniques can greatly influence generator performance [34]. This report describes the performance differences among different aerosol-generating devices. Seemingly small differences in use technique, such as shaking the canister before each puff or failure to do so, can considerably affect puff dose [35]. Physicians, therapists, and patients are not well informed about these important techniques.

For MDIs, lung deposition can be enhanced by (1) gentle exhalation to residual volume rather than to functional residual capacity, (2) slow inhalation (10 L/min) rather that fast inhalation (50 L/min), and (3) breath hold of 10 sec rather than none at end of puff inhalation. These observations were based on measurement of urinary albuterol at 30-min postinhalation, which is considered to reflect lung delivery and to avoid gastrointestinal (GI) tract deposition [36]. The effect of inhalation flowrate through an aerosol device can greatly affect particle size, a factor that may explain in part the reduced deposition with suboptimal flowrates. Failure to quickly achieve optimal inspiratory flowrate via a budesonide Turbuhaler can result in an increase in size from <6.6 microns to

45 microns [37]. For delivery of appropriately sized particles to peripheral airways, a slow inhalation flowrate may be best [38].

INHALATION FLOWRATE. The question of proper flowrate does not need further complication, but it seems children are different. Delivery to children may be different than for adults. This has been the subject of much deliberation over many years. Evidence indicates that an inhaled dose is higher with higher flowrates, which cannot be achieved by small children. However, some information indicates that while larger children, who have higher flowrates, inhale more budesonide via the Turbuhaler, a DPI, the deposition is similar when corrected for weight [39]. Some studies suggest that smaller children may actually achieve higher deposition when calculated on a body weight basis [40]. As with other use techniques, it is essential for all parties, physicians, therapists, and patients to know how to include flowrate control in care.

MDI INHALATION COORDINATION. Both adults and children often have difficulty coordinating the inhalation effort with the timing of the aerosol puff. Evidence indicates considerable intra- and intersubject variability for the inhalation technique [41]. The historically reported deposition fraction into the lung is 5–10% at best. Considerable improvement has been described, using various techniques to improve timing. When uncoached subjects inhaled from an MDI, their deposition fraction is about one-third that achieved by patients taught proper technique (7.2% compared to 22.8%), while use of a breath-actuated MDI improved deposition (20.8%) over that of patients also taught proper technique [42]. Control of MDI firing to deliver the puff at optimal flowrate and time point after beginning inhalation also improves deposition. A device that does this (SmartMist) using conventional MDI canisters has been described, and it achieves approximately double the lung deposition [43]. The deposition fraction can be increased to 48% in adults using an inhalation-synchronized dosimeter, and further increased to 60% by controlling (slowing) inspiratory flow [44]. The problem of patient coordination with MDI use is much discussed.

Spacers. The efficacy of spacers for increasing pulmonary deposition and reducing oropharyngeal drug deposition is well documented [45]. Spacers offer the advantage of (1) particle size reduction by propellant evaporation and (2) reduction in cloud velocity, both reasons for the reduced oropharyngeal deposition and increased pulmonary deposition. Alternatively, spacers can cause particle loss by electrostatic precipitation. Application of antistatic agents or detergents improves the yield of inhalable particles [46] and can improve deposition from 25% to 200%. [47–49]. Metal spacers do not hold a charge and so do not affect deposition [50].

The way in which a spacer is used can also reduce delivery. Multiple puffs delivered to a spacer reduce availability [46,51], as does a delay between the dosing of the spacer and inhaling the dose from the spacer [46,47]. The lung dose of medication from an MDI via a large spacer is generally greater than that via a small spacer [52].

The importance of spacers and all techniques to improve delivery is relative. If the dose delivered "the old way" achieves maximum pharmacodynamic effect, improving delivery is moot [53]. This observation raises other questions about aerosol drug delivery, namely, the effective dose. It is likely that the "dose overkill" concept has been the reason for failure to show differences when some applications were compared. A new, refined device may not be more effective than an older one because the older one delivers such a large dose that, despite inefficiency, it is pharmacodynamically equivalent. At least one study shows no difference in protection from exercise-induced asthma by nedocromil sodium and by sodium cromoglycate via MDI, and use of a spacer did not change results [54].

The "Competition" Between MDIs and DPIs

There has been an intensive effort to develop new ways to deliver aerosols. The DPI devices were developed for the following reasons: (1) They allow aerosol delivery without propellants, (2) they avoid the high velocity of MDI propellants, which leads to excess deposition in the oropharynx; and (3) they do not require the same hand–inspiratory muscle coordination needed for MDIs. Patient performance is still important with DPIs. Inspiratory flow must be properly maintained to achieve optimal performance. Lung deposition falls appreciably using a variety of devices when flow falls very much below the optimal rate of about 60 L/min [55,56]. It is important to recognize that the recommended flowrate varies widely for different DPIs and that adherence to proper flow for each device is important. Acceptance of DPIs in the United States is well behind that in Europe.

There is a place for both of these devices. The deposition efficiency of both can be better than found in early studies of MDIs. Proper use of spacers improves the efficiency of MDIs, and proper inhalation flow is important for both devices. Comparative studies are legion [49,58–65], and sorting the confusing mass of information is difficult.

Young children have difficulties similar to older adults, namely, coordination between hand and inspiratory muscles while using MDIs. Devices have been developed to circumvent this problem. The dry powder inhaler only delivers into an air stream passing though the device as generated by the patient. Similarly, breath-actuated MDIs are made to respond to the beginning of patient inhalation. Some evidence suggests that for small children, the breath-actuated MDIs are easier to trigger than are DPIs [66].

Nebulizers

Nebulizer Generation. Clinicians reviewing articles about aerosol delivery must be sufficiently familiar with all aspects of the process to evaluate laboratory findings. Evaluation of nebulizer performance is a multifaceted process. Newer nuclear scanning methods may improve measurements of regional deposition [67]. More meaningful are clinical studies of efficacy measured either by (3) airflow rates or (4) by long-term patient performance studies. One uncontrolled study reports similar survival over five years in COPD patients using MDIs and nebulizers [68], but controlled studies are needed. Similar studies with better controls would be the most meaningful for the practicing physician, but they are rarely done for aerosol medications, especially bronchodilators.

There is great variability in the output of nebulizers, with lung deposition of older devices reported in the 5–15% range, sometimes lower. Newer devices have promise of better performance. Recent study of a new liquid aerosol generator documented that 53% of the loaded dose reached the lung [69]. Variability of performance using nebulizers has been described [70,71]. Using phantom lung and tissue attenuation methods to measure deposition of ^{99m}Tc-labeled colloidal albumin aerosol, deposition was 4.3 and 6.1%, respectively, for the two methods [68]. Other data show much intersubject and intersubject variability, both with same-day and different-day testing with regard to lung [70–72].

"Generic" Products. Low-cost devices are marketed but can perform much worse with respect to intrapulmonary deposition than more expensive devices [72]. Common nebulizers are ubiquitous, as are compressors to operate them. Aerosol medications are marketed with recommendations for use with specific nebulizers and compressors for optimal results [73]. Nebulizers are commonly used for many weeks to months, even those devices described as "disposable." When disposable devices are washed using saline, they maintain size distribution and output for at least 100 uses but, when not so cleaned, begin to deteriorate after 40 uses [74].

New Devices and Materials. A couple of newer technologies merit brief comment. Pulse nebulization is a technique of pressurizing nebulizers intermittently for 50–800 ms. Evidence indicates that pulse delivery can improve particle delivery [75]. Such devices can deliver quite consistent doses [76].

Porous microsphere technology is another area with considerable potential. Porous microspheres have a large physical diameter but, because they are not solid, have a relatively low aerodynamic diameter, which is the physical property that determines deposition fraction and site. They also have a very large surface area for carrying therapeutic substances. Other potential advantages of these preparations may be extended release capability, better size control, and less susceptibility to hygroscopic size changes. Tests of such spheres using cromolyn sodium, albuterol sulfate, and formoterol fumerate appear to show improved stability, content uniformity, and efficiency of use [77]. Delivery could be via MDIs, but other delivery approaches could be explored.

MDIs vs. Nebulizers. Total delivered dose among devices is further emphasized when comparing MDIs and nebulizers. The clinician is regularly faced with patients who swear by the efficacy of nebulizers over MDIs. Deposition fraction is low for both devices, about 5% in children younger than 4 years and about 10% in children over 4 years old for each type of device. The delivered dose was approximately fivefold higher for the nebulizer, so the mass in the lung was much greater for that device [78]. Most studies comparing MDI to nebulizer bronchodilator efficacy show similar improvement in forced expiratory volume one (FEV1), and better results with MDIs have been demonstrated in some laboratories [79]. Most such studies compare patient expiratory flowrates. For bronchodilators at least, pharmacodynamic studies reported by many authors for several decades have regularly indicated equivalent efficacy.

Ventilator Aerosol Delivery

Delivery of aerosols to patients on ventilators has received much attention since the early 1990s. Some studies of early delivery techniques documented low (2.2%) deposition in the lung, with half retained in the nebulizer, and considerable intersubject variability [80]. While the primary focus of this discussion will be on aerosol delivery to ventilated patients, assessing efficacy of aerosol medications to ventilator patients is very difficult.

The complexity of delivering an aerosol to a patient via a mechanical ventilator is immediately apparent to anyone with even minimal familiarity with particle inhalation. For conventional aerosol therapy, it is generally accepted that good results require patient cooperation. As already noted, achieving high lung deposition is difficult even with the best of devices and very capable patients. With ventilators there is the problem of high particle losses in ventilator hardware before even getting near the endotracheal tube. Delivering a useful quantity to the lung is difficult unless, once again, we return to the concept of "overkill," starting with such a massive quantity that even a small fraction will do the job. A 50% reduction of delivery of aerosol to a ventilated patient was observed when the circuit was humidified, compared to dry [81]. One study attributed the very low delivery to reduced generation, which was a function of circuit humidity (but not temperature) and found (using a mechanical model) that increasing the size of the spacer to allow particles time to evaporate could increase delivery [82].

Evidence suggests that lung deposition of bronchodilators from MDIs via spacers is better than without any spacer and that delivery directly into an endotracheal tube is equivalent to that from a spacer [83].

Delivery to Children with Ventilators and Masks

The delivery problem is magnified in very small children, in whom endotracheal tubes are only a few millimeters in diameter, and ventilator humidity increases the chance of much change in particle size before the particle nears the patient.

Deposition in the lungs of infants from either face mask or ventilator is quite low, whether delivered from MDI/spacer or nebulizer source. Animal studies using a nebulizer to deliver isotope-labeled aerosols to rabbits indicate 1–3% deposition at standard settings, with marked reduction when tidal volume and residence time of aerosol were reduced [84,85]. Two in vitro studies suggest that delivery may be enhanced by increasing the inspiratory time, reducing the respiratory rate, or reducing minute volume [86]. Spacer devices are now used "in-line" in some ventilator circuits. Some evidence suggests that they can improve delivery from an MDI [87], but lung delivery estimated using filter measurements can still be as low as 1.5–2%. Other studies, based on urine excretion (of sodium cromoglycate), show remarkably similar lung depositions, whether delivery to ventilated neonates is by nebulizer or by MDI [88]. Some evidence suggests that deposition may be as much as 30% greater when aerosol delivery is given by pressure-support ventilation [89]. This may be due in part to the patient contribution to the ventilation process in pressure-support mode.

The importance of particle size is well known, and it should be intuitive to anyone knowledgeable about aerosols that a 7.7-μm particle will not reach the lung via a device such as a mask or ventilator. Cystic fibrosis patients inhaled either 3- or 7.7-μm particles via a mask; deposition was <1% for the larger particle and 2% for the smaller particle [90]. Many nebulized aerosols have a broad size distribution so that some of the smaller particles in the cloud will reach the lung, but the vast preponderance of the mass is in the larger particle fraction and will be lost in mask or ventilator hardware. It is not surprising that efficiency is so poor. Information such as this was not new in the 1980s, let alone in the 1990s. There is room for much improvement in this area.

Aerosols in Cystic Fibrosis

Aerosols have played a major role in the management of CF for decades, and their role continues to be important. Many airways are blocked by the inspissated, infected secretions, so delivery beyond the blockage into diseased areas is difficult.

Aerosol delivery is difficult in the best of circumstances, but it becomes especially challenging for sick infants and children, who often cannot perform necessary maneuvers to inhale most efficiently. Nasal masks are used in some of these situations, and lung delivery is very low, in the $0.3-1.6\%$ range for infants and 2.7% for children [91]. Targeting is discussed elsewhere in this chapter and also this book (see Chaps. 3, 7). Targeting of smaller airways is often considered desirable and can be achieved in CF patients as well as others by delivering smaller particles [92]. However, size reduction is also mass reduction (at the third power), so many more particles must be delivered to achieve similar mass to small airways.

Mucolytic Agents

N-*Acetylcysteine.* Mucolytic agents such as *N*-acetylcysteine (NAC) have been used by aerosol delivery in an attempt to aid in sputum clearance. Supplied in sufficient quantity, acetylcysteine will help liquefy tenacious secretions and make their clearance easier. A review of studies on the use of NAC in CF concluded the evidence does not support its use, either via nebulizer or by mouth [93]. Intravenous NAC was tested and found not useful in acute respiratory distress syndrome [94]. In one study, patients with chronic bronchitis who took oral NAC had fewer exacerbations and better symptom improvement than did control patients [95]. In the United States, there is no use of NAC by any route for chronic bronchitis. These data need more examination and further study before any such use might be considered. A newer mucolytic agent, nacystelyn, has been developed for delivery via a dry powder inhaler. Deposition in adults and children with CF was 16% and 23%, respectively [94].

rhDNase. The efficacy of recombinant human deoxyribonuclease aerosol to help liquefy secretions has been documented [97,98] and has come into widespread use among CF patients. Since inhaled organic substances can be antigenic, assessment of rhDNase for immunogenic potential is important. Evidence suggests that antibodies develop in about 9% of subjects but are not associated with side effects [99]. From a different perspective, aerosol rhDNase therapy for 52 weeks leads to a reduction in neutrophil elastase in patients with CF [100]. This is the opposite of what might have predicted, because DNA in sputum should act to inhibit neutrophil elastase, and destruction of DNA could thus cause an increase in neutrophil elastase, an undesirable consequence.

Improvement in pulmonary function with rhDNase using a variety of delivery techniques is reported [101,102]. Decrements in function have been documented after two weeks cessation of use [103].

Not all evidence is favorable. Some evidence suggests that adding rhDNase to therapy in an acute exacerbation of does not improve recovery [104]. No improvement in cough or clearance was noted [102,105], and a retrospective study shows no reduction in hospitalizations or pulmonary function decline after institution of rhDNase [104]. Despite its widespread use, the role of rhDNase in the management of CF may not be fully established.

   Tobramycin.   About 7% of the inhaled dose reaches the lung using an aerosol with MMAD of 5 μm; penetration to the periphery is better with better lung function [106]. Tobramycin is widely used to treat patients with CF. Overall, evidence suggests improved lung function and probably reduced hospitalization when tobramycin is part of maintenance therapy in CF [107,108]. The delivered dose can vary widely. There was a fourfold difference in respirable mass (calculated based on size distribution) when two different nebulizers were compared using different flowrates to deliver tobramycin [34]. Nebulizer device performance is an oft-ignored subject, the assumption being that all are created equal. A study of particle size and device output performance for 14 (eight jet, six ultrasonic) devices found that only three (all jet nebulizers) had bench output characteristics suitable for tobramycin delivery [109]. These rather confusing data indicate a potential for improvement in this treatment modality.

   Amiloride.   Amiloride has been tested for treatment of CF because of the considered potential to reduce sputum tenacity. In pursuit of amiloride as a potentially useful agent, numerous pharmacokinetic and pharmacodynamic studies after inhalation and oral dosing were done [110–113]. Unfortunately, some more recent studies of amiloride have failed to document efficacy [114,115].

   Alpha 1 Antitrypsin in CF.   Alpha 1 antitrypsin (α 1-AT) can inhibit neutrophil elastase in epithelial lining fluid (ELF), restore ELF antineutrophil elastase capacity, and also reverse the inhibitory effect of CF ELF on neutrophil *Pseudomonas* killing [116]. Furthermore, aerosolized secretory leukoprotease inhibitor can reduce neutrophil number and also neutrophil elastase in CF subjects [117]. For these reasons some have suggested a possible role for α 1-AT in CF. This concept requires further exploration before clinical introduction. The treatment is exceedingly expensive, so use without good documentation would be inappropriate.

NEW AEROSOL APPLICATIONS

There are two subjects areas I will include in this discussion: (1) the administration of inhaled medications for systemic delivery, and (2) new aerosol applications for the treatment of lung diseases.

Systemic Absorption of Inhaled Drugs

This topic is included because of its potential growth and development. Interest in this has exploded in the last several years. Absorbed drug can be addressed from several viewpoints: (1) effect of systemically absorbed bronchodilator on bronchodilation (or other lung effect), ordinarily achieved by local deposition, and (2) utilization of the lung as a route for systemic delivery for treatment of nonpulmonary diseases.

Drug Delivery to Obstructed Airways

The controversy over effective drug delivery to obstructed airways continues. Airways that most need effective aerosol penetration cannot achieve it because they are obstructed. This concern is substantiated by the demonstration of lower blood levels, lower fractional improvement in flowrates, and lesser change in systemic effects (heart rate, etc.) after albuterol was inhaled by severe asthmatics, compared to normal subjects or mild asthmatics [118].

Absorption of Drugs Given for Local Lung Effect

β_2-Adrenergic Agonists. Systemic absorption of inhaled adrenergic agonists is a well-described phenomenon. After inhalation of albuterol, 180 μg, by normal subjects, the mean peak level of 1469 $\pm$ 410 pg was attained in an average of 13 minutes [119].

Systemic side effects such as tachycardia with isoproterenol inhalation, mild systolic hypertension and tachycardia with β_2-specific agonists, and the tremor seen with β_2-adrenergic receptor agonists all are caused by hematogenous dissemination of inhaled drug. Absorption of drug from its aerosol deposition site followed by hematogenous delivery to obstructed airways might contribute to the action of β_2-adrenergic agonists [120].

Cromolyn. One would not ordinarily consider cromolyn to have any action other than local, but higher-cromolyn blood correlates with better clinical efficacy [121]. Delivery methods affect cromolyn delivery. Disodium cromoglycate (20 mg) delivered to normal subjects via nebulized aerosol as nebulizer solution only, nebulizer solution with saline, or nebulizer solution plus a beta 2 agonist yielded, respectively, peak levels of 8.8, 17.2, or 24.5 ng/mL [122]. The clinical relevance of these data is not clear.

Inhaled Steroids. Inhaled steroids used in asthma can also be absorbed after aerosol dosing. A major disadvantage of inhaled steroids is that when given in relatively high doses, there is sufficient systemic absorption to cause adrenal suppression. Pharmacological modification that reduces systemic absorption without impairing local anti-inflammatory activity could be important. Evidence examining other inhaled substances suggests that absorption is more rapid from more peripheral sites [123,124] but that total absorption may be quantitatively similar from all sites [124].

The Lung as a Route for Systemic Medication After Aerosol Delivery

The great surface area of the lung (see earlier comments) and its perfusion by the entire cardiac output, as well as the ease of passage of many substances through not only the alveolar wall but airway walls into the capillary circulation, make the lung a potential site for systemic drug delivery. The efficacy of this system is exemplified by the ease of delivery of nicotine in cigarette smoke (as a component of both the gaseous and particulate phases) and of street drugs such as cocaine. For such methods to be clinically useful for medication delivery, (1) the efficacy must be at least as good as, (2) the side effects must not exceed those of, (3) the convenience must at least equal that of, and (4) the cost must be similar to that of conventional management. The list of medications delivered by aerosol for systemic delivery is small, but many new uses are proposed. Aerosolized ergotamine was used successfully for decades to treat migraine headaches. Other medications proposed for aerosol delivery include insulin, other hormones, and nitrates for angina.

Insulin by Aerosol.   Early studies showed that aerosolized insulin had a bioavailability of 57% after delivery via endotracheal tube into animals, about 10-fold higher than after instillation [125]. Human studies documented average time to peak insulin level at 40 min after aerosol inhalation by human diabetics and normalization of blood glucose [126]. Continuing research focuses on delivery systems [127–129] and particle modification [130,131] to enhance efficacy. Success of these new approaches will depend heavily upon their cost and convenience for patients. At this point, systems seem to depend upon nebulization, a distinct disadvantage for active people. Unless patients quickly recognize aerosolized insulin as distinctly superior to current therapy, e.g., subcutaneous insulin, the method will not gain acceptance.

Treatment of Migraine.   Many years ago, ergotamine via metered dose inhaler was used successfully to treat migraine headache. I was made aware of this when I first became interested in medical aerosols by a senior professor of medicine who testified to its efficacy. More recently, sumatriptan nasal spray has been shown to provide significant relief of headaches [132].

Nicotine Aerosol for Smoking Cessation.   The systemic activity of nicotine via cigarette smoke is proven by centuries of social use. Nicotine addiction is the primary reason for cigarette smoking, and nicotine replacement is appealing as a means of reducing cigarette use to ultimately achieve cessation. Nicotine for inhalation and for nasal delivery is available, and studies indicate some improvement in the success of cessation efforts beyond placebo [133,134]. The success of nicotine replacement is usually better when combined with some supportive therapy [135]. Some evidence suggests that replacement using a nicotine vapor inhaler results primarily in oral mucosal absorption, whereas absorption while smoking a cigarette occurs mainly from the lung [136]. Inhaled nicotine substitution for cigarettes has much potential because it most mimics delivery by smoking, giving a rapid rise in blood nicotine level. This quality is regarded by many as important in satiating the nicotine craving of smokers.

Aerosols for Angina. The classic treatment of angina pectoris has been sublingual nitroglycerine. Although nitroglycerine is a known coronary vasodilator, the rapid relief of angina is probably caused by a reduced demand on the heart and the consequent reduced cardiac work. Nitroglycerine in either aqueous or lipophilic base as an oral aerosol has been found effective as a coronary vasodilator, with the action of the aqueous particles somewhat faster in onset [137]. An aerosol form has been tested in Europe and has been found comparable to sublingual nitroglycerine [138–140]. In particular, its efficacy has been found better than nitroglycerine tablets in patients with dry mouth [138]. Isosorbide aerosol has also been reported useful in hypertensive crisis [141]. This modality has gained acceptance and is already in use in some hospitals in the United States.

Aerosol Vaccination. While there was moderate interest in aerosol vaccination 15–20 years ago, progress toward application has been modest. This approach is advantageous because it offers the potential to vaccinate many people efficiently and inexpensively. Seroconversion was documented in only a third of infants given aerosol measles vaccine [142], but other studies suggest very high conversion, up to 100%, in similar age groups [143]. Response seems to depend upon dose and vaccine preparation. The economic advantages of the aerosol approach have been described and are considerable [144]. Whether or not there is a future in aerosol vaccination remains to be seen.

New Applications for Use of Aerosols to Treat Lung Diseases
Alpha 1 Antitrypsin

Alpha 1 antitrypsin (AAT) deficiency leads to lung destruction and the formation of emphysema by uncontrolled neutrophil elastase. Replacement of AAT by recombinant AAT (rAAT) given intravenously (IV) is the currently accepted treatment. Early evaluation of aerosolized AAT documented adequate alveolar fluid AAT and penetration into the lung interstitum [145]. A neutrophil elastase inhibitor, secretory leukocyte protease inhibitor, has also been considered for protection against elastase in CF and patients with AAT deficiency. Delivery to CF patients showed good penetration to well-ventilated areas but little to poorly ventilated areas, a finding that is not surprising [146]. In normal volunteers studied 36 hours after AAT inhalation, the half-life of AAT in bronchoalveolar fluid was 69 hr, the level was twice baseline, and the half-life of antineutrophil elastase activity was 53 hr [147]. It would also be useful to know the level achieved in AAT-deficient individuals. Patients with severe AAT deficiency but with milder pulmonary impairment have been studied by isotope scanning methods and have been found to retain sufficient inhaled AAT in the lung periphery [148]. Eventual clinical application of an aerosol approach to treatment of AAT deficiency will depend upon documentation of efficacy. In rare and slowly progressive disorders, documenting the outcome of any therapy will be a great challenge.

Aerosols in Transplantation

The problems of transplanted organs are legion, and lung transplantation is probably one of the most difficult transplants to maintain. Aerosol applications may play a role. Major problems include transplant rejection, pulmonary hypertension, infection, and progressive bronchial obstruction caused by an immune response in the airways.

During lung transplantation, pulmonary vascular pressure and an intrapulmonary shunt have been shown to respond to inhaled nitric oxide and inhaled aerosolized prostacyclin [149,150]. Aerosolized prostacyclin has also been described as an alternative to nitric oxide in the management of reperfusion injury after lung transplantation [150].

Acute and chronic rejection are major problems compromising transplant and patient survival. Many studies indicate that aerosolized cyclosporin A is useful for reducing the risk of acute rejection. The lung concentrates and retains cyclosporin A better after inhalation [152,153]. A number in investigators have found that aerosolized cyclosporin reduces acute rejection in animals [154–157], and some studies suggest efficacy in treating acute [158] and chronic [159,160] rejection in human transplant recipients.

Immunosuppression associated with transplantation makes recipients susceptible to opportunistic infections. Inhaled antimicrobial agents, including pentamidine for *Pneumocystis carinii* prevention [161], colistin for *Pseudomonas* in CF patients awaiting transplant [162], and amphotericin B lipid complex prophylaxis against postransplant fungal infection [163] have all been described. These various studies suggest much potential for aerosolized medications to protect transplanted lungs.

Pulmonary Hypertension

Primary Pulmonary Hypertension. Primary pulmonary hypertension is a highly lethal disease, usually seen in young women and notoriously difficult to treat. Management with oral antihypertensive agents is generally not satisfactory. Continuous infusion of prostacyclin is useful but not curative, and it is costly and inconvenient. In a study of four patients with primary pulmonary hypertension and two with CREST syndrome, the effects of aerosol prostacyclin and its analogue, iloprost, were compared to IV prostacyclin, oxygen, and inhaled NO. Both iloprost and prostacyclin were similarly effective, with the effect of iloprost lasting longer; both were more effective than O_2 or NO. One patient treated for one year with six doses of iloprost daily showed clinical and hemodynamic improvement [164]. Other studies also suggest long-term efficacy [165,166]. Some evidence suggests a greater improvement in cardiac output, oxygenation, and pulmonary artery pressure with aerosol iloprost, compared to NO 40 ppm [167]. There is continuing uncertainty, however, about the long-term efficacy of aerosolized agents, and a recent study found that patients whose intravenous prostacyclin management of pulmonary hypertension had to be stopped because of catheter infection developed right heart failure when switched to aerosol iloprost [168]. Another long-term study failed to show any efficacy over 10 months in patients with severe pulmonary hypertension [169].

Secondary Pulmonary Hypertension. Secondary pulmonary hypertension is seen in some heart transplant candidates, and documenting the potential for reversibility when the primary defect is corrected is important in selecting appropriate heart transplant candidates and liver transplant patients as well. Aerosolized prostacyclin has been shown at least as effective as inhaled NO 40 ppm for this purpose in heart transplant candidates [170], while aerosolized epoprostenol has been shown similarly useful in liver transplant candidates. Delivery of iloprost was faster with an ultrasonic nebulizer but equally efficacious as compared to a jet nebulizer [171]. The role of aerosolized prostacyclin and related medications for pulmonary hypertension and for diagnostic evaluation of transplant candidates remains to be proven. Certainly, a successful aerosol treatment for pulmonary hypertension would be well received because of the inconvenience of the current method of constant infusion via an indwelling catheter. From an economic viewpoint, the market is small, so the chance of recovery of investment in new treatment would be limited.

Surfactant Aerosol

Instillation of surfactant improves outcome in premature infants with neonatal respiratory distress. Loss of surfactant is probably a contributing factor in pathogenesis of acute respiratory distress syndrome in adults, so there has been an interest in the use of surfactant, by either bolus instillation or aerosol, to treat that disorder. Because of the desire to try to improve lung delivery and distribution, there is interest in exploring aerosol delivery. Early, small studies suggested an efficacy of surfactant aerosol for ARDS [172], but more recent, larger controlled trials have failed to document any survival benefit [173,174].

Surfactant aerosol also has been tested in chronic bronchitis; the modest improvement in FEV1 was small, and its expense would not justify use based on these data [175]. In tests of aerosol surfactant in adults with CF treated over 5 days, no improvement was found [176]. Although instilled surfactant has become common practice for the neonatal respiratory distress of premature infants, aerosol delivery is not yet adequately developed. A recent study showed no difference in outcome for spontaneously breathing newborns who inhaled either surfactant or placebo via a CPAP mask [177]. There continues to be great appeal for the use of surfactant in adults because of the apparent success in neonates, but its use should not become practice until well-controlled trials document clinically meaningful efficacy.

Acute Lung Injury

Hypoxemia is a major complication of acute lung injury, and it is often difficult to manage. Mediators such as nitric oxide and prostacyclin can improve oxygenation by increasing blood flow through ventilated areas. Prostaglandin E1 (PGE1) by continuous aerosol via a ventilator has also been shown to improve oxygenation [178]. At the present time the preponderance of the evidence indicates that transient changes in ventilation/perfusion relationships in the lung may improve oxygenation but do not change outcome. Such therapeutic manipulations should be done using appropriate experimental protocols.

Gene Therapy Via Aerosol

Gene therapy delivered by aerosol for lung disease is the goal of intensive research. The primary focus is the treatment of CF. Cationic-lipid-mediated CFTR gene transfer can significantly influence the underlying chloride defect in the lungs of patients with CF [179]. There are many problems to be overcome before clinical applications are practical. Some of these are safety, successful transfer of sufficient genetic material to appropriate tissue, adequate gene expression, maintenance of expression over time, and efficacy of expression. Early work focused on adenovirus as a vector for transfection [180–184]. Complications caused by reactions to adenovirus caused investigators to search for other mechanisms, such as lipid-based particles [185–189]. The liposomal material chosen can significantly affect the mass of aerosol produced [190] and can also influence the effect of the nebulization process on the efficiency of gene transfer [191]. Targeting of specific airway generations is also a consideration, depending upon the gene and the disease of interest [192].

Much work remains in order to bring about the use of gene transfer for the successful management of CF. The final clinical approach may well involve aerosol delivery of vectors.

Aerosols for Cancer

To the pulmonologist accustomed to treating asthma with steroids and broncho-dilators, the concept of aerosol treatment of pulmonary cancers seems strange indeed. Nevertheless, such therapy has been tried in animals and man. Five of seven patients with metastatic tumor to lung responded, one completely, to aerosolized granulocyte macrophage-colony stimulating factor, with no toxicity [193]. Nude mice treated with liposomal aerosol of 9-nitrocamptothecin responded with a reduction in pulmonary metastases from subcutaneous xenografts of human cancers and from murine melanoma [194]. These initial suggestions of positive results justify further study.

MISCELLANEOUS ANTIBIOTIC AEROSOLS
Pentamidine Aerosol

Patients with acquired immunodeficiency syndrome (AIDS) are susceptible to infections caused by the protozoan *Pneumocystis carinii*, which causes pneumonia (PCP). There is now good evidence that aerosol pentamidine is useful in treating mild PCP [195] and, even more important, that, used intermittently, it is effective as prophylaxis against PCP [196,197]. Pentamidine aerosol is delivered to the alveolar space, where the *P. carinii* organisms are found.

The deposition fraction of pentamidine is relatively low, around 2–3% of total dose in the nebulizer (Respirgard II); but as a fraction of total lung capacity, it is greater in children, leading to the suggestion that dose could be reduced in children [198]. Other studies indicate that deposition varies significantly, depending on nebulizer chosen, with deposition fraction measuring from 5.3% to 26.4% for the same subjects using different nebulizers [199] and, in other studies, from 2.9% to 14.3% among 12 different nebulizers, both ultrasonic and jet types [200].

Patients who relapse with PCP or who develop their first PCP episode while using pentamidine prophylaxis have pneumonia localized more to the upper lung zones. In patients not using pentamidine aerosol prophylaxis, the disease is diffuse, with perhaps some lower lung zone predominance. There is evidence that disease in the upper zones reflects failure of the pentamidine prophylaxis aerosol because of preferential deposition in as it enters the lower zones [201]. Inhalation of pentamidine in the supine position seems to cause redistribution of the aerosol to the upper zones [202]. In any case, the use of pentamidine aerosol for this purpose has declined greatly in since the early 1990s because of the low cost and proven success of oral trimethoprim/sulfamethoxazole.

Amphotericin B

There are periodic reports about amphotericin B use as an aerosol. One recent study documents successful delivery to the lung and region of a mycetoma [203], but this writer is not aware of any good evidence for the efficacy of amphotericin B by any route for mycetoma. Such use should not become clinical practice without good randomized controlled trials.

Ribavirin Aerosol

Therapy of infants with respiratory syncytial virus infections was studied in double-blind randomized trials. Using the aerosol 12 hr/day, infants improved more rapidly than controls, but viral shedding was similar in both groups [204]. When used for 20 hr/day, treated infants improved more rapidly than controls with respect to severity of illness, oxygen saturation, and viral shedding [205]. Knight and colleagues [206] estimated that a useful quantity of drug was retained for 3 days after a 23-hr/day treatment.

Ribavirin seems to be effective, but the lengthy administration that has been used is a disadvantage. There is now evidence that shorter courses (two hours three times per day) of ribavirin are as useful as standard therapy (18 hours per day) [207]. Aerosolized ribavirin has been used with variable success for children ventilated for bronchiolitis caused by RSV [208–210]. The more recent evidence casts some doubt on the efficacy of this aerosol treatment. Ribavirin aerosol has also been used for treatment or prophylaxis following bone marrow transplantation [211,212], but controlled trials are needed to better clarify efficacy. Considering the magnitude of this problem, definitive trials to clearly define efficacy would be welcome.

FINAL THOUGHTS
Science

The clinical science of aerosol generation and delivery is much advanced since the early 1970s, and much of this progress has come since the early 1990s. We know how to get therapeutic particles into the lung much better. What we know less clearly is the contribution this knowledge is or could be making to the patients. Almost all studies of aerosol efficacy examine short-term outcomes. For the patient, long-term consequences are more important. Does the patient live better and longer? And can the improvement be accomplished for an acceptable cost. A 15% improvement in FEV1 measured four hours after a bronchodilator dose is probably not worth considering unless there is not much change in daily function, less need for acute emergency and hospital-based health care, and in longevity.

The question of performance differences among various devices should be addressed on a level much broader than whether a device produces a better size distribution, greater lung penetration, or even better or better particle distribution as measured by isotope scanning. This is not to say that these questions are not important, but, rather, to say that the final answer to drug efficacy does not end with such studies of with short-term efficacy. Long-term outcome is the final determinant of utility of new aerosol modalities, and more such studies are badly needed.

These questions of efficacy are especially important as new aerosol therapies are evaluated. Of special importance is the need for careful evaluation of aerosol treatments for acute lung injury, i.e., for patients in respiratory failure who are on a mechanical ventilator in an intensive care unit (ICU). Application of new therapies such as aerosol surfactant, various vasodilators, and others should not be adopted until clear proof of improved outcome is documented.

All of the questions of efficacy are important from two perspectives. Such approaches divert attention from the main problems. Also, many medications are very expensive, so the benefit should be clearly documented if the cost is to be justified.

Economics

The cost of care, especially in the outpatient setting in the United States, can be very high, especially for older persons on Medicare and for the working poor. Marketing of a product the efficacy of which is based on poorly selected measurement criteria does not serve the patient well. Many times, expensive medications are given by desperate physicians to desperate patients despite modest efficacy. In reality, few are well served by this process except the pharmaceutical industry. The tendency is enhanced by the current practice in the United States of television advertising of medications to the public. There is no way such an approach can properly inform patients. The motive is profit first, and this, in the opinion of this writer, is unacceptable. I was told in the early 1960s, when considering medicine as a career, to take care of the patients and the income would take care of itself. This is still true.

Practicing physicians face daily the economic hardships faced by patients who must pay for medications from limited incomes. Patients with chronic diseases in particular are especially vulnerable. Patients with asthma and COPD often carry several metered-dose inhalers and also take oral anti-inflammatory medications as well. In addition, many have other problems, such as diabetes or cardiovascular disease, that may be heavily treated by prescription medication. The monthly cost is great. Many pharmaceutical companies have compassionate use programs, but the paperwork for qualification is a burden for patients, and overworked clinic staff often bear the load. A company representative speaking to a group of pulmonary physicians was pleased that his company could bring an MDI to their institution for $60 instead of the $70 charged by the competition. Any price improvement is of course helpful, but patients who could not afford $70 also could not afford $60, and many cannot afford $15, especially when there are so many other prescriptions to be bought.

This matter is to some extent dealt with by generic MDIs. Although good equivalency information is not easy to find for all generics, some does exist supporting generic equivalency [213]. More such clarification is needed. That all devices are not equivalent has already been mentioned [72].

Education

Better education of physicians and clinic/hospital staff is necessary if the new methods for aerosol delivery are to be brought to the patient. Good patient education is a time-consuming but necessary final part of the application of inhaled medications to the therapeutic armamentarium. These efforts should allow the clinician to bring to the patient the best evidence-based management, which will really change performance and lengthen life.

SUMMARY

The future for therapeutic aerosols is bright. The proliferation of information describing better delivery of medications is an important advance. The new applications for aerosol treatment of lung diseases is encouraging, and interest in using the lung as an absorption membrane for systemic drug delivery is especially exciting. The need for excellent science is always of the highest importance and should stimulate all who are interested in this subject to redouble their efforts to advance the field.

REFERENCES

1. Scudder JM. On the use of medicated inhalations in the treatment of disease of the respiratory organs. Moore, Wilstach, and Baldwin, Cincinnati, OH, 1867.
2. Gandieva B. Postgrad Med J 1975; 51(suppl. 7):13–20.
3. Conference on the scientific basis of respiratory therapy. Am Rev Respir Dis 1974; 110(6):Part 2.
4. Rogers DF, Ganderton D. Respir Med 1995; 89:253–261.
5. Task Group on Lung Dynamics. Deposition and retention models for internal dosimetry of the human respiratory tract. Health Phys 1966; 12:173–207.

6. Gerrity TR, Lee PS, Hass FJ, Marinelli A, Werner P, Lourenco RV. J Appl Physiol 1979; 47(4):867–873.

7. Gerrity TR. In: Byron PR, ed. Respiratory Drug Delivery. Boca Raton, FL: CRC Press, 1990:1–38.

8. Weibel ER. Morphometry of the Human Lung. New York: Academic Press, 1963.

9. Weibel ER. Physiol Rev 1973; 53(2):419–495.

10. Gehr P, Bachofen M, Weibel ER. Respir Physiol 1978; 32:121–140.

11. Agnus GE, Thurlbeck WM. J Appl Physiol 1972; 32(2):483–485.

12. Schlesinger RB, Lippmann M. Am Ind Hyg Assoc J 1972; 33(4):237–251.

13. Martonen T, Hofmann W. Rad Prot Dosimetry 1986; 15:225–232.

14. Hammersley JR, Olson DE, Hiller FC. Am Rev Respir Dis 1990; 141:A522.

15. Smaldone GC, Messina MS. J Appl Physiol 1985; 59:509–514.

16. Lee Z, Berridge MS, Finlay WH, Hearld DL. Int J Pharm 2000; 199(1):7–16.

17. Zanen P, Go LT, Lammers JW. Eur J Clin Pharmacol 1998; 54(1):27–30.

18. Morrow PE. Phys Rev 1986; 66(2):330–376.

19. Hiller FC. J Aerosol Med 1991; 4:1–23.

20. Rees PJ, Clark TJH, Moren F. Eur J Respir Dis 1982; 63(suppl. 119):73–78.

21. Clay MM, Pavia D, Clarke SW. Thorax 1986; 41(9):364–368.

22. Hickey AJ, Gonda I, Irwin WJ, Fildes FJT. J Pharm Sci 1990; 79(11):1009–1014.

23. Otani Y, Wang CS. Aerosol Sci Technol 1984; 3:155–166.

24. Hiller FC, Mazumder MK, Wilson JD, Bone RC. J Pharm Sci 1980; 69(3):334–337.

25. Smith G, Hiller C, Mazumder M, Bone R. Am Rev Respir Dis 1980; 121(3):513–517.

26. Ferron GA. J Aerosol Sci 1977; 8:251–267.

27. Chan HK, Phipps PR, Gonda I, Cook P, Fulton K, Young L, Bautovich G. Eur Respir J 1994; 7(8):1483–1489.

28. Peng C, Chow AH, Chan CK. Pharm Res 2000; 17(9):1104–1109.

29. Dhand R, Goode M, Reid R, Fink JB, Fahey PJ, Tobin MJ. Am J Respir Crit Care Med 1999; 160(4):1136–1141.

30. Clark DJ, Gordon-Smith J, McPhate G, Clark G, Lipworth BJ. Thorax 1995; 51(3):325–326.

31. Newman SP, Steed KP, Reader SJ, Hooper G, Zierenberg B. J Pharm Sci 1996; 85(9):960–964.

32. Leach CL, Davidson PJ, Boudreau RJ. Eur Respir J 1998; 12(6):1346–1353.

33. Newman S, Pitcarin G, Steed K, Harrison A, Nagel J. J Allergy Clin Immunol 1999; 104(6):S253–S257.

34. Coates AL, MacNeish CF, Meisner D, Kelemen S, Thebert R, MacDonald J, Vadas E. Chest 1997; 111(50):1206–1212.

35. Thorsson L, Edsbacker S. Eur Respir J 1998; 12(6):1340–1345.

36. Hindle M, Newton DA, Chrystyn H. Thorax 1993; 48(6):607–610.

37. Everard J, Devadason SG, Le Souef PN. Respir Med 1999; 91(10):624–628.

38. Cheg JK, Chrystyn H. Respir Med 2000; 94(1):51–56.

39. Devadason SG, Everard ML, MacEarlan C, Roller C, Summers QA, Swift P, Borgstrom L, Le Souef PN. Eur Respir J 1997; 10(9):2023–2028.

40. Coates AL, Allen PD, MacNeish CF, Ho SL, Lands LC. Chest 2001; 119(4):1123–1130.
41. Borgstrom L, Bengtsson T, Derom E, Pauwles R. Int J Pharm 2000; 193(2):227–230.
42. Newman SP, Weisz AW, Talaee N, Clarke SW. Thorax 1991; 46(10):712–716.
43. Farr SJ, Rowe AM, Rubsamen R, Taylor G. Thorax 1995; 50(6):639–644.
44. Hakkinen AM, Uusi-Heikkila H, Jarvinen M, Saali K, Karhumakli L. Clin Physiol 1999; 19(3):269–274.
45. Matthys H, Umile A. Drugs Exp Clin Res 1997; 23(56):183–189.
46. O'Callaghan C, Lynch J, Cant M, Robertson C. Thorax 1993; 48(6):603–606.
47. Clark DJ, Lipworth BJ. Thorax 1996; 51(10):981–984.
48. Anhoj J, Bisgaard H, Lipworth BJ. Br J Pharmacol 1999; 47(3):333–336.
49. Wildhaber JH, Janssens HM, Peirart F, Dore ND, Devadason SG, LeSouef PN. Pediatr Pulmonol 2000; 29(5):389–393.
50. Kenyon CJ, Thorsson L, Borgstrom L, Newman SP. Eur Respir J 1998; 11(3):606–610.
51. Rau JL, Restrepo RD, Deshkpande V. Chest 1996; 109(4):969–974.
52. Lipworth BJ, Clark DJ, Bari. J Clin Pharmacol 1998; 46(1):45–48.
53. Fowler SJ, Wilson AM, Griffiths EA, Lipworth BJ. Chest 2001; 119(4):1018–1020.
54. Commis A, Valletta EA, Sette L, Andreoli LA, Boner AL. Eur Respir J 1993; 6(4):523–526.
55. Borgstrom L, Bondesson E, Moren F, Trofast E, Newman SP. Eur Respir J 1994; 7(1):69–73.
56. Borgstrom L. J Aerosol Med 1994; 7(suppl. 1):S49–S53.
57. Pitcairn GR, Lim J, Hollingworth A, Newman SP. J Aerosol Med 1997; 10(4):295–306.
58. Melchor R, Biddiscombe MF, Mak VH, Short MD, Spiro SG. Thorax 1993; 48(5):506–511.
59. Borgstrom L, Derom E, Stahl E, Wahlin-Boll E, Pauwels R. Am J Respir Crit Care Med 1996; 153(5):1636–1640.
60. Bateman ED, Silins V, Bogolubov M. Respir Med 2001; 95(2):136–146.
61. Vidgren M, Arppe J, Vidgren P, Hyvarinen L, Vainio P, Silvasti M, Tukiainen H. Pharm Res 1994; 11(9):1320–1334.
62. Lipworth BJ, Clark DJ. Eur J Clin Pharmacol 1997; 53(1):47–49.
63. Toogood JH, White FA, Baskerville JC, Fraher LJ, Jennings B. J Allergy Clin Immunol 1997; 99(2):186–193.
64. Newman SP, Pitcairn GR, Hirst PH, Bacon RE, O'Keefe E, Reiners M, Hermann R. Eur Respir J 2001; 16(1):178–183.
65. Newman SP, Hirst PH, Pitcarin GR. Curr Opin Pul Med 2000; 7(suppl. 1):S12–S14.
66. Ruggins NR, Milner AD, Swarbrick A. Arch Dis Child 1993; 68(4):477–480.
67. Coates AL, Dinh L, MacNeish DF, Rollin T, Gagnon S, Ho SL, Lands LC. J Aerosol Med 2000; 13(3):169–178.
68. O'Driscoll BR, Berstein A. Respir Med 1996; 90(9):561–566.
69. Farr SJ, Warren SJ, Lloyd P, Okikawa JK, Schuster JA, Rowe AM, Rubsamen RM, Taylor G. Int J Pharm 2000; 198(1):63–70.

70. Thomas SH, O'Doherty MJ, Page CJ, Nunan TO. Clin Sci 1991; 81(6):767–775.
71. Katz SL, Ho SL, Coates AL. Chest 2001; 119(1):250–255.
72. Botha AS, Houlder AE, Wade L. S Afr Med J 1994; 84(2):63–68.
73. Standaert TA, Bohn SE, Aitken ML, Ramsey B. J Aerosol Med 2001; 14(1):31–42.
74. Standaert TA, Morlin GL, Williams-Warren J, Joy P, Pepe MS, Weber A, Ramsey BW. Chest 1998; 114(2):577–586.
75. Gradon L, Sosnowski TR, Podolec Z. Int J Occup Saf Ergon 1999; 5(1):31–42.
76. Miller NC, Morken MA, Schultz RK. J Aerosol Med 1995; 8(4):357–363.
77. Dellamary LA, Tarara TE, Smith DJ, Woelk CH, Adractas A, Costello ML, Gill H, Weers JG. Pharm Res 2000; 17(2):168–174.
78. Wildhaber JH, Dore ND, Wilson JM, Devadason SG, LeSouef PN. J Pediatr 1999; 135(1):28–33.
79. Yuksel B, Greenough A. Respir Med 1994; 88(3):229–233.
80. Thomas SH, O'Doherty MJ, Fidler HM, Page CJ, Treacher DF, Nunan TO. Thorax 1993; 48(2):154–159.
81. Fink JB, Dhand R, Grychowski J, Tobin MJ. Am J Respir Crit Care Med 1999; 59(1):63–68.
82. Lange CR, Finlay WH. Am J Respir Crit Care Med 2000; 161(5):1614–1618.
83. Fuller HD, Dolovich MB, Turpie FH, Newhouse MT. Chest 1994; 105(1):214–218.
84. Cameron D, Arnot R, Clay M, Sliverman M. Pediatr Pulmonol 1991; 10(3):208–213.
85. Fok TF, Monkman S, Dolovich M, Gray S, Coates G, Paes G, Rashid F, Newhouse M, Kirpalani H. Pediatr Pulmonol 1996; 21(5):301–309.
86. O'Doherty MJ, Thomas SH, Page CJ, Treacher DF, Nunan TO. Am Rev Respir Dis 1992; 146(2):383–388.
87. Everard ML, Stammers J, Hardy JG, Milner AD. Arch Dis Child 1992; 67(7 Spec. No.):826–830.
88. Grigg J, Arnon S, Jones T, Clarke A, Silverman M. Arch Dis Child 1992; 67(1 Spec. No.):25–30.
89. Fauroux B, Itti, Pigcot J, Isabey D, Meignan M, Ferry G, Lofaso F, Willemot JM, Clement A, Harf A. Am J Respir Crit Care Med 2000; 162(6):2265–2271.
90. Mallol J, Rattray S, Walker G, Cook D, Robertson CF. Pediatr Pulmonol 1996; 21(5):276–281.
91. Chua HL, Collis GG, Newbury AM, Chan K, Bower GD, Sly PD, Le Souef PN. Eur Respir J 1994; 7(12):2185–2191.
92. Laube BL, Jashnani R, Dalby RN, Zeitlin PL. Chest 2000; 118(4):1069–1076.
93. Duijvestijn YC, Brand PL. Acta Paediatr Esp 1999; (1): 38–41.
94. Domenighetti G, Suter PM, Schaller MD, Ritz R, Perret CJ. Crit Care 1997; 12(4):177–182.
95. Stey C, Steurer J, Bachmann S, Medici TC, Tramer MR. Eur Respir J 2000; 16(2):253–262, Aug.
96. Vanderbist F, Wery B, Baran D, Van Gansbeke B, Schoutens A, Moes AJ. Drug Dev Ind Pharm 2001; 27(3):205–212.
97. Ramsey BW, Astley SJ, Aitken JL, Burke W, Colin AA, Dorkin HL, Eisenberg JD, Gibson RI, Harwood IR, Schidlow DV. Am Rev Respir Dis 1993; 148(1):145–151.

98. Ranasinha C, Assoufi B, Shak S, Christiansen D, Fuchs H, Empey D, Geddes D, Hodson M. Lancet 1993; 342(8865):199–202.

99. Eisenberg JD, Aitken ML, Korkin HL, Harwood IR, Ramsey BW, Schidlow DV, Wilmott RW, Wohl ME, Fuchs HJ, Christiansen DH, Smith AL. J Pediatr 1997; 13(1 Pt 1):118–124.

100. Costello CVM, O'Connor CM, Finlay GA, Shiels P, FitzGerald MX, Hayes JP. Thorax 1996; 51(6):619–623.

101. Fiel SB, Fuchs HJ, Johnson C, Gonda I, Clark AR. Chest 1995; 108(1):153–156.

102. Laube BL, Auci RM, Shields DE, Christiansen DH, Lucas MK, Fuchs HJ, Rosenstein BJ. Am J Respir Crit Care Med 1996; 153(2):752–760.

103. Diot P, Palmer LB, Smaldone A, DeCelie-Bermana J, Grimson R, Smaldone GC. Am Rev Respir Crit Care Med 1997; 156(50):1662–1668.

104. Wilmott RW, Amin RS, Colin AA, DeVault A, Dozor AJ, Eigen HI, Johnson C, Lester LA, McCoy K, Mckean LP. Am J Respir Crit Care Med 1996; 153(6 Part 1): 1914–1917.

105. Robinson M, Hemming AL, Moriarty C, Eberl S, Bye PT. Pediatr Pulmonol 2000; 30(1):16–24.

106. Milla CE. Thorax 1998; 53(12):1014–1017.

107. Mukhopadhyay S, Staddon GE, Eastman C, Palmer M, Davies ER, Carswell F. Respir Med 1994; 88(3):203–211.

108. Touw DJ, Brimicombe RW, Hodson JE, Heijerman HG, Bakker W. Eur Respir J 1995; 8(9):1594–1604.

109. Le Brun PP, De Boer AH, Gjaltema D, Hagedoorn P, Heijerman HG, Frijlink HW. Int J Pharm 1999; 189(2):205–214.

110. Thomas SH, O'Doherty MJ, Graham A, Page CJ, Blower P, Geddes DM, Nunan TO. Thorax 1991; 46(10):717–721.

111. Jones KM, Liao E, Hohneker K, Turpin S, Henry MM, Sleinger K, Hsyu PH, Boucher RC, Knowles MR, Duker GE. Pharmacotherapy 1997; 17(2):263–270.

112. Hoffman T, Senier I, Bittner P, Huls G, Schwandt HJ, Lindemann H. J Aerosol Med 1997; 10(2):147–158.

113. Noone PG, Regnis JA, Liu X, Brouwer KL, Robinson M, Edwards L, Knowles MR. Chest 1997; 112(5):1283–1290.

114. Bowler IM, Kelman B, Worthington D, Littlewood JM, Watson A, Conway SP, Smye SW, James SL, Sheldon TA. Arch Dis Child 1995; 73(5):427–430.

115. Graham A, Hasani A, Alton EW, Martin GP, Marriott C, Hodson ME, Clarke SW, Geddes DM. Eur Respir J 1993; 6(9):1243–1248.

116. McElvaney NG, Nakamura H, Birrer P, Heber CA, Wong WL, Alphonso M, Baker JB, Catalano MA, Crystal RG. J Clin Investig 1992; 90(4):1296–1301.

117. McElvaney NG, Hubbard RC, Birrer P, Chernick MS, Caplan DB, Frank MM, Crystal RR. Lancet 1991; 337(8738):392–394.

118. Lipworth BJ, Clark DJ. Thorax 1997; 52(12):1036–1039.

119. Anderson PJ, Zhou X, Breen P, Gann L, Logsdon TW, Compadre CM, Hiller FC. J Pharm Sci 1998; 87(7):841–844.

120. Zimment I. Respiratory Pharmacology and Therapeutics. Philadelphia: W. B. Saunders, 1978:28.

121. Kato Y, Muraki K, Fujitaka M, Sakura N, Ueda K. Ann Allergy, Asthma, Immunol 1999; 83(6 Pt 1):553–558.

122. Kato Y, Muraki K, Fujitaka M, Sakura N, Ueda K. Br J Clin Pharmacol 1999; 48(2):154–157.

123. Dahl AR, Felicetti SA, Muggenburg BA. Fundam Appl Toxicol 1983; 3(4):293–297.

124. Herrmann DR, Olsen KM, Hiller FC. (Abstract), Am Rev Respir Dis 1989; 139(suppl):A334.

125. Colthorp P, Farr SJ, Taylor G, Smith IJ, Wyatt D. Pharm Res 1992; 9(6):764–768.

126. Laube BL, Benedict GW, Dobs AS. J Aerosol Med 1998; 11(3):153–173.

127. Jendle J, Karlberg BE, Persliden J, Franzen L, Arborelius M, Jr. J Aerosol Med 1995; 8(3):243–254.

128. Farr SJ, McElduff A, Mather LE, Okikawa J, Ward ME, Gonda I, Licko V, Rubsamen RM. Diabetes Technol Ther 2000; 2(2):185–197.

129. Brunner GA, Balent B, Ellmerer M, Schaupp L, Siebenhofer A, Jendle JH, Okikawa J, Pieber TR. Diabetologia 2001; 44(3):305–308.

130. Edwards DA, Hanes J, Caponetti G, Hrkach J, Ben-Jebria A, Eskew ML, Mintzes J, Deaver D, Lotan N, Langer R. Science 1997; 276(5320):1868–1871.

131. Bustami RT, Chan HK, Dehghani F, Foster NR. Pharm Res 2000; 17(11):1360–1366.

132. Peikert A, Becker WJ, Ashford EA, Dahlof C, Hassani H, Salonen RJ. Eur J Neurol 1999; 6(1):43–49.

133. Jones RL, Nguyen A, Man SF. Psychopharmacology (Berl) 1998; 137(4):345–350.

134. Blondal T, Franzon M, Westin A. Eur Respir J 1997; 10(7):1585–1590.

135. Hjalmarson A, Franzon M, Westin A, Wiklund O. Arch Intern Med 1994; 154(22):2567–2572.

136. Lunell E, Molander I, Ekberg K, Wahren J. Eur J Clin Pharmacol 2000; 55(10):737–741.

137. Gansser RE, Schneeweiss A, Weiss M, KF. Cardiovasc Drugs Ther 1990; 4(2):475–480.

138. Sato H, Koretsune Y, Taniguchi T, Fukui S, Shimazu T, Sugii M, Matsuyama T, Karita M, Hori M. Arzneim-Forsch 1997; 47(2):128–131.

139. Udvardi G. Ther Hung 1994; 42(1):45–47.

140. Kethelyi J. Ther Hung 1992; 40(4):173–176.

141. Rubio-Guerra AF, Vasrgas-Ayala G, Lonzano-Nuevo JJ, Narvaes-Rievera JL, Rodriguez-Lopez L, Caballero-Gonzalez FJ. Angiology 1999; 50(2):137–142.

142. Khanum S, Uddin N, Garelick H, Mann G, Tomkins A. Lancet 1987;(8525)150–153.

143. Sabin AB, Flores Arechiga A, Fernandez de Castro J, Sever JL, Madden DL, Shekarchi I, Albrecht P. J Am Med Assoc 1983; 249(19):2651–2662.

144. Sabin AB. Eur J Epidemiol 1991; 7(1):1–22.

145. Hubbard RD, Crystal RG. Lung 1990; 168(suppl):565–578.

146. Stolk J, Camps J, Feitsma HI, Hermans J, Dijkman JH, Pauwels EK. Thorax 1995; 50(6):645–650.

147. Vogelmeier C, Kirlath I, Warrington S, Banik N, Ulbrich E, Du Bois RM. Am J Respir Crit Care Med 1997; 155(2):536–541.

148. Kropp J, Wencker M, Hotze A, Banik N, Hubner GE, Wunderlich G, Ulbrich E, Konietzko N, Biersack HJ. J Nucl Med 2001; 42(5):744–751.

149. Della Rocca G, Coccia C, Costa MG, Pompei L, Di Marco P, Vizza CD, Venuta F, Rendina EA, Pietropaoli P, Cortesini R. Transplant Proc 2001; 33(1–2): 1634–1636.

150. Rocca GD, Goccia C, Pompei L, Ruberto F, Venuta F, Ge Giacomo T, Pietropaoli P. J Cardiothorac Vasc Anesth 2001; 15(2):224–227.

151. Fiser SM, Cope JT, Kron IL, Kaza AK, Long SM, Kern JA, Tribble CG, Lowson SM. J Cardiothorac Vasc Anesth 2001; 121(5):981–982.

152. Letsou GV, Safi HJ, Reardon MJ, Ergenoglu M, Li Z, Klonaris CN, Balsdin JC, Gilbert BE, Waldrep JC. Ann Thorac Surg 1999; 68(6):2004–2008.

153. Blot F, Faurisson F, Bernard N, Sellam S, Friard S, Tavakoli R, Carbon C, Stern M, Bisson A, Pocidalo JJ, Caubarrere I. Transplantation 1999; 68(2):191–195.

154. Dowling RED, Zenati M, Burckart GJ, Yousem SA, Schaper M, Simmons RL, Hardesty RL, Griffith BP. Transplantation 1990; 108(2):198–204.

155. Keenan RJ, Duncan AJ, Yousem SA, Zenati M, Schaper M, Dowling RD, Alarie Y, Burchart GJ, Griffith BP. Transplantation 1992; 53(1):20–25.

156. Blot F, Tavakoli R, Sellam S, Epardeau B, Faurisson FF, Bernard N, Becquemin MN, Frachon I, Stern M, Pocidalo JJ. J Heart Lung Transplant 1995; 14(6 Pt 1): 1162–1172.

157. Mitruka SN, Pham SM, Zeevi A, Li S, Cai J, Burckart GJ, Yousem SA, Keenan RJ, Griffith BP. J Thorac Cardiovasc Surg 1998; 115(1):28–36.

158. Keenan RJ, Iacono S, Dauber JH, Zeevi A, Yousem SA, Ohori NP, Burckart GJ, Kawai A, Smaldone GC, Griffith BP. J Thorac Cardiovasc Surg 1997; 113(2):335–340.

159. Iacono AT, Keenan RJ, Duncan SR, Smaldone GC, Dauber JH, Paradis IL, Ohori NP, Grgurich WF, Burckart GJ, Zeevi A, Griffith BP. Am J Respir Crit Care Med 1996; 153(4 Pt 1):1451–1455.

160. Iacono AT, Smaldone GC, Keenan RJ, Diot P, Dauber JH, Zeevi A, Burckart GJ, Griffith BP. Am J Respir Crit Care Med 1997; 155(5):1690–1698.

161. Nathan SD, Ross DJ, Qakowski P, Kass RM, Koener SK. Chest 1994; 105(2):417–420.

162. Bauldoff GS, Nunley DR, Manzetti JD, Dauber JH, Keenan RJ. Transplantation 1997; 64(5):748–752.

163. Palmer SM, Drew RH, Whitehouse JD, Tapson VF, Davis RD, McConnell RR, Kanji SS, Perfect JR. Transplantation 2001; 72(3):545–548.

164. Olschewski H, Walmrath D, Schermuly R, Ghofrani A, Grimminger F, Seeger W. Ann Intern Med 1996; 124(9):820–824.

165. Stricker H, Domenighetti G, Fiori G, Mombelli G. Schweiz Med Wochenschr 1999; 129(24):923–927.

166. Hoeper MM, Schwarze M, Ehlerding S, Adler-Schuermeyer A, Spiekerkoetter E, Niedermeyer J, Hamm M, Fabel H. N Engl J Med 2000; 342(25):1866–1870.

167. Hoeper MM, Olschewski H, Ghofrani HA, Wilkens H, Winkler J, Borst MM, Niedermeyer J, Fabel H, Seeger W. J Am Coll Cardiol 2000; 35(1):176–182.
168. Schenk P, Petkov V, Madl C, Kramer L, Kneussl M, Ziesche R, Lang I. Chest 2001; 119(1):296–300.
169. Machherndl S, Kneussl M, Baumgartner H, Schneider B, Petkov V, Schenk P, Lang IM. Eur Respir J 2001; 17(1):8–13.
170. Haraldsson A, Kieler-Jensen N, Nathorst-Westfelt U, Bergh CH, Ricksten SE. Chest 1998; 114(3):780–786.
171. Gessler T, Schmehl T, Hoeper MM, Rose F, Ghofrani HA, Olschewski H, Grimminger F, Seeger W. Eur Respir J 2001; 17(1):14–19.
172. Todisco T, Cosmi E, Dottorini M, Baglioni S, Eslami A, Fedeli L, Palumbo R. J Aerosol Med 1992; 5(2):113–122.
173. Weg JG, Balk RA, Tharratt RS, Jenkinson SG, Shah JB, Zaccardelli D, Horton J, Pattishall EN. J Am Med Assoc 1994; 272(18):1433–1438.
174. Anzueto A, Baughman RP, Guntupalli KK, Weg JG, Wiedemann HP, Raventos AA, Lemaire F, Long W, Zaccardelli DS, Pattishall EN. N Engl J Med 1996; 334(22):1417–1421.
175. Anzueto A, Jubran A, Ohar JA, Piquette CA, Rennard SI, Colice G, Pattishall EN, Barrett J, Engle M, Perret KA, Rubin BK. J Am Med Assoc 1997; 278(17):1426–1431.
176. Griese M, Bufler P, Teller J, Reinhardt D. Eur Respir J 1997; 10(9):1989–1994.
177. Berggren E, Liljedahl M, Winbladh B, Andreasson B, Curstedt T, Robertson B, Schollin J. Acta Paediatr 2000; 89(4):460–464.
178. Meyer J, Theilmeier G, Van Aken H, Bone HG, Busse H, Waurick R, Hinder F, Brooke M. Anesth Analg 1998; 86(40):753–758.
179. Alton EW, Stern M, Farley R, Jaffe A, Chadwick SL, Phillips J, Davies J, Smith SN, Browning J, Davies MG, Hodson ME, Durham SR, Li D, Jeffery PK, Scallan M, Balfour R, Eastman SJ, Cheng SH, Smith AE, Meeker D, Geddes DM. Lancet 1999; 353(9157):947–954.
180. Sene C, Bout A, Imler JL, Schultz H, Willemot JM, Hennebel V, Zurcher C, Valerio D, Lamy D, Pavirani A. Hum Gene Ther 1995; 6(12):1587–1593.
181. Katkin JP, Gilbert BE, Langston C, French K, Beaudet AL. Hum Gene Ther 1995; 6(8):985–995.
182. Bellon G, Michel-Calemard L, Thouvenot D, Jagneaux V, Poitevin F, Malcus C, Accart N, Layani MP, Aymard M, Bernon H, Bienvenu J, Courtney M, Doring G, Gilly B, Gilly R, Larny D, Levrey H, Morel Y, Paulin C, Perraud F, Rodillon L, Sene C, So S, Touraine-Moulin F, Pavirani A. Hum Gene Ther 1997; 8(1):15–25.
183. McDonald RJ, Lukason MJ, Rabbe OG, Canfield DR, Burr EA, Kaplan JM, Wadsworth SC, St George JA. Hum Gene Ther 1997; 8(4):411–422.
184. Lerondel S, Vecellio None L, Faure L, Sizaret PY, Sene C, Pavirani A, Diot P, Le Pape A. J Aerosol Med 2001; 14(1):95–105.
185. McvLachlan G, Davidson DJ, Stevenson BJ, Dickinson P, Davidson-Smith H, Dorin JR, Porteous DJ. Gene Ther 1995; 2(9):614–622.
186. McLachlan G, Ho LP, Davidson-Smith H, Samways J, Davidson H, Stevenson BJ, Carothers AD, Alton EW, Middleton PG, Smith SN, Kallmeyer G, Michaelis U,

Seeber S, Naujoks K, Greening AP, Innes JA, Dorin JR, Porteous DJ. Gene Ther 1996; 3(12):1113–1123.

187. Chadwick SL, Kingston HD, Stern M, Cook RM, O'Conner BJ, Lukasson M, Balfour RPR, Rosenberg M, Cheng SH, Smith AE, Meeker DP, Geddes DM, Alton EW. Gene Ther 1997; 4(9):937–942.

188. Eastman SJ, Tousignant J, Lukason MJ, Chu Q, Cheng SH, Scheule RK. Hum Gene Ther 1998; 9(1):43–52.

189. Gautam A, Densmore CL, Waldrep JC. Gene Ther 2001; 8(3):254–257.

190. Saari M, Vidgren MT, Koskinen MO, Turjanmaam VM, Nieminen MM. Int J Pharm 1999; 181(1):1–9.

191. Densmore CL, Giddings TH, Waldrep JC, Kinsey BM, Knight V. J Gene Med 1999; 1(4):251–264.

192. Cipolla DC, Gbonda L, Shak S, Kovesdi I, Crystal R, Sweeney TD. Hum Gene Ther 2000; 11(2):361–371.

193. Anderson PM, Markovic SN, Sloan JA, Clawson ML, Wylam M, Arndt CA, Smithson WA, Burch P, Gornet M, Rahman E. Clin Cancer Res 1999; 5(9):2316–2323.

194. Knight V, Kleinerman ES, Waldrep JC, Giovanella BC, Gilbert BE, Koshkina NV. Ann N Y Acad Sci 2000; 922:151–163.

195. Montgomery AB, Debs RB, Luce JM, Corkery KJ, Turner J, Brunette EN, Lin ET, Hopewell PC. Lancet 1987; 2:480–483.

196. Girard PM, Landman R, Gaudebout C, et al. Lancet 1989; (18651): 1348–1353.

197. Leoung GS, Feigal DW, Montgomery AB, et al. N Engl J Med 1990; 323:769–775.

198. O'Doherty MJ, Thomas SH, Gib D, Page CJ, Harrington C, Duggan C, Nunan TO, Bateman NT. Thorax 1993; 48(3):220–226.

199. Ilowite JS, Baskin MI, Sheetz MS, Abd AG. Chest 1991; 99(5):1139–1144.

200. Thomas SH, O'Doherty MJ, Page CJ, Nunan TO, Bateman NT. Eur Respir J 1991; 4(5):616–622.

201. Jules-Elysee KM, Stover DE, Zaman MB, Bernard EM, White DA. Ann Intern Med 1990; 112:750–757.

202. O'Doherty MJ, Thomas SH, Page CJ, Bradbeer C, Nunan JO, Bateman NT. Chest 1990; 97:1343–1348.

203. Diot P, Rivoire B, Le Pape A, Lemarie E, Dire D, Furet Y, Breteau M, Smaldone GC. Eur Respir J 1995; 8(8):1263–1268.

204. Taber LH, Knight V, Gilbert BE, McClung HW, Wilson SZ, Norton HJ, Thurston JM, Gordon WH, Atmar RL, Schlaudt WR. Pediatrics 1983; 72:613–618.

205. Hall CB, McBride JT, Walsh EE, Bell DM, Gala CL, Hildreth S, Ten Eyck LG, Hall WJ. N Engl J Med 1983; 308:1443–1447.

206. Knight V, McClung HW, Wilson SZ, et al. Lancet 1981; 2(8253):945–949.

207. Englund JA, Piedra PA, Ahn YM, Gilbert BE, Hiatt P. J Pediatr 1994; 125(4):635–641.

208. Guerguerain AM, Gautheir M, Lebel HM, Farrell CA, Lacroix J. Am J Respir Crit Care Med 1999; 160(3):829–834.

209. Meert KL, Sarnaik AP, Gelmini MJ, Lieh-Lai MW. Crit Care Med 1994; 22(4):566–572.

210. Smith DW, Frankel LR, Mathers LH, Tang AT, Ariagno RL, Prober CG. N Engl J Med 1991; 325(1):24–29.
211. Ghosh S, Champlin RE, Englund J, Giralt SA, Rolston D, Raad I, Jacobson K, Neumann J, Ippoliti C, Mallik S, Whimbey E. Bone Marrow Transplant 2000; 25(7):751–755.
212. Adams R, Christenson J, Petersen F, Beatty P. Bone Marrow Transplant 1999; 24(6):661–664.
213. Chege JK, Chrystyn H. Thorax 1994; 49(11):1162–1163.

14

Aerosolized Pentamidine for Treatment and
Prophylaxis of *Pneumocystis carinii*
Pneumonia in Patients with Acquired
Immunodeficiency Syndrome

Anthony J. Hickey

University of North Carolina, Chapel Hill, North Carolina, U.S.A.

A. Bruce Montgomery

Corus Pharma Inc., Seattle, Washington, U.S.A.

INTRODUCTION

Since the first edition of this book was published there have been substantial
advances in the treatment of human immunodeficiency virus (HIV) infection and
the corollary acquired immunodeficiency syndrome (AIDS). Multiregimen
antiretroviral therapy has allowed HIV/AIDS to be managed in a manner that was
impossible in 1992. The development of successful treatments for HIV/AIDS and
the effectiveness of antimicrobials, trimethoprim/sulfamethoxazole or dapsone,
in the treatment of *Pneumocystic carinii* pneumonia (PCP) have reduced

pentamidine aerosol therapy to a second-line approach. However, this remains a valuable therapy for treatment of PCP.

The clinical experiences obtained from caring for the increased incidence of PCP in patients with AIDS has led to the conclusion that current oral and intravenous therapies, albeit effective, have significant short- and long-term adverse reactions that often limit use. Two approaches for effective and less toxic antipneumocystosis therapy and prophylaxis are possible: new agents and targeted delivery of known agents. This chapter summarizes the significant studies on aerosolized pentamidine isethionate, which is targeted to the lungs.

AEROSOLIZED PENTAMIDINE RATIONALE AND EXPERIMENTAL ANIMAL STUDIES

Pentamidine is an aromatic diamidine that was initially synthesized in the 1930s in a search for hypoglycemic agents. Because of its antiprotozoal activity, pentamidine has been used extensively for treatment and chemoprophylaxis of African trypanosomiasis. The exact mechanism of action of pentamidine is not known; in vitro, it has been found to interfere with folate metabolism, anaerobic glycolysis, oxidative phosphorylation, and nucleic acid replication [1]. Pentamidine usually is given parenterally in a dose of 4 mg/kg/day as the isethionate salt, the only preparation available in the United States [1]. Administration must be parenteral because gastrointestinal absorption is poor. Adverse reactions to pentamidine appear to be dose dependent, in that a 3-g total dose, which usually is reached in the second week of parenteral therapy, frequently causes toxicity [2].

Unlike common prokaryotic pathogens that cause bacterial pneumonia, *P. carinii* has been a taxomonic enigma. Until recently it was regarded as an extracellular protozoan that inhabits predominantly the alveolar spaces, with close approximation to the surfaces of alveolar epithelial cells and alveolar macrophages [3]. Extrapulmonary *P. carinii* infections are rare, suggesting that the alveolar environment is usually necessary for growth of the pathogen [3]. More recently *P. carinii* has been redesignated a fungus [4]. Because of this intra-alveolar location of *P. carinii*, aerosolization of pentamidine should provide an effective, site-specific, and, hence, less systemically toxic method of therapy or prophylaxis [4]. Studies of aerosolized pentamidine in rats with PCP document efficacy and suggest that the half-life of the drug is long, probably weeks, with increased clearance in ill animals [5–7]. Debs and colleagues [5] reported negligible clearance in 48 hr in normal mice; in rats, the elimination half-life from the lungs may be as long as a month. A study of tissue concentrations after parenteral administration in AIDS patients confirmed that the half-life is long [8].

However, exact alveolar concentrations are unknown because analyses of tissue levels from humans are impractical before death.

AEROSOL DEVICES USED TO DELIVER PENTAMIDINE

Pentamidine can cause bronchospasm and airway irritation in humans [9]. This appears to be caused by the pentamidine moiety itself, because similar irritation is seen in nonisethionate salts of pentamidine. Because *P. carinii* habitats the alveolus and because of the potential adverse effects of pentamidine on the airways, pentamidine ideally should be aerosolized in a small particle, between 1 and 2 μm. Studies that make in vitro comparisons of nebulizers cannot be valid unless the particle sizes are identical. The present state of knowledge cannot allow determination of the most effective device because not all the devices have been comparatively tested in humans [10,11]. The optimal particle size for alveolar deposition is between 1 and 3 μm, with 1 μm achieving more peripheral distribution and less airway distribution [12–14]. However, 19% of particles as small as 2 μm still impact in the tracheobronchial regions. The ideal device should have a particle size of 1–2 μm with a high output. Particles between 0.5 and 1 μm have relatively less alveolar deposition than particles between 1 and 2 μm. Other features, such as reservoirs, flows, and external filters, may also be important [9]. However, any nebulizer with particle sizes, on average, greater than 8 μm would not deliver adequate drug to the alveoli.

Commercially available nebulizers that might be used in the United States to aerosolize pentamidine are of two types: ultrasonic and jet. Included in the ultrasonic class are the Microinhaler (Siemens), FisoNeb (Fisons, New Bedford, MA), Pulmosonic (DeVilbiss, Somerset, PA), Portosonic (DeVilbiss). Included among the jet nebulizers are Respirgard II (Marquest Medical Products, Englewood CO), Aerotech II (Cadema, Middletown, NY), and Centimist (Marquest).

The Microinhaler has been largely abandoned because of the large particle size of nearly 20 μm and is now unavailable to the United States [9].

The FisoNeb and Pulmosonic nebulizers both operate at a frequency of 1.3 MHz that generates a mass median aerodynamic diameter (MMDA) of 4–6 μm [9,10]. The Pulmosonic nebulizer has been reported not to deliver many particles smaller than 2 μm and, therefore, is unsuitable for pentamidine administration [10]. The Portosonic (DeVilbiss) device is a 2.3-MHz ultrasonic nebulizer and may offer the combination of less than 2-μm MMAD and a high output. In any study using ultrasonic nebulizers, the output and particle size of each device need to be periodically sampled, because the frequency of the piezoelectric crystal may alter with age [10]. Any MMADs between 0.5 and 2 μm are available. The Respirgard nebulizer II has one-way valves that control a drug reservoir, allow entrainment of room air in patients whose minute ventilation is high, act as a baffle to decrease particle size, and direct expired air to a filter that scavenges remaining drug and prevents environmental contamination. The Centimi nebulizer is a similar device, with a larger reservoir and no expiration filter. The Aerotech II nebulizer has internal baffles in the jet nebulizer and, therefore, may allow recycling of the drug; however, it has a higher flowrate and lacks a reservoir, so much of the drug may not be available for inhalation in patients with normal minute ventilation. Nevertheless, in a direct comparison between the Respirgard II and the Aerotech II nebulizers, the latter delivered 2.5–5 times more drug [15,16]. The increased concentration of pentamidine may actually exceed the tolerance of patients; anecdotal reports of severe coughing with pentamidine doses greater than 100 mg led a 40-mg dose to be used in now-abandoned prophylaxis studies. This dose would probably not be as effective as a 300-mg dose delivered with the Respirgard II device, but it would be less expensive.

Despite their availability, neither dry powder nor metered-dose inhalers have been used to deliver aerosolized pentamidine. The use of metered-dose inhalers may be problematic because these devices are better suited for frequent delivery of small doses rather than intermittent delivery of the large doses that have been therapeutically successful in prophylaxis of PCP. Dry powder devices may produce an increased incidence of cough due to airway deposition.

HUMAN PHARMACOKINETIC DATA FOR PENTAMIDINE

A pharmacokinetic study that allows estimates of the amount of pentamidine needed in both therapy and prophylactic trials using the Respirgard II device has been conducted in eight patients with diffuse alveolar infiltrates undergoing fiberoptic bronchoscopy for suspected PCP [14]. Bronchoalveolar lavage (BAL) sediment and supernatant concentrations of pentamidine were compared 18–24 hr after administration of 4 mg/kg IV ($n = 3$) and aerosolized ($n = 5$) pentamidine isethionate to different groups of patients. An aerosol containing 300 mg pentamidine isethionate in 6 mL distilled water was inhaled for 35–40 minutes. In patients with diffuse alveolar infiltrates, significantly higher concentrations of aerosolized pentamidine reached the airspaces than did the intravenous form of the drug. The BAL pentamidine concentrations in sediment were 9.34 ± 1.74 ng/mL after IV administrations vs. 705 ± 242 ng/mL after aerosol (mean $\pm$ SEM, $p < 0.05$). Serum pentamidine levels were low or undetectable after aerosolization. The large variation in BAL levels after aerosol but not intravenous administration suggests that the variability is due to aerosol deposition and not to BAL technique. Levels remain high; in the first patient to receive 12 monthly 300-mg treatments, a repeated BAL 31 days after the last treatment revealed 1,462 ng/mL in the sediment (B. Montgomery, unpublished data). Nevertheless, BAL cannot be used to provide an absolute alveolar concentration, because the total amount of alveolar fluid in the lungs cannot be determined. In addition, BAL fluid is contaminated by fluid in the airways. Conte and colleagues [17] conducted a similar study and also noted these limitations.

Despite the information about the pharmacokinetics of aerosolized pentamidine, how the drug is cleared from the lung is unknown. Some systemic absorption occurs and, therefore, this suggests the possibility of long-term systemic toxicity [14,17,18]. Furthermore, the moiety on pentamidine that causes a long pulmonary half-life has not been determined. Elucidation of this moiety may lead to development of novel long-lasting aerosol hybrid agents for other lung diseases. Studies of serial pentamidine levels in bronchial epithelial lining fluid after aerosol administration have shown that drug levels decreased rapidly within 2 weeks and were followed by a slow elimination rate [19].

AEROSOLIZED PENTAMIDINE THERAPY FOR ACTIVE *PNEUMOCYSTIS CARINII* PNEUMONIA

The overall rate of PCP prophylaxis failure has decreased significantly since 1995, coincident with the era of highly active antiretroviral therapy (HAART) [20].

Four pilot and three controlled studies using aerosolized pentamidine were conducted (Tables 1 and 2) [17,18,21–23]. Montgomery et al. [18] studied one group of AIDS patients with PCP who had received no prior therapy [18] and a second group that was intolerant to standard therapy [22]. Of the 25 patients, 23 recovered. Relapses occurred in only three patients during a mean follow-up of more than 1 year. No adverse systemic reactions were observed with aerosolized

TABLE 1 Aerosolized Pentamidine Studies for Mild-to-Moderate PCP in Patients with AIDS

Study group	n	Nebulizer type	ADR requiring drug change (%)	Failures (%)	Deaths (%)	Ref.
First episode	15	Respirgard II	0	14	7	18
Intolerant to other agents	10	Respirgard II	0	0	0	21
Mixed	13	Ultravent	0	31	0	17
Mixed	11	System 22	9	72	9	22
Mixed	16	Respirgard II	0	19	0	22

PCP = *Pneumocystis carinii* pneumonia; AIDS = acquired immunodeficiency syndrome; ADR = adverse drug reaction.

TABLE 2 Controlled Comparative Trails of Aerosolized Pentamidine for Mild-to-Moderate PCP in Patients with AIDS

Group	n	Planned duration of therapy (days)	ADR requiring drug change, n (%)	Failures, n (%)	Deaths, n (%)	Ref.
Aerosolized PTN	11	21	0	5 (15)	2 (18)	23
Intravenous PTN	10	21	2 (20)	0	0	
Aerosolized PTN	17	14	0	8 (47)	1 (6)	24
Intravenous PTN	21	14	2 (10)	4 (19)	0	
Aerosolized PTN	127	21	13 (10)	44 (34)	6 (5)	25
IV/PO TMP–SMX	127	21	64 (50)	22 (17)	14 (11)	

PCP = *Pneumocystis carinii* pneumonia; AIDS = acquired immunodeficiency syndrome; ADR adverse drug reaction; TMP–SMX = trimethoprim sulfamethoxazole.
All groups used Respirgard II nebulizer for aerosolized pentamidine.

pentamidine in either group. Coughing was noted in patients with a history of bronchospasm or smoking, but this was managed successfully with an aerosolized bronchodilator [22]. Conte et al. [17] also studied the effects of inhaled or reduced-dose pentamidine treatment of PCP in AIDS patients. Nine of the 13 patients with mild PCP had a satisfactory response to inhaled aerosolized pentamidine; three patients could not be evaluated because of early withdrawal, and one patient had treatment failure. Two of the nine evaluable patients had neutropenia, but those patients had been receiving zidovudine and had low pretreatment leukocyte counts. Other mild adverse reactions included cough, bronchospasm, rash, and elevated temperature. The fourth study was done by Miller et al. [22], who initially reported little success with aerosolized pentamidine using one type of nebulizer but had better results using a nebulizer that generated smaller particles. Soo Hoo and colleagues [23], in a small unblinded randomized trial, reported that all 10 patients with mild-to-moderate PCP responded to intravenous pentamidine, whereas only 6 of 11 responded to aerosolized pentamidine (Table 2). Likewise, in another unblinded comparative trial, Conte and colleagues [24] reported that 15 of 17 patients responded to aerosolized pentamidine, whereas 17 of 21 patients responded to intravenous pentamidine. They reported a high incidence of relapse in the aerosolized pentamidine group, but the duration of treatment was only 2 wk. Of note, neither of these trials was blinded, and decisions on change of therapy or clinical relapse were made in an open fashion. The only large blinded comparative trial was conducted by Montgomery and colleagues [25], who compared aerosolized pentamidine to TMP–SMX in mild-to-moderate PCP of 247 patients; 14 died who were randomized to the TMP–SMX arm, whereas only six died who were in the aerosolized pentamidine arm ($p = 0.07$) Clinical response was slower with aerosolized pentamidine, but toxicity rates were high with TMP–SMX. Relapse occurred more often in the aerosolized pentamidine group unless posttherapy prophylaxis was used. In conclusion, aerosolized pentamidine is equal to TMP–SMX in preventing death and superior in the incidence of toxicity; however, clinical response takes longer in sicker patients. These results highlight the need for large randomized trials to evaluate novel therapies, because small trials can be misleading, and response may not correlate with preventing mortality.

CHEMOPROPHYLAXIS FOR *PNEUMOCYSTIS CARINII* PNEUMONIA
Patients at Risk for *Pneumocystis carinii* Pneumonia

Asymptomatic primary infection from *P. carinii* usually occurs in childhood, with pneumonia occurring from recrudescence in the setting of immunosuppression. Historically, the PCP usually occurred in settings of immunosuppression from either childhood malnutrition, chemotherapy, or congenital immunodeficiencies [26,27]. The overwhelming current cause for immunosuppression is infection from the human immunodeficiency virus (HIV). In people infected with HIV, significant risk for PCP can be quantified by the presence of other opportunistic infections, by symptoms, or by the CD4 lymphocyte count [28–30]. The most obvious and highest-risk group for PCP is patients who have experienced a prior episode; prophylaxis in this group is called secondary prophylaxis. The risks of recurrent PCP have been assessed by historical case control studies and ongoing clinical trials of zidovudine (Table 2) [31,32]. Analysis of 201 consecutive patients with first-episode PCP at San Francisco General Hospital (SFGH) in the prezidovudine era has shown that of the 61 (30%) who relapsed with PCP, 18% did so at 6 mo, 46% at 9 mo, and 65% at 18 mo [31]. Hence, most patients with a second episode of PCP are expected to relapse within 18 mo. Although zidovudine does decrease the risk of PCP slightly, the incidence of PCP over time does not differ greatly in patients taking zidovudine from the SFGH historical controls (Table 2) [33]. In fact, the absolute incidence of recurrent PCP in patients taking zidovudine may have been increased because of longer survival times [33,34].

Identification of HIV-infected individuals at high risk for PCP who have not had an initial bout is more problematic. At least 20% of AIDS patients will never have an episode of PCP, and the number of HIV-infected individuals is large compared to those who have had PCP. Nevertheless, both clinical and immunological status, have been used to determine risk. The initial determinants of risk were case reviews of patients presenting with PCP [28]. In addition to having prodromal symptoms, these patients commonly experience weight loss, hairy leukoplakia, and mucocutaneous candidiasis. In these persons, PCP usually occurs when an absolute CD4 lymphocyte count normally between 800 and 1,000 cells/mm^3 decreases to less than 200 cells/mm^3 [28,29]. These studies could not determine what percentage of unprophylaxed HIV-infected patients with similar symptoms and immunological status would develop PCP. Recently, however, in the Multicenter AIDS Cohort Study (MACS) of 1,660 homosexual males, the incidence of PCP with a baseline of less than 200 CD4 cells/mm^3 was more than 1% a month in the first year (Table 2) [30]. The initial occurrence rate of PCP among persons with a baseline CD4 count between 201 and 350 CD4 cells/mm^3 was low, this may reflect a real finding or a referral bias of relatively healthy survivors into the study. The CD4 lymphocyte count of less than 200 cells/mm^3 is not infallible in the MACS study or other studies. For example, in a prospective trial of TMP–SMX, in the placebo arm of patients with Kaposi's sarcoma, 3 of 16 developed PCP with a CD4 count of greater than 200 cells/mm^3 [29]. The MACS study also confirmed that fever, oral candidiasis, and weight loss were independent factors for increased risk of PCP [30].

Aerosolized Pentamidine

Aerosolized pentamidine prophylaxis has been studied in two large clinical trials in North America and in one large trial in Europe. The first trial was the San Francisco Community Consortium study conducted by Leoung and colleagues, who observed 408 patients with either prior PCP ($n = 250$), Kaposi's sarcoma ($n = 59$), or other AIDS-related diagnosis or complex ($n = 129$). Patients were randomized to receive either 30, 150, or 300 mg aerosolized pentamidine using the Respirgard II nebulizer system [35]. The 30- and 150-mg doses were administered every 2 wk; the 300-mg dose was given every 4 wk. Pentamidine at a dose of 300 mg every 4 wk was significantly better than 30 mg given biweekly in three analyses: intention to treat, analysis of patients on drug, and analysis of patients on drug with histological confirmation of PCP. The regimen consisting of 300 mg every 4 wk also tended to be superior than that of 150 mg every 2 wk. The study was conducted for 18 months, with a mean follow-up approaching 1 yr [35] (Table 3).

The second study was a double-blinded comparative trial of secondary prophylaxis comparing 60 mg aerosolized pentamidine given every 2 wk after five weekly loading bases to placebo using a handheld FisoNeb ultrasonic nebulizer with a 5-μm MMAD particle size [36,37]. The study was intended to run 6 mo, but it was terminated early, with a mean follow-up of only 3.7 mo. Aerosolized pentamidine significantly reduced the reoccurrence rate of PCP as compared to controls in this study [37,38].

Comparing the relapse rate of the 60-mg dose given every 2 wk after four weekly loading doses in the second study to the 300-mg dose given every 4 wk in the first study would best be done by a prospective trial. However, in the patients with one episode of PCP, the life table reoccurrence rate at 6 mo with the 60-mg regimen using the FisoNeb nebulizer was 10%, compared to 4% with the 300-mg regimen using the Respirgard II nebulizer, suggesting an advantage to the 300-mg regimen [37]. Because of the short duration of the second study, no longer-term comparisons could be made at that time.

Based on these data, the Food and Drug Administration (FDA) approved the 300-mg dose of pentamidine delivered by the Respirgard II nebulizer every 4 wk as PCP prophylaxis in any HIV-infected patient with a prior episode of PCP or a CD4 count of less than 200 cells/mm^3. The San Francisco study did not prove a dose response in the primary-prophylaxis patients, most likely because of the small numbers of events, but the trends parallel the secondary-prophylaxis group. The FDA approval for primary prophylaxis was based on inference, accepting proven efficacy in secondary prophylaxis, proven safety in primary prophylaxis, and recognizing recent studies documenting significant PCP risk in HIV-infected patients with low CD4 cell counts [37].

TABLE 3 Kaplan–Meier Estimates of Proportion with PCP in HIV-Infected Persons

Ref.	Study group	Prophylactic drug	N	Cumulative (%)		
				6 mo	12 mo	36 mo
Primary occurrence (CD4 cells/mm³ at entry)						
31	0–200	None	78	8.3	17.9	38.2
30	201–350	None	231	0.4	3.7	24.1
30	351–500	None	391	0	1.3	9.5
34	Variable	AP ± AZT*	171	1.0	5.0	NA
Reoccurrence						
31	Early AIDS patients	None	201	18	46	NA
32	AZT dose-response trial[a]	AZT	318	32	68	NA
36	AP study[b]	AP ± AZT	237	4.0	20	NA

PCP = *Pneumocystis carinii* pneumonia; HIV = human immunodeficiency virus; NA = not available because HIV disease has significant mortality over this time range, the proportions after 1 yr present very small sample sizes, and data are unreliable. All proportions are calculated with censoring at time of death or withdrawal.

All references are preliminary communications; except changes in data with confirmation and follow-up or both.

[a] The higher relapse rate on zidovudine (AZT) may be artifactual because of delay to start zidovudine therapy from episode of PCP.

[b] Represent confirmed episodes of PCP on a 300-mg dose of aerosolized pentamidine every 4 wk.

The European trial studied patients without a history of PCP. In this primary-prophylaxis trial, 223 patients seropositive for HIV were randomized to receive 300 mg pentamidine isethionate or 300 mg sodium isethionate by Respirgard II nebulizer every 28 days [38]. Another entry criterion was a CD4 cell count of less than 200 cells/mm^3. The study was terminated with a mean follow-up of about 1 yr, when 23 cases of PCP had occurred in the placebo group and eight cases in the treatment group. These investigators concluded that aerosolized pentamidine was about 60–70% effective in preventing the first episode of PCP. However, three of the eight events in the treated group occurred in the first 2 mo of the study, suggesting that the patients may have had prodromal PCP at the time of randomization or that a loading dose may be appropriate. This study confirmed the wisdom of the early FDA approval of primary prophylaxis without specific data in this patient group.

Aerosolized pentamidine does not provide perfect prophylaxis. Nevertheless, most relapses are mild, with a case fatality rate of less than 5% [36]. Lowery and colleagues reviewed the radiographic pattern of relapse in patients on a 30-mg dose of aerosolized pentamidine and found a striking increase in upper lobe relapses, a finding that correlates with the predicted deposition of most of the drug in the lower lobes [39]. The use of a higher, 300-mg dose may ameliorate this problem, but breathing patterns that encourage apical deposition, such as occasional exhalation to residual volume and supine position, may also decrease apical reoccurrence [40,41]. Contraindicated is breath holding at increased lung volumes, which would decrease apical deposition.

Comparisons of the performance of two nebulizers in the delivery of pentamidine and their effectiveness in a community-based clinical trial have been reported [42]. The systems employed were the Respirgard II and the Fisoneb. Both systems provided comparable protection against PCP. The study supported the effectiveness of aerosolized pentamidine as a solid second-line prophylaxis for HIV-infected individuals who are tolerant to trimethoprim/sulfamethoxazole or dapsone.

ADVERSE REACTIONS AND EFFECTS OF AEROSOLIZED PENTAMIDINE

Inadequate experience has been obtained to determine the incidence of the infrequent adverse reactions that will be associated with aerosolized pentamidine therapy for acute PCP. In case reports, bronchial bleeding has been reported with high-dose therapy in one center [43]. This was associated with an invasive procedure and has not been seen in the large prospective treatment trial. Case reports of hypoglycemia, rash, and conjunctivitis have also been reported [44,45]. The conjunctivitis is not unexpected; it would be the direct consequence of improper administration of the aerosol to the eyes, because it is well known that pentamidine is irritating to the airways [46].

The systemic side effects of aerosolized pentamidine when used as prophylaxis reported to date occur at a frequency of less than 1% and include mild hypoglycemia and pancreatitis [36]. Airway irritation with cough (10–20%) or bronchospasm (1–2%) occurs commonly [36]. The cough apparently responds to bronchodilators [36]. The long-term pulmonary effects of aerosolized pentamidine do not appear to cause permanent airflow obstruction or decreases in diffusing capacity [36]. Pneumothoraxes are not uncommon in all patients who have had PCP, but those receiving aerosolized pentamidine have an incidence of about 4% a year, not different than historical controls [47,48]. Aerosolized pentamidine does not appear to cause additive or synergistic toxicity to zidovudine but is synergistic in reducing the incidence of PCP [34]. Extrapulmonary infection with *P. carinii* is rare, even if aerosolized pentamidine prophylaxis is used. The total incidence in the San Francisco studies was less than 1 in 200. Most, but not all, cases have been reported in patients who have a history of PCP. Usual sites include the eye, ear canal, liver, and spleen. The presence of extrapulmonary pneumocystosis should be considered when evaluation of patients on aerosolized pentamidine reveals unexplained systemic signs and symptoms [36].

Complications due to pentamidine administration used in prophylaxis following bone marrow transplantation have been observed [49]. Indeed, aerosolized pentamidine was associated with increased risk of other infections and decreased survival rate.

CONCLUSIONS

Aerosolized pentamidine has become one of the major drugs used in the treatment and prophylaxis of patients with HIV infection. Prophylaxis of PCP in patients with HIV infection who are immunosuppressed has now been established as the standard of care, similar to the universal adoption of prophylaxis in immunosuppressed children in the early 1990s. It is not clear whether aerosolized pentamidine or TMP–SMX is the optimal prophylaxis in HIV-infected patients [50]. The largest studies have been conducted with aerosolized pentamidine; comparative trials are now needed between agents as well as dose-response trials with each agent to determine the dosage schedule that has optimal balance between efficacy and safety. By their very nature, trials will need to be large and will be expensive. The finding that a 300-mg dose given once a month is effective indicates that placebo control studies in high-risk groups at this time are probably unethical. Future studies will need to use this dose as a control when testing alternative dosage regimens or nebulizers.

REFERENCES

1. Pearson RD, Hewlett EL. Ann Intern Med 1985; 103:782–786.
2. Waskin H, Stehr-Green JK, Helmick CG, et al. J Am Med Assoc 1988; 260:345–347.
3. Hughes WT. *Pneumocystis carinii* Pneumonia, Vol. 1. Boca Raton, FL: CRC Press, 1987:105–125.
4. Kovacs JA, Gill VJ, Meshnick S, Masur H. J Am Med Assoc 2001; 286:2450–2460.
5. Debs RJ, Blumenfeld W, Brunette EN, et al. Antimicrob Agents Chemother 1987; 31:37–41.
6. Debs RJ, Straubinger RM, Brunette EN, et al. Am Rev Respir Dis 1987; 135:731–737.
7. Girard PM, Brun-Pascaud M, Farinotti R, et al. Antimicrob Agents Chemother 1987; 31:978–981.
8. Donnelly H, Bernard EM, Rothkotter H, et al. J Infect Dis 1988; 157:985–989.
9. Corkery KJ, Luce JM, Montgomery AB. Respir Care 1988; 33:676–696.
10. Newman SP, Pellow PGD, Clarke SW. Chest 1987; 92:991–994.
11. O'Doherty MJ, Thomas S, Page C, et al. Lancet 1988; 2:1283–1286.
12. Raabe G. In: Witschi H, Neltesheim P, eds. Mechanisms in Respiratory Toxicology. Boca Raton, FL: CRC Press, 1982:27–76.
13. Newman SP. Chest 1985; 88(suppl):152S–160S.
14. Montgomery AB, Debs RJ, Luce JM, et al. Am Rev Respir Dis 1988; 137:477–478.
15. Smaldone GC, Fuhrer J, Steigbigel RT, McPeck M. Am Rev Respir Dis 1991; 143:727–737.
16. Smaldone GC, Perry RJ, Deutsch DG. J Aerosol Med 1988; 1:113–126.
17. Conte JE, Hollander H, Golden JA. Ann Intern Med 1987; 107:495–498.
18. Montgomery AB, Debs RJ, Luce JM, et al. Lancet 1987; 2:480–483.
19. Yamamoto H, Koisumi T, Miyahara T, et al. Respiration 2001; 68:506–508.
20. Wei CC-Y, Gardner S, Rachlis A, et al. Chest 2001; 119:1427–1433.
21. Montgomery AB, Debs RJ, Luce JM, et al. Chest 1989; 95:747–750.
22. Miller RF, Godfrey-Fausset P, Semple SJ. Thorax 1989; 565–569.
23. Soo Hoo GW, Mohsenifar Z, Meyer RD. Ann Intern Med 1990; 113:195–202.
24. Conte JE, Chernoff D, Feigal DW, Joseph P, McDonald C, Golden JA. Ann Intern Med 1990; 113:203–209.
25. Montgomery AB, Edison RE, Sattler F, et al. Sixth International Conference on AIDS, San Francisco, 1990.
26. Hughes WT, Kuhn S, Chaudhary S, et al. N Engl J Med 1977; 297:1419–1426.
27. Hughes WT, Rivera GK, Schell MJ, Thornton D, Lott L. N Engl J Med 1987; 316:1627–1632.
28. Masur H, Ognibenc FP, Shelnamer J, et al. Twenty-Eighth Interscience Conference on Antimicrobial Agents and Chemotherapy, Los Angeles, 1988:307.
29. Fischl MA, Dickinson GM, La Voie L. J Am Med Assoc 1988; 259:1185–1189.
30. Phair J, Munoz A, Detels R, Rinaldo C, Saah A. Abstracts of the Fifth International Conference on AIDS, Montreal, Vol. 1, 1989:299.
31. Rainer CA, Feigal DW, Leoung G, et al. Abstracts of Third International Conference on AIDS, Washington, DC, 1987:189.

32. ACTG Administrative Report. Abstract Protocol 002, Clinical Trials Coordinating Center. Meeting of the ACTG Principle Investigators, Bethesda, MD, July 7–8, 1988.

33. Fischl MA, Richman DD, Grieco MH. N Engl J Med 1987; 317:185–191.

34. Montgomery AB, Leoung GS, Wardlaw LA, et al. Am Rev Respir Dis 1989; 139:250.

35. Leoung GS, Feigal DW, Montgomery AB, et al. N Engl J Med 1990; 323:769–775.

36. Montaner JSG, Lawson LM, Gervais A, et al. Ann Intern Med 114:948-953.

37. United States Food and Drug Administration. Transcript of Antiinfective Advisory Subcommittee Meeting on May 1, 1989. U.S. Government Printing Office, Washington, DC.

38. Hirschel B, Lazzarin-Chopard P, et al. N Engl J Med 1991; 324:1079–1083.

39. Lowery S, Fallat R, Feigal DW, et al. Abstracts from the Fourth International Conference on AIDS, 1988:419.

40. Abd AG, Nierman DM, Ilowite JS, Pierson RN, Loomis-Bell AL. Chest 1994; 94:329–331.

41. Baskin MI, Abd AG, Ilowite JS. Am Rev Respir Dis 1989; 139:A248.

42. Mcivor RA, Berger P, Pack L, et al. Chest 1996; 110:141–146.

43. Miller RF, Semple SJG. (Letter) Lancet 1988; 2:1488.

44. Karboski JA, Godley BJ. (Letter) Ann Intern Med 1988; 108:490.

45. Leen CLS, Mandal BK. (Letter) Lancet 1988; 2:1250–1251.

46. Lindley DA, Schleupner CJ. (Letter) Ann Intern Med 1988; 109:988.

47. Leoung GS, Wardlaw L, Montgomery AB, Abrams DI, Feigal DW, S.F. County Community Consortium. Abstracts of the Fifth International Conference on AIDS, Montreal, 1989:299.

48. Mann J, Montgomery AB, Luce JM, et al. Am Rev Respir Dis 1989;139–148.

49. Vasconcelles MJ, Bernardo MV, King C, et al. Biol Blood Marrow Transplant 2000; 6:35–43.

50. Centers for Disease Control. MMWR (no. SS:1-9) 1989.

15

The Application of Aerosolized Antimicrobial Therapies in Lung Infections

Dennis M. Williams
University of North Carolina, Chapel Hill, North Carolina, U.S.A.

INTRODUCTION

The inhalation of antimicrobial agents to treat infections in the lung has been of interest for decades [1]. As early as the 1950s, extemporaneously prepared antimicrobial agents were aerosolized to treat pneumonia. These preparations were often crude and not well tolerated by patients. Dosage, formulation procedures, and stability assessment in these early reports were not consistent. Although some successes were reported, the potential benefit of this route of administration was not fully appreciated until the 1980s.

A number of antibiotics have been used as aerosol therapies. Examples include beta lactam agents, polymycin antimicrobials, neomycin, gentamicin, and tobramycin. Many of the early efforts were reported as case studies, and observations and data regarding safety and efficacy were lacking. Controlled clinical trials were not conducted until the middle of the 1980s. More recent evaluations have focused on the role of inhaled tobramycin used as suppressive therapy for cystic fibrosis patients colonized with *Pseudomonas aeruginosa*.

Currently, there is a paucity of antimicrobial products delivered by aerosolization. Pentamidine and tobramycin are the only two agents approved for use in the United States as aerosolized antimicrobial therapies. However, interest in using the lung as a site of delivery of therapeutic agents has continued to evolve, and several therapies are under investigation for both local and systemic effects [2].

The delivery of antibiotics to the lower airway through aerosolization offers several theoretical advantages over systemically administered therapy [3,4]. It allows for direct deposition at the site of infection, resulting in high concentrations that may be beneficial in eradicating bacteria. The risk of adverse or toxic effects may be lower as a result of this method of administration.

Much of the interest in aerosol therapy has focused on the management of patients with cystic fibrosis and has extended beyond the use of aerosolized antibiotics to various proteins and biotechnological therapies. The use of these therapies is discussed elsewhere in this publication (see Chs. 16, 17). Recent advances in the use of antibiotics directed against bacterial infections and technologic improvements of delivery systems has spurred additional research into the use of antifungal and antiviral therapies as well [5].

Although antimicrobial therapies have been delivered by aerosolization for over five decades, much is still unknown or not well understood. For example, there are few data to help guide dosing of these therapies. For optimal benefit, an understanding of the clinical utility, as well as the physiologic, physical, chemical, and delivery considerations is essential [6].

RATIONALE FOR AEROSOLIZED ANTIBIOTIC THERAPY

The continuing interest in inhaled antibiotic therapy is based on several factors, including the following: The lung is a frequent site of infection; achieving adequate antimicrobial concentrations in lung tissue may be difficult; and systemic antimicrobial therapies may have dose-limiting toxicities in other organ systems. The rationale for the use of aerosolized antibiotics is to maximize the therapeutic effect against bacteria in the lung by direct delivery of the agent to the site of infection. This may allow a lower dose to be administered, which may minimize the risk of systemic toxicity while maintaining efficacy.

The search for useful inhaled antibiotics has been driven, in part, by a concern about the adequacy of systemic antimicrobial therapy for respiratory infections. Some agents, including aminoglycoside antibiotics, exhibit limited penetration into respiratory tract secretions. In fact, aminoglycosides may achieve sputum concentrations that are 12% of related serum concentrations. In addition, cystic fibrosis patients are often colonized with mucoid strains of *Pseudomonas aeruginosa*. This phenotype is associated with a further reduction in penetration of antibiotics.

In some cases, enzymes present in the respiratory secretions inactivate the antibiotic. Based on these factors, systemic aminoglycosides are sometimes dosed aggressively to achieve adequate concentrations in the lung. This increases the risk of systemic toxicity, including nephrotoxicity and ototoxicity. Conversely, concerns about potential toxicities may limit dosage regimens and duration of therapy.

The potential benefit of aerosolized antibiotic therapy is dependent on three factors: characteristics of the disease, aerosol delivery system, and properties of the antimicrobial agent [5]. Diseases that are likely to respond better cause infection in the airway without significant parenchymal or systemic involvement (e.g., cystic fibrosis). There is a significant need for research and scientific advances in the area of aerosol delivery of these therapies. Delivery systems that produce reliable, consistent, and reproducible aerosols are essential. Formulation of drug products requires attention to integrity, stability, tolerability, and overall suitability for aerosolization.

It is important to note that although aerosolization of antibiotic therapy has resulted in significantly higher sputum concentrations, systemic treatment is clearly more effective than this topical route of delivery. This suggests that factors other than sputum concentrations are important in the overall efficacy of therapy.

Although a potential advantage of inhaled antibiotic therapy is the achievement of high concentrations in the sputum, there is substantial variability reported, which may reflect differences in collection and bioassay techniques. There is no clear relationship between systemic and inhaled doses of individual agents. Currently, the decisions about inhaled doses should be made on data specific for an individual agent. In trials with the commercially available inhaled tobramycin product, sputum concentrations of 1200 μg per mL were measured 10 minutes after the dose. Measured concentrations exceeded 25 times the minimum inhibitory concentration (MIC) for the most resistant isolate in 95% of subjects evaluated [7].

Aerosol Deposition of Antimicrobial Agents

Four primary physical factors of an aerosol affect pulmonary deposition. These include particle size, hygroscopicity, viscosity, and surface tension. The characteristics are described in detail elsewhere [8]. This brief overview addresses principles relevant to aerosolized antibiotics.

To achieve benefit from aerosolized antibiotic therapy, an adequate amount of medication must reach the site of infection [3,4,8]. Optimal particle size for deposition in the lower respiratory tract and alveoli lies between 1 and 5 micrometers (μm). For alveolar deposition, particle sizes of 1–2 μm are optimal. Particle diameters of 3 and 4 μm reach the lower airway, while 5-μm particles deposit in the central airways. Particles below this range are likely exhaled, and larger particles deposit in the oropharynx. Removal of deposited particles from the airway surface occurs by absorption, mucociliary clearance, or expectoration of produced sputum.

The pattern of deposition of inhaled particles in a normal lung is dependent on particle size, flow rate, and airway anatomy (branching). There are also patient specific variables that influence aerosol deposition. These include respiratory rate, tidal volume, and other anatomical features. The presence of airflow obstruction characteristic of some lung diseases will affect deposition.

PHARMACEUTICAL CHARACTERISTICS OF AEROSOLIZED ANTIBIOTICS

There are several relevant pharmaceutical factors that should be considered in formulating drug products for aerosol administration to the lung. The purpose of early investigations was to assess potential benefit of aerosolized antibiotics, and they often used crude formulations in which the stability and integrity of the product were not known. In formulating products, consideration should be given to drug-specific characteristics such as pH, stability, tonicity, particle size, and taste. Additionally, the inhalation system used to deliver the dose is an important consideration.

In addition to these various characteristics, patient-specific factors can affect delivery of aerosolized antimicrobials to the lung. Patient breathing technique and several physiologic variables affect ultimate deposition, including age, breathing pattern, ventilation volumes, and the presence of disease [9].

Chemical properties that may affect drug absorption from the airway surface into the systemic circulation include molecular weight, protein binding, and lipophilicity [8], although the extent of absorption is highly variable [10]. However, the extent of absorption into the systemic circulation is felt to be minimal. More research is warranted to evaluate the impact of other patient variables on systemic exposure resulting from inhaled therapies.

The ideal agent for administration by aerosolization to treat infection in the lung would be safe and effective. It should exhibit no local adverse effects and have little or no systemic absorption. The agent should exhibit good activity against the bacteria causing infection and minimize the risk for resistance. Finally, the product should be stable chemically during storage and administration and have an acceptable taste and odor.

OVERVIEW OF CYSTIC FIBROSIS

Cystic fibrosis is a heterogeneous, autosomal recessive genetic disease associated with abnormal exocrine gland function, which affects multiple organs, including the gastrointestinal, pulmonary, and reproductive systems. Cystic fibrosis is caused by mutations in the cystic fibrosis transmembrane regulator gene, which is associated with abnormal ion transport in epithelial cells. Due to early recognition and advances in treatment, the median survival in patients has increased from under 2 years to over 30 years of age.

Lung disease is the major cause of morbidity and mortality in cystic fibrosis, accounting for the majority of deaths [11]. At least 50% of patients are hospitalized at least once a year for treatment of a pulmonary exacerbation. Recurrent infections are associated with a progressive decline in lung function leading to respiratory failure.

Patients with cystic fibrosis experience a chronic progressive loss of lung function associated with infection, inflammation, and tissue destruction. The most common bacteria implicated in lung infections associated with cystic fibrosis are *Haemophilus influenzae, Staphylcoccus aureus*, and *Pseudomonas aeruginosa* [12]. *Pseudomonas aeruginosa* is found in the lower respiratory tract of nearly 70% of cystic fibrosis patients by age 17 years [11], and over 90% of patients have at least one culture positive for *P. aeruginosa* during their lifetime. Chronic pulmonary infection caused by *P. aeruginosa* contributes to a progressive decline in lung function and the development of obstructive lung disease. Additionally, lung function declines more rapidly once colonization with *P. aeruginosa* has occurred. When colonization with *P. aeruginosa* is present, the organism is commonly a mucoid phenotype that is more resistant to antibiotic penetration. Thus, antimicrobial therapy directed against this organism plays a central role in the management of acute exacerbation and potentially on a chronic basis.

Currently, the primary role of aerosolized antibiotics is for patients with cystic fibrosis. Patients with cystic fibrosis experience frequent and recurrent lung infections as a result of their disease. Aminoglycosides, including tobramycin, exhibit good activity against gram-negative bacteria that are frequently implicated in these infections, including *P. aeruginosa.*

POTENTIAL ROLE OF AEROSOLIZED ANTIBIOTICS

Although of interest for over five decades, our understanding of the role of this therapeutic strategy improved significantly during the last 10 years. Evaluations have focused on patients with cystic fibrosis. Potential clinical applications include the use of these therapies as primary or adjunctive therapy during acute exacerbations of lung infection in patients with chronic disease; suppressive regimens designed to reduce the frequency and severity of exacerbations, as well as the associated decline in lung function due to recurrent infections; and to delay or prevent the onset of chronic infection.

Aminoglycosides are the most widely studied class of aerosolized antibiotic therapies. Since they retain bioactivity when aerosolized and are poorly absorbed across epithelium, they can achieve and maintain high concentrations in bronchial and alveolar fluids with minimal potential for toxicity.

Although most recent studies have evaluated aerosolized aminoglycosides, other antimicrobial therapies are used as aerosolized therapy in patients infected with multiresistant organisms. Polymyxin antimicrobials are polypeptides that are poorly absorbed across mucosal membranes. These agents are not absorbed to a clinically significant extent, which limits their application to intravenous use or decontamination of the gastrointestinal tract. When used systemically, these agents carry a significant risk of neurotoxicity and nephrotoxicity. These agents have retained good activity against gram-negative organisms; therefore, their use as aerosolized therapy has been explored.

A worldwide survey of cystic fibrosis centers, including four in the United States [13], indicated that the use of aerosolized antibiotics was being considered on an increasing basis. In the survey, suppressive therapy was more likely to be used in older age groups (≥ 19 years), with half the centers surveyed indicating that they were prescribed in at least 50% of their patients. Although this survey is relatively recent, it is likely this trend has continued to increase and has extended to younger patients, and additional evidence has likely been reported.

Although not well studied, the use of aerosolized antibiotics may have additional applications in other clinical situations, including bronchiectasis, pneumonias, and management of patients following lung transplantation.

CLINICAL TRIALS AND EXPERIENCE

Initial trials of aerosolized antimicrobial therapy with penicillin were published six decades ago [14]. Sporadic reports about the benefit of these therapies continued to appear for the next 30 years as case reports or uncontrolled observations.

These trials evaluated different therapies and utilized several differences in study design, making comparisons difficult. Additionally, the goals of therapy and the endpoints that were measured differed significantly. Controlled studies evaluating the use of inhaled antibiotics began to appear in the 1980s. These studies addressed primarily their use as suppressive therapy, and many were performed in patients with cystic fibrosis.

There are a few reports in the literature about the use of aerosolized antibiotics in patients without cystic fibrosis; however, not many data are available about efficacy, and these observations are not randomized, controlled clinical trials. The review of the literature that follows focuses on patients with cystic fibrosis. In September 1999, a consensus document was published that summarized recommendations for the use of aerosolized antibiotics in patients with cystic fibrosis based on the current evidence [14].

Use During Acute Exacerbations

A few studies have investigated the role of inhaled aminoglycosides used with systemic antimicrobials for treatment of an acute pulmonary exacerbation [15,16] and studied patients with cystic fibrosis who were experiencing an acute pulmonary exacerbation. In the first study [15], aerosolized tobramycin (80 mg three times daily) was added to two weeks of intravenous tobramycin and ticarcillin for 12 subjects. The control group ($n = 16$) received the intravenous therapy alone. After two weeks of therapy, there were no differences between the groups in lung function, severity scores, various vital sign measures, or time to discharge from the hospital. Although a bacterial response (eradication of *Pseudomonas*) favored the inhaled group at 2 weeks ($p = .03$), recolonization occurred in all cases within $1-2$ months after treatment of the exacerbation.

In the second study [16], 62 subjects were treated with intravenous ceftazidime and amikacin. The treatment group also received aerosolized amikacin 100 mg twice daily. Treatments were given for an average of 15 days, and subjects were reevaluated four to six weeks after hospital discharge. During treatment, transient improvements in several outcome measures were noted (e.g., x-ray score, inflammation indices, and percentage underweight); however, there were no differences in any measure at the final evaluation point. As in the earlier study, eradication of bacteria from sputum was also transient.

Although there has been interest in the role of aerosolized aminoglycosides in the management of acute exacerbations of lung disease in patients with cystic fibrosis, there are no quality data to support this practice. Results from these studies suggest minimal benefit from the addition of aerosolized antibiotic therapy added to traditional combination intravenous therapy during treatment of acute pulmonary exacerbations of cystic fibrosis. Any improvements that occurred were temporary, with no apparent long-term benefit. Currently, there is no established role for aerosolized antimicrobial therapy, either alone or in combination with systemic therapy, when treating an acute exacerbation [14].

Use in Delaying or Preventing Acquisition of *Pseudomonas*

Colonization with *P. aeruginosa* is a sentinel event in the course of cystic fibrosis. Chronic infection with this organism is associated with progressive loss of lung function attributed to chronic inflammation and recurrent pulmonary exacerbations. Thus, there is interest in strategies that may delay the acquisition of this organism.

Oral ciprofloxacin has been used in combination with aerosolized colistin as well as a combination of aerosolized colistin and tobramycin to delay the onset of *P. aeruginosa* colonization. Although favorable results were reported, these studies used historical controls, and the concomitant use of oral antibiotics limits interpretation of the role of the aerosolized therapy. Not many data exist on the pharmacokinetic or pharmacodynamic behavior of colistin aerosolized [17–19].

Another recent report suggested promise about the role of aerosolized antibiotics in delaying acquisition of *P. aeruginosa* [20]. In this report, children with cystic fibrosis, who were determined to be at risk for bacterial colonization with *P. aeruginosa*, inhaled 80–120 mg of gentamicin twice daily. A total of 28 children were identified and evaluated in a retrospective manner. Twelve of these patients were followed for at least two years on therapy and were compared to 16 subjects who stopped therapy prematurely due to poor adherence or side effects. None of the patients who continued aerosolized gentamicin acquired *P. aeruginosa* during the observation period, while 7 of 16 patients in the control group exhibited positive cultures ($p = .01$) The authors concluded that aerosolized gentamicin therapy may be beneficial in delaying acquisition of *P. aeruginosa*, although a prospective controlled clinical trial is warranted.

To date, the data are sparse, and the use of aerosolized antibiotics to prevent or delay the acquisition of *P. aeruginosa* cannot be recommended [14].

Role as Suppressive Therapy in Reducing Exacerbation Frequency and Improving Pulmonary Function

The majority of clinical trials with inhaled antibiotics have evaluated the role of suppressive therapy between acute exacerbations in patients with cystic fibrosis. The first report evaluating the role of an aminoglycoside as suppressive therapy appeared over 20 years ago. Aerosolized carbenicillin and gentamicin was reported to result in modest improvement in lung function in 20 adult patients with cystic fibrosis [21]. Subsequently, other investigators concluded that minor benefit was achieved with this route of administration [22]. Generally, improvements in lung function or a reduced rate of decline in lung function were reported.

A meta-analysis published in 1996 [23] combined the preceding results with other research and concluded that the use of nebulized antibiotic therapy against *Pseudomonas* was beneficial in reducing the number of exacerbations requiring systemic antibiotics, reducing the bacterial load in the sputum, and improving lung function. The only concern identified was the potential for an increase in resistance of *P. aeurginosa*. This analysis comprised five trials that met the criteria for quality, and it included beta lactams, aminoglycosides, and polymyxin agents.

Colistin has been evaluated as suppressive therapy in patients with cystic fibrosis. In an uncontrolled case series, the use of colistin inhaled twice daily reduced the frequency of isolation of *Pseudomonas* in the sputum [24]. In another controlled trial, 40 subjects inhaled either colistin 1 million units twice daily or a saline control. After 90 days, the rate of decline in forced vital capacity was lower in subjects using colistin and the drug was tolerated [25]. In the most recent published paper, 20 patients with cystic fibrosis awaiting lung transplantation were treated with aerosolized colistin 75 mg twice daily based on the presence of multiresistant *Pseudomonas* in their sputum [26]. Although the study was not randomized, they were compared to 10 patients who did not receive colistin treatment. There was no difference in lung function detected between groups; however, the colistin-treated patients had sensitive organisms detected more rapidly ($p = .007$) than control patients.

Since the early 1990s, most of the research interest has focused on the role of aerosolized aminoglycosides as suppressive therapy for cystic fibrosis patients colonized with *P. aeruginosa*. In addition to the carbenicillin and gentamicin study mentioned previously [21], earlier studies reported mild to moderate benefit in reducing the frequency of exacerbations and improving lung function with inhaled aminoglycosides. However, as noted, these studies often had poor controls and small numbers of patients.

The major study that stimulated interest in the development of a commercially available inhaled tobramycin product was published in 1993 [27]. In this trial, 71 cystic fibrosis patients with stable pulmonary disease were enrolled in a double-blind, placebo-controlled crossover study in which tobramycin 600 mg was nebulized (ultrasonic nebulizer) three times daily. This dose was based on a preliminary study, which showed that sputum concentrations would exceed 10 times the MIC of *P. aeruginosa* isolates. This concentration has been shown to overcome the competitive binding of tobramycin reported in the sputum of patients with cystic fibrosis.

Pulmonary function improved significantly in patients receiving the tobramycin compared to placebo (3.72% increase compared to 5.97% decrease; $p > .001$) within the first 28 days, and the difference persisted for the duration of the study. In addition, a 100-fold reduction in the sputum density of *P. aeruginosa* was observed.

These findings prompted the development and evaluation of the currently available form of inhaled tobramycin, which is sterile and free of preservatives. The benefit of maintenance therapy with this inhaled tobramycin is supported by the results from two 24-week, multicenter, randomized, double blind, placebo-controlled clinical trials [6]. In these studies, patients with cystic fibrosis were at least six years of age, with an FEV_1 between 25% and 75% predicted. All subjects had evidence of colonization with *Pseudomonas aeruginosa*. Exclusion criteria included an elevated serum creatinine or colonization with *Burkholderia cepacia*, which is typically resistant to tobramycin. Subjects in the active treatment arm received inhaled tobramycin 300 mg twice daily through nebulization, while control subjects inhaled a saline placebo. In each group, the nebulized treatment was administered in 28-day cycles (28 on, 28 off).

Patients receiving inhaled tobramycin ($n = 258$) showed significant improvement in lung function compared to the placebo group ($n = 262$). Reported average improvement in FEV_1 from baseline after 24 weeks was 7% to 11% for tobramycin treated subjects versus 0% to 1% for placebo ($p < .001$). Inhaled tobramycin also significantly reduced the presence of *P. aeruginosa* in sputum during treatment cycles. The average number of hospital days was reduced from 8.1 days for control subjects to 5.1 days in the active treatment group ($p = .001$), and the average number of days of parenteral therapy was lower (9.6 days vs. 14.1 days; $p = .003$) during the 24-week study.

A follow-up to these pivotal studies was published in 2002 [28]. One hundred twenty-eight subjects continued in open-label trials for up to 2 years at the conclusion of the controlled studies. Evidence suggests that the clinical benefit of therapy continued to be exhibited. Patients receiving inhaled tobramycin had improvements in FEV_1 of 14.3% compared to 1.8% in placebo patients, and active treatment significantly reduced sputum density of *P. aeruginosa* ($p = .0001$).

Based on the clinical evidence of benefit from inhaled antibiotic suppressive therapy, the consensus conference recommendation [14] supports the use of the commercially available inhaled tobramycin on a cyclic schedule in cystic fibrosis patients colonized with *P. aeruginosa*. Other inhaled antibiotics may provide benefit as suppressive therapy as well, although the most compelling data support inhaled tobramycin.

COMMERCIAL PRODUCT

Tobramycin solution for inhalation has approval from the Food and Drug Administration (FDA) for maintenance therapy in patients with cystic fibrosis and who are colonized with *Pseudomonas aeruginosa*. The commercially available formulation is a 300 mg per 5 mL. It is a sterile, preservative-free product that is pH adjusted to 6.0. According to the labeling, this product should be used with a specific nebulizer, the Pari C Plus.

The evidence for maintenance therapy with inhaled tobramycin comes from well-controlled clinical trials that reported beneficial outcomes for this therapy. Recommendations are based on evidence suggesting clinical benefits including improved pulmonary function, reduced requirements for hospitalization, and less frequently required systemic therapy against *Pseudomonas*.

The dose of the inhaled tobramycin product is 300 mg by nebulization twice daily. It should be used as cyclic therapy as four weeks on alternating with four weeks off.

SAFETY CONSIDERATIONS WITH AEROSOLIZED ANTIMICROBIAL THERAPY

Generally, aerosol administration of antimicrobial therapies is considered safe; however, respiratory and nonrespiratory side effects occur frequently. Some patients experience bronchoconstriction associated with administration. This has been reported when the parenteral form of gentamicin and tobramycin was aerosolized, and may be attributed to other components of the products, including preservatives [29,30]. Cutaneous rashes have developed rarely, and a sore throat may occur.

With aminoglycosides, systemic therapy is associated with a risk of ototoxicity and nephrotoxicity. However, no toxicity has been reported in several well-controlled trials of inhaled tobramycin in which subjects received repetitive courses [31,32].

After deposition, antimicrobial therapies are cleared from the lung by various mechanisms, including mucociliary clearance, coughing, and absorption into the systemic circulation. The drug is then metabolized or eliminated, depending on its properties. The systemic concentrations are severalfold less that what would be achieved with parenteral therapy and would not be expected to cause toxicity. However, more research is warranted to evaluate the impact of patient characteristics on systemic exposure to inhaled antimicrobial therapies. In the clinical trials of the commercially available inhaled tobramycin preparation, the mean concentration achieved one hour after inhalation was approximately 1 μg/mL.

There are few data from which to draw conclusions about the safety of other inhaled antibiotics. Aerosolized colistin has been generally well tolerated in published reports. The most frequent adverse event reported has been chest tightness associated with administration in some patients. Systemic use of colistin carries the risk for nephrotoxicity and neurotoxicity. Additional research about the safety of aerosolized colistin is warranted.

Similarly, information about the safety of inhaled beta lactams is lacking. One concern that has not surfaced in the limited reports is the potential for hypersensitivity reactions based on the prevalence of this problem in the general population. Again, investigations into the risks and benefits of these therapies by aerosolization are needed.

RESISTANCE CONCERNS

The use of antimicrobial therapies through aerosolization avoids many of the toxicities associated with systemic therapy with aminoglycosides or polypeptide agents. However, the risk for promoting antibiotic resistance is a concern. The emergence of highly resistant organisms has been reported with repeated courses of systemic antimicrobial agents for pulmonary infection [33–35].

To date, data on the potential for this problem have been equivocal, with some studies showing no increase in risk and others showing an association, although the resistance pattern did not persist when aerosol therapy was discontinued.

Resistant *Pseudomonas* species have been reported with prolonged use or repetitive courses of inhaled tobramycin. After three months of treatment with aerosolized tobramycin 600 mg three times daily, the percentage of patients growing a pseudomonal isolate with a tobramycin MIC of 8 or more increased from 29% to 73% [32]. In studies with the commercially available product where cyclic therapy was administered, the tobramycin MIC $\geq$ 16 against *Pseudomonas aeruginosa* was higher in the treatment group compared to placebo (23% vs. 8%) [36].

With the commercially available tobramycin product, an increase in the MIC for *Pseudomonas* was increased in 15% of subjects receiving treatment compared to 3% with placebo. The importance of this finding is unclear, since the pseudomonal isolates with the highest density were not the ones with the highest MIC.

Additionally, there is a question about the relevance of the MICs used in the clinical laboratory, since much higher concentrations of the antibiotic are present in bronchial and alveolar fluids when aerosol therapy is administered. Additional research is needed to clarify the relationship between the MIC of pseudomonal isolates and the clinical response when aerosol therapy is administered.

In addition to the impact on *P. aeruginosa* MICs, the use of inhaled tobramycin is also associated with an increased rate of isolation of fungus in the sputum, including *Candida albicans* and *Aspergillus* species [32]. The increased presence of these fungi did not appear to be associated with deterioration in clinical status. The chronic use of inhaled tobramycin has not been associated with an increased risk of colonization or infection with other bacteria, including *Burkholderia cepacia, Stenotrophomonas maltophilia*, and *Alcaligenes xylosoxidans*.

DELIVERY DEVICE CONSIDERATIONS

Historically, nebulized drug therapy has focused on the administration of bronchodilator therapy. These treatments were often titrated to effect; thus, differences in qualitative and quantitative performance between nebulizers were not considered. The administration of aerosolized antimicrobial therapy, as well as other biotechnologic agents, requires greater precision and consistency in delivery.

Jet and ultrasonic nebulizers have been used to aerosolize antimicrobial therapy. Jet nebulizers used compressed air or oxygen passed through a liquid to produce an aerosol gas. With ultrasonic devices, a piezoelectric element vibrates to generate small aerosol particles. Both systems have advantages and limitations related to their components and technique of use. These are discussed in more detail elsewhere in this text (see Chs. 8, 12).

Commercially available nebulizers have different performance characteristics, including aerosol output and the mean size and range of particle sizes generated [5,37]. The volume of fluid being nebulized and the flowrates generated also influence output.

Currently available nebulizers deliver approximately 10% of the dose to the airways and alveoli. The remainder either remains within the device, deposits in the upper airway, or is exhaled or swallowed [38].

A multicenter, randomized crossover study to evaluate the delivery of aerosolized tobramycin to the lower respiratory tract was conducted with two jet nebulizer systems [39]. The subjects ($n = 68$) with cystic fibrosis inhaled single doses of the commercial formulation of inhaled tobramycin delivered by three different nebulizers. The investigators reported that the Sidestream and the Pari LC jet nebulizer delivered tobramycin to achieve median sputum concentrations of $393\,\mu g/g$ and $452\,\mu g/g$, respectively. Concentrations in the target range of $128–2000\,\mu g/g$ were achieved in 93% and 87% of subjects, respectively. These concentrations were selected because they represent a tenfold increase over the MIC 90 for isolates and a tenfold increase over the most resistant strains identified ($256\,\mu g/mL$). The authors concluded that either nebulizer system was clinically useful in delivering adequate concentrations to the lower airway of patients with cystic fibrosis. Of interest, the ultrasonic nebulizer (Ultrasonic Neb 99/1000) resulted in a median concentration of $1359\,\mu g/g$ and exceeded $2000\,\mu g/g$ in 30% subjects, which the investigators suggested was unnecessarily high.

In the studies conducted in support of the commercially available inhaled tobramycin product, aerosol therapies were delivered using a PARI LC Plus nebulizer and a Pulmo-Aide compressor. Currently, the commercial product is labeled for use with the PARI LC Plus nebulizer.

Some progress has been made in developing alternative devices for the delivery of inhaled antimicrobial therapies. Colistin has been formulated in a dry powder inhaler and evaluated in healthy individuals and patients with cystic fibrosis [40]. Peak serum concentrations of colistin were 2.5–5 times higher when 25 mg of colistin sulfate dry powder was inhaled compared to 160 mg of colistin sulfomethate delivered by nebulization. Some patients experienced a decrease in pulmonary function and severe cough with the dry powder; however, the investigators felt that this may be improved with a reduction in dose.

Although these results are very preliminary, they suggest that this inhalation delivery system is promising.

CONCLUSIONS

Initial experiences with aerosolized antimicrobial therapies appeared in the literature more than 50 years ago. Until the early 1990s, the quality of the evidence supporting this strategy in the management of lung infections was poor. Recently, results from well-controlled clinical trials have established a role for inhaled antibiotics, particularly aminoglycosides, as suppressive therapy for patients with cystic fibrosis. Cyclic therapy with inhaled tobramycin reduces the frequency of pulmonary exacerbations and improves lung function.

Much of the success in this area can be attributed to enhancements in our understanding of this route of drug administration and to advances in drug delivery technology and formulations of products for aerosol administration. There is much to learn about the potential benefits of delivering therapeutic aerosols to the lung for local and systematic effects.

REFERENCES

1. Smith AL, Ramsey B. Aerosol administration of antibiotics. Respiration 62(suppl 1):19–24, 1995.
2. Gonda I. The ascent of pulmonary drug delivery. J Pharm Sci 89:940–945, 2000.
3. Fiel SB. Aerosolized antibiotic treatment for cystic fibrosis. RT, J Respir Care Prac 11:79, 1998.
4. Smaldone GC, Palmer LB. Aerosolized antibiotics: current and future. Respir Care 45(6):667–675, 2000.
5. O'Riordan TG. Inhaled antimicrobial therapy: from cystic fibrosis to the flu. Respir Care 45(7):836–845, 2000.
6. Prober CG, Walson PD, Jones J. Technical report: precautions regarding the use of aerosolized antibiotics. Pediatrics 106(6):e89, 2000.
7. Ramsey BW, Pepe MS, Quan JM, Otto KL, Montgomery AB, Williams-Warren J, Vasilkev-K M, Borowitz D, Bowman CM, Marshall BC, Marshall S, Smith AL. Intermittent administration of inhaled tobramycin in patients with cystic fibrosis. N Engl J Med 340:23–30, 1999.
8. Suarez S, Hickey AJ. Drug properties affecting aerosol behavior. Respir Care 45(6):652–666, 2000.
9. Clay MM, Pavia D, Newman SP, Clarke SW. Factors influencing the size distribution of aerosols from jet nebulizers. Thorax 38:755–759, 1983.
10. Touw DJ, Jacobs FA, Brimicome RW, Heijerman HG, Bakker W, Briemer DD. Pharmacokinetics of aerolized tobramycin in adult patients with cystic fibrosis. Antimicrob Agents Chemother 41:184–187, 1997.

11. Cystic Fibrosis Foundation. Patient Registry 1998 annual data report. Bethesda, MD: The Foundation, 1999.

12. Burns JL, Ramsey BW, Smith AL. Clinical manifestation and treatment of pulmonary infections in cystic fibrosis. Adv Pediatr Infect Dis 8:53–66, 1993.

13. Borsje P, DeJongste JC, Mouton JW, Tiddens HAWM. Aerosol therapy in cystic fibrosis: a survey of 54 CF centers. Pediatr Pulmonol 30:368–376, 2000.

14. Campbell PW, Saiman L. Use of aerolized antibiotics in patients with cystic fibrosis. Chest 116:775–788, 1999.

15. Stephens D, Garey N, Isles A. Efficacy of inhaled tobramycin in the treatment of pulmonary exacerbations in children with cystic fibrosis. Pediatr Infect Dis J 2:209–211, 1983.

16. Schaad RB, Wedgwood-Kruko J, Suter S. Efficacy of inhaled as adjunct to intravenous combination therapy (ceftazidime and amikacin) in cystic fibrosis. J Pediatr 111:599–665, 1987.

17. Valerius NH, Koch C, Hoiby N. Prevention of chronic *Pseudomonas aeruginosa* colonization in cystic fibrosis by early treatment. Lancet 338:725–726, 1991.

18. Frederiksen B, Koch C, Hoiby N. Antibiotic treatment of initial colonization with *Pseudomonas aeruginosa* postpones chronic infection and prevents deterioration of pulmonary function in cystic fibrosis. Pediatr Pulmonol 23:330–335, 1997.

19. Vasquez C, Municio M, Corera M. Early treatment of *Pseudomonas aeruginosa* colonization in cystic fibrosis. Acta Paediatr 82:308–309, 1993.

20. Heinzl B, Eber E, Oberwaldner B, Haas G, Zach MS. Effects of inhaled gentamicin prophylaxis on acquisition of *Pseudomonas aeruginosa* in children with cystic fibrosis: a pilot study. Pediatr Pulmonol 33:32–37, 2002.

21. Hodson ME, Penketh ARL, Batten JC. Aerosol carbenicillin and gentamicin treatment of *Pseudomonas aeruginosa* infection in patients with cystic fibrosis. Lancet 2:1137–1139, 1981.

22. Stead RJ, Hodson ME, Batten JC. Inhaled certazidime compared with gentamicin and carbenicillin in older patients with cystic fibrosis infected with *Pseudomonas aeruginosa*. Br J Dis Chest 81:273–279, 1987.

23. Mukhopadhyay S, Singh M, Cater JI, Ogston S, Franklin M, Olver RE. Nebulized antipseudomonas antibiotic therapy in cystic fibrosis: a meta-analysis of benefits and risks. Thorax 51:364–368, 1996.

24. Littlewood JM, Miller MG, Ghoneim AT. Nebulized colomycin for use in early *Pseudomonas* colonization in cystic fibrosis. Lancet 1:865, 1985.

25. Jensen T, Pedersen SS, Garne S. Colistin inhalation therapy in cystic fibrosis patients with chronic *Pseudomonas aeruginosa* lung infections. J Antimicrob Chemother 19:831–838, 1987.

26. Bauldoff GS, Nunley DR, Manzetti JD. Use of aerosolized colistin sodium in cystic fibrosis awaiting lung transplantation. Transplantation 64:748–752, 1997.

27. Ramsey BW, Dorkin HL, Eisenberg JD. Efficacy of aerosolized tobramycin in patients with cystic fibrosis. N Engl J Med 328:1740–1746, 1993.

28. Moss RB. Long-term benefit of inhaled tobramycin in adolescent patients with cystic fibrosis. Chest 121:55–63, 2002.

29. Nikolaizik WH, Jenni-Galovic V, Schoni MH. Bronchial constriction after nebulized tobramycin preparations and saline in patients with cystic fibrosis. Eur J Pediatr 155:608–611, 1996.

30. Melani AS, Di Gregorio A. Acute respiratory failure due to gentamicin aerosolization. Monaldi Arch Chest Dis 53:274–276, 1998.

31. Steinkamp G, Trummler B, Gappa M. Long-term tobramycin aerosol therapy in cystic fibrosis. Pediatr Pulmonol 6:91–98, 1989.

32. Smith AL, Ramsey BW, Hedges DL. Safety of aerosol tobramycin administration for 3 months to patients with cystic fibrosis. Pediatr Pulmonol 7:265–271, 1989.

33. Burns JL, Ramsey BW, Smith AL. Clinical manifestations and treatment of pulmonary ifections in cystic fibrosis. Adv Pediatr Infect Dis 8:53–66, 1993.

34. MacDonald NE. *Pseudomonas aeruginosa* and cystic fibrosis: antibiotic therapy and the science behind the magic. Can J Infect Dis 335–342, 1997.

35. Saiman L, Mehar F, Niu WW. Antibiotic susceptibility of multiply resistant *Pseudomonas aeruginosa* isolated from patients with cystic fibrosis, including candidates for transplantation. Clin Infect Dis 23:532–537, 1996.

36. Burns JL, Van Dalfsen JM, Shawar RM. Effect of chronic intermittent administration of inhaled tobramycin on respiratory microbial flora in patients with cystic fibrosis. J Infect Dis 179:1190–1196, 1999.

37. Coats AL, MacNeish CF, Meisner D. The choice of jet nebulizer, nebulizing flow, and addition of albuterol affects the output of tobramycin aerosols. Chest 111:1206–1212, 1997.

38. Iliwite JS, Gorvoy JD, Smaldone GC. Quantitative deposition of aerosolized gentamicin in cystic fibrosis. Am Rev Resp Dis 136:1445–1449, 1987.

39. Eisenberg J, Pepe M, Williams-Warren J, Vasiliev M, Montgomery AB, Smith AL, Ramsey RW. A comparison of peak sputum tobramycin concentration in patients with cystic fibrosis using jet and ultrasonic nebulizer systems. Chest 111:955–962, 1997.

40. Le Brun PPH, De Boer AH, Mannes GPM, de Fraiture DMI, Brimicombe RW, Touw DJ, Vinks AA, Frijlink HW, Heijerman GM. Dry powder inhalation of antibiotics in cystic fibrosis therapy: part 2. Inhalation of a novel colistin dry power formulation: a feasibility study in healthy volunteers and patients. Eur J Pharmaceut Biopharmaceut 54:25–32, 2002.

16

Gene Delivery to the Lung

Justin Hanes, Michelle Dawson, Yah-el Har-el, Junghae Suh, and Jennifer Fiegel
Johns Hopkins University, Baltimore, Maryland, U.S.A.

INTRODUCTION

Pharmaceutical treatments for pulmonary disease may one day include gene transfer therapies for cystic fibrosis (CF), emphysema, oxygen injury, lung cancer, and general inflammatory pulmonary conditions [1]. In 2002, over six hundred clinical trials utilizing gene therapy were completed, ongoing, or pending in 2001, of which roughly 10% targeted lung diseases [2].

A variety of delivery systems and routes of administration have been used for gene delivery to the lung. Viruses are the most common vectors, but lipids and polymeric vectors are gaining in popularity. Routes of administration include: (1) systemic administration, in which the gene carrier may become trapped in the capillary network of the lung; (2) intratracheal (i.t.) instillation of a suspension containing the gene of interest; and (3) inhalation of aerosolized material carrying the therapeutic gene, either as droplets or dry powders. Systemic administration provides direct access to blood vessel endothelial cells, while instillation and inhalation provide direct access to epithelial cells at the air/lung interface. Systemic delivery to the lung may offer a method to bypass the diseased lung yet still reach the target site to achieve a therapeutic result [3,4]. Intratracheal instillation allows for only small doses of material and has a distribution within the lung independent of particle size [5]. It is an invasive technique plagued with low and uneven coverage of lung surfaces [1]. Inhalation requires optimization of inhaler and/or particle characteristics to achieve proper aerosolization and deposition. Deposition within the lung following inhalation is also subject to patient variability [5]. Even so, inhalation of aerosolized material is the most common method of delivery to the respiratory tract, owing to the ease of administration combined with a more uniform distribution [6].

Several important barriers must be overcome before efficient gene therapy in the lung can be realized. A gene entering the lung via inhalation will first encounter the fluid lining the lung surfaces. The innate immunity of the lung surfaces, including an adhesive mucous layer in the upper respiratory tract, surfactant proteins that function specifically in host defense, and alveolar macrophages in the deep lung, provides a formidable barrier to gene delivery. Genes successfully traversing the mucosal barrier encounter cellular barriers that must be overcome before protein translation can occur. Intracellular barriers to gene expression include cellular uptake, endosomal release, nuclear localization, nuclear uptake, and gene transcription, which may require vector/DNA unpacking. Naked DNA has been an inefficient method of gene therapy in the lung, owing to its poor ability to bypass these barriers.

Finally, controlled/targeted deposition of DNA-containing aerosols in various regions of the lung can be achieved by designing aerosols with appropriate physical and chemical attributes. Physical attributes of the particles, such as size, density, and shape, as well as patient-controlled effects, including tidal volume and respiratory rate, significantly affect regional deposition. In addition, proper deaggregation of particles is necessary for predictable and reproducible deposition within the respiratory tract.

This chapter is designed to provide an overview of the important barriers to gene delivery in the lung, but it is not intended as an exhaustive review. We do not attempt to summarize the recent preclinical or clinical aerosol gene therapy literature, nor do we attempt to cover all potential gene carriers. Instead, we were guided by the principle that advances in the basic knowledge related to gene vector design, transport barriers in the lung, and regional targeting should lead to the developing of more efficient carriers for pulmonary gene delivery. For complementary reviews on the topics discussed herein, the reader is referred to Refs. 7–14.

OVERVIEW OF GENE VECTOR SYSTEMS

DNA vectors consist of two major components: the gene expression system and the carrier. The gene expression system contains regulatory sequences and a nucleic acid sequence that codes for the therapeutic protein. Expression of the therapeutic gene is controlled by promoter regions to regulate protein expression [15]. Some promoters are tissue-specific, which allows one level of control over targeting gene expression [16]. In viral vectors, a portion of the viral genome is replaced by sequences coding for the therapeutic protein. Nonviral vectors generally use plasmid DNA (pDNA).

The gene carrier is typically composed of a viral capsid or, in the case of nonviral delivery systems, a lipid, polymer, protein, peptide, or multivalent cation. For recent reviews of nonviral gene carriers, the reader is referred to Refs. 10 and 17. The carrier is meant to protect DNA from degradation by enzymes and/or low pH, found in various body fluids, the extracellular matrix, cytoplasm, and lysosomes [17]. Carriers can also be modified to target specific cells using receptor–ligand interactions (for reviews see Refs. 18 and 19). Some vector strategies used for gene delivery are illustrated in Fig. 1.

The ideal method of DNA delivery should maintain the integrity of the gene and yield high gene expression in the target tissue without compromising the safety of the patient. Genetically engineered viruses, commonly used in clinical and preclinical pulmonary gene therapy protocols, are based on vectors that have evolved over millions of years to produce high levels of gene expression. As a result, viral vectors are easily the most advanced and most effective in terms of gene delivery. Of the 600 completed, ongoing, or pending gene therapy clinical trials recorded in September 2001, 72% involved a viral vector [2]. Cationic liposomes were the next most popular vector (13%). Unfortunately, some viral vectors have been associated with inflammatory immune responses [20–25], which can be detrimental to the health of patients suffering from lung diseases such as cystic fibrosis, chronic obstructive pulmonary disorder, and asthma. A clinical trial involving an adenovirus gene vector injected into the hepatic blood vessel resulted in the death of a teenage boy due to acute respiratory distress syndrome (ARDS) in September 2000. Analysis showed that the vector caused systemic inflammatory response syndrome (SIRS), which is associated with ARDS [26]. In the wake of this tragedy, there has been an increased focus on the development of safer gene delivery systems to complement the highly efficient viral vectors.

Viral Vectors

Adenoviruses (Ad), adeno-associated viruses (AAV), and retroviruses, are amongst those viruses currently in gene therapy clinical trials [2]. Viral vectors have evolved several mechanisms that facilitate cell uptake and delivery

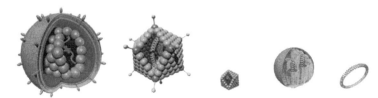

	Retroviruses	Adenoviruses	Adeno-Associated Viruses	Liposomes	"Naked" DNA
Some Potential Advantages	Integrates gene into host chromosomes, offering chances for long-term stability	Most do not cause serious disease; large capacity for foreign genes	Integrates genes into host chromosomes; cause no known human diseases	Have no viral genes, so do not cause disease	Same as for liposomes; expected to be useful for vaccination
Some Drawbacks of Existing Vectors	Genes integrate randomly, so might disrupt host genes; many infect only dividing cells	Genes may function transiently, owing to lack of integration or to attack by the immune system	Small capacity for foreign genes	Less efficient than viruses at transferring genes to cells	Inefficient at gene transfer; unstable in most tissues of the body

FIGURE 1   Schematic: example drawing of a few gene delivery vectors. A. Retrovirus, B. adenovirus, C. adeno-associated virus, D. liposomes, E. naked DNA. Polyplex not shown. (Reprinted from Ref. 295. Courtesy of Slim Films.)

to the nucleus. Many viral vectors, including Ad and AAV, can transduce most cells, including nondividing lung epithelial cells, while retroviruses target proliferating cells, such as tumors [27–29].

The AAV and retroviruses integrate their genomic material into the host genome, which carries the risk of activating oncogenes or deactivating tumor suppressor genes [29,30]. This risk must be weighed against the advantage of stable gene expression. Adenoviruses induce both a humoral and a cell-mediated immune response, making chronic therapy difficult [20–25]. Viral vectors also have a DNA packing size limit; for example, AAV can accommodate ~4 kilobase (kb) pairs of DNA [5]. The coding region of the CFTR gene (4.5 kb) narrowly makes the size cutoff of many viral vectors, limiting potentially beneficial modifications to the gene expression system. Modifications aimed to make viral vectors safer also may reduce the DNA packaging limit [5]. To address this potential shortcoming, the CFTR gene has been spliced into multiple parts and delivered in multiple vectors [31–34]. Finally, it is noteworthy that viral vectors have exhibited reduced efficiency following nebulization [35–38]. Even with these limitations, viral vectors will remain the predominant mode of gene delivery in the lung until the efficiency of synthetic systems is significantly improved. For recent reviews of viral gene therapy, see Refs. 39–41.

Synthetic Gene Vectors

Without evolution working to carefully hone and optimize the delivery process, man-made delivery vectors suffer from lower efficiencies compared to nature's DNA viruses. However, nonviral vectors, including cationic liposomes and cationic polymers, are gaining popularity because they are easy to make and to mass-produce, there is no size limit on the DNA to be delivered, there are fewer immunological and safety implications, and they can be targeted by the attachment of cell-specific ligands [17–19,42]. However, basic knowledge of the relationship between vector structure and efficiency, and critical in vivo mechanisms involved in gene delivery with synthetic carriers is still scarce [43]. As discussed in this and subsequent sections, improved knowledge pertaining to the "bottlenecks" to efficient nonviral gene delivery is critical to the further improvement of the biological performance of these systems.

Cationic Liposomes

Since the pioneering work of Felgner and coworkers [44], cationic lipid/DNA lipoplexes have been used to deliver a variety of genes to the lungs of animals and humans [4,36–38,45–48,50–59]. Lipoplexes are made by the interaction of negatively charged DNA with cationic lipids or liposomes. Two common cationic lipids are dioleoyltrimethylammonium propane (DOTAP) and dioleoxipropyltrimethylammonium (DOTMA), which are both two-chain amphiphiles whose acyl chains are linked to a propyl ammonium group through an ester or ether bond, respectively. Lipids with the more stable ether linkage have exhibited higher toxicity than those with a labile ester linkage [15,61] but DOTMA has been shown to have ten-fold higher transfection efficiency than DOTAP [115]. Marshall et al. found that gene expression in the lung after intratracheal (i.t.) administration of cationic lipid:DNA lipoplexes in mice was dependent on the structure of the lipid [55]. They synthesized a series of lipids in which they varied the cationic headgroup, the hydrophobic anchor, and the linker between the two and found that the lipids whose structure resembled a "T-shape" had higher efficiency than linear lipids. Lipids used in gene carries differ in hydrophobicity, degradability of their linker group, and the positive valence of the polar headgroup, all of which translate into variable transfection efficiencies of the vector [43,50].

Cationic lipids are often mixed with neutral lipids, such as cholesterol, dioleoylphosphatidylethanolamine (DOPE), and dioleoylphosphatidylcholine

(DOPC). Neutral lipids are used to facilitate the formation of liposomes and to ease disassembly of the lipoplexes after internalization [62]. The choice of neutral lipid is also important; for example, cationic liposomes made with DOTAP:DOPE have shown higher transfection efficiency in mammalian cell culture than those made with DOTAP:DOPC [63]. Although in vivo work has shown lower transfection efficiency of DOTAP:DOPE than DOTAP alone following i.v. administration in mice [115].

DNA association with lipids may increase its permeability through the cell membrane due to membrane fusion [15,44] or endocytosis involving clathrin- and nonclathrin-coated vesicles [49,64,65]. Lipids also may protect DNA from degradation [62,66,67]. However, high doses of cationic lipoplexes can trigger an inflammatory response, which may be increased by the inherent immunogenicity of the condensed bacteria-derived pDNA [54]. In addition, lipoplexes are relatively unstable in many physiological environments [68], which may limit their efficacy in vivo compared to in vitro cell culture. Sanders and coworkers showed that DOTAP:DNA lipoplexes released pDNA upon contact with mucus components at concentrations comparable to those of cystic fibrosis (CF) patients [69]. In another study, cationic liposome–mediated gene delivery was prevented by coating cell monolayers with sputum from patients with cystic fibrosis before transfection [48]. Meyer and colleagues found that neither DOTMA-DOPE nor DOTAP liposomes enhanced gene expression over naked DNA in the murine airways [56]. Another study showed similar levels of transfection between DOTAP:DNA and naked DNA in the mouse airways following i.t. administration, but there were higher levels of transfection with lipoplexes made from DORI analogues [50]. Finally, similar to viral vectors, cationic lipids exhibit reduced transfection efficiency following nebulization [35–38]. A review of cationic lipid complexation with DNA can be found in Refs. 43, 60, and 70; a review of lipoplexes for CF can be found in Ref. 71.

Cationic Polymers

Polyplex (cationic polymer/DNA complex) formation is driven largely by electrostatic interactions of negatively charged DNA with cationic polymers, such as poly-L-lysine (PLL) [72,73], polyethylenimine (PEI) [74–77], poly(methacrylate) [78,79], poly(amidoamine) [80] and dendrimers [81–83], which serve to condense the DNA. Cationic polymers are capable of protecting DNA from degradation by nucleases [84], and the complexes enter cells either via adsorptive endocytosis [49,85] or by receptor-mediated endocytosis [86]. Cationic polymers have been used to deliver DNA to the lungs of animals and humans [59,87–98]. In a study including linear and branched PEIs, dendrimers, and a conjugate of Pluronic P123, Gebhart and Kabanov found that the difference in transfection efficiency could not be related to the structural differences of the cationic compound [99].

PEI/DNA polyplexes were found to maintain functional stability and provide 10-fold higher transfection efficiency in vivo than lipoplexes following nebulization [89]. Interestingly, PEI/DNA was more efficient in providing in vivo gene expression in the lungs compared to the nasal passageways [89]. Linear PEI (L-PEI) has achieved higher levels of transfection than 25 kDa molecular weight branched PEI following instillation in rats [96]. However, as with some viral and most synthetic systems, gene expression is typically transient [213]. Additionally, cationic polymers can be cytotoxic at high doses. Reviews of cationic polymer complexation with DNA can be found in Refs. 10, 75, and 101.

Preparation and Characterization of Lipoplexes and Polyplexes

There is relatively little physical understanding of why certain preparation conditions of nonviral gene vectors generate better gene expression than others [68]. This deficiency has hindered the development of nonviral gene delivery vectors, since relatively few reports quantitatively evaluate DNA complex structure and composition, especially as it relates to gene delivery efficiency. Some structural and physical characteristics, including shape, size, and zeta potential, have been studied for various synthetic DNA delivery systems and have, in some instances, been related to transfection efficiency.

Shape. Lin et al. demonstrated a correlation between lipoplex structure and transfection efficiency [102]. Liposomes that formed hexagonal structures were more efficient in gene delivery than those that formed a lamellar, owing to improved fusion with mouse cell membranes (both endosomal and plasma membranes), whereas lamellar structures remained stable inside the cell. This correlation of structure and transfection efficiency was used to explain the increased efficiency of DOTAP:DOPE liposomes (hexagonal structures) compared to DOTAP:DOPC liposomes (lamellar structures) [102].

Polyplexes, made with cationic polymers such as PEI and PLL, have been reported to be both spherical and toroidal in shape [103]. The distinction between the two may be due to the visualization technique and sample preparation procedures [103]. Gebhart and Kabanov found that some polymers formed large aggregates when complexed with DNA, one of which (25K PEI) had high transfection efficiency, while the others did not [99]. Tang et al. studied PEI, dendrimers, and PLL and found that the type of polymer plays a role in aggregation and that models predicting electrostatic stability do not adequately describe the aggregation of polyplexes [103].

Size. Vector size has a marked effect on transport across several barriers to gene delivery in the lung, including mucus lining the airways and intracellular barriers. The ultimate size of the vector depends on a variety of parameters, including DNA and condensing agent concentrations, solvent choice and concentration, and the specific choice of condensing agent and its molecular weight [104,105]. The size of DNA condensates is nearly independent of plasmid size when the plasmid is between 400 and 50,000 bp for a variety of agents capable of condensing DNA, including cationic lipids, cationic polymers, and multivalent cations [104,106,107]. The cationic polymer, PEI, has been reported to condense and efficiently deliver yeast artificial chromosome (YAC) DNA that was up to 2.3 megabase (Mb) pairs [108]. PEI/DNA polyplexes measured using transmission electron microscopy (TEM) and atomic force microscopy (AFM) have been reported to be between 20–100 nm in diameter [75,109], while measurements using dynamic light scattering (DLS) reported polyplex sizes between 40 and 750 nm [103,110,111].

Interestingly, larger PEI/DNA complexes were more effective transfection agents than smaller particles over a range of PEI molecular weights in one study [111]. A possible explanation was that the "proton sponge" effect, as discussed later, may be more efficient with larger complexes. Larger particles may also sediment to interact with cells more readily under in vitro culture conditions [112]. Enhanced transfection with larger vectors was also seen with lipid-DNA lipoplexes in CHO cells [113]. However, the opposite was found with linear PEI (L-PEI) in vivo. Smaller complexes led to higher levels of gene expression in adult and newborn mice, which correlated to their diffusivity through tissue [100]. In this study, L-PEI DNA complexes were shown to cross the endothelial cell barrier following intravenous administration and preferentially transfect pulmonary cells [92]. Cationic lipids, on the other hand, show some expression in pulmonary cells following intravenous administration but preferentially transfected endothelial cells [51,53,114,115], perhaps due to their reduced stability compared to polyplexes.

Surface Charge. DNA polyplexes with a positive surface charge have been found to translocate preferentially to the nucleus of cells [116–118]. One hypothesis is that high charge density endows the carriers with properties similar to nuclear localization sequences that are made up of cationic amino acids [119]. Another explanation may be that, following endocytosis, particles are delivered to the perinuclear region of cells as part of the normal cellular processing of endosomes [118]. Negatively charged complexes have more unbound phosphate groups (from DNA) than positive groups (from condensing species), such that the DNA is not fully condensed and may not be fully protected from degradation. Negatively charged complexes also are not taken up by cells as efficiently as neutral or positively charged complexes. As a result, negatively charged vectors provide lower transfection efficiency in general. Finally, as discussed more fully later, small neutral particles diffuse through the mucus barrier most rapidly [120], which may be a prerequisite to high transfection efficiency in the lung.

Density. Density of synthetic gene carriers [Eq. (1)] was recently correlated with transfection efficiency for both lipoplexes [121,122] and polyplexes [123,124], where R_g is the mean-square radius of gyration. Carrier density for nearly equal-sized vectors is a measure of the amount of DNA packed into each carrier. Therefore, higher-density vectors deliver more DNA per carrier particle that successfully reaches the cell nucleus. Also, high-density vectors may provide improved protection of DNA from degradation.

$$\mathrm{complex/density} = \frac{\mathrm{molar\ mass}}{2.87\,\pi R_g^3} \qquad (1)$$

Recently, we systematically varied PEI/DNA preparation parameters, including PEI molecular weight, N/P ratio, solution pH, and ionic strength, in order to determine their effect on vector size, molar mass, and density [124]. The molar mass of PEI/DNA polyplexes made with 25-kDa molecular weight PEI varied nonmonotonically with the N/P ratio, with a maximum value at $N/P = 6$. The maximum polyplex molar mass occurred at an N/P ratio near the transition between negatively and positively charged complexes, possibly due to reduced charge repulsion. Since these polyplexes typically had similar diameters but vastly different molar masses, their densities varied depending on N/P ratio and PEI molecular weight. Polyplexes made with and N/P ratio of 6 contained 60 times more DNA per complex than those made with $N/P = 10$. PEI/DNA complex molar mass changed by an additional order of magnitude over the range of PEI molecular weights studied when $N/P = 6$ and varied by two orders of magnitude when $N/P = 10$, but the geometric size and charge remained approximately the same [125]. The densest PEI/DNA polyplexes were those of PEI molecular weight and N/P ratio reported in the literature to have the highest transfection efficiencies [126].

Stability. Current protocols for nonviral delivery systems call for the preparation of the vector at the bedside, due to their aggregation over time [127–129]. Specifically, aggregation of some lipoplex formulations stored as liquids reduced their transfection efficiency [130,131]. Electron microscopy was used to show that PEI/DNA complexes did not aggregate, but vectors made with poly-L-lysine and dendrimers did in one study [103].

Recently, van Zanten and coworkers showed that PLL/DNA and PEI/DNA polyplexes maintain their size over long periods of time but decrease in molar mass quickly [121–125], suggesting that liquid storage of these polyplexes may reduce their efficacy.

PHYSIOLOGICAL BARRIERS TO GENE DELIVERY IN THE LUNG

Efficient gene delivery is significantly limited by the multitude of barriers that serve to protect the lung against particle and bacterial insult. The upper airways are protected by the mucociliary escalator, a thick mucus layer (8–10 μm) that works in concert with ciliated epithelial cells to efficiently sweep particles out of the lungs into the mouth [132]. The liquid layer is extremely thin (average thickness <0.2 μm) in the alveolar regions of the lung [133]; however, an army of alveolar macrophages rapidly phagocytose most particles following deposition in this region [134]. Diseases such as cystic fibrosis and alpha-1-antitrypsin disease induce changes in lung physiology that include thickening of mucus secretions, inflammation, and bacterial colonization, which may further reduce the efficiency of gene delivery to the lungs.

Mucus

Mucus is the most frequently cited extracellular barrier to the delivery of genes to the cells of the upper respiratory tract [120,135]. Kitson et al. found a 25-fold increase in transfection efficiencies with lipoplexes in mucus-depleted tissues compared to those that were mucus covered [136]. Respiratory mucus lines the luminal side of the tracheobronchial tree from the entrance of the trachea to the terminal bronchioles, humidifying inspired air and trapping small particles and microorganisms until they can be transported out of the lungs. The continuous flow of dry air into the lungs dehydrates mucus at the air–liquid interface, forcing mucus to partition into two layers: a viscous superficial "gel" layer (0.5–2.0 μm) covering an aqueous periciliary "sol" layer (7–10 μm) [132]. Inhaled particles that become trapped in the mucus gel layer are removed by mucociliary transport [132]. Beating cilia extending from the mucus sol layer sweep the mucus gel layer from the lungs into the pharynx. The continual motion of cilia at the interface of the sol and gel layers creates a slippage plane, which aids in clearing mucus and maintaining an unstirred gel layer [120,132].

An improved understanding of the relationship between mucus properties and particle transport is critical to the design of DNA carriers for delivery in the nondistal airways of the lung. Important properties of the mucus gel layer, including viscosity, elasticity, adhesivity, permeability, and clearance rate, can be affected by disease, inflammation, bacterial infection, and the addition of chemical substances [120,137–139]. For example, cystic fibrosis (CF) is a genetic disease characterized by reduced clearance of thick airway secretions. Mucus from cystic fibrosis patients is denser and more highly glycosylated than in normal patients [138]. The addition of chemical agents (including polylysine salts, surfactants, and DNase) can reduce the viscosity of CF mucus, thereby increasing the clearance rate of airway secretions [140]. DNA vector design should, therefore, be guided by the nature and functionality of airway mucus in the relevant disease state [138]. For example, in cases where the mucosal layer is a rate-limiting step to gene delivery, the addition of adjuvants that decrease the viscosity of mucus may increase gene transfer to airway epithelial cells [88].

Composition and Structure of Mucus

The primary constituents of mucus are glycoproteins and water ($\sim 95\%$). Mucus glycoproteins (sialomucins, fucomucins, and sulfomucins) are composed of four to five mucin subunits, each with molecular weight of ~ 500 kDa [138,141]. Subunits are composed of a highly glycosylated protein backbone with nonglycosylated protein ends [141,142]. Subunits are attached at their nonglycosylated regions by disulphide bonds and are cross-linked with other glycoproteins by protein–carbohydrate lectin bonds and carbohydrate–carbohydrate noncovalent bonds [120,141,142]. Several other constituents interact with mucus glycoproteins to form a dense network, including phospholipids, cellular and serum macromolecules, neutrophil-derived DNA and F-actin, alginate, electrolytes, microorganisms, and sloughed cells [142]. Concentrations of various constituents are dependent on the anatomical location as well as the physiological and pathophysiological condition of the mucus donor [142]. Each of these factors contributes to the unique microstructure of mucus, which should be understood prior to the development of gene vectors capable of passing efficiently through the mucosal barrier. Hydrophobic interactions between mucin polymers cause mucus to form a fine network. In cervical mucus, this network consists of a fine mesh with interfiber spacings of approximately 100 nm within a macroporous mesh of interfiber spacings approximately 500 nm [143]. A similar network structure has been observed in CF sputum [144] (Fig. 2).

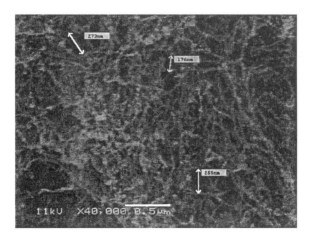

FIGURE 2 Scanning electron microscopic image of CF sputum, showing the pores in the biopolymer network. Bar $= 0.5$ μm. (Reprinted from Ref. 144. Courtesy of the *American Journal of Respiratory Critical Care Medicine*.)

Viscoelastic and Rheological Properties of Mucus

Disease conditions such as CF, chronic obstructive pulmonary disease (COPD), and emphysema generally result in an increase in the viscoelasticity of mucus, owing in part to reduced liquid content and an increased percentage of highly branched glycoproteins [145]. The viscoelasticity of mucus is closely regulated (in the normal lung) to provide the proper elasticity to resist gravitational flow while minimizing viscosity to attain rapid mucociliary transport [120]. Mucociliary transport is responsible for clearing matter from the upper conducting airways, via the larynx, to the gut [146]. For mucociliary transport to work efficiently, the viscosity of mucus should be sufficient to support a load without hindering the ability of cilia to move it toward the mouth. Mucus velocity has been estimated in vitro by measuring the velocity of tracer particles on depleted frog palates, incised tracheal tissues, or intact airways using fiber-optic bronchoscopy [147]. The rate of mucociliary transport in humans is $5-10$ cm/min [120]. This rate may be affected, however, by diseases or inhalation of mucolytic agents.

Changes in the viscoelasticity of mucus gels alter the mucus clearance rate and, hence, particle transport efficiency. An increase in viscosity [148], or a decrease in elasticity [132,149] of mucus gels leads to slower mucociliary clearance rates, allowing particles a longer time to penetrate mucus.

However, mucus permeability is reduced as viscosity increases, owing to the increased viscous drag and steric obstruction from multiple mucus-particle interactions [120,145,150]. One might expect that an increase in elasticity of mucus gels would lead to caging of particles moving through the mesh [151], thereby reducing particle permeability. However, Sanders and coworkers related variations in the elastic modulus (G') of mucus samples to particle transport and found that the percentage of particles ($124-270$ nm) transported through mucus increased with increasing elasticity ($G' > 100$ Pa) [144] (Fig. 3). This unexpected finding was explained by a possible increase in the heterogeneity of the mucus mesh, allowing larger pores for particle transport as elasticity increased.

The rheological properties of mucus forming important to particle transport through the mucosal barrier, including viscosity and elasticity, are dependent on the shear rate along the tracheobronchial tree. Shear is imposed by ciliary motion and coughing [152]. Mucus acts as a thixotropic gel, meaning its viscosity increases with increasing shear rate initially and then begins to decrease [138,153]. The critical shear rate for respiratory mucus, at which viscosity begins to decrease, is approximately $1 \sec^{-1}$ [153]. By modeling the tracheobronchial regions of the lungs as cylindrical tubes, average shear rates were estimated as $0.91 \sec^{-1}$ (large bronchi), $0.78 \sec^{-1}$ (medium bronchi), and $0.25 \sec^{-1}$ (small bronchi) [152]. Thus, mucus acts elastically at physiological shear rates in

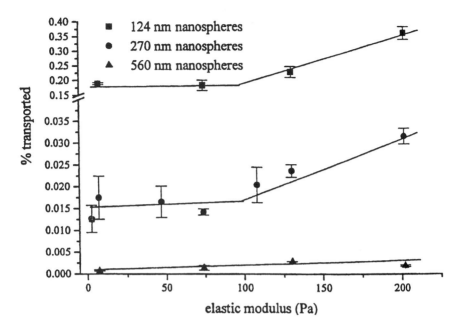

FIGURE 3 Percentages of nanospheres that diffused through 220-µm-thick layers of CF and COPD (gray circle) sputum and into the acceptor compartment of the diffusion chamber system after 150 min as a function of the elastic moduli of the sputum samples ($n = 4$ for each data point). (Reprinted form Ref. 144. Courtesy of the *American Journal of Respiratory and Critical Care Medicine.*)

the upper airways, thereby maintaining the shape of mucus fibers and the structure of the mucus fiber networks [152].

Particle Transport Through Mucus

Investigations of diffusion through mucus gels demonstrated that small molecules (e.g., testosterone with molecular weight 401 Da) diffuse rapidly through mucosal barriers, while large molecules become trapped, owing, in part, to steric hindrance [120,144]. Particle diffusion through mucus is related to interfiber spacing, decreasing approximately as the square root of mucin concentration [120]. The cutoff size for particles able to diffuse efficiently through mucus gels with high mucin concentration (e.g., thick colonic mucus) has been reported as 100 nm [120] (Fig. 3). Gene vectors are often larger than 100 nm, which may significantly limit their ability to permeate the mucosal layer and transfect cells. Mucus from cystic fibrosis patients was found to provide a size-dependent barrier to particle transport, with the smallest latex particles (124 nm) studied diffusing most efficiently and the largest latex particles (560 nm) becoming completely trapped in CF sputum [144].

If the translocation of particles through mucus were only a function of particle size, virus-sized latex particles (< 100 nm) would diffuse through mucus readily ($D_{mucus}/D_{pbs} \sim 1$, where D is diffusivity) (Fig. 4). However, latex particles adhere strongly to mucin fibers via hydrophobic interactions, resulting

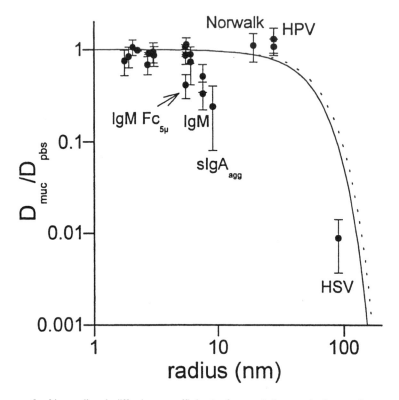

FIGURE 4 Normalized diffusion coefficients for proteins and viruses in mucus. $D_{muc}/D_{pbs} \pm$ SD is plotted for particles with molecular weights 15 kDa–20 mou. For a particle that diffuses in mucus as fast as it diffuses in saline, $D_{muc}/D_{pbs} = 1$. The lines drawn on the graph are the ratio predicted by Amsden's obstruction-scaling model, developed for modeling covalently cross-linked hydrogels. The *solid line* uses a mucin fiber radius of 3.5 nm and a mesh fiber spacing of 100 nm. The *dotted line* takes into account the 20% dilution of the mucus samples by increasing the mesh fiber spacing by 10%. (Reprinted from Ref. 151. Courtesy of the Biophysical Society.)

in a sharp reduction of their diffusion rates through mucus [120,154] (Fig. 5). Surface charge may also be a factor in the translocation of particles through mucus [154]. The high density of negatively charged carboxyl and sulphate groups on the surface of mucus fibers bind positively charged particles [120]. Viruses may avoid the viscid nature of mucus by maintaining a surface that is densely coated equally with negative and positive charges [120]. The high density of negative charges reduces viral interaction with mucus fibers, while the positive charges aid entry into the mucus gel and glycocalyx [120].

Effects of Mucus Degrading Agents on Particle Transport

The prolonged retention of viscous airway secretions in the diseased lung (e.g., CF and COPD) can lead to recurring bacterial infections, resulting in a viscous, more purulent sputum [155]. Increased mucus viscoelasticity may be attributed to extensive disulphide and lectin bonding, poor hydration, and/or excess concentrations of extracellular DNA or actin [155]. In these situations, therapeutics have been used to reduce the viscosity of airway secretions to improve the rate of mucociliary clearance.

Mucolytic agents, such as N-acetylcysteine [88], guaifenesin [156], and diothiothreitol (DTT) [157], are used clinically and/or in vitro to reduce mucus viscosity. Lytic agents, such as recombinant human deoxynuclease I (rhDNase I, or Pulmozyme$^{®}$) and Gelsolin$^{®}$ have also been effective in clearing viscous

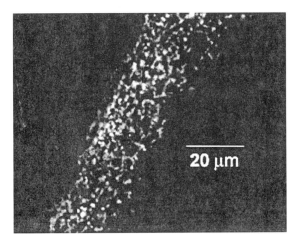

FIGURE 5 Fluorescent image of 200-nm carboxylated polystyrene microspheres in CF mucus collected by expectoration from an 18-year-old Caucasian male. Mucus fibers are bundled together, forming a thick mucus cord, which can be visualized owing, in part, to the adhesion of fluorescent microspheres.

airway secretions [155]. Pulmozyme® enzymatically degrades extracellular DNA in human sputum [139]. Gelsolin® severs noncovalent bonds between polymerized monomers of actin filaments. Gelsolin® may scavenge actin filaments released during the inflammation process, increasing the effectiveness of DNase I [158]. Finally, the application of pulmonary surfactant to canine airways increased the mucus transport velocity nearly 400% in one study [147]. The affect of using mucus-altering agents as adjuncts in gene delivery was investigated: the addition of mucus-altering agents produced similar transgene expression to mechanical mucus depletion [88].

Pulmonary Surfactant

Pulmonary surfactant, synthesized by type II alveolar cells and nonciliated epithelial cells (Clara cells), is a surface-active material that reduces the surface tension in the lungs. The main components of surfactant are phospholipids, neutral lipids, serum proteins, and surfactant proteins, including SP-A, SP-B, SP-C, and SP-D [159]. Surfactant proteins play integral roles in lowering surface tension and maintaining host defense [159]. SP-B and SP-C are hydrophobic proteins involved primarily in the adsorption and spreading of surfactant phospholipids at the air–liquid interface. SP-A (specific for mannose, glucose, galactose, and fucose) and SP-D (specific for maltose, mannose, and glucose) are hydrophilic proteins that act as the first line of host defense to inhaled pathogens. SP-A and SP-D are members of the collectin subgroup of mammalian C-type lectins that function in host immunity by binding carbohydrate ligands on the surface of invading particles, marking the complexes for destruction by alveolar macrophages [8,160,161]. SP-A stimulates the chemotaxis of alveolar macrophages and enhances their binding to viral and bacterial invaders [8,162]. SP-D binds to alveolar macrophages, polymorphonuclear cells, and various viral, fungal, and bacterial components, thereby playing a role in the regulation of inflammation [163]. As a result, surfactant proteins may reduce the efficiency of gene delivery when DNA vectors contain carbohydrate moieties [8]. For more information on the role of surfactants in the lung, see Refs. 159 and 164.

Alveolar Macrophages

Gene therapy targeted to the alveolar regions of the lung or to the systemic circulation via the alveoli may be limited by the actions of alveolar macrophages (AMφ). AMφ phagocytose and digest bacteria and other invaders, leading to cytokine secretion and inflammation [165,166]. The inhibitory effects of AMφ on transfection efficiencies with viral and liposomal gene vectors have been demonstrated [167,168]. Transfection efficiencies in gene therapy trials for cystic fibrosis have been dramatically reduced in comparison to in vitro studies [167]. The inflammatory response has been implicated as a potential reason for the reduced expression levels, with a 10-fold increase in the AMϕ population and a 1000-fold increase in the polymorphonuclear neutrophil population [167]. However, macrophages may also serve as potential targets of gene therapy. Cytokine gene therapy in the lung with interferon-γ (IFN-γ) increased AMϕ phagocytic and destructive capacity against bacteria, parasites, and fungi [166]. Murine studies have demonstrated that IFN-γ plays a key role in normal host defense from a number of pulmonary pathogens, including *Pseudomonas, Histoplasma, Candida, Mycoplasma, Hemophilus, Legionella, Chlamydia,* and *Pneumocytis* [166].

INTRACELLULAR BARRIERS TO GENE DELIVERY

DNA vectors that deposit in the appropriate lung region and successfully transverse the mucosal barrier encounter a new set of barriers at the cellular level (Fig. 6). Vectors must first gain access to the interior of target cells either nonspecifically, as in adsorptive endocytosis [49,85], or specifically, as in

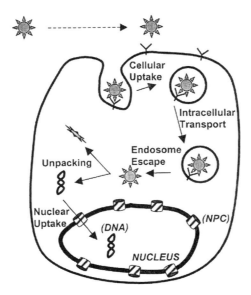

FIGURE 6 Intracellular barriers to gene delivery include cellular uptake, intracellular transport, endosome escape, vector unpacking, and nuclear uptake. The gene carrier illustrated here has targeting moieties on the vector surface that are specific for cell surface receptors. The dotted arrow represents the prerequisite step of bypassing physiological barriers of the lung, such as the mucosal layer, and reaching the target cell surface.

receptor-mediated endocytosis [86].They must subsequently break free of their endosomal compartments by physically disrupting the lipid bilayer that separates the DNA vectors from the cytoplasm [10,17,169]. Alternatively, vectors may induce a phenomenon termed the "proton-sponge effect," which indirectly disrupts endosomes due to osmotic forces [74]. A step in the intracellular DNA trafficking process that may precede or follow endosomal escape is transport to the perinuclear region [118]. DNA vectors must ultimately deliver their cargo into the nucleus, either by physically transporting DNA through the nuclear pore complex (NPC) or by releasing DNA at the door of the NPC, allowing free DNA to gain access. Finally, DNA must be available to the transcription machinery of the cell in order to synthesize the desired protein.

The need to overcome intracellular barriers may require improved methods of determining rate-limiting steps for specific gene carriers, which will lead to the rational design of new carriers. To this end, our lab uses multiple-particle tracking (MPT) to investigate quantitatively the motion of nanometer-sized DNA delivery vehicles [170].

Cellular Uptake

Adsorptive endocytosis is a common method of uptake for nonviral DNA vectors, as seen under in vitro conditions [49,85]. Unfortunately, this method only passively targets cells, resulting in gene carriers adsorbing onto cells with surface glycoproteins that provide proper adhesive environments [171,172]. Viral DNA vectors, on the other hand, enter cells specifically and efficiently through the use of receptor–ligand interactions [173]. To impart nonviral DNA vectors with cellular uptake capabilities similar to viruses, various ligands have been attached to the vector surface, both covalently and noncovalently [86]. Attached ligands bind to their complementary cell surface receptors, resulting in enhanced rates of uptake and improved target cell specificity [174]. Examples of ligands used for active targeting include transferrin [175,176], epidermal growth factor (EGF) [174], and the integrin-binding RGD sequences [177,178]. RGD peptides associated with cationic liposomes were used to transfer genes into human cystic fibrosis and noncystic fibrosis tracheal epithelial cells in vitro [179]. Use of the RGD sequence enhanced uptake via endocytosis and resulted in a 10-fold increase in gene expression.

The ability to modify the surface of gene carriers with relative ease is an advantage of nonviral systems. Viruses have a specific repertoire of surface receptors that may induce endocytosis [173], and it is not trivial to attach foreign ligands to viral gene carriers to modify their target cell specificity. Recently, however, bifunctional molecules that bind adenoviruses at one end and integrins at the other have been used to alter the specificity of the viruses [180].

Ligand attachment to DNA carriers may not only affect cellular uptake but may also have important implications on their intracellular trafficking [181]. Ligand choice should, therefore, consider intracellular trafficking in addition to target cell specificity and increased uptake.

High levels of intracellular DNA do not always correlate with high levels of protein production [182], suggesting that cellular uptake is not always a major bottleneck in gene delivery. However, this may be specific to cell and/or gene carrier type. For example, differentiated airway epithelial cells exhibited lower uptake than their poorly differentiated counterparts and, therefore, had lower expression of the cationic liposome-delivered gene [65]. Another study showed that adenovirus-mediated gene delivery into well-differentiated cultured airway epithelial cells was inefficient, due to a lack of adenovirus fiber-knob receptors and aVb3/5 integrins on the cells as well as to the low level of apical plasma membrane uptake [183]. Limited apical membrane uptake was also implicated as a potential explanation for low efficiencies in cationic lipid-mediated gene delivery to human primary cultures of ciliated airway epithelia [184].

Endosome Escape

DNA vectors entering the cell via endocytosis must escape the membrane-bound vesicle prior to gene uptake by the nucleus. Methods to enhance endosome escape often lead to significant improvements in transfection efficiency, thereby highlighting this barrier as one of the crucial bottlenecks in the gene delivery process for some cell type/gene carrier combinations. One method of endosome escape involves DNA vector fusion to the endosomal lipid bilayer, leading to the release of its cargo into the cytoplasm. This mechanism has been hypothesized for lipid-based delivery systems [185,186].

Another possible method of endosome escape is the "proton-sponge" hypothesis [74]. Nonviral DNA vectors that are able to accept protons at physiological pHs, such as polyethylenimine (PEI), act as a buffering agent within endosomes. As a result, more protons are pumped into the endosome, accompanied by an influx of chloride ions (to maintain the appropriate membrane potential) and water (due to osmotic pressure), which may lead to endosome rupture.

Lysosomotropic agents, such as chloroquine and sucrose, have been used to enhance DNA/vector release into the cytoplasm in vitro [187]. Viral DNA vectors have evolved the ability to escape acidified endosomes. To mimic this property, replication-defective adenoviruses were administered with transferrin-polylysine DNA vectors, resulting in greater gene expression [188,189]. More recently, endosomolytic structures have been attached to DNA vectors in lieu of using whole viruses. HA-2, the fusogenic peptide of the influenza virus hemagglutinin, has been used with transferrin-polylysine [190] and Lipo-fectamine® [191] to enhance the escape of these DNA vectors from endosomes. Similarly, melittin, the component in bee sting venom that destabilizes membranes, has been conjugated to PEI and shown to improve endosome escape [192].

Synthetic polymers, such as poly(propylacrylic acid), have also been designed with the ability to disrupt membranes [193–195]. These polymers are pH-sensitive and were designed to destabilize membranes when within acidic environments such as endosomes.

Transport to the Perinuclear Region

DNA transport to the nuclear region of the cell is poorly characterized [10,75] but is believed to involve movement through endosomes [49,85] and diffusion of vectors [75]. Gene carriers that escape endosomes may need to diffuse through the cytoplasm to reach the nucleus [75]. Diffusion of gene carriers through the cytoplasm has not yet been investigated; however, a study of the diffusion of naked DNA segments using fluorescence recovery after photobleaching (FRAP) demonstrated that the cytoplasm can be a critical barrier to nuclear gene delivery [196]. The involvement of cytoskeletal elements in the intracellular transport of gene carriers is highly probable [118], especially since transport of endosomes requires such structures. Intracellular transport of liposomes has been shown to involve microtubules [197], since microtubule depolymerization by nocodazole and stabilization by taxol both prevented perinuclear accumulation of the carriers. Our lab showed that PEI/DNA nanocomplexes also utilized microtubules for rapid transport to the perinuclear region in Cos-7 cells [118].

The method by which a DNA vector is trafficked intracellularly may have important implications on the efficiency of gene delivery. If DNA vectors are trafficked to sites far from the nucleus, gene delivery will be hindered by the diffusion-limited cytoplasm. PEI and polylysine are both cationic polymers with the ability to condense DNA; however, they have been shown to traffic to different intracellular destinations [198] and result in different transfection efficiencies [199]. In addition, particles of different chemistries were routed differently by the same cell type [200]. Understanding the intracytoplasmic transport of DNA vectors will be critical if higher-efficiency vectors are to be engineered.

Nuclear Uptake

Nuclear entry has been described as a formidable barrier to gene delivery [201–203]. Transport of DNA into this target organelle most likely involves the nuclear pore complex, which has an inner channel size of 9 nm, as determined by electron microscopy [204]. Molecules less than 40–45 kDa diffuse freely through the

NPC, but anything larger must have specific signals, such as nuclear localization sequences to facilitate transport [119].

Several attempts to improve nuclear uptake have been explored. The nuclear localization sequence (NLS) derived from the SV40 large-tumor antigen has been attached to a double-stranded DNA fragment, resulting in enhanced gene expression [205]. The NLSs are thought to enhance nuclear uptake via NPCs (see Ref. 119 for a comprehensive review of NLSs and the biology of NPCs). Adenovirus hexon proteins that mediate translocation of viral genes into the nucleus, through a mechanism separate from NLS-dependent pathways, have also been exploited. PEI/DNA complexes with covalently attached hexon proteins showed 10-fold increase in gene expression in HepG2 cells in vitro [206]. As an alternate approach, a dexamethasone–psoralen conjugate (DR9NP), a steroid derivative, has been complexed with DNA to enhance nuclear uptake [207]. Psoralen binds DNA, and dexamethasone (the steroid) binds its complementary cytoplasmic glucocorticoid receptor. Subsequent to receptor binding, the complex is transported into the nucleus. This novel method resulted in enhanced gene expression in both dividing and nondividing cells.

Gene delivery into mitotic cells is generally more efficient than in quiescent cells since the nuclear envelope breaks down in the dividing cells, allowing for foreign genes to gain nuclear access [208]. The mitotic activity of the target cells, therefore, may dictate the need for special methods to facilitate nuclear entry. Gene delivery to cells in the lung may involve both quiescent and mitotic cells since lung epithelial cells undergo mitosis periodically.

Transcription and Nuclear Persistence

Once DNA successfully enters the nucleus, the DNA carrier must unpack sufficiently for the desired protein to be transcribed and translated [209]. Premature release of DNA by the carrier may result in its degradation by enzymes in lysosomes and the cytoplasm [17]. Delayed unpacking, however, may prevent transcription [209]. For example, liposome unpacking prior to nuclear entry may be necessary for gene transcription, since microinjection of these gene carriers into the nucleus hindered gene expression [117]. PEI, however, did not prevent gene expression when PEI complexes were microinjected into the nucleus [117]. It is unclear at what point in the gene delivery process DNA must unpack from its vector. Schaffer et al. found that higher short-term gene expression resulted when lower-molecular-weight polylysine was used as a DNA vector [209]. Complexes using low-molecular-weight polylysine dissociated more readily from DNA than the longer polymer chains, hypothetically allowing the transcription machinery to have faster access. Whether the DNA vector unpacks the cargo DNA outside of the nucleus or enters the nucleus prior to unpacking may depend on the vector type [198] and may affect transfection outcome.

Our group [210] and others [211,212] have recently designed biodegradable gene-carrying polymers. Degradable cationic polymers condense DNA and subsequently release it at a predetermined rate, thereby increasing delivery of free DNA to or within the cell nucleus. This type of system may be especially important when vector unpacking is a rate-limiting step. Our group has recently discovered PEI/DNA complexes in the perinuclear region within minutes after they are added to cells [118]. This adds support to the hypothesis that DNA unpacking may be a major barrier to efficient transfection, at least with some cell type/gene carrier combinations.

Plasmid DNA delivered by nonviral vectors does not generally recombine with the host chromosome, limiting the danger of improper insertions [213]. However, the extrachromosomal plasmid DNA is often susceptible to intranuclear degradation over time [213], resulting in transient gene expression. Also, the transcription of genes delivered by certain viruses, such as retroviruses and adenoviruses, have been shown to be silenced through methylation [214]. The prevention of methylation with 5-azacytidine, an inhibitor of DNA methyltransferase, allowed for an extended period of gene expression [214]. The stability and persistence of the delivered gene will help determine the profile of protein production and ultimately the effectiveness of the gene therapy.

Steps taken to understand the intracellular barriers to gene delivery have led to the rational modification and improvement of carriers. Quantitative methods, such as multiple-particle tracking, to assess to the intracellular transport of gene carriers promise to add valuable insight that may ultimately lead to nonviral carriers rivaling the efficiencies seen in viral systems.

Multiple Particle Tracking (MPT)

After cellular uptake by endocytosis, the gene carrier must traverse the expansive and molecularly crowded cytoplasm to reach the nucleus. Unfortunately, the biophysical and biological mechanisms underlying the intracellular transport of gene carriers remain largely unknown, which limits our ability to make rational modifications to gene carriers for improved gene delivery. Nuclear translocation is a critical bottleneck in gene delivery [201–203]; however, it is unclear whether this limitation is owed to difficulty in gene carrier transport to the nucleus through the crowded cytoplasm, to the transport through the nuclear membrane, or to something else completely.

Quantitative investigations of the intracellular transport of synthetic gene carriers are currently undocumented. Confocal microscopy and electron microscopy (EM) have been used often to qualitatively study intracellular trafficking of nonviral systems [85,116,215–219], allowing the locations of complexes to be determined, over time. FRAP has recently been used to quantify overall rates of DNA molecules in the cytoplasm [196]. With these ensemble transport techniques, however, information such as the rates of individual particle movements, the mode of transport (such as random versus directed or active), and the trajectory and directionality of the transport remains elusive.

Using MPT [170], our group recently showed that the intracellular transport of PEI/DNA nanocomplexes involves active (i.e., nonrandom) transport to the perinuclear space of Cos-7 cells within 30 minutes [118]. The implication is that reaching the nucleus is not a rate-limiting step in PEI-mediated gene delivery, at least in Cos-7 cells. Comparison with other cell types and DNA vectors is currently under way to determine whether intracytoplasmic transport to the nucleus is a critical barrier to efficient gene delivery. Actively transported complexes moved several orders of magnitude faster [as measured by mean square displacement (MSD)] than complexes undergoing random thermal motion. For example, many actively transported complexes can travel $10\,\mu m$ in less than one minute, whereas the average diffusive PEI/DNA nanocomplex ($D_{ove} = 0.0008\,\mu m^2/s$), would take 8.7 h to travel the same $10\,\mu m$.

Actively transported PEI/DNA nanocomplexes exhibited an average velocity of $0.2\,\mu m/sec$ [118], a value on the same order of magnitude as motor-protein driven motion. Transport was revealed to be microtubule dependent, because both active transport and perinuclear accumulation were abolished upon microtubule depolymerization. Experiments utilizing MPT to quantify the other intracellular barriers to gene delivery are under way.

TARGETING LUNG REGIONS BY CONTROLLED AEROSOLIZATION OF PARTICLES

Efficient gene delivery by inhalation is significantly limited by the tortuous physiology of the lungs. Aerosolized droplets and particles inhaled into the lung deposit in various parts of the respiratory tract, dependent on their physical and chemical properties and the properties of the airstream in which they are entrained (Table 1). The lung itself, whether healthy or diseased, adult or child, may also affect deposition. Deposition occurs when a particle collides with the fluid lining of the respiratory tract. Targeting deposition to specific lung regions may increase the safety and efficiency of the DNA delivery system [5]. Once aerosol is deposited on the lung surface, the aerosol systems that can quickly traverse the mucus network and enter the cell nucleus are needed.

TABLE 1   Targeting Aerosols to the Lung Via Inhalation

Target region	Particle diameter range (μm)	Primary deposition mechanisms	Inhalation method	Potential target diseases for gene therapy
Extrathoracic	$d_a > 8$	Impaction	High inspiratory flow velocity	Cancer
Tracheobronchial	$d_a = 4-6$ (limited extra-thoracic deposition) $d_a = 6-8$ (some extrathoracic deposition)	Impaction and sedimentation	Slow inspiratory flowrate	CF, COPD, emphysema, cancer
Alveolar	$d_a = 2-5$	Sedimentation and diffusion	Slow inspiratory flowrate	Vaccines, cancer cytokine therapy (asthma, inflammation)
			High tidal volume Breath holding 2-6 sec	
	$d_a = 0.02-0.05$	Diffusion		

Aerosol Deposition

Three primary mechanisms govern the deposition of aerosols in the respiratory tract: inertial impaction, sedimentation, and diffusion (Fig. 7). Early work by Landahl and coworkers showed that both sedimentation and inertial impaction in the mouth, throat, and lungs uniquely depend on the particle aerodynamic diameter [220]. Deposition by diffusional transport is independent of particle density and limited primarily to particles with geometric diameters smaller than 0.5 μm [221].

Aerodynamic diameter is the key parameter used to determine the expected depth a particle ($d > 0.5\,\mu$m) will travel into the lung prior to deposition.

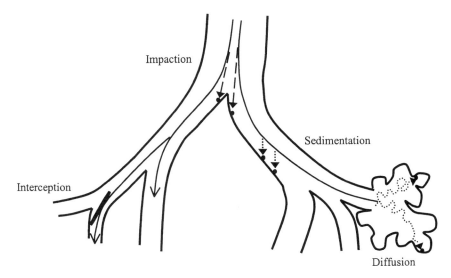

Interception

FIGURE 7   Primary deposition mechanisms of inhaled particles in the respiratory tract.

The quantitative relationship for the aerodynamic diameter (d_a) of a particle is [222]:

$$d_a = \frac{d\sqrt{\frac{\rho}{\rho_a}}}{\gamma} \tag{2}$$

where d = geometric diameter, ρ = particle bulk density (g/cm^3), ρ_a = water mass density (1 g/cm^3), and γ = shape factor = 1 for a sphere. Therefore, an aerosolized particle with a geometric diameter of 1 μm and a density of 1 g/cm^3 will deposit in the respiratory tract in the same manner as a 10-μm particle with a density of 0.01 g/cm^3.

Particles with aerodynamic diameters between 0.02–0.05 μm and 2–5 μm that are inhaled via the mouth are capable of efficient alveolar deposition [221,223–226] (Fig. 8). Aerodynamic diameters of 1–3 μm are appropriate for particle deposition in the alveolar region when the particles are inhaled via the nose [227]. Aerodynamic diameters between 4 and 10 μm are appropriate for deposition in the bronchial region. Finally, particles of aerodynamic diameter larger than 8 μm deposit primarily in the upper airways or mouth and throat (extrathoracic region), while a significant percentage of those less than 1 μm are exhaled [228]. Due to this region-specific deposition, particles can be targeted to various areas in the lung by engineering particle aerodynamic diameter. For example, particles with an aerodynamic diameter of approximately 4–10 μm

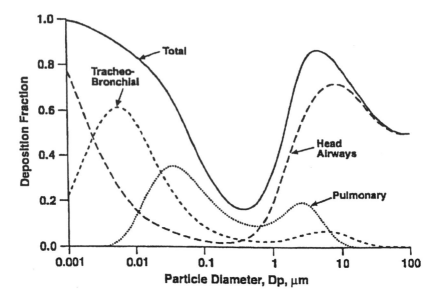

FIGURE 8 Particle deposition in the human respiratory tract as a function of particle aerodynamic diameter. (Reprinted from Ref. 226. Courtesy of Medical Physics Publishing.)

may be used as therapeutic vectors for bronchial delivery to treat lung disorders such as cystic fibrosis [229–231].

A particle's shape can have a significant effect on its deposition in the airways. For example, the aerodynamic diameter of a rod-shaped particle is roughly 2–3 times that of a spherical particle with a diameter equal to the width of the rod (independent of rod length) [232,233]. Therefore, long fibers with small diameters can deposit well in the deep lung [234,235]. Deposition of rod-shaped particles often results from another mechanism called interception (235–237). Interception occurs when a particle's center of mass follows an airstream in the lung but the particle still impacts a wall owing to its elongated shape. Deposition by interception is especially important in small airways, where the dimensions of the airspace are comparable to the lengths of the rods [236].

Inertial Impaction

Deposition by inertial impaction occurs when particles of sufficient momentum cannot follow the abrupt directional changes in the airways. The particles instead follow their original direction, causing them to impact the airway walls when the air ducts change direction. The probability that a particle of diameter d and density ρ will diverge from an airstream of velocity u is characterized by the Stokes number [238]:

$$\mathrm{Stk} = \frac{\rho d^2 u}{18\eta G} = \frac{d_a^2 u}{18\eta G} \tag{3}$$

where η is the fluid viscosity and G is a constant that characterizes the geometry of the structure in which the particles are traveling. Therefore, deposition by impaction increases in proportion to $(d_a^2 u)$. Inertial impaction is most significant for particles with large mass (determined by particle size and density) and/or velocity (determined by the respiratory flow velocity). Inertial impaction occurs mostly in the upper lung regions, since flowrates are high and changes in flow direction occur abruptly. Forced breathing increases particle velocity, thereby shifting particle deposition patterns towards the upper airways.

Sedimentation Due to Gravity

Sedimentation occurs when particles of sufficient mass are acted on by gravity. The settling velocity of a particle due to gravity is determined by Stokes' Law [232,239]:

$$v = \frac{\rho d^2 g C_s}{18\eta\gamma} = \frac{d_a g C_s}{18\eta} \tag{4}$$

where ρ and d are the particle density and diameter, respectively, g is the gravitational constant, η is the fluid viscosity, and C_s is the slip correction factor that corrects Stokes' Law for the assumption that the air velocity at the particle surface is zero (which does not hold for particles smaller than 10 μm) [222]. The probability of gravitational deposition is proportional to the particle settling distance and, therefore, increases in proportion to $(t * d_a^2)$. Deposition owing to gravitational settling is significant for particles with aerodynamic diameters larger than 0.5 μm [221] and occurs primarily in the lower bronchial and alveolar regions, due to the significantly decreased velocities compared to the upper airways. Long residence times within the airways and low air velocities—for example, during breath holding—increase particle deposition by sedimentation.

Diffusion

Deposition by random diffusion occurs as a consequence of thermally driven Brownian motion. The root mean square displacement (Δ) of a particle moving by diffusion is given by [240]:

$$\Delta = \sqrt{4 D_p t} \tag{5}$$

where D_p is its diffusivity and t is the residence time of the particle in the lung. For a particle with diameter d in a fluid of viscosity η, D_p is given by the Stokes–

Einstein equation:

$$D_p = \frac{\kappa T C_s}{3 \pi \eta d} \tag{6}$$

where κ is the Boltzmann constant, T is the absolute temperature, and C_s is the slip correction factor. Combining Eqs. (5) and (6), one finds diffusional transport is proportional to $(t/d)^{0.5}$, where t is the residence time of the particle in the lung and d is the geometric diameter of the particle. Note that diffusional transport is independent of particle density, such that aerodynamic diameter is not a significant parameter in deposition by diffusion. Therefore, increasing particle residence time and decreasing geometric size increases the probability that a particle will deposit by diffusional transport. However, diffusion is only an effective deposition mechanism for submicrometer-sized particles ($<0.5\,\mu m$) [221]. Additionally, low flowrates are necessary for diffusion to be significant; therefore, deposition by diffusion occurs mainly in the alveolar region of the lung, where velocities are typically on the order of 0–0.3 cm/sec (compared, for example, to velocities of 390 cm/sec in the trachea. 52–430 cm/sec in the bronchi, and 1.9–14 cm/sec in the bronchioles at a flowrate of 60 L/sec) [241]. Increasing tidal volume (at a given flowrate) and/or breath holding both increase the residence time of particles within the smaller airways, thus increasing diffusional deposition [242–244].

Effect of Airway Disease on Deposition

Deposition patterns within the lung are influenced by individual differences in anatomy as well as different patient inhalation techniques. To deposit in the lungs, particles must traverse a complex lung structure that varies in geometry and environment from patient to patient. Partial obstructions and irregularities of the airway surface disrupt deposition and create uneven particle distributions in the lung [245,246]. Lung morphology can be complicated further by airway obstruction, infection, and/or inflammation caused by diseased states such as cystic fibrosis and chronic obstructive pulmonary disease [247–250]. In such cases, deposition patterns are often shifted, with enhanced deposition in the central airways and reduced deposition in the alveolar region [251–254].

Aerosol Aggregation Phenomena

Aggregation of aerosol particles can have detrimental effects on their predicted deposition pattern in the lung, since aggregates will deposit in the lungs as if they had the aerodynamic diameter of a larger particle. Therefore, proper deaggregation of particles is important for predictable and reproducible deposition within the respiratory tract.

Whether in a dry state or suspended in a liquid, particles can aggregate significantly. Surface free energy is the driving force for particle aggregation [255]. The extent of aggregation can be controlled by altering particle physical and chemical characteristics or by addition of excipients [256–258]. We give a brief overview of particle aggregation/deaggregation phenomena below (see Refs. 259 and 260 for more extensive discussions).

Adhesion Forces

Three primary adhesive forces are responsible for the aggregation of aerosols: van der Waals, electrostatic, and capillary [232,261] (Fig. 9). For dry powders, all three forces may play important roles. Interactions between particles in suspension include only van der Waals and electrostatic forces.

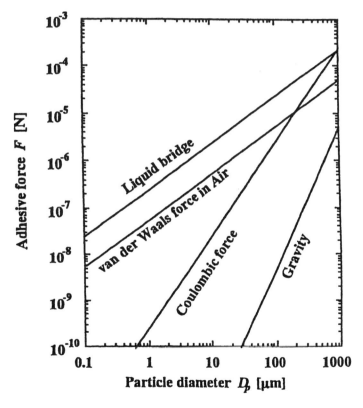

FIGURE 9 Comparison of primary adhesion forces between aerosol particles. (Reprinted from Ref. 261. Courtesy of Marcel Dekker, Inc.).

The van der Waals (VDW) attractive forces are the principal forces between dry, noncharged spherical aerosol particles [262] and may reduce stability and cause flocculation of suspended particles. The VDW forces arise from the attractive forces between permanent dipoles (Keesom forces), induced dipoles (London forces), and dipole-induced dipoles (Debye forces). For nonpolar or slightly polar compounds, the force of attraction between two particles with diameter d separated by a distance h (where $h < d$) is:

$$F_{VDW} = \frac{Ad}{24h^2} \tag{7}$$

where the Hamaker constant, A, is dependent on the particle surface chemistry and surface roughness, the fluid surrounding the particles, and the separation distance between the particle surfaces [263,264].

Two types of electrostatic forces are important for small particles: the electrostatic image (coulomb) force and the electric double-layer force. Electrostatic forces can accumulate during particle formulation and/or use in an inhaler [265]. However, it has been shown that electrostatic forces do not play an important role in the adhesion of dry uncharged particles, since VDW forces dominate [266]. In addition, large nonequilibrium charges on dry particles are necessary for electrostatic forces to become significant. Suspended particles can acquire a surface charge by interactions with molecules such as surfactants, the suspending liquid, and water.

Coulomb forces result from the interaction between a charged surface and another charged or neutral surface. These forces can be attractive or repulsive, depending on the charge of each surface, and are relevant for particles with diameters larger than 5 µm [267]. For two-point electric charges separated by a distance h, Coulomb's Law gives:

$$F_{coulomb} = \frac{q_1 q_2}{4\pi\varepsilon_0 h^2} \tag{8}$$

where q_1 and q_2 are the electric charges on the particles and ϵ_0 is the dielectric constant of the medium. For particles in contact, with $h \ll d$:

$$F_{coulomb} = \pi \frac{\sigma_1 \sigma_2}{4\varepsilon_0} d^2 \tag{9}$$

where σ_1 and σ_2 are the surface charge densities of the particles and d is the diameter of the particles.

Electric double-layer forces result from the contact between two compounds of different contact potential. In a dry environment, electric double-layer forces are only significant for particles less than 5 µm in diameter [267]. Lewis acid–base interactions, determined by the chemical composition of the surface, may be used to alter the adhesion of particles. However, if capillary bridges are present between the particles in a dry environment, electric forces cannot develop [268]. For particles in suspension, the electric double layer forms when counterions in the solution balance the charge on the particle surface. The resultant forces are important for the stability of colloidal systems [255]. Two similarly charged surfaces will repel each other unless the distance between the surfaces is decreased to a critical distance, whereupon the surfaces will become adherent [255].

Capillary forces develop when liquid bridges are formed in small gaps between two surfaces. Above a critical relative humidity, capillary forces are the dominant attractive force between aerosol particles [269,270]. The magnitude of this force depends on other parameters as well, such as particle surface chemistry and size. For two particles attached by a liquid bridge, the adhesive force is [260]:

$$F_{cap} \approx 2\pi R \gamma_L \tag{10}$$

where R is the radius of the particles and γ_L is the liquid surface tension.

Designing Aerosols for Improved Dispersion

Atomization. The main mechanism used for deaggregation of aerosol particles is the atomization process. Various mechanisms, such as a turbulent airstream and ultrasonication, are used in inhaler devices to separate dry particles or create fine liquid droplets. Methods of aerosol generation and the characterization of the various inhalers are available elsewhere [264].

Inhalation Flowrate. Particles that do not deaggregate upon atomization must separate within the oropharyngeal cavity to avoid excessive deposition in the mouth and throat. Increasing inspiratory flowrate can significantly help separate aggregated particles. By numerical simulation, Li et al. determined that dry particles less than 10 μm in diameter have little chance of deaggregation in the mouth and throat at flowrates of 30 L/min or less [52]. Flow rates of 60 L/min or higher were necessary for these particles to separate and may be required for particles to deposit in the deep lung [271]. Their results were consistent with the high flowrates needed for proper function of dry powder inhalers [272].

Physical Properties of Aerosols. Physical properties of aerosols, including size, shape, and surface roughness, are important factors in determining aerosol deaggregation [273]. Traditionally, aerosols under investigation for therapeutic purposes were small, dense particles or droplets. However, large, low-density particles with aerodynamic diameters between 2 and 5 μm have more recently shown considerable potential for alveolar deposition and systemic delivery [263,274]. Particle aggregation due to van der Waals forces is greatly reduced with larger particles, resulting in an increase in aerosolization efficiency [275]. The number of contact points between particles per unit volume is smaller for larger particles, thus decreasing the net interparticle force. Similarly, hollow, porous particles dispersed in a propellant (for use in a metered-dose inhaler) possessed decreased interparticle attractive forces, which improved their delivery efficiency to the lung [276,277].

Particles that are elongated or have flat edges tend to align along their long axis, thereby increasing their contact area and adhesive force [278]. Similarly, irregularly shaped particles typically have a decrease in adhesion force due to a reduction in their contact area [268]. A rough surface tends to decrease the force of adhesion in the absence of capillary forces, due to a reduced area of surface contact [279–281]. However, if surface asperities become too large, interparticle adhesion may increase, owing to an increase in surface contact area as smaller particles nest within the asperities [268].

Chemical Properties of Aerosols. Surface chemical properties of aerosol particles can also be tailored to improve deaggregation [273]. Hygroscopic particles absorb water when inhaled into the humid airways [282–284], increasing particle size and density in the process, as well as creating the potential for capillary bridge formation between particles. Hygroscopic growth can be reduced by the use of hydrophobic additives [285] or compounds with low aqueous solubility [286,287].

The adsorption or incorporation of molecules, such as surfactants and polymers, can create a steric repulsion that prevents aggregation [288–290]. This can also increase suspension stability, important for metered-dose inhaler formulations [291]. Lung surfactant coating on the surface of poly(lactic-*co*-glycolic) acid microparticles has been shown to dramatically improve dry powder aerosol performance by reducing particle–particle interactions [134,292].

New Polymers for Controlled Delivery Via the Lung. New materials can be created to tailor particle surface properties. In addition, producing materials that can achieve sustained release is important in gene therapy, since gene expression is often inadequately brief [213]. Toward this end, we have recently synthesized a new family of biodegradable poly(ether-anhydrides) composed of monomers with FDA approval for other uses: 1,3-bis(carboxyphenoxy)propane (CPP), sebacic acid (SA), and poly(ethylene glycol) (PEG) [229,293]. Sebacic acid is a flexible monomer that allows polymerization of high-molecular-weight polymers and imparts improved solubility and mechanical strength to the polymers; CPP is a hydrophobic monomer, which adds control over degradation time scales of the polymer (higher amounts of CPP in the polymer led to longer release times); PEG allows control of the hydrophilicity of polymer particulates, which in turn significantly improves particle aerosolization efficiency by decreasing aggregation due to VDW forces [262]. PEG may also create a steric repulsion that does not allow particles to come into direct contact, thereby reducing adhesion forces. The new polymers were used to encapsulate plasmid DNA into exceptionally large (~ 5–$15\,\mu m$) and light ($<0.4\,g/cm^3$)

aerosol carriers for controlled delivery to the lung [293]. Particles were made with aerodynamic diameters appropriate for targeted delivery to either the upper airways or the deep lung. By changing the ratio of monomers in backbone, we were able to control the degradation and erosion of the polymer, thereby controlling the release of DNA for up to one week in a continuous fashion.

In a related study, PEI was used to complex *LacZ* plasmid DNA and the resulting complexes were encapsulated within porous polymeric microparticles with properties suitable for efficient inhalation [294]. Microparticle sizes were between 1 and 10 μm, but their density was much lower, leading to aerodynamic diameters in the range appropriate for delivery to the lung. Time-resolved multiangle laser light scattering (TR-MALLS) was used to show that 150 nm PEI/DNA complexes were encapsulated and subsequently released for more than 75 days in vitro. Released complexes were capable of transfection over the entire period of release in both HeLa and Cos-7 cells. The longest previous release of active DNA from biodegradable microparticles was only 21 days and used naked DNA.

REFERENCES

1. Patapoff TW, Gonda I. Inhalation delivery and formulation issues in gene therapy in the respiratory tract. In Inhalation Delivery of Therapeutic Peptides and Proteins; Adjei AL, Gupta PK, eds. Marcel Dekker: New York, 1997; 493–514.

2. http://www.wiley.com/genetherapy/clinical/index.html (The Journal of Gene Medicine), 2001.

3. Stewart MJ, Plautz GE, Del Buono L, Yang ZY, Xu L, Gao X, Huang L, Nabel EG, Nabel GJ. Gene transfer in vivo with DNA–liposome complexes: safety and acute toxicity in mice. Hum Gene Ther 1992, 3, 267–275.

4. Zhu N, Liggitt D, Liu Y, Debs R. Systemic gene expression after intravenous DNA delivery into adult mice. Science 1993, 261, 209–211.

5. Thompson MM, Weiner-Kronish JP. General issues in gene delivery via the lung. In Inhalation Delivery of Therapeutic Peptides and Proteins; Adjei AL, Gupta PK, eds. Marcel Dekker: New York, 1997; 475–491.

6. Driscoll KE, Costa DL, Hatch G, Henderson R, Oberdorster G, Salem H, Schlesinger RB. Intratracheal instillation as an technique for the evaluation of respiratory tract toxicity: uses and limitations. Toxicol Sci 2000, 55, 24–35.

7. Suzuki M, Matsuse T, Isigatsubo Y. Gene therapy for lung diseases: development in the vector biology and novel concepts for gene therapy applications. Curr Mol Med 2001, 1, 67–79.

8. Vadolas J, Williamson P, Ioannou P. Gene therapy for inherited lung disorders: an insight into pulmonary defense. Pulmon Pharmacol Ther 2002, 15, 61–72.

9. Albelda SM, Wiewrodt R, Zuckerman JB. Gene therapy for lung disease: hype or hope? Ann Intern Med 2000, 132, 649–660.

10. Pouton CW, Seymour LW. Key issues in non-viral gene delivery. Adv Drug Deliv Rev 2001, 46, 187–203.
11. Garcia-Contreras L, Hickey AJ. Pharmaceutical and biotechnological aerosols for cystic fibrosis therapy. Adv Drug Deliv Rev 2002, 54, 1491-1509.
12. Flotte TR, Laube BL. Gene therapy in cystic fibrosis. Chest 2001, 120, 124S–131S.
13. Rolland AP. From genes to gene medicines: recent advances in nonviral gene delivery. Crit Rev Ther Drug Carrier Syst 1998, 15, 143–198.
14. Anwer K, Bailey A, Sullivan SM. Targeted gene delivery: a two-pronged approach. Crit Rev Ther Drug Carrier Syst 2000, 17, 377–424.
15. Felgner JH, Kumar R, Sridhar CN, Wheeler CJ, Tsai YJ, Border R, Ramsey P, Martin M, Felgner PL. Enhanced gene delivery and mechanism studies with a novel series of cationic lipid formulations. J Biol Chem 1994, 269, 2550–2561.
16. Tomlinson E, Rolland AP. Controllable gene therapy: pharmaceutics of non-viral gene delivery systems. J Control Release 1996, 39, 357–372.
17. Luo D, Saltzman WM. Synthetic DNA delivery systems. Nat Biotechnol 2000, 18, 33–37.
18. Micheal SI, Curiel DT. Strategies to achieve targeted gene delivery via the receptor-mediated endocytosis pathway. Gene Ther 1994, 1, 223–232.
19. Vyas SP, Singh A, Sihorkar V. Ligand-receptor-mediated drug delivery: an emerging paradigm in cellular drug targeting. Crit Rev Ther Drug Carrier Syst 2001, 18, 1–76.
20. Crystal RG, McElvaney NG, Rosenfeld MA, Chu CS, Mastrangeli A, Hay JG, Brody SL, Jaffe HA, Eissa NT, Danel C. Administration of an adenovirus containing the human CFTR cDNA to the respiratory tract of individuals with cystic fibrosis. Nat Genet 1994, 8, 42–51.
21. Engelhardt JF, Ye X, Doranz B, Wilson JM. Ablation of E2A in recombinant adenoviruses improves transgene persistence and decreases inflammatory response in mouse liver. Proc Natl Acad Sci USA 1994, 91, 6196–6200.
22. Yang Y, Nunes FA, Berencsi K, Furth EE, Gonczol E, Wilson JM. Cellular immunity to viral antigens limits E1-deleted adenoviruses for gene therapy. Proc Natl Acad Sci USA 1994, 91, 4407–4411.
23. Yei S, Mittereder N, Wert S, Whitsett JA, Wilmott RW, Trapnell BC. In vivo evaluation of the safety of adenovirus-mediated transfer of the human cystic fibrosis transmembrane conductance regulator cDNA to the lung. Hum Gene Ther 1994, 5, 731–744.
24. Yei S, Mittereder N, Tang K, O'Sullivan C, Trapnell BC. Adenovirus-mediated gene transfer for cystic fibrosis: quantitative evaluation of repeated in vivo vector administration to the lung. Gene Ther 1994, 1, 192–200.
25. Yang Y, Li Q, Ertl HC, Wilson JM. Cellular and humoral immune responses to viral antigens create barriers to lung-directed gene therapy with recombinant adenoviruses. J Virol 1995, 69, 2004–2015.
26. Hollon T. Researchers and regulators reflect on first gene therapy death. Nat Med 2000, 6, 6.

27. Crystal RG. Gene therapy strategies for pulmonary disease. Am J Med 1992, 92, 44S–52S.

28. Johnson LG, Boucher RC. Gene therapy for lung disease. In Inhalation Delivery of Therapeutic Peptides and Proteins; Adjei AL, Gupta PK, eds. Marcel Dekker: New York, 1997; 515–553.

29. Mastrangeli A, Danel C, Rosenfeld MA, Stratford-Perricaudet L, Perricaudet M, Pavirani A, Lecocq JP, Crystal RG. Diversity of airway epithelial cell targets for in vivo recombinant adenovirus-mediated gene transfer. J Clin Invest 1993, 91, 225–234.

30. Weitzman MD, Kyostio SR, Kotin RM, Owens RA. Adeno-associated virus (AAV) Rep proteins mediate complex formation between AAV DNA and its integration site in human DNA. Proc Natl Acad Sci USA 1994, 91, 5808–5812.

31. Sun L, Li J, Xiao X. Overcoming adeno-associated virus vector size limitation through viral DNA heterodimerization. Nat Med 2000, 6, 599–602.

32. Yan Z, Zhang Y, Duan D, Engelhardt JF. Trans-splicing vectors expand the utility of adeno-associated virus for gene therapy. Proc Natl Acad Sci USA 2000, 97, 6716–6721.

33. Duan D, Yue Y, Yan Z, Engelhardt JF. A new dual-vector approach to enhance recombinant adeno-associated virus-mediated gene expression through intermolecular cis activation. Nat Med 2000, 6, 595–598.

34. Duan D, Yue Y, Engelhardt JF. Expanding AAV packaging capacity with trans-splicing or overlapping vectors: a quantitative comparison. Mol Ther 2001, 4, 383–391.

35. Crook K, McLachlan G, Stevenson BJ, Porteous DJ. Plasmid DNA molecules complexed with cationic liposomes are protected from degradation by nucleases and shearing by aerosolisation. Gene Ther 1996, 3, 834–839.

36. Eastman SJ, Tousignant JD, Lukason MJ, Murray H, Siegel CS, Constantino P, Harris DJ, Cheng SH, Schedule RK. Optimization of formulations and conditions for the aerosol delivery of functional cationic lipid, DNA complexes. Hum Gene Ther 1997, 8, 313–322.

37. Eastman SJ, Lukason MJ, Tousignant JD, Murray H, Lane MD, St George JA, Akita GY, Cherry M, Cheng SH, Scheule RK. A concentrated and stable aerosol formulation of cationic lipid. DNA complexes giving high-level gene expression in mouse lung. Hum Gene Ther 1997, 8, 765–773.

38. Eastman SJ, Tousignant JD, Lukason MJ, Chu Q, Cheng SH, Scheule RK. Aerosolization of cationic lipid. pDNA complexes–in vitro optimization of nebulizer parameters for human clinical studies. Hum Gene Ther 1998, 9, 43–52.

39. Friedmann T. The Development of Human Gene Therapy; Cold Spring Harbor Laboratory Press: Cold Spring Harbor, NY, 1999.

40. Mizuguchi H, Kay MA, Hayakawa T. Approaches for generating recombinant adenovirus vectors. Adv Drug Deliv Rev 2001, 52, 165–176.

41. Burton EA, Bai Q, Goins WF, Glorioso JC. Targeting gene expression using HSV vectors. Adv Drug Deliv Rev 2001, 53, 155–170.

42. Rojanasakul Y, Wang LY, Malanga CJ, Ma JK, Liaw J. Targeted gene delivery to alveolar macrophages via Fc receptor-mediated endocytosis. Pharm Res 1994, 11, 1731–1736.

43. Pedroso de Lima MC, Simoes S, Pires P, Faneca H, Duzgunes N. Cationic lipid-DNA complexes in gene delivery: from biophysics to biological applications. Adv Drug Deliv Rev 2001, 47, 277–294.

44. Felgner PL, Gadek TR, Holm M, Roman R, Chan HW, Wenz M, Northrop JP, Ringold GM, Danielsen M. Lipofection: a highly efficient, lipid-mediated DNA-transfection procedure. Proc Natl Acad Sci USA 1987, 84, 7413–7417.

45. Stribling R, Brunette E, Liggitt D, Gaensler K, Debs R. Aerosol gene delivery in vivo. Proc Natl Acad Sci USA 1992, 89, 11277–11281.

46. Logan JJ, Bebok Z, Walker LC, Peng S, Felgner PL, Siegal GP, Frizzell RA, Dong J, Howard M, Matalon ?, et al. Cationic lipids for reporter gene and CFTR transfer to rat pulmonary epithelium. Gene Ther 1995, 2, 38–49.

47. Yoshimura K, Rosenfeld MA, Nakamura H, Scherer EM, Pavirani A, Lecocq JP, Crystal RG. Expression of the human cystic fibrosis transmembrane conductance regulator gene in the mouse lung after in vivo intratracheal plasmid-mediated gene transfer. Nucleic Acids Res 1992, 20, 3233–3240.

48. Cangrico AE, Conary JT, Meyrick BO, Brigham RL. Aerosol and intravenous transfection of human alpha, L-antitryp gene to lungs of rabbits. Am J Respir Cell Mol Biol 1994, 19, 24–29.

49. Zabner J, Fasbender AJ, Moninger T, Poellinger KA, Welsh MJ. Cellular and molecular barriers to gene transfer by a cationic lipid. J Biol Chem 1995, 270, 18997–19007.

50. Balasubramaniam RP, Bennett MJ, Aberle AM, Malone JG, Nantz MH, Malone RW. Structural and functional analysis of cationic transfection lipids: the hydrophobic domain. Gene Ther 1996, 3, 163–172.

51. Li S, Huang L. In vivo gene transfer via intravenous administration of cationic lipid–protamine–DNA (LPD) complexes. Gene Ther 1997, 4, 891–900.

52. Li WI, Edwards DA. Aerosol particle transport and deaggregation phenomena in the mouth and throat. Adv Drug Deliv Rev 1997, 26, 41–49.

53. Liu Y, Mounkes LC, Liggitt HD, Brown CS, Solodin I, Health TD, Debs RJ. Factors influencing the efficiency of cationic liposome-mediated intravenous gene delivery. Nat Biotechnol 1997, 15, 167–173.

54. Yew NS, Wang KX, Przybylska M, Bagley RG, Stedman M, Marshall J, Scheule RK, Cheng SH. Contribution of plasmid DNA to inflammation in the lung after administration of cationic lipid:pDNA complexes. Hum Gene Ther 1999, 10, 223–234.

55. Marshall J, Nietupski JB, Lee ER, Siegel CS, Rafter PW, Rudginsky SA, Chang CD, Eastman SJ, Harris DJ, Scheule RK, Cheng SH. Cationic lipid structure and formulation considerations for optimal gene transfection of the lung. J Drug Target 2000, 7, 453–469.

56. Meyer KB, Thompson MM, Levy MY, Barron LG, Szoka FC. Intratracheal gene delivery to the mouse airway: characterization of plasmid DNA expression and pharmacokinetics. Gene Ther 1995, 2, 450–460.

57. Alton NFW, Middleton PG, Caplen NJ, Smith SN, Steel DM, Munkonge FM, Jeffery PK, Geddes DM, Hart SL, Williamson R, Fasold KI, Miller AD, Dickinson P, Stevenson BJ, Molachlan G, Dorin JR, Porteous DJ. Noninvasive liposome-mediated gene delivery can correct the ion transport defect in cystic fibrosis mutant mice. Nat Genet 1993, 5, 135–142.

58. Alton EW, Stern M, Farley R, Jaffe A, Chadwick SL, Phillips J, Davies J, Smith SN, Browning J, Davies MG, Hodson ME, Durham SR, Li D, Jeffery PK, Scallan M, Balfour R, Eastman SJ, Cheng SH, Smith AE, Meeker D, Geddes DM. Cationic lipid-mediated CFTR gene transfer to the lungs and nose of patients with cystic fibrosis: a double-blind placebo-controlled trial. Lancet 1999, 353, 947–954.

59. Bragonzi A, Boletta A, Biffi A, Muggia A, Sersale G, Cheng SH, Bordignon C, Assael BM, Conese M. Comparison between cationic polymers and lipids in mediating systemic gene delivery to the lungs. Gene Ther 1999, 6, 1995–2004.

60. Felgner PL, Tsai YJ, Sukhu L, Wheeler CJ, Manthorpe M, Marshall J, Cheng SH. Improved cationic lipid formulations for in vivo gene therapy. Ann NY Acad Sci 1995, 772, 126–139.

61. Scheule RK, St George JA, Bagley RG, Marshall J, Kaplan JM, Akita GY, Wang KX, Lee ER, Harris DJ, Jiang C, Yew NS, Smith AE, Cheng SH. Basis of pulmonary toxicity associated with cationic lipid-mediated gene transfer to the mammalian lung. Hum Gene Ther 1997, 8, 689–707.

62. Harvie P, Wong FM, Bally MB. Characterization of lipid DNA interactions. I. Destabilization of bound lipids and DNA dissociation. Biophys J 1998, 75, 1040–1051.

63. Farhood H, Serbina N, Huang L. The role of dioleoyl phosphatidylethanolamine in cationic liposome mediated gene transfer. Biochim Biophys Acta 1995, 1235, 289–295.

64. Friend DS, Papahadjopoulos D, Debs RJ. Endocytosis and intracellular processing accompanying transfection mediated by cationic liposomes. Biochim Biophys Acta 1996, 1278, 41–50.

65. Matsui H, Johnson LG, Randell SH, Boucher RC. Loss of binding and entry of liposome–DNA complexes decreases transfection efficiency in differentiated airway epithelial cells. J Biol Chem 1997, 272, 1117–1126.

66. Xu Y, Szoka FC, Jr. Mechanism of DNA release from cationic liposome/DNA complexes used in cell transfection. Biochemistry 1996, 35, 5616–5623.

67. Xu Y, Hui SW, Frederik P, Szoka FC, Jr. Physiochemical characterization and purification of cationic lipoplexes. Biophys J 1999, 77, 341–353.

68. Lee LK, Mount CN, Shamlou PA. Characterization of the physical stability of colloidal polycation–DNA complexes for gene therapy and DNA vaccines. Chem Eng Sci 2001, 56, 3263–3272.

69. Sanders NN, De Smedt SC, Cheng SH, Demeester J. Pegylated GL67 lipoplexes retain their gene transfection activity after exposure to components of CF mucus. Gene Ther 2002, 9, 363–371.

70. Safinya CR. Structures of lipid–DNA complexes: supramolecular assembly and gene delivery. Curr Opin Struct Biol 2001, 11, 440–448.

71. Cheng SH, Scheule RK. Airway delivery of cationic lipid:DNA complexes for cystic fibrosis. Adv Drug Deliv Rev 1998, 30, 173–184.

72. Kwoh DY, Coffin CC, Lollo CP, Jovenal J, Banaszczyk MG, Mullen P, Phillips A, Amini A, Fabrycki J, Bartholomew RM, Brostoff SW, Carlo DJ. Stabilization of poly-L-lysine/DNA polyplexes for in vivo gene delivery to the liver. Biochim Biophys Acta 1999, 1444, 171–190.

73. Wagner E, Ogris M, Zauner W. Polylysine-based transfection systems utilizing receptor-mediated delivery. Adv Drug Deliv Rev 1998, 30, 97–113.

74. Boussif O, Lezoualc'h F, Zanta MA, Mergny MD, Scherman D, Demeneix B, Behr JP. A versatile vector for gene and oligonucleotide transfer into cells in culture and in vivo: polyethylenimine. Proc Natl Acad Sci USA 1995, 92, 7297–7301.

75. Kircheis R, Wightman L, Wagner E. Design and gene delivery activity of modified polyethylenimines. Adv Drug Deliv Rev 2001, 53, 341–358.

76. Demeneix B, Behr J, Boussif O, Zanta MA, Abdallah B, Remy J. Gene transfer with lipospermines and polyethylenimines. Adv Drug Deliv Rev 1998, 30, 85–95.

77. von Harpe A, Petersen H, Li Y, Kissel T. Characterization of commercially available and synthesized polyethylenimines for gene delivery. J Control Release 2000, 69, 309–322.

78. Cherng JY, van de Wetering P, Talsma H, Crommelin DJ, Hennink WE. Effect of size and serum proteins on transfection efficiency of poly ((2-dimethylamino)ethyl methacrylate)-plasmid nanoparticles. Pharm Res 1996, 13, 1038–1042.

79. van de Wetering P, Cherng JY, Talsma H, Crommelin DJ, Hennink WE. 2-(Dimethyllamino)ethyl methacrylate–based (co)polymers as gene transfer agents. J Control Release 1998, 53, 145–153.

80. Jones NA, Hill IR, Stolnik S, Bignotti F, Davis SS, Garnett MC. Polymer chemical structure is a key determinant of physicochemical and colloidal properties of polymer–DNA complexes for gene delivery. Biochim Biophys Acta 2000, 1517, 1–18.

81. Haensler J, Szoka FC, Jr. Polyamidoamine cascade polymers mediate efficient transfection of cells in culture. Bioconjug Chem 1993, 4, 372–379.

82. Bielinska A, Kukowska-Latallo JF, Johnsson J, Tomalia DA, Baker JR, Jr. Regulation of in vitro gene expression using antisense oligonucleotides or antisense expression plasmids transfected using starburst PAMAM dendrimers. Nucleic Acids Res 1996, 24, 2176–2182.

83. Kukowska-Latallo JF, Bielinska AU, Johnson J, Spindler R, Tomalia DA, Baker JR, Jr. Efficient transfer of genetic material into mammalian cells using Starburst polyamidoamine dendrimers. Proc Natl Acad Sci USA 1996, 93, 4897–4902.

84. Bielinska AU, Kukowska-Latallo JF, Baker JR, Jr. The interaction of plasmid DNA with polyamidoamine dendrimers: mechanism of complex formation and analysis of alterations induced in nuclease sensitivity and transcriptional activity of the complexed DNA. Biochim Biophys Acta 1997, 1353, 180–190.

85. Remy-Kristensen A, Clamme JP, Vuilleumier C, Kuhry JG, Mely Y. Role of endocytosis in the transfection of L929 fibroblasts by polyethylenimine/DNA complexes. Biochim Biophys Acta 2001, 1514, 21–32.

86. Varga CM, Wickham TJ, Lauffenburger DA. Receptor-mediated targeting of gene delivery vectors: insights from molecular mechanisms for improved vehicle design. Biotechnol Bioeng 2000, 70, 593–605.

87. Ferrari S, Pettenazzo A, Garbati N, Zacchello F, Behr JP, Scarpa M. Polyethylenimine shows properties of interest for cystic fibrosis gene therapy. Biochim Biophys Acta 1999, 1447, 219–225.

88. Ferrari S, Kitson C, Farley R, Steel R, Marriott C, Parkins DA, Scarpa M, Wainwright B, Evans MJ, Colledge WH, Geddes DM, Alton EW. Mucus-altering agents as adjuncts for nonviral gene transfer to airway epithelium. Gene Ther 2001, 8, 1380–1386.

89. Densmore CL, Orson FM, Xu B, Kinsey BM, Waldrep JC, Hua P, Bhogal B, Knight V. Aerosol delivery of robust polyethyleneimine–DNA complexes for gene therapy and genetic immunization. Mol Ther 2000, 1, 180–188.

90. Gautam A, Densmore CL, Waldrep JC. Pulmonary cytokine responses associated with PEI-DNA aerosol gene therapy. Gene Ther 2001, 8, 254–257.

91. Gautam A, Densmore CL, Golunski E, Xu B, Waldrep JC. Transgene expression in mouse airway epithelium by aerosol gene therapy with PEI-DNA complexes. Mol Ther 2001, 3, 551–556.

92. Goula D, Becker N, Lemkine GF, Normandie P, Rodrigues J, Mantero S, Levi G, Demeneix BA. Rapid crossing of the pulmonary endothelial barrier by polyethylenimine/DNA complexes. Gene Ther 2000, 7, 499–504.

93. Orson FM, Kinsey BM, Hua PJ, Bhogal BS, Densmore CL, Barry MA. Genetic immunization with lung-targeting macroaggregated polyethyleneimine-albumin conjugates elicits combined systemic and mucosal immune responses. J Immunol 2000, 164, 6313–6321.

94. Rudolph C, Lausier J, Naundorf S, Muller RH, Rosenecker J. In vivo gene delivery to the lung using polyethylenimine and fractured polyamidoamine dendrimers. J Gene Med 2000, 2, 269–278.

95. Zou SM, Erbacher P, Remy JS, Behr JP. Systemic linear polyethylenimine-(L-PEI)-mediated gene delivery in the mouse. J Gene Med 2000, 2, 128–134.

96. Uduehi AN, Stammberger U, Frese S, Schmid RA. Efficiency of nonviral gene delivery systems to rat lungs. Eur J Cardiothorac Surg 2001, 20, 159–163.

97. Uduehi AN, Stammberger U, Kubisa B, Gugger M, Buehler TA, Schmid RA. Effects of linear polyethylenimine and polyethylenimine/DNA on lung function after airway instillation to rat lungs. Mol Ther 2001, 4, 52–57.

98. Fasbender A, Zabner J, Chillon M, Moninger TO, Puga AP, Davidson BL, Welsh MJ. Complexes of adenovirus with polycationic polymers and cationic lipids increase the efficiency of gene transfer in vitro and in vivo. J Biol Chem 1997, 272, 6479–6489.

99. Gebhart CL, Kabanov AV. Evaluation of polyplexes as gene transfer agents. J Control Release 2001, 73, 401–416.

100. Goula D, Remy JS, Erbacher P, Wasowicz M, Levi G, Abdalkan B, Demeneix BA. Size, diffusibility and transfection performance of linear PEI/DNA complexes in the mouse central nervous system. Gene Therapy 1998, 5, 712–717.

101. Segura T, Shea LD. Materials for nonviral gene delivery. Annu Rev Mater Res 2001, 31, 25–46.

102. Lin AJ, Slack NL, Ahmad A, Koltover I, George CX, Samuel CE, Safinya CR. Structure and structure–function studies of lipid/plasmid DNA complexes. J Drug Target 2000, 8, 13–27.

103. Tang MX, Szoka FC. The influence of polymer structure on the interactions of cationic polymers with DNA and morphology of the resulting complexes. Gene Ther 1997, 4, 823–832.

104. Bloomfield VA. DNA condensation. Curr Opin Struct Biol 1996, 6, 334–341.

105. Bloomfield VA. DNA condensation by multivalent cations. Biopolymers 1997, 44, 269–282.

106. Bloomfield VA. Condensation of DNA by multivalent cations: considerations on mechanism. Biopolymers 1991, 31, 1471–1481.

107. Widom J, Baldwin RL. Cation-induced toroidal condensation of DNA studies with $Co3+$ (pH_3). J Mol Biol 1980, 144, 431–453.

108. Marschall P, Malik N, Larin Z. Transfer of YACs up to 2.3 Mb intact into human cells with polyethylenimine. Gene Ther 1999, 6, 1634–1637.

109. Godbey WT, Wu KK, Mikos AG. Poly(ethylenimine) and its role in gene delivery. J Control Release 1999, 60, 149–160.

110. Kircheis R, Schuller S, Brunner S, Ogris M, Heider KH, Zauner W, Wagner E. Polycation-based DNA complexes for tumor-targeted gene delivery in vivo. J Gene Med 1999, 1, 111–120.

111. Ogris M, Steinlein P, Kursa M, Mechtler K, Kircheis R, Wagner E. The size of DNA/transferrin–PEI complexes is an important factor for gene expression in cultured cells. Gene Ther 1998, 5, 1425–1433.

112. Boussif O, Zanta MA, Behr JP. Optimized galenics improve in vitro gene transfer with cationic molecules up to 1000-fold. Gene Ther 1996, 3, 1074–1080.

113. Ross PC, Hui SW. Lipoplex size is major determinant of in vitro lipofection efficiency. Gene Ther 1999, 6, 651–659.

114. McLean JW, Fox EA, Baluk P, Bolton PB, Haskell A, Pearlman R, Thurston G, Umemoto EY, McDonald DM. Organ-specific endothelial cell uptake of cationic liposome–DNA complexes in mice. Am J Physiol 1997, 273, H387–H404.

115. Song YK, Liu F, Chu S, Liu D. Characterization of cationic liposome-mediated gene transfer in vivo by intravenous administration. Hum Gene Ther 1997, 8, 1585–1594.

116. Godbey WT, Wu KK, Mikos AG. Tracking the intracellular path of poly(ethylenimine)/DNA complexes for gene delivery. Proc Natl Acad Sci USA 1999, 96, 5177–5181.

117. Pollard H, Remy JS, Loussouarn G, Demolombe S, Behr JP, Escande D. Polyethylenimine but not cationic lipids promotes transgene delivery to the nucleus in mammalian cells. J Biol Chem 1998, 273, 7507–7511.

118. Suh J, Wirtz D, Hanes J. Efficient active transport of gene nanocarriers to the cell nucleus. DNAs 2002, 100, 3878–3882.

119. Jans DA, Chan CK, Huebner S. Signals mediating nuclear targeting and their regulation: application in drug delivery. Med Res Rev 1998, 18, 189–223.

120. Cone RA. Mucus. In Mucosal Immunology; 2nd ed; Orga PL, ed. Academic Press: San Diego, 1999; 43–64.

121. Lai E, Van Zanten JH. Evidence of lipoplex dissociation in liquid formulations. J Pharm Sci 2002, 91, 1225–1232.

122. Lai E, van Zanten JH. Real-time monitoring of lipoplex molar mass, size and density. J Control Release 2002, 82, 149–158.

123. Lai E, van Zanten JH. Monitoring DNA/poly-L-lysine polyplex formation with time-resolved multiangle laser light scattering. Biophys J 2001, 80, 864–873.

124. Har-el Y, van Zanten JH, Hanes J. PEI/VEGF DNA polyplexes: effects of serum and solvent on vector size, molar mass, and transfection efficiency, in preparation.

125. Har-el Y, van Zanten JH, Hanes J. Effect of formulation parameters on PEI/VEGF DNA polyplex physical properties determined using time-resolved multiangle laser light scattering, in preparation.

126. Lemkine GF, Demeneix BA. Polyethylenimines for in vivo gene delivery. Curr Opin Mol Ther 2001, 3, 178–182.

127. Nabel EG, Gordon D, Yang ZY, Xu L, San H, Plautz GE, Wu BY, Gao X, Huang L, Nabel GJ. Gene transfer in vivo with DNA–liposome complexes: lack of autoimmunity and gonadal localization. Hum Gene Ther 1992, 3, 649–656.

128. Nabel GJ, Nabel EG, Yang ZY, Fox BA, Plautz GE, Gao X, Huang L, Shu S, Gordon D, Chang AE. Direct gene transfer with DNA–liposome complexes in melanoma: expression, biologic activity, and lack of toxicity in humans. Proc Natl Acad Sci USA 1993, 90, 11307–11311.

129. Caplen NJ, Alton EW, Middleton PG, Dorin JR, Stevenson BJ, Gao X, Durham SR, Jeffrey PK, Hodson ME, Coutelle C, et al. Liposome-mediated CFTR gene transfer to the nasal epithelium of patients with cystic fibrosis. Nat Med 1995, 1, 39–46.

130. Gustafsson J, Arvidson G, Karlsson G, Almgren M. Complexes between cationic liposomes and DNA visualized by cryo-TEM. Biochim Biophys Acta 1995, 1235, 305–312.

131. Li B, Li S, Tan Y, Stolz DB, Watkins SC, Block LH, Huang L. Lyophilization of cationic lipid-protamine-DNA (LPD) complexes. J Pharm Sci 2000, 89, 355–364.

132. Quraishi MS, Jones NS, Mason J. The rheology of nasal mucus: a review. Clin Otolaryngol 1998, 23, 403–413.

133. Bastacky J, Lee CY, Goerke J, Koushafar H, Yager D, Kenaga L, Speed TP, Chen Y, Clements JA. Alveolar lining layer is thin and continuous: low-temperature scanning electron microscopy of rat lung. J Appl Physiol 1995, 79, 1615–1628.

134. Hanes J, Edwards DA, Evora C, Langer R. Particles incorporating surfactants for pulmonary drug delivery. U.S. Patent No. 5,855,913, 1999.

135. Sanders NN, Van Rompaey E, De Smedt SC, Demeester J. Structural alterations of gene complexes by cystic fibrosis sputum. Am J Respir Crit Care Med 2001, 164, 486–493.

136. Kitson C, Angel B, Judd D, Rothery S, Severs NJ, Dewar A, Huang L, Wadsworth SC, Cheng SH, Geddes DM, Alton EW. The extra- and intracellular barriers to lipid and adenovirus-mediated pulmonary gene transfer in native sheep airway epithelium. Gene Ther 1999, 6, 534–546.

137. Willits RK, Saltzman WM. Synthetic polymers alter the structure of cervical mucus. Biomaterials 2001, 22, 445–452.

138. Khanvilkar K, Donovan MD, Flanagan DR. Drug transfer through mucus. Adv Drug Deliv Rev 2001, 48, 173–193.

139. Gonda I. Inhalation therapy with recombinant human deoxyribonuclease I. Adv Drug Deliv Rev 1996, 19, 37–46.

140. Rubin B. Emerging therapies for cystic fibrosis lung disease. Chest 1999, 115, 1120–1126.

141. Silberberg A. Models of Mucus Structure; Raven Press: New York, 1988.

142. Sanders N, De Smedt S, Demeester J. The physical properties of biogels and their permeability for macromolecular drugs and colloidal drug carriers. J Pharm Sci 1999, 89, 835–849.

143. Yudin AI, Hanson FW, Katz DF. Human cervical mucus and its interaction with sperm: a fine-structural view. Biol Reprod 1989, 40, 661–671.

144. Sanders NN, De Smedt SC, Van Romaey E, Simoens P, De Baets F, Demeester J. Cystic fibrosis sputum: a barrier to the transport of nanospheres. Am J Respir Crit Care Med 2000, 162, 1905–1911.

145. Bhat PG, Flanagan DR, Donovan MD. Drug diffusion through cystic fibrotic mucus: steady-state permeation, rheologic properties, and glycoprotein morphology. J Pharm Sci 1996, 85, 624–630.

146. Wu-Pong S, Byron P. Airway to biophase transfer of oligonucleotides. Adv Drug Del Rev 1996, 19, 47–71.

147. Rubin B. Therapeutic aerosols and airway secretions. J Aerosol Med 1996, 9, 123–130.

148. Lele BS, Hoffman AS. Mucoadhesive drug carriers based on complexes of poly(acrylic acid) and PEGylated drugs having hydrolysable PEG-anhydride-drug linkages. J Control Release 2000, 69, 237–248.

149. Zahm JM, Galabert C, Chaffin A, Chazalette JP, Grosskopf C, Puchelle E. Improvement of cystic fibrosis airway mucus transportability by recombinant human DNase is related to changes in phospholipid profile. AM J Respir Crit Care Med 1998, 157, 1779–1784.

150. De Smedt S, Meyvis E, van Oostveldt P, Blonk J, Hennink W, Demeester J. The diffusion of macromolecules in dextran methacrylate solutions and gels as studied by confocal scanning laser microscopy. Macromolecules 1997, 30, 4863–4870.

151. Olmsted SS, Padgett JL, Yudin AI, Whaley KJ, Moench TR, Cone RA. Diffusion of macromolecules and virus-like particles in human cervical mucus. Biophys J 2001, 81, 1930–1937.

152. Banerjee R, Bellare J, Puniyani R. Effect of phospholipid mixtures and surfactant formulations on rheology of polymeric gels, simulating mucus, at shear rates experienced in the tracheobronchial tree. Biochem Eng J 2001, 7, 195–200.

153. Girod S, Zahm JM, Plotkowski C, Beck G, Puchelle E. Role of the physiochemical properties of mucus in the protection of the respiratory epithelium. Eur Respir J 1992, 5, 477–487.

154. Norris D, Sinko P. Effect of size, surface charge, and hydrophobicity on the translocation of polystyrene microspheres through gastrointestinal mucin. J Appl Polym Sci 1996, 63, 1481–1492.

155. Mrsny R, Daugherty A, Short S, Widmer R, Siegel M, Keller G. Distribution of DNA and alginate in purulent cystic fibrosis sputum: implications to pulmonary targeting strategies. J Drug Targeting 1996, 4, 233–243.

156. Sisson JH, Yonkers AJ, Waldman RH. Effects of guaifenesin on nasal mucociliary clearance and ciliary beat frequency in healthy volunteers. Chest 1995, 107, 747–751.

157. Lusuardi M, Donner C. Glycoproteins; Raven Press: New York, 1998.

158. Vasconcellos CA. Reduction in viscosity of cystic fibrosis sputum in vitro by gelsolin. Science 2002, 263, 969–971.

159. Cruewels L, Golde L, Haagsman H. The pulmonary surfactant system: Biochemical and clinical aspects. Lung 1997, 175, 1–39.

160. LeVine AM, Whitsett JA. Pulmonary collectins and innate host defense of the lung. Microbes Infect 2001, 3, 161–166.

161. van Iwaarden JF, Pikaar JC, Storm J, Brouwer E, Verhoef J, Oosting RS, van Golde LM, van Strijp JA. Binding of surfactant protein A to the lipid A moiety of bacterial lipopolysaccharides. Biochem J 1994, 303, 407–411.

162. LeVine AM, Whitsett JA, Hartshorn KL, Crouch EC, Korfhagen TR. Surfactant protein D enhances clearance of influenza A virus from the lung in vivo. J Immunol 2001, 167, 5868–5873.

163. Pruitt K, Rahemtulla B, Rahemtulla F, Russell M. Innate Humoral Factors. In Mucosal Immunology; Orga PL, ed. Academic Press: San Diego, 1999; 65–88.

164. Pryhuber GS. Regulation and function of pulmonary surfactant protein B. Mol Genet Metab 1998, 64, 217–228.

165. Tabata Y, Ikada Y. Effect of the size and surface charge of polymer microspheres on their phagocytosis by macrophage. Biomaterials 1988, 9, 356–362.

166. Dinghua L, Lancaster J, Mahesh S, Nelson S, Stoltz D, Bagby G, Odom G, Shellito J, Kolls J. Activation of alveolar macrophages and lung host defenses using transfer of the interferon-gamma gene. Am J Physiology 1997, 272, L852–L859.

167. Baatz JE, Zou Y, Korfhagen TR. Inhibitory effects of tumor necrosis factor-alpha on cationic lipid-mediated gene delivery to airway cells in vitro. Biochim Biophys Acta 2001, 1535, 100–109.

168. Zsengeller Z, Otake K, Hossain SA, Berclaz PY, Trapnell BC. Internalization of adenovirus by alveolar macrophages initiates early proinflammatory signaling during acute respiratory tract infection. J Virol 2000, 74, 9655–9667.

169. Zuber G, Dauty E, Nothisen M, Belguise P, Behr JP. Towards synthetic viruses. Adv Drug Deliv Rev 2001, 52, 245–253.

170. Apgar J, Tseng Y, Fedorov E, Herwig MB, Almo SC, Wirtz D. Multiple-particle tracking measurements of heterogeneities in solutions of actin filaments and actin bundles. Biophys J 2000, 79, 1095–1106.

171. Mislick KA, Baldeschwieler JD. Evidence for the role of proteoglycans in cation-mediated gene transfer. Proc Natl Acad Sci USA 1996, 93, 12349–12354.

172. Mounkes LC, Zhong W, Cipres-Palacin G, Heath TD, Debs RJ. Proteoglycans mediate cationic liposome–DNA complex–based gene delivery in vitro and in vivo. J Biol Chem 1998, 273, 26164–26170.

173. Baranowski E, Ruiz-Jarabo CM, Domingo E. Evolution of cell recognition by viruses. Science 2001, 292, 1102–1105.

174. Schaffer DV, Lauffenburger DA. Optimization of cell surface binding enhances efficiency and specificity of molecular conjugate gene delivery. J Biol Chem 1998, 273, 28004–28009.

175. Zenke M, Steinlein P, Wagner E, Cotten M, Beug H, Birnstiel ML. Receptor-mediated endocytosis of transferrin–polycation conjugates: an efficient way to introduce DNA into hematopoietic cells. Proc Natl Acad Sci USA 1990, 87, 3655–3659.

176. Wagner E, Zenke M, Cotten M, Beug H, Brinstiel ML. Transferrin–polycation conjugates as carriers for DNA uptake into cells. Proc Natl Acad Sci USA 1990, 87, 3410–3414.

177. Erbacher P, Remy JS, Behr JP. Gene transfer with synthetic virus-like particles via the integrin-mediated endocytosis pathway. Gene Ther 1999, 6, 138–145.

178. Scott ES, Wiseman JW, Evans MJ, Colledge WH. Enhanced gene delivery to human airway epithelial cells using an integrin-targeting lipoplex. J Gene Med 2001, 3, 125–134.

179. Colin M, Harbottle RP, Knight A, Kornprobst M, Cooper RG, Miller AD, Trugnan G, Capeau J, Coutelle C, Brahimi-Horn MC. Liposomes enhance delivery and expression of an RGD-oligolysine gene transfer vector in human tracheal cells. Gene Ther 1998, 5, 1488–1498.

180. Kim J, Smith T, Idamakanti N, Mulgrew K, Kaloss M, Kylefjord H, Ryan PC, Kaleko M, Stevenson SC. Targeting adenoviral vectors by using the extracellular domain of the coxsackie-adenovirus receptor: improved potency via trimerization. J Virol 2002, 76, 1892–1903.

181. Fajac I, Grosse S, Briand P, Monsigny M. Targeting of cell receptors and gene transfer efficiency: a balancing act. Gene Ther 2002, 9, 740–742.

182. James MB, Giorgio TD. Nuclear-associated plasmid, but not cell-associated plasmid, is correlated with transgene expression in cultured mammalian cells. Mol Ther 2000, 1, 339–346.

183. Pickles RJ, McCarty D, Matsui H, Hart PJ, Randell SH, Boucher RC. Limited entry of adenovirus vectors into well-differentiated airway epithelium is responsible for inefficient gene transfer. J Virol 1998, 72, 6014–6023.

184. Fasbender A, Zabner J, Zeiher BG, Welsh MJ. A low rate of cell proliferation and reduced DNA uptake limit cationic lipid-mediated gene transfer to primary cultures of ciliated human airway epithelia. Gene Ther 1997, 4, 1173–1180.

185. Zelphati O, Szoka FC, Jr. Mechanism of oligonucleotide release from cationic liposomes. Proc Natl Acad Sci USA 1996, 93, 11493–11498.

186. Hafez IM, Maurer N, Cullis PR. On the mechanism whereby cationic lipids promote intracellular delivery of polynucleic acids. Gene Ther 2001, 8, 1188–1196.

187. Ciftci K, Levy RJ. Enhanced plasmid DNA transfection with lysosomotropic agents in cultured fibroblasts. Int J Pharm 2001, 218, 81–92.

188. Curiel DT, Agarwal S, Wagner E, Cotten M. Adenovirus enhancement of transferrin-polysine-mediated gene delivery. Proc Natl Acad Sci USA 1991, 88, 8850–8854.

189. Cotten M, Wagner E, Zatloukal K, Phillips S, Curiel DT, Birsnstiel ML. High-efficiency receptor-mediated delivery of small and large (48-kilobase gene constructs using the endosome-disruption activity of defective or chemically inactivated adenovirus particles. Proc Natl Acad Sci USA 1992, 89, 6094–6098.

190. Plank C, Oberhauser B, Mechtler K, Koch C, Wagner E. The influence of endosome-disruptive peptides on gene transfer using synthetic virus-like gene transfer systems. J Biol Chem 1994, 269, 12918–12924.

191. Subramanian A, Ma H, Dahl KN, Zhu J, Diamond SL. Adenovirus or HA-2 fusogenic peptide-assisted lipofection increases cytoplasmic levels of plasmid in nondividing endothelium with little enhancement of transgene expression. J Gene Med 2002, 4, 75–83.

192. Ogris M, Carlisle RC, Bettinger T, Seymour LW. Melittin enables efficient vesicular escape and enhanced nuclear access of nonviral gene delivery vectors. J Biol Chem 2001, 276, 47550–47555.

193. Cheung CY, Murthy N, Stayton PS, Hoffman AS. A pH-sensitive polymer that enhances cationic lipid-mediated gene transfer. Bioconjung Chem 2001, 12, 906–910.

194. Pack DW, Putnam D, Langer R. Design of imidazole-containing endosomolytic biopolymers for gene delivery. Biotechnol Bioeng 2000, 67, 217–223.

195. Murthy N, Robichaud JR, Tirrell DA, Stayton PS, Hoffman AS. The design and synthesis of polymers for eukaryotic membrane disruption. J Control Release 1999, 61, 137–143.

196. Lukacs GL, Haggie P, Seksek O, Lechardeur D, Freedman N, Verkman AS. Size-dependent DNA mobility in cytoplasm and nucleus. J Biol Chem 2000, 275, 1625–1629.

197. Hasegawa S, Hirashima N, Nakanishi M. Microtubule involvement in the intracellular dynamics for gene transfection mediated by cationic liposomes. Gene Ther 2001, 8, 1669–1673.

198. Godbey WT, Barry MA, Saggau P, Wu KK, Mikos AG. Poly(ethylenimine)-mediated transfection: a new paradigm for gene delivery. J Biomed Mater Res 2000, 51, 321–328.

199. Gonzalez H, Hwang SJ, Davis ME. New class of polymers for the delivery of macromolecular therapeutics. Bioconjugate Chemistry 1999, 10, 1068–1074.

200. Oh YK, Swanson JA. Different fates of phagocytosed particles after delivery into macrophage lysosomes. J Cell Biol 1996, 132, 585–593.

201. Tachibana R, Harashima H, Shinohara Y, Kiwada H. Quantitative studies on the nuclear transport of plasmid DNA and gene expression employing nonviral vectors. Adv Drug Deliv Rev 2001, 52, 219–226.

202. Nakanishi M, Akuta T, Nagoshi E, Eguchi A, Mizuguchi H, Senda T. Nuclear targeting of DNA. Eur J Pharm Sci 2001, 13, 17–24.

203. Pouton CW. Nuclear import of polypeptides, polynucleotides and supramolecular complexes. Adv Drug Deliv Rev 1998, 34, 51–64.

204. Goldberg MW, Allen TD. High-resolution scanning electron microscopy of the nuclear envelope: demonstration of a new, regular, fibrous lattice attached to the baskets of the nucleoplasmic face of the nuclear pores. J Cell Biol 1992, 119, 1429–1440.

205. Zanta MA, Belguise-Valladier P, Behr JP. Gene delivery: a single nuclear localization signal peptide is sufficient to carry DNA to the cell nucleus. Proc Natl Acad Sci USA 1999, 96, 91–96.

206. Carlisle RC, Bettinger T, Ogris M, Hale S, Mautner V, Seymour LW. Adenovirus hexon protein enhances nuclear delivery and increases transgene expression of polyethylenimine/plasmid DNA vectors. Mol Ther 2001, 4, 473–483.

207. Rebuffat A, Bernasconi A, Ceppi M, Wehrli H, Verca SB, Ibrahim M, Frey BM, Frey FJ, Rusconi S. Selective enhancement of gene transfer by steroid-mediated gene delivery. Nat Biotechnol 2001, 19, 1155–1161.

208. Brunner S, Sauer T, Carotta S, Cotten M, Saltik M, Wagner E. Cell cycle dependence of gene transfer by lipoplex, polyplex and recombinant adenovirus. Gene Ther 2000, 7, 401–407.

209. Schaffer DV, Fidelman NA, Dan N, Lauffenburger DA. Vector unpacking as a potential barrier for receptor-mediated polyplex gene delivery. Biotechnol Bioeng 2000, 67, 598–606.

210. Fu J, Krauland E, Har-el Y, Hanes J. Biodegradable cationic poly(aspartic anhydride-co-ethylene glycol): Synthesis, characterization, and self-assembly with plasmid DNA, submitted to Macromolecules.

211. Lynn DM, Langer R. Degradable poly(beta-amino esters): synthesis, characterization, and self-assembly with plasmid DNA. J Am Chem Soc 2000, 122, 10761–10768.

212. Lim YB, Han SO, Kong HU, Lee Y, Park JS, Jeong B, Kim SW. Biodegradable polyester, poly[alpha-(4-aminobuty1)-L-glycolic acid], as a nontoxic gene carrier. Pharm Res 2000, 17, 811–816.

213. Kamiya H, Tsuchiya H, Yamazaki J, Harashima H. Intracellular trafficking and transgene expression of viral and nonviral gene vectors. Adv Drug Deliv Rev 2001, 52, 153–164.

214. Hong K, Sherley J, Lauffenburger DA. Methylation of episomal plasmids as a barrier to transient gene expression via a synthetic delivery vector. Biomol Eng 2001, 18, 185–192.

215. Ishii T, Okahata Y, Sato T. Mechanism of cell transfection with plasmid/chitosan complexes. Biochim Biophys Acta 2001, 1514, 51–64.

216. Labat-Moleur F, Steffan AM, Brisson C, Perron H, Feugeas O, Furstenberger P, Oberling F, Brambilla E, Behr JP. An electron microscopy study into the mechanism of gene transfer with lipopolyamines. Gene Ther 1996, 3, 1010–1017.

217. Briane D, Lesage D, Cao A, Coudert R, Lievre N, Salzmann JL, Taillandier E. Cellular pathway of plasmids vectorized by cholesterol-based cationic liposomes. J Histochem Cytochem 2002, 50, 983–991.

218. Lappalainen K, Miettinen R, Kellokoski J, Jaaskelainen I, Syrjanen S. Intracellular distribution of oligonucleotides delivered by cationic liposomes: light and electron microscopic study. J Histochem Cytochem 1997, 45, 265–274.

219. El Ouahabi A, Thiry M, Schiffmann S, Fuks R, Nguyen-Tran H, Ruysschaert JM, Vandenbranden M. Intracellular visualization of BrdU-labeled plasmid DNA/cationic liposome complexes. J Histochem Cytochem 1999, 47, 1159–1166.

220. Landahl H. On the removal of air-borne droplets by the human respiratory tract I. The lung. Bull Math Biophys 1950, 12, 43–56.

221. Schulz H. Mechanisms and factors affecting intrapulmonary particle deposition: implications for efficient inhalation therapies. Pharm Sci Technol Today 1998, 1, 336–344.

222. Crowder TM, Rosati JA, Schroeter JD, Hickey AJ, Martonen TB. Fundamental effects of particle morphology on lung delivery: predictions of Stokes' law and the particular relevance to dry powder inhaler formulation and development. Pharm Res 2002, 19, 239–245.

223. Lippmann M, Albert RE. The effect of particle size on the regional deposition of inhaled aerosols in the human respiratory tract. Am Ind Hyg Assoc J 1969, 30, 257–275.

224. Lippmann M. Recent advances in respiratory tract particle deposition. In Occupational and Industrial Hygiene: Concepts and Methods; Esmen NA, Mehlman MA, eds. Princeton Scientific: Princeton, NJ, 1984; Vol. VIII, 75–103.

225. Heyder J, Gebhart J, Rudolf G, Schiller CF, Stahlhofen W. Deposition of particles in the human respiratory tract in the size range 0.005–15 μm. J Aerosol Sci 1986, 17, 811–825.

226. Snipes MB. Biokinetics of inhaled radionuclides. In Internal Radiation Dosimetry; Raabe OG, ed. Medical Physics: Madison, WI, 1994; 181–204.

227. Task Group on Lung Dynamics. Deposition and retention models for internal dosimetry of the human respiratory tract. Health Phys 1966, 12, 173–207.

228. Darquenne C, Brand P, Heyder J, Paiva M. Aerosol dispersion in human lung: comparison between numerical simulations and experiments for bolus tests. J Appl Physiol 1997, 83, 966–974.

229. Fu J, Fiegel J, Krauland E, Hanes J. New polymeric carriers for controlled drug delivery following inhalation or injection. Biomaterials 2002, 23, 4425–4433. pulmonary drug delivery, Biomaterials, Published Online, June 18, 2002.

230. Newman SP, Woodman G, Clarke SW. Deposition of carbenicillin aerosol in cystic fibrosis: effects of nebulizer system and breathing pattern. Thorax 1988, 43, 318–322.

231. Regnis JA, Robinson M, Bailey DL, Cook P, Hooper P, Chan HK, Gonda I, Bautovich G, Bye PT. Mucociliary clearance in patients with cystic fibrosis and in normal subjects. Am J Respir Crit Care Med 1994, 150, 66–71.

232. Hinds WC. Aerosol Technology: Properties, Behavior, and Measurement of Airborne Particles; 2nd ed; Wiley: New York, 1999.

233. Stoeber W. Dynamic shape factors of nonspherical aerosol particles. In Assessment of Airborne Particles; Mercer TT, Morrow PE, Stoeber W, eds. Charles C Thomas: Springfield, IL, 1972; 249–289.

234. Timbrell V. Deposition and Retention of Fibers in the Human-Lung. Ann Occup Hyg 1982, 26, 347–369.
235. Asgharian B, Yu CP. Deposition of inhaled fibrous particles in the human lung. J Aerosol Med 1988, 1, 37–50.
236. Timbrell V. Human exposure to asbestos: dust controls and standards. The inhalation of fibrous dusts. Ann NY Acad Sci 1965, 132, 255–273.
237. Gonda I. Targeting by deposition. In Pharmaceutical Inhalation Aerosol Technology; Hickey AJ, ed. Marcel Dekker: New York, 1992; 61–82.
238. Schultz H, Brand P, Heyder J. Particle Deposition in the Respiratory Tract. Particle–Lung Interactions; Marcel Dekker: New York, 2000; 229–290.
239. Raabe OG. Aerosol aerodynamic size conventions for inertial sampler calibration. J Air Poll Control Assoc 1976, 26, 856–860.
240. Einstein A. On the kinetic molecular theory of thermal movements of particles suspended in a quiescent fluid. Ann Phys 1905, 17, 549–560.
241. Lippmann, M. Regional deposition of particles in the human respiratory tract. In: D.H.K. Lee, H.L. Falk, S.O. Murphy, S.R. Geiger (eds.), Handbook of Physiology, Reaction to Environmental Agents. Bethesda, MD: American Physiological Society, 1977.
242. Martonen TB, Katz IM. Deposition patterns of aerosolized drugs within human lungs: effects of ventilatory parameters. Pharm Res 1993, 10, 871–878.
243. Gebhart J, Heyder J, Stahlhofen W. Use of aerosols to estimate pulmonary air-space dimensions. J Appl Physiol 1981, 51, 465–476.
244. Palmes ED, Wang CS, Goldring RM, Altshuler B. Effect of depth of inhalation on aerosol persistence during breath holding. J Appl Physiol 1973, 34, 356–360.
245. Kim CS, Eldridge MA. Aerosol deposition in the airway model with excessive mucus secretions. J Appl Physiol 1985, 59, 1766–1772.
246. Smaldone GC, Messina MS. Enhancement of particle deposition by flow-limiting segments in humans. J Appl Physiol 1985, 59, 509–514.
247. Anderson PJ, Blanchard JD, Brain JD, Feldman HA, McNamara JJ, Heyder J. Effect of cystic fibrosis on inhaled aerosol boluses. Am Rev Respir Dis 1989, 140, 1317–1324.
248. Kavanaugh RE, Unadkat JD, Smith AL. Drug disposition in cystic fibrosis. In Cystic Fibrosis; Davis PB, ed. McGraw-Hill: New York, 1993; 91–136.
249. Martonen T, Katz I, Cress W. Aerosol deposition as a function of airway disease: cystic fibrosis. Pharm Res 1995, 12, 96–102.
250. Brand P, Meyer T, Sommerer K, Weber N, Scheuch G. Alveolar deposition of monodisperse aerosol particles in the lung of patients with chronic obstructive pulmonary disease. Exp Lung Res 2002, 28, 39–54.
251. Gagnadoux F, Diot P, Marchand S, Thompson R, Dieckman K, Lemarie E, Varaigne F, Maurage C, Baulieu JL, Rolland JC. Pulmonary deposition of colistin aerosols in cystic fibrosis. Comparison of an ultrasonic nebulizer and a pneumatic nebulizer. Rev Mal Respir 1996, 13, 55–60.
252. Kuni CC, Budd JR, Regelmann WE, Ducret RP, Boudreau RJ. Comparison of Tc-99m DTPA aerosol ventilation studies with pulmonary function testing in cystic fibrosis. Clin Nucl Med 1993, 18, 15–18.

253. Laube BL, Chang DY, Blask AN, Rosenstein BJ. Radioaerosol assessment of lung improvement in cystic fibrosis patients treated for acute pulmonary exacerbations. Chest 1992, 101, 1302–1308.

254. Marshall LM, Francis PW, Khafagi FA. Aerosol deposition in cystic fibrosis using an aerosol conservation device and a conventional jet nebulizer. J Paediatr Child Health 1994, 30, 65–67.

255. Podczeck F. Particle–Particle Adhesion in Pharmaceutical Powder Handling; Imperial College Press: London, 1998.

256. Zeng XM, Martin GP, Tee SK, Marriott C. The role of fine particle lactose on the dispersion and deaggregation of salbutamol sulphate in an air stream in vitro. Int J Pharm 1998, 176, 99–110.

257. Tee SK, Marriott C, Zeng XM, Martin GP. The use of different sugars as fine and coarse carriers for aerosolized salbutamol sulphate. Int J Pharm 2000, 208, 111–123.

258. French DL, Edwards DA, Niven RW. The influence of formulations on emission, deaggregation, and deposition of dry powders for inhalation. J Aerosol Sci 1996, 27, 769–783.

259. Staniforth JN. Particle interactions in dry-powder formulation of aerocolloida suspensions. In: Proceedings of the Second Respiratory Drug Delivery Symposium, College of Pharmacy, The University of Kentucky, Keystone, CO, 1990, pp. 26–30.

260. Hickey AJ, Concessio NM, Van Oort MM, Platz RM. Factors influencing the dispersion of dry powders as aerosols, Pharm Tech 58 + , 1994.

261. Gotoh K, Masuda H, Higashitani K. Powder Technology Handbook; 2nd ed; Marcel Dekker: New York, 1997.

262. Visser J. Van der Waals and other cohesive forces affecting powder fluidization. Powder Technol 1989, 58, 1–10.

263. Edwards DA, Ben-Jebria A, Langer R. Recent advances in pulmonary drug delivery using large, porous inhaled particles. J Appl Physiol 1998, 85, 379–385.

264. Hickey AJ. Inhalation Aerosols; Marcel Dekker: New York, 1996; Vol. 96.

265. Bennett FS, Carter PA, Rowley G, Dandiker Y. Modification of electrostatic charge on inhaled carrier lactose particles by addition of fine particles. Drug Dev Ind Pharm 1999, 25, 99–103.

266. Marlow WH. Survey of aerosol interactive forces. In Aerosol Microphysics I: Particle Interaction; Marlow WH, ed. McGraw-Hill: New York, 1980; 116–156.

267. Khilnani A. Cleaning semiconductor surfaces: facts and foibles. In Particles on Surfaces 1: Detection, Adhesion, and Removal; Mittal KL, ed. Plenum Press: New York, 1988; 17–35.

268. Zimon AD. Adhesion of Dust and Powder; 2nd ed; Consultants Bureau: New York, 1982.

269. Podczeck F, Newton JM, James MB. Variations in the adhesion force between a drug and carrier particles as a result of changes in the relative humidity of the air. Int J Pharm 1997, 149, 151–160.

270. Finlay WH. The Mechanisms of Inhaled Pharmaceutical Aerosols; Academic Press: San Diego, 2001; 221–276.

271. Li W-I, Perzl M, Heyder J, Langer R, Brain JD, Englmeier K-H, Niven RW, Edwards DA. Aerodynamics and aerosol particle deaggregation phenomena in model oral-pharyngeal cavities. J Aerosol Sci 1996, 27, 1269–1286.

272. Timsina MP, Martin GP, Marriott C, Ganderton D, Yianneskis M. Drug delivery to the respiratory tract using dry powder inhalers. Int J Pharm 1994, 101, 1–13.

273. Neumann BS. The flow properties of powders. In Advances in Pharmaceutical Science; Bean HS, Beckett AH, Carless JE, eds. Academic Press: London, 1967; Vol. 2, 181–221.

274. Edwards DA, Hanes J, Caponetti G, Hrkach J, BenJebria A, Eskew ML, Mintzes J, Deaver D, Lotan N, Langer R. Large porous particles for pulmonary drug delivery. Science 1997, 276, 1868–1871.

275. Batycky RP, Hanes J, Langer R, Edwards DA. A theoretical model of erosion and macromolecular drug release from biodegrading microspheres. J Pharm Sci 1997, 86, 1464–1477.

276. Hirst PH, Pitcairn GR, Weers JG, Tarara TE, Clark AR, Dellamary LA, Hall G, Shorr J, Newman SP. In vivo lung deposition of hollow porous particles from a pressurized metered-dose inhaler. Pharm Res 2002, 19, 258–264.

277. Duddu SP, Sisk SA, Walter YH, Tarara TE, Trimble KR, Clark AR, Eldon MA, Elton RC, Pickford M, Hirst PH, Newman SP, Weers JG. Improved lung delivery from a passive dry powder inhaler using an engineered PulmoSphere powder. Pharm Res 2002, 19, 689–695.

278. Podczeck F, Newton JM, James MB. The influence of physical properties of materials in contact on the adhesion strength of particles of salmeterol base and salmeterol salts to various substrate materials. J Adhesion Sci Technol 1996, 10, 257–268.

279. Maugis D. On the contact and adhesion of rough surfaces. J Adhesion Sci Technol 1996, 10, 161–175.

280. Podczeck F, Newton JM, James MB. The adhesion force of micronized Salmeterol Xinafoate particles to pharmaceutically relevant surface materials. J Phys D: Appl Phys 1996, 29, 1878–1884.

281. Tabor D. Surface forces and surface interactions. J Colloid Interfac Sci 1977, 58, 2–13.

282. Broday DM, Georgopoulos PG. Growth and deposition of hygroscopic particulate matter in the human lungs. Aerosol Sci Technol 2001, 34, 144–159.

283. Peng CG, Chow AHL, Chan CK. Study of the hygroscopic properties of selected pharmaceutical aerosols using single particle levitation. Pharm Res 2000, 17, 1104–1109.

284. Morrow PE. Factors determining hygroscopic aerosol deposition in airways. Physiol Rev 1986, 66, 330–376.

285. Hickey AJ, Gonda I, Irwin WJ, Fildes FJ. Effect of hydrophobic coating on the behavior of a hygroscopic aerosol powder in an environment of controlled temperature and relative humidity. J Pharm Sci 1990, 79, 1009–1014.

286. Chan HK, Gonda I. Aerodynamic properties of elongated particles of cromoglycic acid. J Aerosol Sci 1989, 20, 157–168.

287. Chan HK, Gonda I. Respirable form of crystals of cromoglycic acid. J Pharm Sci 1989, 78, 176–180.

288. Somasundaran P, Xiang Y, Krishnakumar S. Role of conformation and orientation of surfactants and polymers in controlling flocculation and dispersion of aqueous and nonaqueous suspensions. Colloids Surf A 1998, 133, 125–133.

289. Coombes AGA, Tasker S, Lindblad M, Holmgren J, Hoste K, Toncheva V, Schacht E, Davies MC, Illum L, Davis SS. Biodegradable polymeric microparticles for drug delivery and vaccine formulation: the surface attachment of hydrophilic species using the concept of poly(ethylene glycol) anchoring segments. Biomaterials 1997, 18, 1153–1161.

290. Lin W, Garnett MC, Davies MC, Bignotti F, Ferruti P, Davis SS, Illum L. Preparation of surface-modified albumin nanospheres. Biomaterials 1997, 18, 559–565.

291. Farr SJ, McKenzie L, Clarke JG. Drug–Surfactant Interactions in Apolar Systems; Interpharm Press: Buffalo Grove, IL, 1994; Vol. 221.

292. Hanes J, Evora C, Ben-Jebria A, Edwards DA, Langer R. Porous Dry-Powder PLGA Microspheres Coated with Lung Surfactant for Systemic Insulin Delivery via the Lung. Proceed Inter Symp Control Rel Bioact Mater 1997, 24, 57–58.

293. Fu J, Fiegel J, Hanes J. Synthesis and characterization of PEG-based ether-anhydride terpolymers: novel polymers for pulmonary drug delivery. Submitted to Macromolecules.

294. Har-el Y, Janardhana D, Hanes J. Enhanced transfection efficiency through long-term delivery of PEI/DNA nanocomplexes from porous PLGA microspheres. In preparation.

295. Friedman T. Overcoming the obstacles to gene therapy. Scientific American 1997, 96–101.

17

Recent Advances Related to the Systemic Delivery of Therapeutic Molecules by Inhalation

David A. Edwards, André X. Valente, Jonathan Man, and Nicolas Tsapis
Harvard University, Cambridge, Massachusetts, U.S.A.

INTRODUCTION

The years since the early 1990s have seen many new scientific and engineering developments related to the therapeutic inhalation technology, especially for systemic delivery of drugs to the lungs. From novel inhaler to novel particle design [1], these developments have focused largely on improving the efficiency of the delivery of inhaled drugs to the lungs while limiting inhaler system user complexity. In the most successful delivery systems, lung deposition efficiencies, measured relative to the nominal dose of drug in the inhaler, have increased from approximately 10% to 60% [1], and delivery reproducibility has improved as well. Nevertheless, while early reports of inhaled insulin bioavailability in animals suggested numbers as high as 50% [2] and sustained pharmacodynamic action following deposition in the lungs of several days [3], published results from the most advanced human insulin trials [4] show relative biopotencies of less than 5%, and no public data have yet emerged from the clinic to confirm the feasibility of long-acting insulin delivery through the lungs. These circumstances point to the need for continued scientific and technological innovation if inhaled delivery of drugs for systemic application is to achieve widespread commercial use.

This chapter focuses on two recently published studies in the *Proceedings of the National Academy of Sciences* [5,6] related to inhalation delivery systems for the treatment of diseases modulated by the systemic circulation. We attempt to critically examine the results in the context of current technology and discuss their implications on the challenges facing the inhalation drug delivery field today.

BACKGROUND

By far the most compelling current case for an inhaled therapeutic delivery system is that of insulin. There are presently over 100 million diabetics in the world, with diabetes at the origin of a vast array of other medical complications, including renal, ophthalmologic, neuralgic, and cardiovascular diseases [7–9]. Financially, an estimated one-eighth of U.S. health care costs are diabetes related. Including indirect costs, the cost associated with diabetes in the United States is on the order of $90 billion annually [7]. The trend is for these numbers to increase, because many Type II diabetics are acquiring the more serious Type I symptoms, at least in part due to inadequate glucose control [7]. Five companies or consortiums are presently developing in-the-clinic inhaled insulin delivery systems. Inhale Therapeutics, of San Carlos, CA, in a joint collaboration with Pfizer and the insulin supplier Aventis, is furthest along the development path. With a product in a post–Phase III stage, this trio currently intends to file a new drug application (NDA) with the Food and Drug Administration (FDA) in 2003. The drug delivery company Alkermes, of Cambridge, MA, together with the world's largest insulin producer, Eli Lilly, is in post–Phase I testing. Likewise for Aradigm from Hayward, CA, in Phase II testing via a joint collaboration with insulin supplier Novo Nordisk. With each of the three major world insulin suppliers (Eli Lilly, Aventis, and Novo Nordisk) developing its own inhalation technology, other biotechnology companies, such as PDC (Elmsford, NY) and Aerogen (Sunnyvale, CA), are pursuing late Phase I inhaled insulin programs with smaller insulin suppliers.

The most recently published clinical data from the Inhale Therapeutics/Pfizer/Avenits collaboration, based on a clinical study involving 334 patients over a period of 12 weeks, showed that the overall quality-of-life scale and subscales of health perceptions, symptom interference, depression, positive affect, life satisfaction, psychological well-being, and cognitive function all improved with inhaled insulin therapy relative to the standard therapy based on multiple daily injections [10]. In another published study (2000) by the same group [4], improved patient satisfaction correlated in Type 1 and Type 2 diabetics with improved glycemic control for the inhaled insulin patients relative to those receiving multiple daily injections. Clouding these encouraging findings were the bioefficacy data from this same Phase 2 clinical study, which showed equivalent changes in glycosylated haemoglobin (HbA_{1c}) and glucose control with mean daily inhalations of approximately 366 international units of insulin versus approximately 15.9 international units of mean daily (mealtime) injections of regular insulin [4], implying a relative biopotency of 4.3%. This result oddly followed earlier published clinical data with the same Inhale® system showing biopotency, after a single administration of inhaled insulin to normal human subjects, in the range of 10–11% [11]. The AerX® [11] and AIR [12] systems have each produced good insulin biopotencies (above 10% in the first 10 hours after administration) in normal and/or diabetic human subjects, although it is too early to comment on how their results will compare with the Inhale® system in late-stage clinical trials. Other systemically targeted therapeutic molecules that have been clinically administered in recent years by inhalation include interferon-alpha, interferon-gamma, leuprolide acetate, alpha-1-antitrypsin, and heparin [13]. Due to the demanding cost and supply issues surrounding development of these drug products, only a few of these are currently progressing through the clinic. These include alpha-1-antitrypsin for emphysema, through collaborations between Inhale Therapeutics and Aventis (using the Inhale® system), and growth hormone, through collaboration between Alkermes and Eli Lilly & Co. (using the AIR® system). None of the systemically targeted drugs currently in the clinic appear to be designed for achieving sustained drug delivery action.

INCREASING BIOAVAILABILITY: THE CASE FOR ETHANOL

The commercial need to improve relative bioavailability for systemic-targeted inhalation therapies relates to both basic economics and safety. Increased bioavailabilities obviously translate into smaller masses of drug product per therapeutic dose and potentially lesser negative side effects. Given the relatively high delivery efficiencies achievable with the best inhaler systems, one path toward achieving higher bioavailabilities is the use of the chemical enhancers [14]. The goal of the chemical enhancers, such as those used for marketed transdermal drug delivery systems, has traditionally been to increase the permeability of target epithelia by influencing tight junctions, plasma membrane partitioning, or some other barrier property, improving the efficiency of drug entry into the bloodstream while possibly raising questions of long-term safety, particularly severe in the case of nasally inhaled insulin [15]. An Astra-funded clinical study [11] of enhancer-assisted insulin delivery through the lungs incorporated bile salts in a dry powder aerosol formulation to enhance insulin penetration. This strategy improved inhaled biopotency from 7.6% to 12.5% [11]. More recently, PDC produced bioengineered insulin particles in dry powder form with diketopiperazine derivatives [16]. These absorption enhancers significantly enhanced the rate of insulin absorption and the overall insulin biopotencies [16].

An approach published in 2001 based on research out of the Klibanov laboratory at MIT is to use ethanol [5]. Ethanol, isopropanol, and other alcohols have long been used successfully as penetration enhancers for medical applications. Ethanol is one of the first molecules to have been used as a transdermal enhancer, because its effects are so easily and well characterized and its systemic and local toxicities are understood. It is currently contained in commercial delivery systems for estradiol [17] and other bioactive molecules. Ethanol and isopropanol have been used in a variety of studies based on their effects on drug transport. More applications can be found in the patent literature [18].

Klibanov and coworkers [5] showed that insulin can be stored in ethanol and delivered by nebulization to the lungs of rats. Pharmocokinetic and pharacodynamic analyses showed increased serum levels of insulin and altered glucose levels (see, e.g., Fig. 1). It was also shown that breathing nebulized ethanol had no discernible acute toxicity. Other reported advantages or attributes of delivering insulin from ethanol solutions included:

1. Ethanol can stabilize the tertiary and quaternary structure of proteins.
2. Ethanol can act as a biocide and limit microbial contamination of the suspension.
3. Higher dosing can be achieved with ethanol because the amount of drug in suspension is not limited by solubility.
4. The nonpolar nature of ethanol can allow inclusion of large quantities per volume of lipophilic drugs.
5. Ethanol can act as an enhancer of drug permeation, similar to transdermal systems.

The last point, related to degree of absorption enhancement obtained by the ethanol—if any—was not in fact clarified by this study for no positive control (i.e., insulin delivery from an aqueous solution) was performed.

Assuming ethanol can be shown to lead to substantially improved insulin absorption from the lungs, a few key questions will still need to be answered before this technology will translate into a practical therapeutic advance:

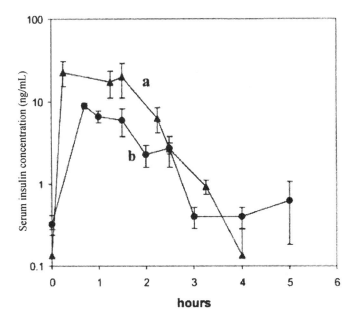

FIGURE 1 Serum insulin concentrations as a function of time after 40 minutes inhalation of 10 mg/mL suspension of insulin in absolute ethanol. The solid lines refer to the test animals, and the dashed lines represent the control animals. (From Ref. 5.)

1. What are the acute and chronic toxicity limits of inhaled ethanol in humans?
2. How can an inhalation delivery system be designed to safely deliver macromolecules and other drugs for systemic administration through the lungs, given the safety profile of ethanol, while maintaining user simplicity?
3. How long after delivery of ethanol to the lungs do lung epithelia remain especially permeable?
4. What is the molecular weight or other drug molecule–specific dependence on ethanol absorption?

Whether or not ethanol proves a key to substantially improving inhaled protein bioavailabilities in humans, research related to bioavailability enhancement is likely to be followed closely by those aiming to fully exploit the commercial potential of inhaled delivery systems for systemic application.

INCREASING DURATION OF THERAPEUTIC ACTION: THE CASE FOR NANOPARTICLES

Various attempts to achieve sustained drug action in the lungs following drug deposition via aerosol have led to promising results in animals but so far disappointing results in humans. These include the use of liposomes [19], polymers [20], and surfactants [21] and the modulation of particle size through the lowering of particle density [22]. Among the factors working against long action of drugs in the lungs are natural clearance mechanisms related to airway mucocilia and macrophages that remove drug particles within less than a day after deposition.

A 2002 study [6] that may point the way to solving the lung clearance problem involved the production of dry powder aerosol particles of aerodynamic diameter 1–5 microns that dissolve in the lungs into polymeric nanoparticles capable of releasing drug over long periods of time. The goal of the "Trojan" particles (i.e., particles designed to efficiently deliver to the lungs particles possessing dimensions and mass too small to otherwise deposit effectively in the lungs) is to aerosolize effectively from a simple inhaler in a dry powder form and then to release particles whose dimensions are sufficiently small to avoid mucociliary and phagocytic clearance until the particles have delivered their therapeutic payload. The hypothesis of this new drug delivery system is that, since nano-, or "ultrafine", particles, once deposited, often remain in the lung-lining fluid until dissolution (assuming they are soluble), escaping both phagocytic *and* mucociliary clearance mechanisms [23,24], deposition of drug-bearing nanoparticles in the lungs may offer the potential for sustained drug action and release throughout the lumen of the lungs.

The particles were made by spray-drying of an ethanol–water cosolvent into the form of large porous particles, characterized by geometric sizes greater than 5 μm and mass densities around 0.1 g/cm^3 or less, this physical structure having achieved recent popularity as carriers of drugs to the lungs for local and systemic applications [25].

Figure 2 illustrates the kinds of particles made in this study. Here, polystyrene nanoparticles (170-nm diameter) were prepared in an ethanol cosolvent and spray-dried to produce large thin-walled particles with a wall thickness of approximately 400 nm, or 3 layers of nanoparticles. The study showed that such particles aerosolize effectively from a small inhaler and redisperse into nanoparticles once in solution. Nanoparticle aggregates were made with a variety of different materials and through many different spray-drying conditions, suggesting that these large porous nanoparticle systems are robust and functional as aerosols.

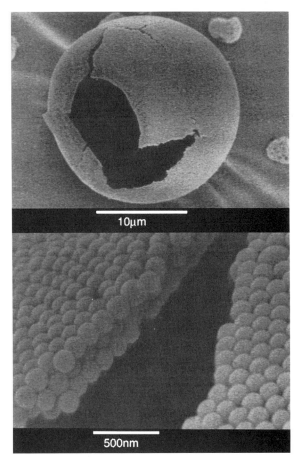

FIGURE 2 A hollow "Trojan" particle formed of polystryrene nanoparticles that spontaneously assemble into ordered arrays following spray-drying from a colloidal suspension. This particle, shown at two different magnifications, is sufficiently large and massive to enter the lungs and deposit prior to exhalation. Upon deposition, the particle can dissolve into nanoparticles, which by virtue of their small size can avoid the lungs' natural clearance systems (phagocytosis and mucociliary clearance). Such "large porous nanoparticle" (LPNP) aggregates may provide an important new drug delivery system for the sustained release of drugs for diseases such as asthma, chronic obstructive pulmonary disease, and tuberculosis. (From Ref. 6.)

The authors did not, however, incorporate drug into their particles or examine drug delivery properties in an animal model, thus it remains to be seen how effective these particles will be at actually achieving sustained drug release in the lungs. It is probable that the "noncleared" lifetime of the particles following deposition in the lungs will be highly dependent on the actual size of the nanoparticles; i.e., that smaller nanoparticle size will translate into longer potential lifetime in the lungs. However, achieving sustained drug release from very small particles is extremely challenging, particularly given the relative shortness of diffusion path lengths involved. Moreover, high drug load will also work against sustained release of drugs. Thus these large porous nanoparticle delivery systems will almost certainly have an optimal "duration of action" window, driven largely by nanoparticle size and drug load, though lacking experimental release data it is hard to know what this window of duration will actually be.

In any case such novel "Trojan" particle systems open up a new avenue of material property research for inhaled drug delivery systems and may help progress the goal of achieving long-action therapies through inhalation, for important diseases such as tuberculosis and diabetes.

SUMMARY

Delivery of drugs by inhalation to the systemic circulation will very likely become a health care reality by 2010. Starting most probably with insulin for diabetes, it may include growth hormone for growth deficiency, morphine for pain, and potentially some others. Should the field of inhalation delivery systems continue to advance appropriately, this new therapy may grow even more dramatically to lead to new therapies that replace current oral delivery therapies involving poorly absorbed compounds or compounds possessing a negative toxicity profile via the oral route. Two important areas of research that need urgent attention include the enhancement of drug absorption via the lungs, particularly for large proteins, and the enhancement of drug duration of action. Possibly the two technological advances described in this review will help point the way to achieving these goals. Should ethanol succeed as a chemical enhancer, it will help clarify the mechanism of absorption and perhaps lead to other ways of addressing absorption enhancement; likewise, should nanoparticles permit day-long (or greater) duration of action, they will likely illuminate other avenues for achieving the same end, perhaps more simply and with greater dose flexibility.

The inhalation drug delivery field, while still awaiting the first therapy approval, is poised to grow even more dramatically than since the early 1990s, but this requires continued and diligent scientific advance.

REFERENCES

1. Edward D, Dunbar C. Bioengineering of therapeutic aerosols. Annual Reviews of Bioengineering 4:93–107, 2002.
2. Patton J. Inhaled insulin. Adv Drug Deliv Rev 19:3–36, 1996.
3. Edwards DA, Hanes J, Caponetti G, Mintzes J, Hrkach J, Lotan N, Langer R. Large porous particles for pulmonary drug delivery. Science 276:1868–1871, 1997.
4. Rave KM, Heise T, Pfützner A, Stiner S, Heinemann L. Results of a dose–reponse study with a new pulmonary insulin formation and inhaler. Diabetes 49(Suppl. 1):305, 2000.
5. Choi WS, Murthy GGK, Edwards DA, Langer R, Klibanov AM. Inhalation delivery of proteins from ethanol suspensions. Proc Natl Acad Sci 98(20):11103–11107, 2001.
6. Tsapis N, Bennet D, Jackson B, Weitz D, Edwards DA. Trojan Particles: large porous nanoparticle systems for drug delivery. Proc Natl Acad Sci 99:12001–12005, 2002.
7. American Diabetes Association. Diabetes: Vital Statistics, Alexandria, VA, 1996.
8. National Diabetes Data Group. Diabetes in America: Diabetes Data Compiled. Bethesda, MD: National Institutes of Health, 1985.
9. Deckert T, Poulsen JE, Larsen M. Prognosis of diabetics with diabetes onset before the age of thirty-one. Diabetologia 14:363–377, 1978.
10. Rave K, Heise T, Pfützner A, Steiner S, Heinemann L. Results of a dose–response study with a new pulmonary insulin formulation and inhaler. 60th Scientific Sessions ADA; San Antonio, TX, 2000.
11. Heinemann L, Traut T, Heise T. Time-action profile of inhaled insulin. Diabet Med 14(1):63–72, 1997.
12. Osborn C, Batycky R, Verma A, Illerperuma A. Time–action profile of a new rapid-acting inhaled insulin with high biopotency. 61st Scientific Sessions ADA; Philadelphia, 1998.
13. Wolff RK. Safety of inhaled proteins for therapeutic use. J Aerosol Med 11:197–219, 1988.
14. Heinemann L, Klappoth W, Rave K, Hompesch B, Linkeschowa R, Heise T. Intra-individual variability of the metabolic effect of inhaled insulin together with an absorption enhancer. Diabetes Care 23(9):1343–1347, 2000.
15. Hilsted J, Madsbad S, Hvidberg A, Rasmussen MH, Krarup T, Ipsen H, Hansen B, Pedersen M, Djurup R, Oxenboll B. Intranasal insulin therapy: the clinical realities. Diabetologia 38:680–684, 1995.
16. Steiner S, Rave K, Heise T, Harzer O, Flacke F, Pfützner A, Heinemann L. Technosphere™/insulin: bioavailability and pharmacokinetic properties in healthy volunteers. Diabetologia 43(Suppl. 1):771, 2000.
17. Good WR, Powers MS, Campbell P, Schenkel L. A new transdermal delivery system for estradiol. J Control Release 2:89–97, 1985.
18. Santus GC, Baker RW. Transdermal enhancer patent literature. J Control Release 25(1–2):1–20, 1993.
19. Gregoriadis G. Engineering liposomes for drug discovery: progress and problems. Tibtech 13:527–537, 1995.

20. Deaton AT, Jones LD, Dunbar CA, Hickey AJ, Williams DM. Generation of gelatin aerosol particles from nebulized solutions as model drug carrier systems. Pharm Dev Technol 7(2):147–153, 2002.

21. Ben-Jebria A, Chen DH, Eskew ML, Vanbever R, Langer R, Edwards DA. Large porous particles for sustained protection from carbachol-induced bronchoconstriction in guinea pigs. Pharm Res 16(4):555–561, 1999.

22. Edwards DA, Ben-Jebria A, Langer R. Recent advances in pulmonary drug delivery using large, porous inhaled particles. J Appl Physiol 85(2):379–385, 1998.

23. French DL, Edwards DA, Niven RW. The influence of formulation on emission, deaggregation and deposition of dry powders for inhalation. J Aerosol Sci 27(5):769–783, 1996.

24. Kawaguchi H, Koiway N, Ohtsuka Y, Miyamoto M, Sasakawa S. Phagocytosis of latex-particles by leukocytes. 1. Dependence of phagocytosis on the size and surface-potential of particles. Biomaterials 7(1):61–66, 1986.

25. Edwards DA. Delivery of biological agents by aerosols. AIChE J 48(1):2–6, 2002.

18

Modulated Drug Therapy with Inhalation Aerosols: Revisited

Ralph Niven
Discovery Laboratories, Inc., Redwood City, California, U.S.A.

INTRODUCTION

A number of elegant devices have been developed in recent years that can deliver an aerosol to the deep lungs with high efficiency, but what can be influenced *after* deposition has occurred? Presently, there is little flexibility in aerosol formulations that will allow for manipulation of in vivo performance, and there remains an inadequate body of literature discussing the concept [1]. Despite this situation there is certainly more than ample justification for pursuing the topic, as specified in Table 1.

In a previous incarnation of this chapter, emphasis was placed on the *feasibility* of modulating pulmonary drug delivery. This version looks beyond feasibility and critically examines several formulation strategies that have been pursued since the early 1990s. Before proceeding, however, it is beneficial to mention topics that will be neglected. Clearance mechanisms and kinetics will not be mentioned, for they were covered at length in the first edition. The mathematics certainly hasn't changed, and, although our understanding of lung

TABLE 1   Reasons for Modulating Release of Drug in the Lungs

Optimization of drug combinations
Life cycle management of existing therapeutics
Limiting acute toxicity caused by the actions of the drug or in response to it
Minimizing toxicity arising from high initial levels of drug in the circulation
Limiting irritation due to the chemical action of a specific drug
Reducing the clearance rate of a drug of short pulmonary half-life
Taste-masking of drug deposited in the oral cavity
Improved targeting of drug load to macrophages
Tendency of some drugs to intrinsically exhibit extended "release" due to limited solubility
Improving in vivo stability due to chemical or biological degradation mechanisms
Influencing the potential for an immune response to the drug or components

biology has evolved, no earth-shattering developments in the way we analyze drug clearance have emerged. There is also the emergence of gene therapy, and many studies have aerosolized lipid–DNA complexes with the objective of sustaining the expression and "release" of protein therapeutics in the lungs. However, gene therapy is hardly a "classical" controlled delivery system and is beyond the scope of this chapter. Finally, the use of absorption enhancers to promote uptake will also be avoided because the vast majority, if not all, appear to exert their action by causing varying degrees of damage to the surrounding tissue.

SALTS AND PRECIPITATES
Salts

Surprisingly little work has been published since the early 1990s on the use of salt forms to enhance the performance of inhaled drugs. The concept is not novel and has not been ignored in years past [2–5]. Specific efforts were even made by Byron and coworkers in several publications [6–8] to demonstrate the influence of salt type on the dissolution of fluorescein in the lungs. Unfortunately, these observations appear not to have been exploited to a greater extent. Most of the work involving inhaled salts has revolved around inhalation toxicology of inorganic compounds found in the workplace or the environment. Perhaps this lack of pharmaceutical manipulation is a reflection of the de-emphasis of the pharmaceutical sciences within pharmacy curricula, in particular, those of the areas of physical chemistry [9], or, more simply, there have been numerous other avenues to pursue, which indeed there have. But surely the creation of drug salts is a less complex undertaking relative to creating dosage forms containing microspheres or liposomes, areas that have received far greater attention? Perhaps interest will be reinvigorated with the emergence of sensitive tools to analyze thermodynamic transformations, polymorphs, crystallites, and solvates of drugs [10–15]. Furthermore, the general recognition of the importance of surface characteristics [16] should ignite some enthusiasm toward altering these properties through manipulation of the salt.

Precipitates

The use of coprecipitates and complexes has, in contrast, received significant attention in recent years. This has been enabled by an increased use of spray-drying [17–19], the introduction of supercritical fluid extraction techniques [20,21] and related methods, such as spray-freeze-drying [19,22]. Together, these approaches allow investigators to generate an almost infinite variety of solid particulates. Spray-drying in particular is a versatile method of producing almost ideal particulates for inhalation in a single step [17,19,23]. In addition to solutions, suspensions and emulsions can readily be spray-dried; depending upon the components, the medium [24], and the spray-drying conditions [25,26], composite particles of unique character can be produced. A fairly recent example of extended release supported by pharmacodynamic data has been published by Ben-Jebria et al. [27], where spray-dried porous particles composed of lactose (18%), DPPC (60%), albumin (18%), and albuterol (4%) (by mass) were shown to extend the duration of action of albuterol in guinea pigs given periodic carbochol challenges. The results demonstrated that resistance to bronchoconstriction could be maintained for at least 16 hours (Fig. 1). However, the interpretation of the data emphasizes the porous characteristics of the particles and less so the composition. That is, it was thought that the clearance of the large, porous particles would be diminished relative to small, nonporous particles. Unfortunately, the study lacked a true control of nonporous particles of similar composition, and thus the relative importance of particle morphology versus particle composition has not been addressed.

The effort that leads to optimization of the particle morphology is largely one of trial and error, and there is no simple means to describe the distribution of components within individual particulates. Clearly, if the majority of an active component (API) is in the interior of a particle, then the dissolution or release characteristics are likely to differ from particles where the API is predominantly on the surface. The *surface* distribution of proteins and polymers within spray-dried particles has been studied using electron spectroscopy for chemical analysis that involves analyzing the energy signature of electrons scattered from surfaces while being bombarded by x-rays [11,28–31]. Conclusions can then be drawn

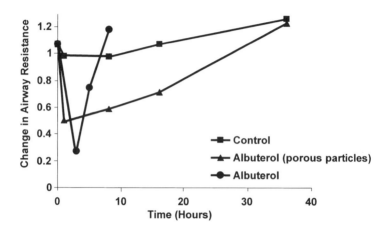

FIGURE 1   Response of guinea pig airways to periodic carbochol challenges after pretreatment with dry powder formulations containing albuterol.

about the overall distribution by comparing the initial presprayed bulk composition with the final surface composition. Taking this one step further, it should also be possible to garner some information about the release characteristics of composite particles. For instance, if there is an excess of drug at the surface then a "burst" effect is to be expected.

Surface changes are highly relevant for inhalation powders since they are customarily composed of particulates of high surface area relative to their volume. This has great significance to their aerosolization characteristics and is an area of current interest [16,32–37]. But almost any change of surface where we are dealing with micron-sized particles will also manifest during dissolution, and it seems reasonable to state that changes in the salt types or use of precipitated complexes, whether via spray-drying, milling, or supercritical fluid processing, can be better exploited for pulmonary applications.

The emphasis within the text is upon extending the effects of drugs in the lungs, but equally, modulated drug delivery applies to poorly soluble drugs where enhanced dissolution is desirable. A good example is Elan Pharmaceutical's NanoCrystal® technology that could be used to enhance aerosol delivery of poorly water-soluble drug compounds. This technology involves the use of a proprietary milling process with which to generate submicron-particle-size distributions and thus to capitalize on increases in dissolution that occur through increasing the overall particle surface area. Alternatively, composites with surfactant agents might also be expected to dissolve and spread more rapidly than the drug alone. In fact, the surfactant lining layer may contribute to the dissolution of hydrophobic drugs presented to the lung surface, as has been seen for budesonide [38].

COATED PARTICLES

A popular approach for tablets and granules is the application of coating materials [39]. These generally consist of natural or synthetic polymers, such as methacrylate, methylcellulose mixtures, and cellulose acetate phthalate (Aquacoat®), materials that would have dubious merits if employed for inhalation therapy. However, there have been a number of studies with aerosol powders demonstrating that release of probes can be markedly influenced after application of a coating agent. Notably, a study by Pillai et al. [40] using paraffin-coated particles was able to demonstrate a marked reduction in the absorption half-life of fluorescein and pentamidine. Related studies by Hickey et al. [7,41,42] have shown that the hygroscopic properties of aerosolized powders are altered when coated with fatty acids. It seems reasonable to expect that these materials would also influence the dissolution behavior in the lungs. The hydrophobic coatings constituted approximately 10% of the final particle mass, which is not substantive relative to the "drug" content when compared to the meager "payloads" offered by microspheres and liposomes, but there will always be the question of how much coating is necessary to achieve marked changes in dissolution and to what extent payload will be sacrificed. Fortunately, this may not be as much as first envisioned. Nanocoat Technologies Inc. (www.nano-sphere.com) is developing a technology that involves vapor deposition of minute quantities of biodegradable polymer (e.g., PLGA or PLA) using pulsed laser ablation. This approach has been used to efficiently coat the surface of hydrophobic drugs. Layer depths as small as 10 nm can have a profound effect on the dissolution of the "encapsulated" drug. Example data, using micronized particles of rifampicin, are shown in Fig. 2. This technology illustrates that of the various factors influencing dissolution, the *thoroughness* of the coverage can also play an important role.

LIPOSOMES AND LIPIDS

Around 1990, the pulmonary delivery of liposomes was largely an academic exercise [43–46] and at best at an early stage of commercial development [47]. However, these and earlier efforts demonstrated the utility of liposomes, and interest has continued to flourish. This has been reinforced by greater acceptance of the dosage form, since there are now several injectable liposomal products on the market [e.g., Ambisome®, Fungisome®, Myocet®]. The specific use of lipid-based vehicles to deliver plasmid-based DNA has attracted much attention [48–51]. These developments have indirectly helped improve the quality and variety of

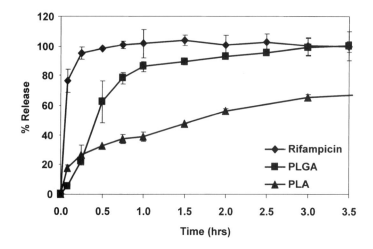

FIGURE 2   In vitro release profiles of rifampicin and rifampicin coated with PLGA or PLA.

lipids now available, and for similar reasons better analytical technology to study liposome characteristics and biology has emerged.

Nebulization can cause disruption or "processing" of multilameller vesicles [52]. Fortunately, these issues can be addressed, and, through manipulation of the composition, buffer and environment liposomes have been aerosolized without causing loss of entrapped drug [53–55]. Liposomes have also been prepared as spray-dried and lyophilized powders [56–59]. The former may be aerosolized directly as a powder, but in both cases reconstitution in an aqueous environment results in liposome formation. However, it is not understood if this is just spontaneous reformation of original liposomes (pre-spray-drying) or the creation of de novo liposomes in an aqueous environment.

With respect to safety and the use of phospholipids, no NDA-supporting chronic inhalation studies have been conducted except for those found in commercial pulmonary surfactants. These studies presumably will have involved intratracheal instillation and *not* aerosolization, since the primary indication is respiratory distress syndrome of the newborn. Nevertheless, the fact that these products are available suggests that synthetic versions of natural lipids such as dipalmitoyl phosphatidylcholine (DPPC) and dipalmitoyl phosphatidylglycerol (DPPG) are likely to be well tolerated. This assumption has been supported from subchronic aerosol studies in mice [60] and acute single-dose aerosol studies in man, the latter involving soy-derived phosphatidylcholines [61].

A variety of other small molecules and proteins have also been incorporated with liposomes. In all cases, modulation of absorption or the response has been distinguished due to the presence of the phospholipids. A brief discussion on selected molecules now follows.

The potential of liposomes as extended delivery vehicles for beta-agonists has been investigated [62–65]. The rationale is logical because the short duration of action of compounds like terbutaline and albuterol requires frequent dosing (1–2 actuations four times daily). A less frequent dosing regime would be welcomed by patients and may lead to better compliance and less abuse of these drugs. Results with metoproterenol proved disappointing, but animals receiving albuterol [64] and terbutaline [63] resisted a challenge from a bronchocontstricting agent for an extended period relative to the drug alone. To some degree, interest in this approach has waned with the introduction of longer-acting beta-2 agonists such as salmeterol [66] and formoterol [67]. However, these newer drugs do not satisfy the need for immediate relief that the short-acting beta-agonists can provide.

An intriguing 1996 study conducted by Li and Mitra [68] examined the length of the acyl side chain of the lipids on the absorption of insulin from the lungs and observed an unusual parabolic relationship between glucose lowering and the length of the acyl side chain (Fig. 3). In a 2001 paper [69] they expand on this finding and note that DPPC mixtures with insulin produce higher circulating levels of insulin than liposomes alone after intratracheal instillation. Together, these results highlight the importance of phospholipid type *and* structure on biological effects.

Cyclosporine A is indicated for the prophylaxis of organ rejection associated with allogeneic transplants. It has not been indicated for lung allografts, because systemic therapy does not provide the necessary level of imunosuppression at tolerable doses [70]. It is poorly water-soluble and has been formulated in various solvents, including alcohol, oil, and even Cremophor EL. Issues concerning inhaled therapy relate to the narrow therapeutic index of the drug, the high doses that will be necessary for transplant rejection, possible irritation in sensitive and diseased tissue, the increased risk of infection and, importantly, the identification of a suitable formulation [71]. Although cyclosporine has been nebulized using nonaqueous intravenous formulations [72,73], this is hardly an optimized medium. Not surprisingly, cyclosporine has been successfully formulated as a liposome aerosol [70] and has been tested in normal volunteers [74]. Some irritation was noted, which appears to have been related to the drug and not the lipids. This apparently was lessened through the use of a face mask. The pharmacokinetics of the liposome formulation has been studied in dogs via inhalation, and, as expected, lung concentrations were substantially higher than those of the other major organs [75].

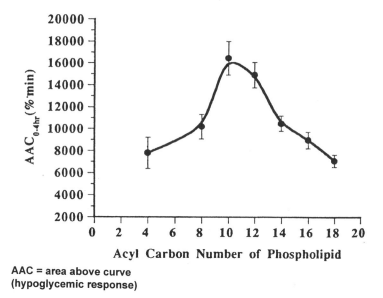

AAC = area above curve
(hypoglycemic response)

FIGURE 3   Influence of the length of the phospholipid acyl side chain on the pulmonary absorption of insulin.

Various glucocorticoids have also attracted attention for delivery using liposomes as a vehicle [71,76–81]. These are highly potent molecules normally delivered from pressurized metered-dose inhalers or dry powder inhalers for treatment of asthma. Young children with asthma or infants with inflammatory lung conditions cannot be treated using pMDIs or DPIs. The alternative is to use a nebulizer, but this has, until recently, required that the drug be soluble in an aqueous environment—an issue for all the major inhaled steroids. Dilauryl PC in combination with beclomethasone diproprionate has been evaluated using a variety of nebulizers [76], with a view to identifying those devices best suited for aerosol delivery. A subsequent adult volunteer study was completed, and no adverse responses were reported after using reservoir doses of 1 mg beclomethasone and 25 mg dilauryl PC/mL. Dexamethasone entrapped in liposomes has also been tested in animal models [81,82] and found to be better retained in the lungs than "free" dexamethasone, signifying that the liposomes have a role in modulating absorption [82]. Triamcinolone acetonide (TA) and the phosphate (TAP) have also been incorporated in DSPC and DSPG lipsomes, where it was found that pulmonary residence time was a function of liposome size for TAP-containing but not the TA-containing liposomes. The conclusions that can be drawn from these studies is that there is a role for lipid-based steroid therapy but that much has yet to be learned about how they should best be formulated and used in the clinical setting. Furthermore, any liposome formulation worthy of commercial development will have to compete with the nebulizer-compatible budesonide suspensions (now available as Pulmicort Respules®) that are now in widespread use [83–86].

Antibiotics have also been aerosolized with lipids [87]. This combination has come about to deliver therapeutic agents that might otherwise not be used because of low solubility or toxicity. There are a variety of antibacterials, antifungals, and antivirals that demonstrate excellent in vitro activity but are not effective because of their systemic toxicity and/or poor penetration into the lung tissue. It is also believed that liposomes might be a means to deliver drug to macrophages harboring infections such as tuberculosis or other mycobacteria [88,89]. However, it has been known for many years that although alveolar macrophages will happily phagocytose liposomes, the phagosomes remain excluded from the cystol [90]. Unless the antibiotic is capable of diffusing across the internalized membranes, the liposome-drug targeting ability is compromised.

The main concern with delivering antibiotics to the lungs is the dose required. Recommended doses of most antibiotics via inhalation (e.g., colistin or tobramycin) are in the range of 250–500 mg daily. The drugs require delivery via nebulizer or some form of continuous delivery device. Drug concentrations as high as possible are necessary to deliver the maximum concentration of antibiotic to the lung surface, to minimize the dosing time, and thus, hopefully, to maximize compliance. Combined with lipids, the absolute mass dosed may exceed gram quantities, amounts that may be intolerable even if successful formulations could be created.

Formulations will increasingly become more complex as the content of the antibiotic is raised within the liposomes [91], and stability is a general concern: Dispersions may exhibit aqueous stability of only a matter of days. This issue has partially been addressed through the use of reconstituted lyophilized preps, and a formulation of anamycin has demonstrated over 3 months' stability in the solid state [56]. Beauloac et al. [58] have taken this one step further by aerosolizing a dry powder of lyophilized liposome-tobramycin to administer to mice infected with *Pseudomonas aeruginosa*. [58]. However, the use of powdered preparations does not address the dosing problem.

The merits of liposome antibiotic therapy vs. antibiotic alone seem rarely to have been compared directly. Studies have shown benefit of using some liposome antifungals [92], but the formulations were either under development or were commercialized as a liposome product for administration by injection [93]. So the debate must continue. Although liposomal formulations can be generated and aerosolized and have proved effective in combination with various drugs, do the benefits ultimately outweigh the issues developing these kinds of formulations [94]?

MICROSPHERES AND NANOSPHERES

Improvements in the techniques and ability to incorporate proteins and peptides, better targeting approaches, and new materials have been developed since the early 1990s, and thus many microsphere-based products are under clinical development for delivery via most routes of administration [22,95,96]. One of their chief advantages is that the duration of drug release can be extended to a greater degree than virtually any other formulation option, although this benefit may be curtailed in the lungs. Other issues surrounding micropshere use have included stability, loading efficiency, and a method of production that has traditionally involved organic solvents [97,98]. There are, however, newer technologies (e.g., Promaxx®—Epic Therapeutics, www. epictherapeutics.com) where processing is conducted entirely in an aqueous environment using water-soluble polymers. Unfortunately, with pulmonary delivery come the added concerns of what materials can be used and whether micropsheres of a size suitable for pulmonary delivery $(1-5\,\mu m)$ can readily be prepared. These general issues have, to date, limited the pulmonary use of microspheres, although those formed using albumin [99,100], lipid [101], or PLGA [102] have been delivered to the lungs, demonstrating the feasibility of using the dosage form.

Can they be used practically in the lungs? Albumin would an ideal biodegradable encapsulating agent, but, to be practical, a low-cost recombinant version of the protein is a prerequisite. Using synthetic spray-dried micropsheres in combination with drugs that would otherwise be cleared rapidly seems logical, especially where the duration of therapy would be short-term rather than of a chronic nature. A nontherapeutic example might be their use as diagnostic contrast agents [103]. This would reduce safety concerns about the accumulation of polymeric material or, say, acidity arising from the biodegradation of commonly employed PLA and PLGA compositions [104,105]. Nevertheless, as long as simpler formulation options exist, the use of a microsphere preparation is unlikely to be developed for pulmonary use in the near term.

POLYMER CONJUGATION

The "PEGylation" of peptides and proteins has proved to be a highly successful means of extending the circulating half-life of a number of proteins after injection. Several are now approved or close to approval, including PEGylated interferon alfa (PEG Intron®, Pegasys®), pegademase, pegasparaginase, and PEGylated rhG-CSF (SD/01). This general interest has not translated to any significant product development for pulmonary delivery, and few feasibility studies have been conducted. PEGylated superoxide dimutase has proved to be a successful oxygen-radical scavenger in a rodent model of oxygen-induced toxicity [106], while PEGylated G-CSF can generate an extended neutropenic response despite limited pulmonary absorption [107]. PEG conjugates of ovalbumin have also been aerosolized to dogs as "desensitizers." Bronchoconstriction to subsequent ovalbumin aerosol challenges were completely blocked [108]. There actually seems no clear reason for not pursuing the use of PEGylation in clinical studies. Two-week toxicity studies in animals using PEG have not exhibited any pathological conditions or responses that would warrant the apparent reticence [109]. Furthermore, where there is a need to restrict absorption and to limit systemic side effects (e.g., certain antibiotics or cytokines), this approach may have merit as a targeted delivery system.

LIMITATIONS AND ISSUES

Unlike the majority of controlled-, sustained-, or extended-release systems in use, the extent of response in the lungs will be limited by intrinsic clearance mechanisms [110]. It will be surprising, but not unwelcome, if any deposited dosage form can extend the effective duration of action much beyond a day. Twenty-four hours would, in fact, be a significant achievement.

Another issue is reproducibility. The formulation may work perfectly in an in vitro test system, but the dosage form requires aerosolization, and lung deposition is a function of the characteristics of the aerosol (dose, mass concentration, droplet/particle size, etc.) and the nature of the inspiratory maneuver, a factor that the patient has control over. These factors can influence performance to a far greater extent than can be "built" into a particle, and thus the term controlled does not seem a defensible objective for pulmonary delivery. The vagaries of the deposition profile and of the amount that will deposit also imply that sustaining a certain drug concentration is a difficult proposition, but the loosest definition extended release, seems an acceptable goal within the boundaries set by the clearance mechanisms.

A basic concern is the limited set of materials that can be safely packaged with a drug. It is the inactive components that impart flexibility to a dosage form. Unfortunately, relatively few materials have been thoroughly evaluated for use in pulmonary products, and only *one* excipient, lactose, is approved for general use. From a pharmaceutical perspective, lactose is less than ideal, being a reducing sugar, a characteristic that can have implications for protein and peptide stability [111,112]. Not surprisingly therefore, various other sugars, such as nonreducing trehalose, are being used with the tacit but reasonable assumption that they are safe. Several others are found in combination with a specific product (e.g., the components of lung surfactant) and thus have been employed in delivery systems. Other, untested compounds that are generally regarded as safe (GRAS) by other routes of administration might also be evaluated. However, the use by one route does not mean that the use via another is appropriate. Despite the efficiency of the clearance mechanisms, there are general concerns that the introduction of polymeric carriers, for example, may result in toxicity through chronic use. This may be via gradual accumulation of poorly absorbed components of limited biodegradability or, if degraded, the byproducts could result in local inflammation. So the context of the use and the characteristics of the proposed material must be carefully weighed. The more adventurous investigators and companies have also begun to explore novel entities such as sugar–lipid conjugates [Quadrant—Elan] that ultimately should expand the choice of materials that can be used in pulmonary products.

The boundary between classification as an excipient or as an active component is not always easy to differentiate. Testing required in stability programs and accompanying documentation must be expanded to satisfy chemistry, manufacturing, and control (CMC) requirements during clinical development. Thus, the additional efforts and costs to develop the formulation must be balanced by the benefits expected from the inclusion of the additives. The state of the excipient must also be considered. Is the dosage form dominated by an amorph or crystalline polymorph of an identical excipient? Will the product be affected by phase transitions occurring at body temperature that would not be seen at room-temperature storage? Does the cellular response to the additive(s) differ from that using the drug alone? Are there acute changes in tonicity after lung deposition? Multiple questions like these may have to be addressed, if not to provide supporting application data, then to provide peace of mind to the developer.

Experimental modeling and analytical testing is an ever-present problem. The lining layer of a human lung consists of an ill-defined steady-state volume of approximately 40 mL spread over a surface area of between 70 and 140 m^2 [113]. Furthermore, the surface of the alveolar lining fluid consists of an ever-changing lipid–protein monolayer [114], whereas within the airways this layer is a complicated mixture of mucopolysaccharides, surfactant, DNA and various proteins [115–117]. It is not a simple matter to mimic such a medium on the bench: Lavage fluid has been used, but this is a highly diluted, variable, and often-contaminated solution (blood, cells) and fails to represent the medium in a physiologically relevant arrangement. Dissolution from a rotating disk or within a standard dissolution apparatus will always generate data, but there is no assurance that this information will predict what may happen in vivo. A number of attempts have been made to resolve, at least in part, this situation. McConville et al. [118] have been exploring the use of modified twin-stage impinger to deposit and monitor drug release, while other attempts have monitored release from aerosol deposits on filters [119]. No approach is ideal, and significantly more work is necessary to establish a test apparatus that can generate data at a reasonable experimental throughput and that investigators can have confidence in.

Why is an in vitro test system needed? Because it is far easier to generate formulations for testing than it is to conduct a thorough evaluation in small-animal models whose relevance to the human lung architecture is tenuous at best [120]. Furthermore, the mode of delivery often dictates the data that will be observed. Intratracheal instillation or insufflation is not representative of aerosol delivery and is difficult to perform reproducibly. The technique is useful for initially determining if a pharmacological response will be observed or if absorption takes place, but no conclusions should be drawn regarding the nature of absorption-vs.-time profiles. In contrast, aerosol delivery is expensive, complicated to set up and monitor, and time consuming. There is also no standardization of models or delivery technique. The upshot is that results cannot be generated rapidly and that even under the best of circumstances data will be highly variable, requiring a large number of animals to statistically discriminate between formulations.

CONCLUSIONS

The concluding remarks made in the first edition of the book highlighted numerous opportunities that were not being realized due to general concerns about safety. Unfortunately, despite the greater awareness of the inhaled route as a mode of delivery, the landscape is still essentially the same. One could also argue that there has not been a compelling economic reason to tackle the safety and formulation questions, which, although difficult, are not insurmountable. Despite this sobering viewpoint and the critical nature of this discourse, there is a promising trend within the field. Efforts under way appear more focused and, rather than emphasizing feasibility, tend to be more product oriented. That is, the choices of drug and components are being made on a rational pharmaceutical basis. Hopefully, this trend will continue and the inherent risks of pursuing modulated pulmonary drug delivery will be rewarded.

REFERENCES

1. Hardy JG, Chadwick TS. Sustained release drug delivery to the lungs: an option for the future. Clin Pharmacokinet 39(1):1–4, 2000.
2. Lewis AJ, et al. The comparative bronchodilator properties of alkyl quaternary salts of promethazine. Int Arch Allergy Appl Immunol 75(3): 282–283, 1984.
3. Scherer PW, et al. Growth of hygroscopic aerosols in a model of bronchial airways. J Appl Physiol 47(3):544–550, 1979.

4. Sciarra JJ, Patel JM, Kapoor AL. Synthetics and formulation of several epinephrine salts as an aerosl dosage form. J Pharm Sci 61(2):219–223, 1972.
5. Chowhan ZT, Amaro AA. Pulmonary absorption studies utilizing in situ rat lung model: designing dosage regimen for bronchial delivery of new drug entities. J Pharm Sci 65(11):1669–1672, 1976.
6. Hickey AJ, Byon PR. Preparation characterization, and controlled release from coprecipitates of fluorescein and magnesiumhydroxide. J Pharm Sci 75(8):756–759, 1986.
7. Hickey AJ, Jackson GV, Fildes FJ. Preparation and characterization of disodium fluorescein powders in association with lauric and capric acids. J Pharm Sci 77(9):804–809, 1988.
8. Niven RW, Byron PR. Solute absorption from the airways of the isolated rat lung. I. The use of absorption data to quantify drug dissolution or release in the respiratory tract. Pharm Res 5(9):574–579, 1988.
9. Wurster DE. Will the Pharm.D. make the pharmaceutics Ph.D. an endangered species? Pharm Dev Technol 2(1):vii–viii, 1997.
10. Yu L. Amorphous pharmaceutical solids: preparation, characterization and stabilization. Adv Drug Deliv Rev 48(1):27–42, 2001.
11. Blomberg E, Claesson PM, Froberg JC. Surfaces coated with protein layers: a surface force and ESCA study. Biomaterials 19(4–5):371–386, 1998.
12. Desai TR, et al. Determination of surface free energy of interactive dry powder liposome formulations using capillary penetration technique. Colloids Surf B Biointerfaces 22(2):107–113, 2001.
13. Bottom R. The role of modulated temperature differential scanning calorimetry in the characterization of a drug molecule exhibiting polymorphic and glass forming tendencies. Int J Pharm 192(1):47–53, 1999.
14. Newell HE, et al. The use of inverse phase gas chromatography to study the change of surface energy of amorphous lactose as a function of relative humidity and the processes of collapse and crystallization. Int J Pharm 217(1–2):45–56, 2001.
15. Rabel SR, Jona JA, Maurin MB. Applications of modulated differential scanning calorimetry in performulation studies. J Pharm Biomed Anal 21(2):339–345, 1999.
16. Buckton G. Characterization of small changes in the physical properties of powders of significance for dry powder inhaler formulations. Adv Drug Deliv Rev 26(1):17–27, 1997.
17. Masters K. Spray Drying Handbook. 5th ed. New York: Halsted Press, 725, 1991.
18. Christensen KL, Pedersen GP, Kristensen HG. Preparation of redispersible dry emulsions by spray drying. Int J Pharm 212(2):187–194, 2001.
19. Maa YF, et al. Protein inhalation powders: spray drying vs spray freeze drying. Pharm Res 16(2):249–254, 1999.
20. Palakodaty S, York P, Pritchard J. Supercritical fluid processing of materials from aqueous solutions: the applications of SEDS to lactose as a model substance. Pharma Res 15(12):1835–1843, 1998.
21. York P. Strategies for particle design using supercritical fluid technologies. Pharm Sci Technol Today 2(11):430–440, 1999.

22. Constantine HR, et al. Protein spray-freeze drying. Effect of atomization conditions on particle size and stability. Pharm Res 17(11):1374–1383, 2000.

23. Vanbever R, et al. Formulation and physical characterization of large porous particles for inhalation. Pharm Res 16(11):1735–1742, 1999.

24. Bain DF, Monday DL, Smith A. Solvent influence on spray-dried biodegradable microspheres. J Microencapsulate 16(4):453–474, 1999.

25. Maa YF, et al. The effect of operating and formulation variables on the morphology of spray-dried protein particles. Pharm Dev Technol 2(3):213–223, 1997.

26. Dunbar CA, Concession NM, Hickey AJ. Evaluation of atomizer performance in production of respirable spray-dried particles. Pharm Dev Technol 3(4):433–441, 1998.

27. Ben-Jebria A, et al. Large porous particles for sustained protection form carbochol-induced bronchoconstriction in guinea pigs. Pharm Res 16(4):555–561, 1999.

28. Kieswetter K, et al. Characterization of calcium phosphate powders by ESCA and EDXA. Biomaterials 15(3):183–188, 1994.

29. Millqvist-Fureby A, Malmsten M, Bergenstahl B. Spray-drying of trypsin—surface characterization and activity preservation. Int J Pharm 188(2):243–253, 1999.

30. Millqvish-Fureby A, Malmsten M, Bergenstahl B. An aqueous polymer two-phase system as carrier in the spray-drying of biological material. J Colloid Interface Sci 225(1)54–61, 2000.

31. Adler M, Unger M, Lee G. Surface composition of spray-dried particles of bovine serum albumin/trehalose/surfactant. Pharm Res 17(7):863–870, 2000.

32. Tee SK, et al. The use of different sugars as fine and coarse carriers for aerosolized salbutamol sulphate. Int J Pharm 208(1–2):111–123, 2000.

33. Zeng XM, et al. The influence of carrier morphology on drug delivery by dry powder inhalers. Int J Pharm 200(1):93–106, 2000.

34. Bosquillon C, et al. Influence of formulation excipients and physical characteristics of inhalation dry powders on their aerosolization performance. J Control Release 70(3):329–339, 2001.

35. de Villiers MM. Influence of cohesive properties of micronized drug powders on particle size analysis. J Pharm Biomed Anal 13(3):191–198, 1995.

36. Fults KA, Miller IF, Hickey AJ. Effect of particle morphology on emitted dose of fatty acid-treated disodium cromoglycate powder aerosols. Pharm Dev Technol 19952(1):67–79, 1995.

37. Suarez S, Hickey AJ. Drug properties affecting aerosol behavior. Respir Care 45(6):652–666, 2000.

38. Pharm S, Wiedmann TS. Note: dissolution of aerosol particles of budesonide in Survanta, a model lung surfactant. J Pharm Sci 90(1):98–104, 2001.

39. Porter SC. Coating of pharmaceutical dosage forms. In: Remington: The Science and Practice of Pharmacy, Gennaro AR, ed. Lippincot Williams & Wilkins: Philadelphia, 2000, pp. 894–902.

40. Pillai RS, et al. Controlled dissolution from wax-coated aerosol particles in canine lungs. J Appl Physiol 84(2):717–725, 1998.

41. Hickey AJ, et al. Effect of hydrophobic coating on the behavior of a hygroscopic aerosol powder in an environment of controlled temperature and relative humidity. J Pharm Sci 79(11):1009–1014, 1990.

42. Hickey AJ, Martonen TB. Behavior of hygroscopic pharmaceutical aerosols and the influence of hydrophobic additives. Pharm Res 10(1):1–7, 1993.

43. Meisner D, Pringle J, Mezei M. Liposomal pulmonary drug delivery. I. In vivo disposition of atropine base in solution and liposomal form following endotracheal instillation to the rabbit lung. J Microencapsul 6(3):379–387, 1989.

44. Jurima-Romet M, Shek PN. Lung uptake of liposome-entrapped glutathione after intratracheal administration. J Pharm Pharmacol 43(1):6–10, 1991.

45. McCalden TA, Porter J, Kamarei A. Aerosol delivery of lipsomes metaproternol sulfate. Pro West Pharmacol Soc 33, 171–173, 1990.

46. Forsgren P, et al. Intrapulmonary deposition of aerosolized Evans blue dye and liposomes in an experimental porcine model of early ARDS. Ups J Med Sci 95(2):117–136, 1990.

47. Fielding RM. The use of inhaled liposome formulations for drug delivery to the lungs and systemic circulation. Proc West Pharmacol Soc 32, 103–106, 1989.

48. Scheule RK, Cheng SH. Airway delivery of cationic lipid: DNA complexes for cystic fibrosis. Adv Drug Deliv Rev 30(1–3):173–184, 1998.

49. Eastman SJ, et al. Optimization of formulations and conditions for the aerosol delivery of functional cationic lipid: DNA complex. Hum Gene Ther 8(3):313–322, 1997.

50. McDonald RJ, et al. Aerosol delivery of lipd:DNA complexes to lungs of rhesus monkeys. Pharm Res 15(5):671–679, 1998.

51. Stribling R, et al. Aerosol gene delivery in vivo. Proc Natl Acad Sci USA 89(23):11277–11281, 1992.

52. Gilbert BE, et al. Small particle aerosols of enviroxime-containing lipsomes. Antiviral Res 9(6):355–365, 1988.

53. Niven RW, Schreier H. Nebulization of liposomes. I. Effect of lipid composition. Pharm Res 7(11):1127–1133, 1990.

54. Niven RW, Speer M, Schreier H. Nebulization of liposomes. II. The effects of size and modeling of solute release profiles. Pharm Res 8(2):217–221, 1991.

55. Niven RW, Carvajal TM, Schreier H. Nebulization of liposomes. III. The effects of operating conditions and local environment. Pharm Res 9(4):515–520, 1991.

56. Zou Y, Priebe W, Perz-Soler R. Lyophilized preliposomal formulation of the non-cross-resistant anthracycline anamycin: effect of surfactant on liposome formation, stability and size. Cancer Chemother Pharmacol 39(1–2):103–108, 1996.

57. Skalko-Basnet N, Pavelin Z, Becirevic-Lacan M. Liposomes containing drug and cyclodextrin prepared by the one-step spray-drying method. Drug Dev Ind Pharm 26(12):1279–1284, 2000.

58. Beaulac C, Sachetelli S, Lagace J. Aerosolization of low phase transition temperature liposomal tobramycin as a dry powder in an animal model of chronic pulmonary infection caused by Pseudomonas aeruginosa. J Drug Target 7(1):33–41, 1999.

59. Schreier H, Hickey AJ, Niven RW. Formulation and in vitro performance of liposome powder aerosols. STP Pharma 4, 1–3, 1994.
60. Myers MA, et al. Pulmonary effects of chronic exposure to liposome aerosols in mice. Exp Lung Res 19(1):1–19, 1993.
61. Thomas DA, et al. Acute effects of liposome aerosol inhalation on pulmonary function in healthy human volunteers. Chest 99(5):1268–1270, 1991.
62. Vyas SP, Sakthivel T. Pressurized pack-based liposomes for pulmonary targeting of isoprenaline—development and characterization. J Microencapsul 11(4):373–380, 1994.
63. Fielding RM, Abra RM. Factors affecting the release rate of terbutaline from liposome formulations after intratracheal instillation in the guinea pig. Pharm Res 9(2):220–223, 1992.
64. McCalden TA, Radhakrishnan R. A comparative study of thebronchodilator effect and duration of action of liposome encapsulated beta-2 adrenergic agonists in the guinea-pig. Pulm Pharmacol 4(3):140–145, 1991.
65. Taylor KM, Newton JM. Liposomes for controlled delivery of drugs to the lung. Thorax 47(4):257–259, 1992.
66. Lotvall J, Svedmyr N. Salmeterol: an inhaled beta 2-agonist with prolonged duration of action. Lung 171(5):249–264, 1993.
67. Bartow RA, Brogden RN. Formoterol. An update of its pharmacological properties and therapeutic efficacy in the management of asthma. Drugs 2(55):303–322, 1998.
68. Li Y, Mitra AK. Effects of phospholipid chain length, concentration, charge, and vescile size on pulmonary insulin absorption. Pharm Res 13(1):76–79, 1996.
69. Mitra R, et al. Enhanced pulmonary delivery of insulin by lung lavage fluid and phospholipids. Int J Pharm 217(1–2):25–31, 2001.
70. Gilbert BE, et al. Characterization and administration of cyclosporine liposomes as a small-particle aerosol. Transplantation 56(4):974–977, 1993.
71. Klyaschitsky BA, Owen AJ. Nebulizer-compatible liquid formulations for aerosol pulmonary delivery of hydrophobic drugs: glucocorticoids and cyclosporine. J Drug Target 7(2):79–99, 1999.
72. Ceyhan B, et al. Effect of inhaled ingredients of a commercial cyclosporin A ampoule on airway inflammation. Respiration 65(1):89, 1998.
73. Ceyhan BB, et al. Effect of inhaled cyclosporin on the rat airway: histologic and bronchoalveoar lavage assessment. Respiration 65(1):71–78, 1998.
74. Gilbert BE, et al. Tolerance of volunteers to cyclosporine A-dilauroylphosphatidylcholine liposome aerosol. Am J Respir Crit Care Med 156(6):1789–1793, 1997.
75. Letsou GV, et al. Pharmacokinetics of liposomal aerosolized cyclosporine A for pulmonary immunosuppressin. Ann Thorac Surg 68(6):2044–2048, 1999.
76. Waldrep JC, et al. Operating characteristics of 18 different continuous-flow jet nebulizers with beclomethasone diproprionate liposome aerosol. Chest 105(1):106–110, 1994.
77. Waldrep JC, et al. Pulmonary delivery of beclomethasone liposome aerosol in volunteers. Tolerance and safety. Chest 111(2):316–323, 1997.

78. Batavia R, et al. The measurement of beclomethasone diproprionate entrapment in liposomes: a comparison of a microscope and an HPLC method. Int J Pharm 212(1):109–119, 2001.

79. Gonzqlez-Rothi RJ, et al. Pulmonary targeting of liposomal triamcinolone acetonide phosphate. Pharm Res 13(11):1699–1703, 1996.

80. Suarez S, et al. Effect of dose and release rate on pulmonary targeting of liposomal Triamcinolone acetonide phosphate. Pharm Res 15(3):461–465, 1998.

81. DiMatteo M, Reasor MJ. Modulation of silica-induced pulmonary toxicity by dexamethasone-containing liposomes. Toxicol Appl Pharmacol 142(2):411–421, 1997.

82. Suntrez ZE, Shek PN. Liposomes promote pulmonaryglucocorticoid delivery. J Drug Target 6(3):175–182, 1998.

83. Hvizdos KM, Jarvis B. Budesonid inhalation suspension: a review of its use in infants, children and adults with inflammatory respiratory disorders. Drugs 60(5):1141–1178, 2000.

84. Shapiro G, et al. Efficacy and safety of budesonide inhalation suspension (Pulmicort Respules) in young children with inhaled steroid-dependent, persistent asthma. J Allergy Clin Immunol 102(5):789–796, 1998.

85. Scott MB, Skoner DP. Short-term and long-term safety of budesonide inhalation suspension in infants and young children with persistent asthma. J Allergy Clin Immunol 104(4 Pt 2):200–209, 1999.

86. Szefler SJ. Meeting needs of infants and young children with asthma: new developments in nebulized corticosteroid therapy. Introduction. J Allergy Clin Immunol 104(4 Pt 2):159–161, 1999.

87. Gilbert BE. Liposomal aerosols in the management of pulmonary infections. J Aerosol Med 9(1):111–122, 1996.

88. Honeybourne D. Antibiotic penetration in the respiratory tract and implications for the selection of antimicrobial therapy. Curr Opin Pulm Med 3(2):170–174, 1997.

89. Barrow WW. Treatment of mycobacterial infections. Rev Sci Tech 20(1):55–70, 2001.

90. Petty HR, McConnell HM. Cytochemical study of liposome and lipid vesicle phagocytosis. Biochim Biophys Acta 735(1):77–85, 1983.

91. Pedroso de Lima MC, et al. Interaction of antimycobacterial and anti-pneumocystis drugs with phospholipid membranes. Chem Phys Lipids 53(4):361–371, 1990.

92. Ruijgrok EJ, Vulto AG, Van Etten EW. Aerosol delivery of amphotericin B Desoxycholate (Fungizone) and liposomal amphotericin B (AmBisome): aerosol characteristics and in-vivo amphotericin B deposiiton in rats. J Pharm Pharmacol 52(6):619–627, 2000.

93. Purcell IF, Corris PA. Use of nebulized liposomal amphotericin B in the treatment of *Aspergillus fumigatus* empyema. Thorax 50(12):1312–1323, 1995.

94. Kulkarni SB, Betageri GV, Singh M. Factors affecting microencapsulation of drugs in liposomes. J Microencapsul 12(3):229–246, 1995.

95. Ravi Kumar MN. Nano and microparticles as controlled drug delivery devices. J Pharm Pharm Sci 3(2):234–258, 2000.

96. Bartus RT, et al. Sustained delivery of proteins for novel therapeutic agents. Science 281(5380):1161–1162, 1998.

97. Cleland JL. Solvent evaporation processes for the production of controlled release biodegradable microsphere formulations for therapeutics and vaccines. Biotechnol Prog 14(1):102–107, 1998.

98. Watts PJ, Davies MC, Melia CD. Microencapsulation using emulsification/solvent evaporation: an overview of techniques and applications. Crit Rev Ther Drug Carrier Syst 7(3):235–259, 1990.

99. Haghpanah M, Marriott C, Martin GP. Potential use of microencapsulation for sustained drug delivery to the respiratory tract. J Aerosl Med 7(2):185–188, 1994.

100. Todisco T, et al. Fate of human albumin micropshere and spherocyte radioaerosols in the human tracheobronchial tree. Lung 168, 665–671, 1990.

101. Bot AI, et al. Novel lipid-based hollow-porous microparticles as a platform for immunoglobulin delivery to the respiratory tract. Pharm Res 17(3):275–283, 2000.

102. O'Hara P, Hickey AJ. Respirable PLGA microspheres containing rifampicin for the treatment of tuberculosis: manufacture and characterization. Pharm Res 17(8):955–961, 2000.

103. Narayan P, Marchant D, Wheatley MA. Optimization of spray drying by factorial design for production of hollow microspheres for ultrasound imaging. J Biomed Mater Res 56(3):333–341, 2001.

104. Martin C, Winet H, Bao JY. Acidity near eroding polylactide-polyglycolide in vitro and in vivo in rabbit tibial bone chambers. Biomaterials 17(24):2373–2380, 1996.

105. Fu K, et al. Visual evidence of acidic environment within degrading poly(lactic-*co*-glycolic acid) (PLGA) microspheres. Pharm Res 17(1):100–106, 2000.

106. Tang G, et al. Polyethylene glycol-conjugated superoxide dismutase projects rats against oxygen toxicity. J Appl Physiol 74(3):1425–1431, 1993.

107. Niven RW, et al. The pulmonary absorption of aerosolized and intratracheally instilled rhG-CSF and monoPEGylated rhG-CSF. Pharm Res 12(9):1343–1349, 1995.

108. Lang GM, et al. Potential therapeutic efficacy of allergen-monomethoxypolyethylene glycol conjugates for in vivo inactivation of sensitized mast cells responsible for common allergies and asthma. Int Arch Allergy Immunol 113(1–3):58–60, 1997.

109. Klonne DR, et al. Two-week aerosol inhalation study on polyethylene glycol (PEG) 3350 in F-344 rats. Drug Chem Toxicol 12(1):39–48, 1989.

110. Niven RW. Delivery of biotherapeutics by inhalation aerosol. Crit Rev Ther Drug Carrier Syst 12(2–3):151–231, 1995.

111. Li S, et al. Effects of reducing sugars on the chemical stability of human relaxin in the lyophilized state. J Pharm Sci 85(8):873–877, 1996.

112. Dubost DC, et al. Characterization of a solid state reaction product from a lyophilized formulation of a cyclic heptapeptide. A novel example of an excipient-induced oxidation. Pharm Res 13(12):1811–1814, 1996.

113. Crapo JD, et al. Cell number and cell characteristics of the normal human lung. Am Rev Respir Dis 126(2):332–337, 1982.

114. Nicholas TE. Pulmonary surfactant: no mere paint on the alveolar wall. Respirology 1(4):247–257, 1996.

115. Jeffery PK, Li D. Airway mucosa: secretory cells, mucus and mucin genes. Eur Respir J 10(7):1655–1662, 1997.

116. Widdicombe JG. Airway liquid: a barrier to drug diffusion? Eur Respir J 10(10):2194–2197, 1997.

117. Rubin BK. Therapeutic aerosols and airway secretions. J Aerosol Med 9(1):123–130, 1996.

118. McConville JT, et al. Use of a novel modified TSI for the evaluation of controlled-release aerosol formulations. I. Drug Dev Ind Pharm 26(11):1191–1198, 2000.

119. Niven, R.W. Engineering and testing of dry powders for inhalation therapy. In: International Society of Aerosols in Medicine. ISAM: Vienna, Austria, 1999.

120. Tyler WS, Julian MD. Gross and subgross anatomy of the lungs, pleura, connective tissue septa, distal airways, and structural units. In: Comparative Biology of the Normal Lung, Parent RA, ed. CRC Press: Boca Raton, FL, 1991, pp. 37–48.

19

Pulmonary Delivery Technology: Recent Advances and Potential for the New Millennium

Andrew R. Clark

Nektar Therapeutics, San Carlos, California, U.S.A.

INTRODUCTION

"Pharmaceutical inhalers" have been used to treat respiratory diseases for centuries. Early therapies included the use of vapors from aromatic plants, balsams, myhrr, and sulfur. However, around the turn of the 19th century, with the advent of liquid nebulizers, these early treatments developed into legitimate pharmaceutical therapies. In the 1920 s adrenaline was introduced as a nebulizer solution, in 1925 nebulized porcine insulin was used in experimental studies in diabetes, and in 1945 pulmonary delivery of the recently discovered penicillin was investigated [1]. By the mid 1950s, steroids had been introduced for the treatment of asthma and nebulizers were enjoying widespread use. In 1956 the pressured metered-dose inhaler (pMDI) was introduced [2], over the past 5 decades, helped by the advances in molecule design and drug discovery, the pMDI has risen to become the main stay of asthma treatment around the globe. However, both the nebulizer and the pMDI have limitations, in terms of both the dose they can deliver and the ease with which they can be used. Thus, in the late 1950s the dry powder inhaler (DPI) was added to the arsenal of aerosol delivery techniques. By the early 1990s these three aerosol delivery modalities had become established technologies and had been used widely across a range of diseases and with a host of molecules.

However, at the start of the 1990s it was obvious to those involved in pulmonary drug delivery that is was going to be an exciting, if not exhausting, decade. With a few notable exceptions, mainly driven by technical limitations, the previous four decades of aerosol therapy had been dominated by chlorofluorocarbon-(CFC)-propelled metered-dose inhalers, and by the late 1980s it was becoming apparent that CFCs were an environmental threat that the global community was no longer prepared to tolerate. In 1991, the work started by Mollina and Rowlands [3] in the early 1970s finally led to the Montreal Protocols [4] and a planned withdrawal of CFCs. This event forced the pharmaceutical industry to look for alternatives to CFCs, and it was responsible, in large part, for the succeeding years of exploration and invention in the pulmonary drug delivery arena.

At about the same time, the emerging biotechnology industry was leading a revolution in protein therapeutics. The large macromolecules produced by recombinant technology had attendant formulation and delivery challenges. Most had to be delivered by either subcutaneous or intravenous injection, and there was, and to a large extent still is, a tremendous need for an alternative, noninvasive delivery route. The realization that the pulmonary epithelium may be one of the most effective noninvasive routes of delivery for macromolecules brought about interest in pulmonary delivery from a new group within the industry. However, the then-current platforms, developed for small-molecule topical therapy, lacked both the efficiency and the reproducibility needed to deliver this new class of molecules to the lung. It was apparent that new technology was needed. The stage was therefore set for a decade of exploration, discovery, and invention, with formulation and device technologies being driven by the need to replace CFCs and the desire to improve efficiency and reproducibility (Fig. 1).

THE INVENTIVE DECADE

Over the last 3 decades there have been two peaks in patent filings in the pulmonary delivery area (Fig. 2). Both of these seem to be related to the work of Molina and Rowlands [3], and both seem to have been driven by the threat that CFCs would be banned and would no longer be available for use in metered-dose inhalers. The first of these occurred in early 1970s. In the U.S. this first "scare" resulted in reformulation efforts for consumer products, but after a brief flurry of pulmonary patents the pharmaceutical industry settled back, oblivious to what

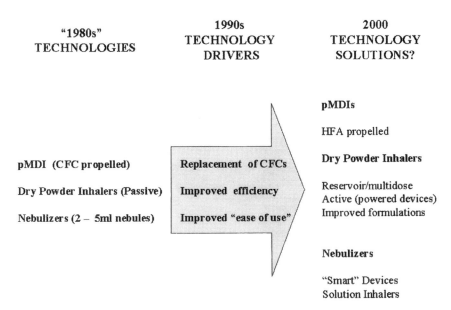

| "1980s"
TECHNOLOGIES | 1990s
TECHNOLOGY
DRIVERS | 2000
TECHNOLOGY
SOLUTIONS? |

pMDIs

HFA propelled

Dry Powder Inhalers

pMDI (CFC propelled)   Replacement of CFCs

Dry Powder Inhalers (Passive)   Improved efficiency   Reservoir/multidose
Active (powered devices)
Nebulizers (2 – 5ml nebules)   Improved "ease of use"   Improved formulations

Nebulizers

"Smart" Devices
Solution Inhalers

FIGURE 1   Technology drivers and "transformation" from conventional to new pulmonary delivery technologies.

was to follow or secure in the knowledge that at least in the short term CFC availability would not be an issue. However, at the start of the 1990s the renewed interest in the role CFCs were playing in the depletion of the ozone layer led to a plan to completely eliminate their manufacture and use [4]. The chemical industry responded by developing molecules with similar physicochemical properties to those of CFCs as replacements for refrigerants and blowing agents. The pharmaceutical industry responded by forming consortia to carry out the pulmonary toxicology on two of these new chemicals, propellants 134a and 227, to enable their use in metered-dose inhalers (IPACT I and IPACT II, respectively [5]). The industry's other response was to look for alternative technologies that could replace metered-dose inhalers. Between 1991 and 2000 over 1300 patents were filed in the pulmonary delivery technology area. These were roughly split between metered-dose inhalers and dry power technologies, with a small but significant number targeted at aqueous delivery. For comparison: in the previous decade, 1981–1990, only 240 patents were filed in those areas.

Metered-Dose Inhalers

As is evident from Fig. 2, the desire to reformulate CFC metered-dose inhalers in order to enable the use of HFA propellants has resulted in a lot of activity in the

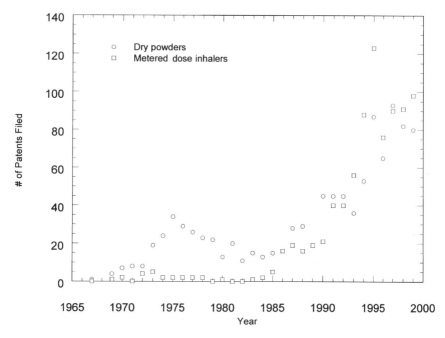

FIGURE 2 Pulmonary technology patent filings per year related to either metered-dose or dry powder inhalers. (Data generated using Aurigin Inc. patent search engine. Numbers may be slight overestimates of total related patents, due to restriction in search terms.)

pMDI area. The major issues that the industry faced at the start of the 1990s were: the need for new materials that were compatible with the new propellants for use in both valve components and filling and packaging lines; the need for new techniques to stabilize MDI suspensions and maintain adequate dose uniformity; toxicology data on the new propellants and valve materials, and a regulatory pathway for approving replacement MDI products.

From a regulatory perspective, the route taken by most of the industry was to design "bioequivalent" products, that is, to formulate existing molecules in HFAs so they exhibited the same performance (emitted-dose and particle-size characteristics) as the CFC products they were to replace. While this approach is logical from a product registration perspective, because it raises fewer clinical issues and concerns, it has been criticized as a lost opportunity for product improvement [6]. Generally speaking, the higher vapor pressures of the HFAs (particularly 134a) have the potential to generate aerosols of higher quality than the "old" CFC formulations. However, except in a few notable instances, potential product improvements have been sacrificed for development costs and time-to-market considerations. Two of the notable exceptions to this have been Qvar, beclomethasone, and Aerospan, flunisolide. Both of these products are based on solution pMDI technology. Deposition data for Qvar [7] indicates that it delivers more than twice the lung dose of the "old" CFC products, with a concomitant reduction in oral deposition. However, the companies that "bit this bullet" and produced new, improved products have had to perform extra clinical trials and generate extra data to support the safety and efficacy of their products in order to enable registration.

The main formulation challenge with HFA pMDI has been the poor solubility of the surfactants that were used in CFC products. Most pMDI formulations are suspensions of fine powder in propellant, and in order to obtain acceptable dose uniformity these suspensions usually require surfactants to stabilize them. The inability to use conventional surfactants has therefore led to a range of diverse formulation approaches. These encompass drug solubilization using cosolvents (Qvar is an example), new surfactants, coating particles with surfactant, and particle engineering (Fig. 3). However, as is the case with most

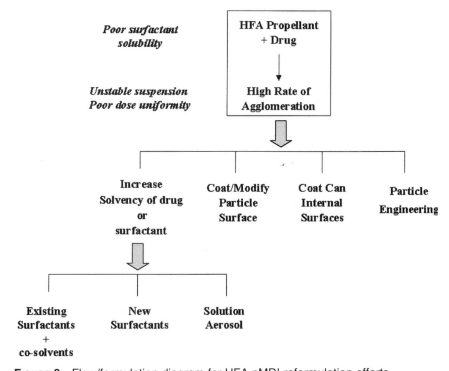

FIGURE 3   Flow/formulation diagram for HFA pMDI reformulation efforts.

formulation technologies, no one technique seems to suit all molecules and no one approach seems to be dominating product development. It likely that products that use most of these approaches will reach the market. Individual product choices will be driven by the technical suitability for a particular molecule and the need to avoid patent infringement and ensure freedom to operate.

As would be expected, the large amount of inventive effort and resultant patent activity have produced a patent minefield. The most prominent patents appear to be those of 3M Laboratories. Inc., and the Schering Corporation. 3M holds a broad patent covering the use of 134a [8] and Schering holds a patent covering the use of 227 [9]. Though the situation is a little simpler in Europe, these patents, or slightly different version of them, are still in force in the United States. It appears that company tactics in the U.S. involve licensing deals rather than direct challenges in the U.S. patent courts.

Despite the technical difficulties and the patent issues just outlined, the future for pMDIs looks bright. It would appear that the pMDI is here to stay, at least for the near term.

Dry Powder Technologies
Devices

There have been two major objectives for dry powder inhaler device design over the last decade. The first (and major) focus has been to design multidose dry powder inhalers that are small, easy to use, and as convenient for the patient as a pMDI. This has resulted in a proliferation of devices where the powder medicament is stored in a bulk reservoir and metered (or dosed) inside the device. Typically these technologies use volumetric metering techniques involving perforated plates, notches, grooves, or some sort of space that can be filled with powder and then moved to a dosing area where the powder can be "extracted" for delivery to the patient. The dose reservoirs generally hold from 50 to 200 doses, and in this respect at least they are similar to a pMDI. However, no matter how worthy the goal, progress has been difficult and success has been more limited than the list of patents in this area would suggest. The main issue with these technologies has been the inability of conventional pharmaceutical powder formulation techniques to produce powders with acceptable flow and dispersion properties (progress on new formulation technologies will be discussed later). This has led to a large number of device concepts simply falling by the wayside due to the technologies' inability to meet reasonable dose uniformity standards [10]. Also, in many cases technology has been abandoned due to a failure to find a sufficient financial incentive to warrant the development time and expense. Applying advanced expensive device technologies to generic asthma molecules is fraught with commercial difficulties.

Only three multiple blister device technologies, where dosing is carried out in the factory and multiple unit doses are stored on disks or tapes, have been commercialized (GSK, Diskhaler, and Accuhaler). This technology overcomes the dose uniformity issues seen with the reservoir devices, but it does limit the number of doses available in a device, simply because of the volume of the packaging space that is required. Even here it has proved difficult and expensive to commercialize some technically viable concepts, with a number of technologies being abandoned [11] or severely delayed in development.

The second area of focus has been the elimination of the flowrate-dependent performance that early dry powder devices exhibit [12]. For example, it is not uncommon for conventional dry powder inhalers to deliver lung doses that vary by a factor of 3 or 4, depending upon how much effort a patient puts into an inhalation. The device-engineering solutions to this problem have been to add an internal power source to supply the energy to disperse the powder. This technique negates the need for inspiratory effort on behalf of the patient, but it does add an additional coordination requirement, i.e., the need for an additional device element to coordinate actuation with inhalation. The dispersion energy sources employed have ranged from purely mechanical solutions, compressed air or small hammers, to battery-powered devices using impellers or ultrasonic transducers. Again progress has generally been slow and difficult, with one electronic device failing after Phase III during the approval process [11].

In addition to these advances, a number of device developments have focused on using the established capsule technologies. These "new designs on an old theme" appear to be have been successful [13], although a number have still to make it through the approval process to the marketing phase.

Figure 4 summarizes the dry powder device landscape, highlighting the various device approaches and plotting a number of successes and failures in each area. Interestingly, no powered devices (active) have yet made it to market (although the Inhale PDS device is in Phase III studies with insulin), and the group of devices that attempted to combine multidose reservoirs with powered aerosol dispersion all seem to have been abandoned. The most successful group have been patient-driven (passive) reservoir devices, where simple powder blend technology and inexpensive engineering have been combined to produce patient-friendly devices with limited, if any, performance enhancement over earlier products. This perhaps should not be too surprising. The largest portion of the pulmonary market is asthma. Most asthma drugs possess reasonably wide therapeutic widows and, as described earlier, the drive to produce products with pMDI-like "handling" characteristics has been far more important than the drive to improve efficiency and reproducibility.

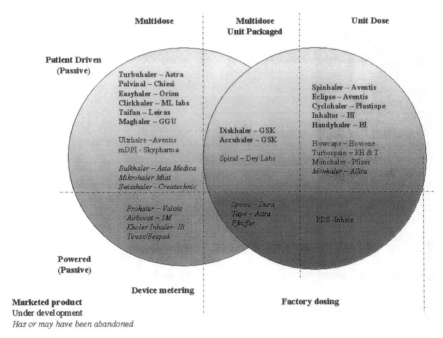

FIGURE 4 Dry powder device "landscape" broken down by energy source, dosing method, and packaging.

Formulations

The second area of dry powder development is dry powder formulation. At the start of the 1990s the need for new powder technologies was evident from the generally poor performance of micronized, spheronized, or blended powders. It was also apparent that, with a few notable exceptions [14], device technology alone could not dramatically improve the performance characteristics of DPI products. That is, with improved powder technology the need for device-engineering solutions to aerosol dispersion problems are somewhat mitigated. Over the years there has been some reluctance to develop new excipients for pulmonary use (because this can be as arduous as developing a new pharmacologically active molecule), and early attempts at improving powders focused on existing generally-regarded-as-safe pulmonary excipients. However, recent advances have clearly demonstrated that new excipients are an essential component of high-performance dry powder delivery technologies. Figure 5 summarizes the route that powder formulation development has been taking since the early 1990s.

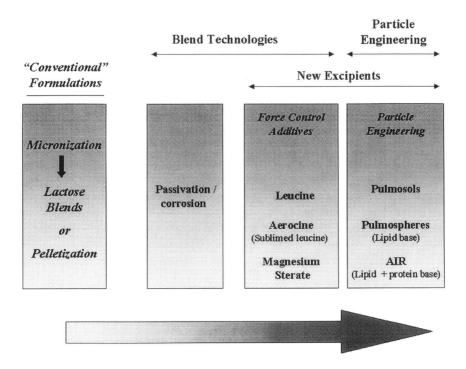

FIGURE 5 Progress toward new excipients and new manufacturing technology for dry powder formulations.

The basic problem that developers have been trying to solve is the need for a dry powder to flow, for dosing and emptying purposes, yet disperse adequately to make an "inhalable' aerosol. In terms of conventional powder technology these two requirements are usually mutually exclusive. Coarse powders flow well but contain very little "respirable" material. Fine powders possess a high "respirable" content but generally exhibit very poor flow properties. The focus then has been on trying to find ways to make these contradictory requirements compatible.

Progress with formulation innovation has focused on two areas. In chronological order they are improving existing blending techniques, followed by new excipients and particle-engineering methods to produce particles that do not require blending.

Blend improvements began with passivation and corrosion of the lactose carrier surface [15]. The idea was to reduce the number of high-energy binding sites on the lactose carrier surface and hence to reduce the energy required to remove the drug particles from the carrier. This approach generally produces modest improvements in performance. However, one of its major advantages is that "fine" excipient particles (small enough to reach the lung) are not required, and hence there are no major toxicology issues. The next step in blend improvement was to use "force additives" and to manufacture blends with multiple components. Conventional powder blends utilize fine drug particles and large sugar carrier particles. With this new "force additive" technology, a third component is added to the blend, with the intent of its occupying the active binding sites on the carrier and acting as a "breakable" bridge between the carrier and the drug. The data suggest this technique can be very effective [16], although a second excipient with a particle size in the range capable of reaching the lung is required, and this has obvious consequences from a toxicology perspective. Blends using magnesium state are now marketed in Europe, and blends using leucine and other amino acids have been reported in the literature [17].

   Published data suggest that the fine-particle "engineering" approach is proving successful from a performance perspective and that it is capable of addressing both overall delivery efficiency and the flowrate-dependence issues without the need for carrier particles or active devices. However, products based on these techniques have yet to reach the market. The approach has been to manufacture particles that include active drug and excipient. By choice of appropriate excipients and judicious selection of manufacturing techniques and conditions, particles with low surface energies and advantageous morphologies and densities can be obtained. The techniques for manufacturing range form coprecipitation to spray-drying. The excipients used include sugars, amino acids, and lipids. The sugar-based systems have been used as both powder-dispersion aids and stabilizers for protein inhalation powders. The most widely reported examples of the lipid-based systems are AIR particles [18], which are ultralow-density particles made by spray-drying lipid and albumin in solution with active drugs, and Pulmospheres [19], where a blowing agent is used to "inflate" particles to produce spongelike structures. These technologies have been extremely successful in generating powders with the required properties for dry powder inhalers. For Pulmospheres, lung deposition as high as 57% of the nominal dose has been reported for a simple passive inhaler [20,21]. However, as stated earlier, these second-generation powder formulations have yet to demonstrate commercial viability.

Nebulizers and Soft Mist Inhalers

At the start of the 1990s the only available aqueous solution-based pulmonary delivery systems were the nebulizers that had their routes in technology developed at the turn of the nineteenth century. From a patient perspective, nebulizer therapy is time consuming, equipment costs are high, and cleaning and maintenance can be problematic; from a pharmaceutical perspective, nebulizers exhibit poor delivery efficiency and high variability [22]. However, nebulizers are capable of delivering high doses of medication to the airways, and patients do not seem to need intensive training to be able to use them effectively. Thus efforts have been made to improve nebulizer design. The first and simplest improvements are entrainment designs, where aerosol generation decreases during expiration, and these designs appear to reduce wasted medication and improve delivery efficiency [23]. More recent designs use valves that respond to the inspiratory cycle and completely stop aerosol generation during the expiration phase [24]. Electronic devices, which synchronize delivery with inspiration, have also been developed. The most advanced of these, Adaptive Aerosol Delivery [25], also counts the number of "actuations" and automatically adjusts the number of delivery cycles so as to deliver a constant dose, regardless of the patients' breathing pattern.

Advances have also been made in atomization technology, with ultrasonic mesh atomizers now being used in some commercial nebulizer devices [26]. The promise for the future is that flow monitoring will be more effectively liked to atomization to control delivery and enhance the efficiency, reproducibility, and ease of use of the next generation of nebulizers. This will enable drug-specific dosing regimes to be developed. However, as nebulizer designs become ever more drug specific they run the risk of being regulated as an intergral part of a drug product and losing their "generic" device status. This would mean much heavier regulation and a loss of the design freedoms they currently enjoy.

In the early part of the 1990s a natural extension to nebulizer technology was conceived. The idea was to deliver an effective dose of medication from an aqueous solution in a small number of breaths and to embody this in a device as small and simple as a pMDI. These soft mist inhaler (SMI) concepts, which began development in the early 1990s, were based on three basic atomizer concepts. The first uses small nozzles and high pressures to dispense and atomize metered volumes of solution; trade-offs can be made between the number of nozzles and the pressure used to extrude the solution through the nozzles, and two technologies at opposite ends of the trade-off spectrum have now emerged [27,28]. The second technology uses multiplexed, ultrasonic-driven nozzles (mesh arrays) to atomize droplets, and specific variants of this technique are currently at different stages of development [29,30]. The third, slightly later, entrant uses electrohydrodynamic atomization [31], and this technology has been used in early studies with cancer therapeutics. Some of these technologies have already demonstrated high delivery efficiencies. For example, the Respimat (formerly BINeb) has shown 50% delivery to the lungs [27], and the Aradigm AERx has reported close to 80% [28]. However, in addition to the device-engineering issues, one of the major challenges has been dealing with the possibility of microbial contamination of the aqueous solution reservoirs and/or mastering aseptic manufacturing techniques for unit-dose devices. Again, as with some dry powder device technologies and the second-generation powder formulations, none of these SMIs have yet made it to market. Although as of summer 2002, Phase III clinical studies with the Respimat had been completed and the AERx was poised to begin Phase III studies with insulin.

Figure 6 summarizes developments in the solution area and illustrates the migration of aqueous solution technology from nebulizer, through "controlled" nebulizer, to SMI technologies. However, it should be remembered that nebulizers still exhibit some unique qualities that will probably ensure their continued use over the coming years.

IMPROVED DELIVERY EFFICIENCIES

So overall, what has all this patent and development activity given us? In terms of performance, great strides appear to have been made. Figure 7 is a compilation of deposition data published from 1980 to 2000. The ordinate is year of publication, and the abscissa is lung delivery efficiency, as measured by gamma scintigraphic techniques. Each point represents the first time a deposition value has been

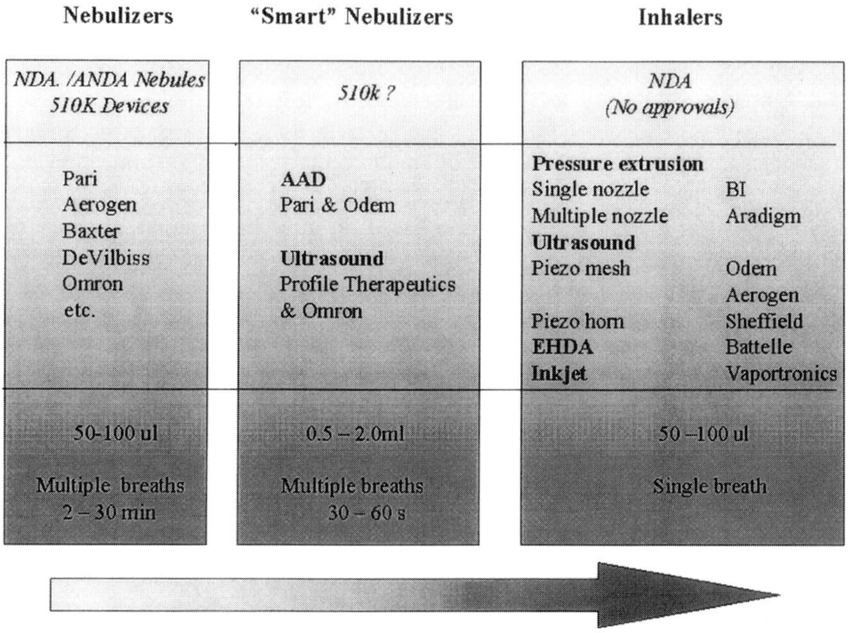

Nebulizers	"Smart" Nebulizers	Inhalers	
NDA. /ANDA Nebules 510K Devices	510k ?	NDA (No approvals)	
Pari Aerogen Baxter DeVilbiss Omron etc.	AAD Pari & Odem Ultrasound Profile Therapeutics & Omron	**Pressure extrusion** Single nozzle Multiple nozzle **Ultrasound** Piezo mesh Piezo horn **EHDA** **Inkjet**	BI Aradigm Odem Aerogen Sheffield Battelle Vaportronics
50-100 ul Multiple breaths 2 – 30 min	0.5 – 2.0ml Multiple breaths 30 – 60 s	50 –100 ul Single breath	

FIGURE 6 Pulmonary "solutions" landscape. Though a large number of solution inhalers are under development, none has yet made it to market. Nebulizers remain the only solution devices currently available.

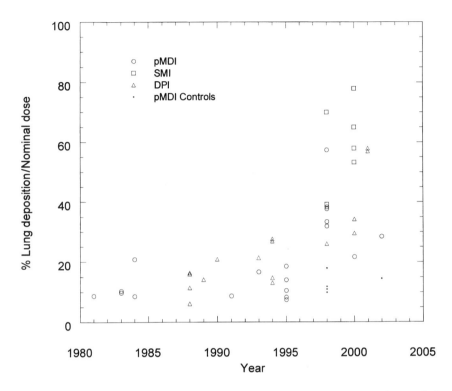

FIGURE 7 Lung deposition for new inhalation technologies over the period 1980–2000. (From Refs. 7, 20, 27, 32–50.)

reported for a new technology. It can be seen that prior to 1995 the average delivery efficiency, i.e., the percentage of the nominal dose delivered to the lungs, for inhalation technologies was around 20%. After 1995 performance improved dramatically. The average deposition values reported in 2000 were around 40–50%, with the highest value being 80%. The only conclusion that can be drawn from these numbers is that the patent activity, which began at the start of the 1990s (Fig. 2), has really led to product performance improvements. However, the reported data are, in general, produced with prototype devices and formulations. Because of the phase lag caused by the long development and registration time frames for pharmaceutical products, this tremendous improvement in product performance has not yet filtered through to market products. An example of this lag is obtained by comparing the patent-filing dates for the SMI technologies, the late 1980s and 1990s, to the publication of clinical data, 1995 onward. There are no SMI data in the early part of the decade of the 1990s.

However, one area where "new" products have made it to market, but where dramatic improvements have deliberately not been realized, is in the replacement HFA pMDIs. As already discussed, with the exception of two or three products, the regulatory and commercial pressures to replace the "old" CFC pMDIs with new HFA pMDIs with similar performance have resulted in possible product improvements that have not been implemented.

The other question that should perhaps be asked going forward is: Where and when do molecules need these improved delivery efficiencies? If local lung delivery is compared to other forms of drug delivery, in terms of the percentage of the nominal dose reaching the site of action, topical lung delivery is, and has always been, the most efficient delivery modality, and one has to ask why it needs improving. There are some obvious instances where it would be advantageous, for example, when oral or gastrointestinal exposure needs to be limited or avoided, where the drug is expensive, or where systemic delivery through the peripheral lung is required. Efficient second-generation pulmonary technologies are therefore here to stay, although they may not be necessary for all molecules.

MACROMOLECULE DELIVERY

As pointed out earlier, one of the main drivers for improvements in pulmonary delivery performance has been the desire to deliver proteins and peptides noninvasively. The pulmonary route offers an ideal opportunity for systemic absorption because its surface area is large and the pulmonary epithelium is thin. In fact, the first attempt to deliver insulin through the lung took place as long ago as 1925. However, putting this sparse early study aside, it wasn't until the beginning of the 1990s, when recombinant technology made protein therapeutics widely available, that researchers really began to tackle the issues related to pulmonary macromolecule delivery. The main challenges were to understand the delivery requirements and to come to grips with the factors that influence and control efficient absorption.

Early work identified deep lung deposition as an imperative to absorption efficiency, and a number of studies have demonstrated higher bioavailabilites (absorption efficiencies) for peripherally deposited aerosols [51]. However, despite a decade of work, the absorption mechanisms that facilitate transfer from the pulmonary epithelium to the blood are still not well understood. Two mechanisms are believed to operate, transcellular and pericellular. There is some evidence that small invaginations called *caveolae* may be involved in transcellular transport, whereas pericellular transport is via leaky tight junctions.

Numerous macromolecules have been investigated in preclinical models [52]; delivery to and through the lung appears to be generally safe [53], and a large number of molecules have made it to trials in man. Figure 8 summarizes the majority of these investigations by clinical development phase. It will be noted that rhDNAse, a topical lung therapy for the treatment of cystic fibrosis, is the only approved pulmonary protein and that a number of other molecules have progressed as far as Phase III studies. At the time of writing, systemic inhaled insulin was in late Phase III trials.

THE FUTURE

So what of the future direction of pulmonary delivery technologies over the next decade? While it is always difficult to foretell the future and any projections are always risky, we can base a guess on observation of the last decade.

For example, aerosol performance, as measured by the percentage of the nominal dose that reaches the lungs, has improved immensely. In fact it has to be asked whether there is any real mileage in trying to improve things any further. With the highest reported deposition values reaching on the order of 80%, there is surely little room for further improvement. It also has to be asked how many current and future molecules really require these staggeringly high lung deposition efficiencies. Outside of the expensive protein therapeutics, systemic delivery, and molecules where oral deposition can lead to unwanted side effects,

Phase I/II	Phase II	Phase III	Approved
SLPI	IL-4R	Insulin (Inhale)	Pulmonary surfactant
α-1-antitrypsin (Inhale)	GM-CSF	Leuprolide	DNase
α-1-antitrypsin (Arriva)	INS-365 (UTP deriv)	KL-4 peptide+lipid	
γ-interferon (NIH)	α-1-antitrypsin (PPL)	gamma-interferon (Intermune)	
ß-interferon	IL-2	SPC+lipid	
INS37217	tgAAV-CF	Insulin (Aradigm)	
α-interferon	PTH 1-34		
IL-1R			
cyclosporine			
calcitonin			
tgAAV-CF (CF)			
VIP			
anti-IgE			
DNA-lipid forms			
growth hormone			
heparin			
insulin (Microdose)			
insulin (Aerogen)			
insulin (Microdose)			
anti-IL-4			
CC10			
lactoferrin			
RASONS			

FIGURE 8 Large-molecule pulmonary development. (Courtesy of Ralph Niven.)

high delivery efficiency is difficult to justify if it adds significant cost to a product. As just discussed, aerosol delivery is already efficient compared to most other pharmaceutical modalities.

A second observation is the length of time and the investment that it takes to develop and commercialize an entirely new aerosol delivery technology. Although difficult to compute, because many of the technologies are still in the development stage or have been completely abandoned, the average is probably close to 6–8 years, even when they are developed with an existing molecule.

A third observation is that the industry successfully rose to the challenge of developing HFA metered-dose inhalers. As a consequence, the pMDI will probably still play a major therapeutic role in this next decade. The 1990s were a decade when the future of the pMDI was uncertain and there was a window of opportunity for new "advanced" aerosol technologies. However, at the end of the decade the window appeared to be closing, and we are left with many advanced technologies, but none that seem to be complete replacements for the pMDI. However, there are new patient-driven multidose powder inhalers that have been commercialized (mainly in Europe), and we are on the verge of seeing a number of new, highly efficient liquid and powder technologies reach the market.

Therapy since the early 1990s has also matured. In asthma, the leading clinical applications of aerosol delivery, steroids and bronchodilators, have become the mainstay therapy. These molecules are effective. However, some are already off patent and experiencing generic competition, and many of the newer molecules will be coming off patent before 2010 [54]. By 2010 a large proportion of the asthma molecule market will be generic, and, although there are new therapeutic approaches under investigation, the commercial hurdle is going to be high. If they are going to compete with what will then be generically priced effective therapies, they will have to demonstrate a significant clinical advantage to be successful.

Finally, pulmonary protein delivery has advanced tremendously since 1990. One local therapy has been approved and a number of others, including insulin, are in the later stages of clinical development. The device platforms that have been developed for these macromolecules have also exhibited higher delivery efficiencies and greater reproducibility than the "old" technologies, and these attributes may well have application in other areas of pulmonary delivery. For example, they may facilitate delivery of small molecules though the lung for a faster onset of action.

So taking all of these observation together, what will the next decade bring? Firstly, many of the new devices and formulation technologies that began development in the 1990s should emerge as products. The time frame for development of new pharmaceutical technologies appears to be close to a decade, and in this respect the next 10 years should see the fruit of all the technology development of the last decade.

These technologies may also bring new pulmonary opportunities, for example, systemic delivery of small molecules and maybe local delivery of cancer therapeutics. The products that do emerge will involve new (or at least new to pulmonary) molecules, and as they become established they may be applied to "old" molecules. However, the burden as always is to justify the technology cost with improved product performance. There may also be significant effort in reducing the cost of the technologies developed in the 1990s to allow their application to cheaper branded generic products. Systemic delivery of macromolecules via the lung should also become a commercial reality soon.

However, it is certain that some of the "old" technologies will still be popular. The pMDI, with its new propellants, is here to stay. It is always tempting when developing a new molecule to take the cheapest and fastest time to market rather than necessarily developing the right product for the market. It has also always been difficult to develop new chemical entities (NCEs) and new delivery technologies together. The balance between the increased risk of product failure and the market risk of not having the "perfect" product is always an interesting trade-off. From a commercial perspective, it is quite often the less risky route (the old technology) that is the correct one to take. For example, development of a nebulizer solution for a new drug is relatively quick and inexpensive. The delivery technology is "generic", and the drug company involved does not have to gain approval for a drug product that includes a device. For small markets where patients will tolerate this form of delivery, it will always be tempting to develop this type of product.

So what of new pulmonary technology through 2010? Well, as expressed earlier, delivery efficiency has been the holy grail of the last decade. I believe that applying these hard-won improvements to molecules will undoubtedly be the new focus. We understand far more about pulmonary delivery and far more about the potential applications of lung delivery than we ever have. Using this knowledge to uncover and develop novel therapeutics that can be delivered using the advanced pulmonary technologies developed since 1990 will probably be the "grail" through 2010.

REFERENCES

1. Nerbrink O. Characterization of aerosol delivery devices and their influences and deposition in humans and animals. PhD dissertation, Karolinska Institute, Stockholm. 2001.
2. Theil CG. From Susie's question to CFC-free: an inventor's perspective on 40 years of MDI development and regulation. In Respiratory Drug Delivery V; Dalby RN, Byron PR, Farr SJ, eds. Interpharm Press: Phoenix, AZ, 1998; 115–119.

3. Molina MJ, Rowlands FS. Stratospheric sink for chlorofluoromethanes: chlorine atom—catalyzed destruction of ozone. Nature 1974, 249, 810–812.

4. Montreal Protocol. Treaty Series, No. 19, Her Majesty's Stationary Office, 1987.

5. Partridge MR, Woodcock AA. Propellants. In: Bisgard H, O'Callaghan C, Smaldone G, eds. Drug Delivery to the Lung. Marcel Dekker, New York, 2002.

6. Everard M. CFC transition: the emperor's new clothes. Each class of drug deserves a delivery system that meets its own requirements. Thorax 55(10), 811–814.

7. Leach CL, Davidson PJ, Boudreau RJ. Improved airway targeting with the CFC-free HFA-beclomethasone metered-dose inhaler compared with CFC-beclomethasone. Eur Respir 1998, 12, 1346–1353.

8. Purewal T, Greenleaf DJ. Medical aerosol formulations. U.S. Patent, No. 5,695,743, 1997

9. Fassberg J, Sequeira JA, Chaudry IA, Kopcha M. Non-chlorofluorocarbon aerosol formulation. U.S. Patent, No. 5,474,759, 1995.

10. Federal Drug Administration. Guidance for Industry: Nasal Spray and Inhalation Solution, Suspension and Spray Drug Products—Chemical, Manufacturing and Control Documentation. Center for Drug Evaluation and Research, Washington, DC, 2002.

11. Schultz R. Caution: past performance is not a predictor of future success. In Respiratory Drug Delivery VIII; Dalby RN, Byron PR, Farr SJ, eds. Interpharm Press: Tucson, AZ, 2002; 79–84.

12. Cark AR. Medical aerosol inhalers: past present and future. Aerosol Sci Tech 1995, 22, 374–391.

13. Borgstrom L, Bisgaard H, O'Callaghan C, Pedersen S. Dry-powder inhalers. In: Bisgard, H., O'Callaghan, C., Smaldone, G., eds. Drug Delivery to the Lung. Marcel Dekker, New York, 2002.

14. Smith AE, Burr JD, Axford GS, Anthony JM. Apparatus and methods for dispensing dry powder medicaments. U.S. Patent, No 5,740,794, 1998.

15. Ganderton D, Kasim NM. Dry powder inhalers. Adv Pharm Sci 1992, 6, 161–191.

16. Morton DA, Green M, Staniforth JN, Whittock A, Begat P, Price R, Young P. The study of force control additives in creating high-performance dry powder inhalation formulations. In: Respiratory Drug Delivery VIII; Dalby RN, Byron PR, Farr SJ, eds. Interpharm Press: Tucson, AZ, 2002; 763–766.

17. Staniforth J, Patel N, Morton D, Tservitas M, Braithwaite P, Parry-Billings M, Shott M, Ganderton D. Biotech—DPI strategies: accomplishing affordable control and effective action. In: Respiratory Drug Delivery VIII; Dalby RN, Byron PR, Farr SJ, eds. Interpharm Press: Tucson, AZ, 2002; 267–276.

18. Edwards DA, Hanes J, Caponetti G, Hrkach J, Ben-Jebria A, Eskew M, Mintzes J, Deaver D, Lotan N, Langer R. Large porous particles for pulmonary drug delivery. Science 1997, 276, 1868–1871.

19. Dellamary LA, Tarara TE, Smith DJ, Woelk CH, Adractas A, Costello ML, Gill H, Weers JG. Hollow porous particles for inhalation. Pharm Res 2000, 17, 168–174.

20. Duddu SP, Sisk SA, Walter YH, Weers JG, Tarara TE, Leung D, Clark AR, Newman SP, Pickford M, Elton RC, Hirst PH. Highly efficient, flow-independent pulmonary

delivery of PulmoSphere budesonide from a dry powder inhaler. Pharm Sci. Abstracts AAPS meeting, 2001.

21. Duddu SP, Sisk SA, Walter YH, Tarara TF, Trimble K, Clark AR, Eldon M, Elton RC, Pickford M, Hirst PH, Newman SP, Weers JG. Improved lung delivery from a passive dry powder inhaler using an engineered PulmoSphere powder. Pharm Res 2002, 19, 689–695.

22. Smaldone G, LeSouef PN. Nebulization: the device and clinical considerations. In: Bisgard H, O'Callaghan C, Smaldone G, eds. Drug Delivery to the Lung. Marcel Dekker, New York, 2002.

23. Keller M, Lintz FC, Walther E. Novel liquid formulation technologies as a tool to design the aerosol performance of nebulizers using air jet (LC plus) or a vibrating membrane principle (E-Flow). In: Drug Delivery to the Lungs. London, Dec 13 and 14, 2001.

24. Mitchell JP, Scarrot PM, Nagel MW, Wiersema KJ, Bates SA, Lusty ME. An in vitro investigation of common nebulizer dosing protocols, comparing a breath-actuated with a conventional pneumatic small volume nebulizer. In: Respiratory Drug Delivery V; Dalby RN, Byron PR, Farr SJ, eds. Interpharm Press: Tucson, AZ, 2002; 627–630.

25. Marsden R, Dood ME, Conway S, Weller PH. Comparison of compliance in cystic fibrosis patients using Halolite Adaptive Aerosol Delivery (AAD) system with conventional high-output nebulizer system. In: Respiratory Drug Delivery V; Dalby RN, Byron PR, Farr SJ, eds. Interpharm Press: Phoenix, AZ, 2002; 557–560.

26. Fink J, McCall A, Simon M, Uster P. Enabling aerosol delivery technology for critical care. In: Respiratory Drug Delivery VIII; Dalby RN, Byron PR, Farr SJ, eds. Interpharm Press: Tucson, AZ, 2002; 323–326.

27. Zierenberg B. Boehringer Ingelhiem nebulizer (BINeb)—a new approach to inhalation therapy. In: Respiratory Drug Delivery V; Dalby RN, Byron PR, Farr SJ, eds. Interpharm Press: Phoenix AZ, 1996; 187–194.

28. Farr S. AERx development of a novel liquid aerosol delivery system: concept to clinic. In: Respiratory Drug Delivery V; Dalby RN, Byron PR, Farr SJ, eds. Interpharm Press: Phoenix AZ, 1996; 175–185.

29. DeYoung L. The Aerodose multidose inhaler—device design and delivery characteristics. In: Respiratory Drug Delivery VI; Dalby RN, Byron PR, Farr SJ, eds. Interpharm Press: Hilton Head, SC, 1998; 91–96.

30. Smart J, Berg E, Nerbrink O, Zuban R, Blakey D, New M. TouchSpray technology: Comparison of the droplet size measured with cascade impaction and laser diffraction. In: Respiratory Drug Delivery V; Dalby RN, Byron PR, Farr SJ, eds. Interpharm Press: Phoenix, AZ, 2002; 525–532.

31. Zimlich WC. The development of a novel electrohydrodynamic (EHD) pulmonary drug delivery device. In: Respiratory Drug Delivery VII; Dalby RN, Byron PR, Farr SJ, eds. Interpharm Press: Tarpon Springs, FL, 2000; 241–246.

32. Newman SP, Brown J, Steed KP, Reader SJ, Kladders H. Lung deposition of fenoterol and flunisolide delivered using a novel device for inhaled medications. Chest 1998, 113, 957–963.

33. Farr SJ, Warren SJ, Lloyd P, Okikawa JK, Schuster JA, Rowe AM, Rubsamen RM, Taylor G. Comparison of in vitro and in vivo efficiencies of a novel unit-dose aerosol generator and a pressurized metered-dose inhaler. Int J Pharm 2000, 198, 63–70.
34. Newman SP, Pavia D, Moren F, Sheahan NF. Deposition of pressurized aerosols in the human respiratory tract. Thorax 1981, 36, 52–55.
35. Dolovich MB, Ruffin RE, Corr D, Newhouse MT. Clinical evaluation of a simple demand inhalation MDI aerosol delivery device. Chest 1983, 84, 36–41.
36. Zimlich WC, Ding JY, Busick DR, Moutvic RR, Placke ME, Hirst PH, Pitcairn GR, Malik S, Newman SP, Macintyre F, Miller PR, Shepherd MT, Lukas TM. The development of a novel electrohydrodynamic pulmonary drug delivery device. In: Respiratory Drug Delivery VII; Dalby RN, Byron PR, Farr SJ, Peart J, eds. Serentec Press: Raleigh, NC, 2000; 241–246.
37. De Young L, Chambers F, Narayan S, Wu C. The Aerodose multidose inhaler device: design and delivery characteristics. In: Respiratory Drug Delivery VI; Dalby RN, Byron PR, Farr SJ, eds. Interpharm Press: Buffalo Grove, In, 1998; 91–95.
38. Pitcairn GR, Lankinen T, Seppälä O-P, Newman SP. Pulmonary drug deliveries from the Taifun dry powder inhaler is relatively independent of the patient's inspiratory effort. J Aerosol Med 2000, 13, 97–104.
39. Newman S, Brown J, Steed K, Reader S, Kladders H. Lung deposition of budesonide inhaled via Turbuhaler: a comparison with Terbutaline sulphate in normal subjects. Eur Respir, J 1998, 7, 69–73.
40. Newman SP, Moren F, Trofast E, Talaee N, Clarke SW. Deposition and clinical efficacy of terbutaline sulphate from Turbuhaler, a new multidose powder inhaler. Eur Respir J 1989, 2, 247–252.
41. Kenyon CJ, Thorsson L, Borgström L, Newman SP. The effects of static charge in spacer devices on glucocorticosteroid aerosol deposition in asthmatic patients. Eur Respir J 1998, 11, 606–610.
42. Hirst PH, Pitcairn GR, Weers JG, Tarara TE, Clark AR, Dellamary LA, Hall G, Shorr J, Newman SP. In vivo lung deposition of hollow porous particles from a pressurized metered-dose inhaler. Pharm Res 2002, 19, 258–264.
43. Farr S, Rowe A, Rubsamen R, Taylor G. Aerosol deposition in the human lung following administration from a microprocessor-controlled pressurized metered-dose inhaler. Thorax 1995, 50, 639–644.
44. Borgström L, Bondesson E, Morén F, Trofast E, Newman SP. Lung deposition of budesonide inhaled via Turbuhaler: a comparison with terbutaline sulphate in normal subjects. Eur Respir J 1994, 7, 69–73.
45. Newman S, Hollingworth A, Clark A. Effect of different modes of inhalation on drug delivery from a dry powder inhaler. Int J Pharm 1994, 102, 127–132.
46. Newman S, Clark A, Talaee N, Clarke S. Lung deposition of 5 mg Intal from a pressurized metered-dose inhaler assessed by radiotracer technique. Int J Pharm 1991, 74, 203–208.
47. Vidgren M, Karkkainen A, Karjalainen P, Paronen P, Nuutinen J. Effect of powder inhaler design on drug deposition in the respiratory tract. Int J Pharm 1988, 42, 211–216.

48. Borgstrom L, Newman S. Total and regional lung deposition of terbutaline sulpahte inhaled via a pressurized MDI or via Turbuhaler. Int J Pharm 1993, 97, 47–53.

49. Vidgren M, Paronen P, Vidgren P, Vainio P, Nutitinen J. Radiotracer evaluation of the deposition of drug particles inhaled from a new powder inhaler. Int J Pharm 1990, 64, 1–6.

50. Thorsson L, Kenyon C, Newman S, Borgstrom L. Lung deposition of budesonide in asthmatics: a comparison of different formulations. Int J Pharm 1998, 168, 119–127.

51. Newman SP, Hirst PH, Pitcairn GR, Clark AR. Understanding regional deposition data in gamma scinitgraphy. In: Respiratory Drug Delivery VI; Dalby RN, Byron PR, Farr SJ, eds. Interpharm Press: Hilton Head, SC, 1998; 9–16.

52. Nivern RW. Delviery of biotherapeutics by inhalation aerosol. Crit Rev Ther Drug Carrier Systems 1995, 12 ((2 and 3)), 151–231.

53. Wolff RK. Safety of inhaled proteins for therapeutic use. J Aerosol Med 1998, 11 ((4)), 197–219.

54. Scala SM, Sanderson IC, Moran JR, Cacciatore KC, Perreault JB. Pharmaceutical Therapeutic Catagories Outlook. SG Cowan, New York, Finance report, 2002.

Index